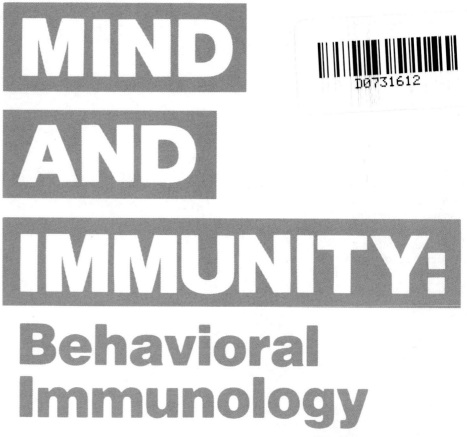

MIND AND IMMUNITY:

Behavioral Immunology

An Annotated Bibliography 1976-1982

Compiled & Edited by

Steven E. Locke

Mady Hornig-Rohan

Published by:

**Institute for the
Advancement of Health**

16 East 53rd Street
New York, N.Y. 10022

Cover photograph:
Electron micrograph of normal human lung
mast cells. These cells have a single-lobed
nucleus and numerous dense granules. The
granules contain potent inflammatory
mediators which can be released by both
allergic and neurohumoral mechanisms.
Photograph provided by Ann Dvorak
and Kathryn Tyne, Department of
Pathology, Beth Israel Hospital, Boston,
Massachusetts.

Second printing, March 1984

Library of Congress Catalog Number 83-81107
ISBN 0-910903-01-8

Published by:
Institute for the Advancement of Health
16 East 53rd Street
New York, N.Y. 10022

With the assistance of:
Elliot Press
27 Camden Road
Auburndale, MA 02166

Designed by
Modi & Beckler Design
New York, N.Y. 10016

Printed in the United States of America

To two pioneers—Hans Selye (1907-1982) and Vernon Riley (1914-1982)—who dedicated their lives to advancing our understanding of the interrelationships of brain, behavior and immunity to disease.

If intelligence is the capacity to adapt to changing circumstances then the central nervous system and the immune system manifest this ability beyond all others. It would be remarkable if each of these supreme exemplars of rapid and subtle adaptation did not tap the other's almost limitless potential for variation but except for the work of a small number of explorers seeking the Northwest Passage between these vast intellectual continents, the interrelationships of these fields has received much less attention than it deserves. It is interesting to note that the First International Congress of Neuroimmunology was held in September, 1982.

Yet even a rapid overview of the material in this volume shows how closely the two systems are linked. While at one time the concept existed that stress might alter immune reactivity through some relatively diffuse activation of the endocrine system or the hypothalamus we now find that there are specific interactions at every level. At one extreme there is modulation of immune responsiveness by the sympathetic system. At the other extreme we find a linkage between cerebral dominance and autoimmunity, differential immune effects of right and left cortical lesions and HLA associations of major psychiatric disorders.

Locke and Hornig-Rohan have performed a signal service in bringing together the information now available on the interactions of the immune and nervous systems, culled from journals in many disciplines and in all languages. They have been sensitive to the fact that the most startling scientific advances occur when conventional disciplinary boundaries are crossed, and that this field will be of relevance not just to immunology, psychiatry and neurology, but to every clinical discipline. It will also have a major impact on embryology, pharmacology, biochemistry and nearly every field of laboratory investigation.

The reader who works through a particular section methodically, or browses at random, will again and again find new vistas opening to him. This may be the last moment in history when it will be possible to obtain a view of the entire landscape. The opportunity should be seized enthusiastically.

Norman Geschwind, M.D.

James Jackson Putnam Professor of Neurology
Harvard Medical School
Professor of Psychology
Massachusetts Institute of Technology

Boston, September 1982

This work grew out of an expressed need for sources of information about the linkages between the nervous and immune systems and a thirst for knowledge about the role of brain and behavior in immunomodulation. The fields represented in the body of research contained in this volume include: psychiatry, psychology, neurology, immunology, endocrinology, rheumatology, dermatology, anatomy, hematology, biochemistry, neuroscience, behavioral and psychosomatic medicine, pharmacology and immunogenetics, to name a few.

The interdisciplinary network involved in this field is awesome and far exceeded our preconceptions. There is no official name for this field and it has no organized structure. It is a fluid network, similar to the very nexus it attempts to define and study. Many years ago, George Solomon and Alfred Amkraut--a psychiatrist and an immunologist--teamed up and coined the term "psychoimmunology" to describe their seminal collaborative research. In 1979, Herbert Spector coined the term "neuroimmunomodulation" and launched a newsletter with that name. Recently, Robert Ader chose the name "Psychoneuroimmunology" as the title for his textbook on the subject--the first of its kind. Popular science magazines such as *Omni* and *Psychology Today* are now referring to psychoneuroimmunology using the acronym "PNI," conferring the scientific equivalent of the special legitimacy usually bestowed by *Time* magazine. A more proper name for this field is "psychoneuroendocrinoimmunology," but we doubt that it will catch on. For simplicity's sake, we favor the term "behavioral immunology."

In 1979, one of the editors (S.E.L.) prepared a partial bibliography titled "Behavioral Immunology (1900-1979): The Relationships of Brain and Behavior to Immune Function," and the notice describing it which appeared in the *Journal of Behavioral Medicine* in 1980 generated a deluge of requests for copies. Thus, it seemed to us that there was a need for a more comprehensive collection.

The decision to produce the bibliography led to several problems. Initially, we had intended to write our own critical annotations for each paper we selected. After beginning that process, however, we quickly realized that such a plan was incompatible with a timely publication. Since we believe strongly in the value of the annotations, we elected to reprint the authors' own abstracts as the most efficient means of providing a summary of each paper cited. We were then faced with the ethical and legal problems connected with the ownership of copyright. Although we believe that our use of the verbatim abstracts constitutes a "fair use" as defined by the U.S. Copyright Code, we requested permission to reprint the abstracts from the copyright holders as a courtesy. When requested by the publishers to seek the authors' approval to reprint abstracts, we attempted to contact the lead author by mail to solicit his or her permission. We are extremely grateful to those publishers and authors whose expeditious responses and generosity have allowed us to make these abstracts available to the reader. However, we remind users of this bibliography that the reprinting of these abstracts in this volume in no way alters the copyright ownership of the abstracts and the articles themselves. Readers should keep in mind that the articles can only be duplicated under the provisions of the Copyright Code. Also, the appearance of the abstracts here does not constitute a permission from the original publisher to photoduplicate the original articles. Finally, readers are advised that, although every effort has been made to reproduce this material accurately, citations and abstracts should be checked against the original publication prior to the use of any direct quotations.

As the scope of the book unfolded, it quickly became apparent that there were hundreds of citations related to both the nervous and immune systems which we felt belonged in a different volume. These papers represent the field of "neuroimmunology" and include immunologic aspects of myasthenia gravis, multiple sclerosis, mental retardation, and viral diseases of the nervous system. We intend to publish these in another volume at a future date. More problematic was our decision to exclude papers relating behavior to blood platelets, coagulation and the complement system when no other immunologic factors were involved. There were simply too many to include them all, so we omitted the whole group rather than mislead the reader who might mistakenly believe our collection was comprehensive.

We chose to include papers reporting on purported relationships between behavioral factors (e.g., personality) and diseases related to immune regulation (e.g., rheumatoid arthritis) even when no immunological measures were obtained. Since the bibliography is intended to be a useful sourcebook for behavioral immunology, we wanted to be comprehensive where possible behavioral-immune links might exist. Unambiguous assignment of papers to chapter headings was difficult. We used our best judgment and elected not to place abstracts in more than one location. Hopefully, the index will compensate for this problem. Finally, against the advice of some colleagues, we chose not to be selective in designating papers for inclusion based on criteria of quality or significance. The editorial responsibility of such a review task was too great a burden and would have precluded publication. Furthermore, the problems inherent in such a selection process without the protection of a blinded, peer-review system are obvious. Hence, we cast as fine a net as we could weave, being forced to limit the final work to references from 1976 to the present due to the sheer numbers of citations caught in our shimmering net. For those interested in older, "classic" papers, the reader is referred to the forthcoming publication, *Classics in Psychoneuroimmunology*, edited by Steven Locke, Robert Ader, Hugo Besedovsky, Nicholas Hall, George Solomon and Terry Strom, to be published by Aldine Press in 1983.

The reader may wish to know the delimiters of our search in order to judge the size of the mesh in our net and to check for possible holes. We used citations from several sources: computer bibliographic data bases (Medlars II, 1976-82; BIOSIS, 1980-82; PsycInfo, 1976-82), book chapter references, and reference bibliographies in both published review papers and original articles. These sources were searched exhaustively for citations falling between 1976 and the fall of 1982. Less complete were published abstracts of papers presented at national or international scientific meetings. This is due to the limited availability of published proceedings from such meetings. Where the abstracts were published in the official journal of the society (e.g., *Psychosomatic Medicine* or *Federation Proceedings*), they were included. Another limitation is that foreign language journals without English abstracts were generally omitted as were some foreign language publications where the paper was unavailable in time for our publication. Foreign citations with English abstracts were included. Occasionally, we were unable to obtain a copy of the text of an abstract in time for inclusion in this edition. Authors wishing to have their omitted abstracts included in future editions should send copies of the abstracts to the editors.

We are eager to learn from users of the bibliography of other papers which should have been included but were inadvertently omitted. A form which can be torn out and mailed has been provided in the back of the book to facilitate such feedback.

S.E. Locke
M. Hornig-Rohan

Acknowledgements

This undertaking could not have been accomplished without the generous assistance of a number of individuals. Citations and suggested sources were provided by Theodore Melnechuk, Edward Shaskan and Bernard Fox. Theodore Melnechuk also gave us ideas about the publishing process, as did Leonard Pace. Warner Slack and Howard Bleich made available to us the considerable resources of the Division of Computer Medicine at the Beth Israel Hospital. The technical expertise of Edna Moody, who custom-tailored the word-processing system to meet our needs, was invaluable. Her willingness to provide on-the-spot training and trouble-shooting are gratefully appreciated. Her colleague Michael McKay was helpful in answering our occasional questions relating to hardware needs. Jamieson Forsyth and Elyse McDonough endured the seemingly endless task of typing abstracts and citations into the computer with skill and enthusiasm. In particular, Jamieson's experience with word-processing systems proved extremely useful in organizing our system for obtaining copyright permissions. Bibliographic searching services and photocopying were competently and expediently carried out by Janice Rand at the Countway Medical Library in Boston, Massachusetts. The Countway Library, an incredible educational resource, graciously provided the use of its facilities without which the project could not have been completed. The artwork, layout and advertising assistance of Judy West is much appreciated. Several reviewers with considerable editorial experience and knowledge of the field provided useful feedback following review of an early draft of this bibliography. These were: Theodore Melnechuk, Robert Ader, George Solomon and Bernard Fox. We are deeply indebted to M. Barry Flint and the Institute for the Advancement of Health for facilitating the timely publication of this work. One of the authors (S.E.L.) was supported in part by a Young Investigator Award (1R23-CA-29155) from the National Cancer Institute, which afforded the opportunity to delve into brain-immune relationships. The Department of Psychiatry at Beth Israel Hospital, by providing a stimulating and supportive academic environment, facilitated the publication of this work. Finally, we wish to express our gratitude to Gilbert Levin, Edith and Raymond Locke, Debra Shapiro, and Jim Hornig-Rohan for personal support and encouragement.

S.E. Locke
M. Hornig-Rohan

The Institute for the Advancement of Health extends special thanks to Ambassador William A. Hewitt and Mrs. William A. Hewitt. Their generous contributions provided important assistance in the publication of this book.

"Well, I don't get angry, okay? I mean I have a tendency to internalize. I can't express anger. That's one of the problems I have. I-I grow a tumor instead."

—Isaac Davis in *Manhattan*,
by Woody Allen and Marshall Brickman

Contents

The Central Nervous System and Immune Function

Neuroanatomy of the immune system

1

Anonymous. **Autoimmunity in left-handers** (research news). *Science.* 1982;217:141-4. (English)

2

Aubert C, Janiaud P, Lecalvez J. **Effect of pinealectomy and melatonin on mammary tumor growth in Sprague-Dawley rats under different conditions of lighting.** *J Neural Transm.* 1980; 47:121-30. (English) (no abstract)

3

Bardos P, Biziere K, De Genne D, Renoux G. **Regulation of natural killer activity by the cerebral neocortex.** In: *Natural Killers: Fundamental Aspects and Role in Cancer.* Human Cancer Immunology, Vol 6. B Serron, RB Herberman (eds.). Amsterdam: Elsevier/North Holland, in press. (English)

An initial study showed that production of lesions in the left cerebral neocortex caused in mice a 50% reduction in the number of splenic Thy-1+ cells and a severe depression of T-cell mediated responses. This study was prompted by the thought that the central nervous system could mediate the influence of sodium diethyldithiocarbamate (DTC) on T cells, through an increased production of selective inducers of prothymocytes, and of the anabolic effect of the agent on emaciated mice. Although natural killer (NK) cells do not possess the full characteristics of T cells, indirect evidence, i.e., the reduction of NK activity after repeated treatment with anti-Thy-1 serum and complement, would suggest that they may correspond to a subpopulation of T cells or, rather, of pre-T cells. It seemed, therefore, of interest to investigate the effect of partial ablation of the left or right cerebral neocortex on the NK activity of mouse spleen cells, and on antibody-dependent cell-mediated cytotoxicity (ADCC) to chicken erythrocytes, which was chosen as a further control for the lack of indirect influence by surgical trauma. We present here an account of our findings which indicate that an intact left cerebral cortex is essential for the expression of NK activity, while this activity is not affected by lesions in the right neocortex.

4

Bardos P, Degenne D, Lebranchu Y, Biziere K, Renoux G. **Neocortical lateralization of NK activity in mice.** *Scand J Immunol.* 1981;13:609-11. (English)

The natural killer (NK) reactivity of mouse spleen cells is controlled by the left brain neocortex and not by the right symmetrical brain area. The finding strongly suggests direct relationships between the central nervous system and the immune system, both involved in biological adaptation for the maintenance of homeostasis and body integrity in relation to the external environment.

5

Besedovsky HO, Del Rey A, Sorkin E, Da Prada M, Keller HH. **Immunoregulation mediated by the sympathetic nervous system.** *Cell Immunol.* 1979;48:346-55. (English)

A postulated immunoregulatory role for the autonomic nervous system was explored utilizing several *in vivo* and *in vitro* approaches. Local surgical denervation of the spleen in rats and general chemical sympathectomy by 6-hydroxydopamine combined with adrenalectomy yielded a similar removal of restraint expressed as enhancement in the number of PFC (plaque-forming cells) in response to immunization. Noradrenaline (norepinephrine) and the synthetic alpha-agonist clonidine which are, respectively, natural and artificial effector molecules of the sympathetic nervous system each strongly suppressed the *in vitro* induced immune response of murine spleen cells to SRBC (sheep red blood cells). Radiometric-enzymatic assay of noradrenaline in the splenic pulp revealed a decrease in the content of this neurotransmitter just preceding the exponential phase of the immune response to SRBC (days 3 and 4) in this site. A dynamic immunoregulatory relationship between the immune and sympathetic nervous system was suggested.

6

Besedovsky HO, Sorkin E, Felix D, Haas H. **Hypothalamic changes during the immune response.** *Eur J Immunol.* 1977;7:323-25. (English)

The immune system is subject to an array of identified autoregulatory processes, but immunoregulation may also have a further basis in a network of immune-neuroendocrine interactions. Two antigens each produced an increase of more than 100% in electrical activity of individual neurones in the ventromedial but not in the anterior nucleus of the rat hypothalamus. Animals that failed to respond to antigen manifested no increase in the firing rate. These findings constitute the first evidence for a flow of information from the activated immune system to the hypothalamus, suggesting that the brain is involved in the immune response.

7

Boranic M. **Central nervous system and immunity** (author's transl). *Lijec Vjesn.* 1980;102:602-8. (Czech)

The immune reactions are controlled to a large extent by intrinsic regulatory mechanisms of the immune apparatus, such as programmed functions of different cell classes and cellular interactions taking place in the lymphatic tissue. But there is also control at the level of the organism as a whole. That is accomplished by hormonal and vegetative nervous mechanisms integrated by the hypothalamus. Experimental lesions of the anterior hypothalamus supress the immune reactivity, whereas lesions of the posterior hypothalamus may stimulate it. Lymphocytes have receptors for hormones and catecholamines at their membranes, the spectrum of which varies with type and maturity of the lymphoid cell. Specificity of the neurohumoral control is thus ensured at each stage of the immune reaction. Differentiation of lymphocytes into mature forms is also promoted by neurohumoral influences. Alterations of the immune reactivity under physical or psychogenic stress is probably accomplished by the operation of neurohumoral mechanisms. The resistance to infectious agents, as a form of immunity, can thus be decreased or increased, depending on the type and duration of stress. Therefore, psychosomatic factors may contribute to the acquisition of infectious diseases, their course, and to the reconvalescence. The recognition of neuroendocrine control over the immune processes has warranted attempts at modification of the immune response by means of drugs that act on central or peripheral synaptic transmission.

8

Brooks WH, Cross RJ, Roszman TL, Markesbery WR. **Neuroimmunomodulation: neuroanatomical basis for impairment and facilitation.** *Ann Neurol.* 1982;12:56-61. (English)

Rats with bilateral electrolytic lesions of specific limbic nuclei show alterations in lymphoid cell number and *in vitro* concanavalin A (Con A) induced lymphocyte activation. A decrease in the number of splenocytes occurs after lesioning in the anterior hypothalamus (AHT;$p<0.001$), ventromedial hypothalamus (VMH;$p<0.02$) and mamillary bodies (MB;$p<0.001$). The number of thymocytes decreases after AHT-lesioning ($p<0.001$) and increases after hippocampal lesions (HC;$p<0.001$). Spleen cell responsiveness to Con A decreases subsequent to AHT-lesioning, whereas, enhanced reactivity occurred after lesion placement in the MB ($p<0.002$), HC ($p<0.001$) and amygdaloid complex (AM;$p<0.001$). Thymocyte mitogen reactivity is increased by lesions of the HC ($p<0.001$) and AM ($p<0.001$). These effects manifest themselves maximally 4 days after lesioning, with a return to normal by day 14. These preliminary data indicate that quantitative and qualitative lymphocyte function are altered by ablation of selected brain nuclei, thereby, suggesting the presence of neural modulation of immune function.

9

Bulloch K, Moore RY. **Innervation of the thymus gland by brainstem and spinal cord in mouse and rat.** *Am J Anat.* 1981;162:157-66. (English)

Central nervous system (CNS) projections to the thymus were studied in the mouse and rat using the horseradish peroxidase (HRP)-retrograde transport method. With discrete HRP injections localized to the thymus, labeled neurons are evident in both medulla and spinal cord. In the medulla the largest population of labeled neurons is present in the retrofacial nucleus. Within this cytoarchitectonically distinct nucleus the majority of neurons are labeled with large thymus HRP injections. In addition to retrofacial nucleus, scattered labeled neurons are found throughout the rostrocaudal extent of the nucleus ambiguus and in the dorsal medullary tegmentum adjacent to the dorsal motor vagus nucleus. With HRP injections restricted to thymus parenchyma, no labeled neurons are evident in the dorsal motor vagus nucleus. Two groups of spinal cord neurons are labeled. In segments C2-C4, neurons localized to the ventral horn are labeled in two distinct columns, one lying laterally in the ventral horn and the other located medially. Labeling of neurons in these segments is distinct from that of large motor neurons located medially in the ventral horn extending from the level of the decussation of the pyramids through the C1 segment. The location and sizes of neurons labeled in these areas following thymus HRP injection are identical in mouse and rat. These observations provide evidence for previously unknown projections from spinal cord and brainstem to the thymus which may play an important role in the regulation of thymic function.

10

Bulloch K. **Neuroendocrine-immune circuitry: pathways involved with the induction and persistence of humoral immunity.** *Diss Abstr Int.* 1981;41:4447-B. (English)

The hypothesis has been put forth that many human as well as murine autosomal recessive diseases, with multiple defects in the nervous, endocrine and immune systems, have their etiology in a disruption of the formation and/or integration of neuroendocrine-immune network. In order to test this hypothesis a thorough study was undertaken of the murine mutant staggerer, reported to have anomalies in these three systems. Since the functional integrity of the thymus gland is crucial to the formation of the hypothalamic-pituitary axis during the perinatal period as well as to immune competence during postnatal development, an anatomical study was first carried out in normal animals to define CNS parasympathetic pathways that may be involved with thymic function. Utilizing horseradish peroxidase (HRP) histochemistry, CNS thymic projections were localized to the brainstem's nucleus ambiguus and the medial ventral horn of the upper cervical spinal cord. Terminal distribution of cholinergic fibers was determined developmentally utilizing acetylcholinesterase (AChE) histochemistry. From this study it was learned that cholinergic vagal fibers entered the thymus prior to birth and may be responsible for prenatal differentiation of the gland. The heaviest distribution of these fibers within the thymus was confined primarily to the corticomedullary boundaries and beneath the capsule. An analysis of the development of catecholamine innervation was undertaken to evaluate the sympathetic aspect of autonomic innervation. Utilizing glyoxylic fluorescent histochemistry it was found that catecholamine (CA) innervation develops postnatally with fibers entering the thymus along the vasculature and septa and forming perivascular plexi within the medulla and among the interlobular septa. In addition, CA free nerve endings were found present within the medulla and cortex. Other delicate CA fibers developed in the cortex in intimate association with a discrete system of cortical autofluorescent (CAF) cells and formed what appeared to be part of a neuroendocrine reflex possibly involved in immune thymic function. An analysis of autonomic innervation of the staggerer thymus revealed CNS neuronal organization consistent with the wildtype mice. However, terminal distribution of the cholinergic fibers was aberrant and indicated an anomaly in prenatal vagal innervation. Sympathetic CA innervation was also found aberrant as was the organization of the CAF cells indicating a disturbance in the neurosecretory reflex arc. Characterization of an aberrant endocrine-dependent behavior, nest-building, in the staggerer mutant indicated that the anomalous prenatal thymic innervation of the vagus may have initiated a perturbation in the neuroendocrine axis resulting in the aberrant patterns of postnatal thymic innervation. In order to ascertain if aberrant autonomic innervation in the thymus influenced immunological competence, a study of antigen-specific humoral and cell-mediated immunity was undertaken in the staggerer mutant. The results from this immunological characterization revealed that a sexual dimorphism in antigen-specific humoral immunity exists in the normal phenotype, whereas it was lacking in the mutant. In an attempt to verify that an endocrine imbalance was responsible for that staggerer's immune phenotype, hormone capsules were implanted in nonmutant mice prior to immunization. This study revealed that: (1) males and females implanted with the same hormone produced a different response to a given antigen when compared to controls and (2) a comparison of the magnitude of this response revealed no differences between males and females and produced a phenotype similar to that found in male and female staggerer mutants. The experimental results presented in this dissertation offer strong evidence supporting a role for thymic innervation in the development and function of the neuroendocrine-immune network and lend further credence to the hypothesis proposed.

11
Cogburn LA, Glick B. **Lymphopoiesis in the chicken pineal gland.** *Am J Anat.* 1981;162:131-42. (English)

Pineal lymphoid development was studied in two breeds of chickens from hatching until sexual maturity. No lymphocytes were found in the pineal prior to 9 days of age (da). Lymphocytes migrate through the endothelium of venules into the pineal stroma. Lymphoid tissue reached its maximal accumulation in 32-da pineal glands of both breeds. At this age, the New Hampshire (NH) breed had a larger proportion of lymphoid volume to total pineal volume (32%) than did pineal glands from White Leghorn (WL) (18%). Averaged over the period 23 to 62 da, NH chickens (a heavy breed) had a lymphoid volume (0.753mm^3) that was about three times greater (p<0.05) than that of the lighter WL breed (0.251 mm^3). Lymphocytes are able to enter cerebrospinal fluid from lymphoid accumulations (LA) embedded in the choroid plexus by migrating between choroid ependymal cells. The 122-da chickens typically lacked lymphoid tissue in the pineal gland with the exception of occasional LA contained in capsular tissue. Surgical bursectomy, thymectomy, or their combination at hatching followed with whole-body irradiation (IR) at

24 hours postsurgery inhibited the initial influx of lymphocytes usually seen in 9-da pineal glands. Also, these treatments prevented formation of germinal centers normally found in the pineal at 3 and 5 weeks and reduced total pineal volume at each age examined. However, pineal lymphoid volume of the surgical-IR group did not differ from control-IR chickens at either 3 or 5 weeks. Pineal glands from birds made agammaglobulinemic (bursa-cell depleted) by cyclophosphamide treatment *in ovo* were devoid of germinal centers, although thin strands of lymphocytes were usually found along venous sinuses. These dissociation studies suggest that the normal expression of lymphoid tissue in the chicken pineal gland is dependent on the bursa and thymus. Furthermore, these observations indicate that the pineal gland should be considered a functional component of the chicken's lymphomyeloid complex.

12
Cross RJ, Brooks WH, Roszman TL, Markesbery WR. **Hypothalamic-immune interactions: effect of hypophysectomy on neuroimmunomodulation.** *J Neurol Sci.* 1982;53:557-66. (English)

Electrolyte destruction of certain nuclei of the brain causes specific structural and functional changes in the immune system. Lesions in the preoptic-anterior hypothalamic area result in thymic involution and a decrease in the number and blastogenic reactivity of splenocytes. In contrast, lesions in the hippocampus increase thymic and splenic mitogenic responsiveness and cellularity. Hypophysectomy abrogates all changes in splenocyte number and function induced by hypothalamic and limbic lesions. The effects of ablating the hippocampus and amygdaloid complex on thymocyte number and function also are abolished. Hypothalamic lesions in hypophysectomized animals result in an increase in the number of thymocytes but suppressed mitogenic activity. These data indicate that neuroimmunomodulation is mediated predominantly but not exclusively by the pituitary gland.

13
Cross RJ, Markesbery WR, Brooks WH, Roszman TL. **Hypothalamic-immune interactions; I--The acute effect of anterior hypothalamic lesions on the immune response.** *Br Res.* 1980;196:79-87. (English)

Rats with electrolytic anterior hypothalamic lesions show changes in lymphoid tissue cellularity and a decrease in the response to concanavalin A (Con A). This effect manifests itself maximally 4 days after lesioning, with a return to normal by day 14. The changes are not mediated through the release of corticosteroids. These data indicate the presence of a neuroendocrine pathway that is capable of modulating immune function.

14
Cross RJ, Markesbery WR, Brooks WH, Roszman TL. **The acute effect of hypothalamic lesions on the immune response** (abstract). *Fed Proc, Am Soc Exp Biol.* 1980;39:1162. (English)

Fischer 344 rats with bilateral electrolytic anterior hypothalamic lesions show changes in lymphoid tissue cellularity (spleen and thymus) and a decrease in the response to Concanavalin A (spleen). This effect manifests itself maximally four days after lesioning, with a return to normal by day fourteen. The suppressed response noted at day four can be abrogated by removal of adherent cells from the spleen cell suspension prior to culturing with Concanavalin A. Addition of varying numbers of adherent cells to non-adherent cells results in progressive suppression of the response. The suppressor activity in the adherent cell population appears to have characteristics best associated with the macrophage. These changes, furthermore, are not mediated through the release of corticosteroids. These data indicate the presence of a neuro-endocrine pathway that is capable of modulating immune function.

15
Cunnane SC, Manku MS, Horrobin DF. **The pineal and regulation of fibrosis: and prostaglandins in fibrosis and regulation of T lymphocytes.** *Med Hypotheses.* 1979;5:403-14. (English)

Pinealectomy leads to increased formation of fibrous tissue in the abdominal cavity, increased skin pigmentation and elevated cholesterol and alkaline phosphatase levels. It also leads to reduced formation and/or action of prostaglandin (PG) E[1] and thromboxane (TX) A[2]. PGE[1] plays an important role in enhancing function of T suppressor lymphocytes which control overactive antibody-producing B lymphocytes. In primary biliary cirrhosis there are increased skin pigmentation, hepatic fibrosis, elevated cholesterol and alkaline phosphatase levels, defective T lymphocytes and hyperactive B lymphocytes. Primary biliary cirrhosis may be a pineal deficiency disease. Serotonin is important in the pineal and the serotonin antagonist methysergide may cause retroperitoneal fibrosis by interfering with pineal function. There is a good deal of other evidence which suggests that melatonin, PGE[1] and TXA[2] are important in the regulation of fibrosis in other situations such as "collagen" diseases, lithium-induced fibrosis and cardiomyopathies. This suggests that enhancement of formation of PGE[1] and of TXA[2] may be of value in diseases associated with excess fibrosis and defective T suppressor cell function. PGE[1] levels may be raised by zinc, penicillin, penicillamine and essential fatty acids. TXA[2] levels may be raised by low dose colchicine. These new approaches to treatment may prove safer and more effective than existing ones. They may be of value in disorders such as cardiomyopathy, Hodgkin's disease and other lymphomas, multiple sclerosis, Crohn's disease, atopy and other diseases in which defective T cell function is suspected.

16
Dann JA, Wachtel SS, Rubin AL. **Possible involvement of the central nervous system in graft rejection.** *Transplantation.* 1979;27:223-6. (English)

Electrolytic lesions were produced in the tuberal hypothalamus and amygdala of male Fischer and female BNLF[1] rats, and in male Fischer and female BNLF[1] rats that had received antecedent hypophysectomies. Skin grafts from Lewis rats survived less well on tuberal-lesioned male Fischer rats than similar grafts on sham-operated and amygdala-lesioned male Fischer rats. Lewis skin graft survival was also curtailed in male Fischer rats that had received hypophysectomies followed by tuberal lesions. These differences were not apparent across the male to female (H-Y) BNLF[1] histocompatibility barrier. We conclude: (1) that tuberal hypothalamic lesions stimulate allograft reactivity in rats, (2) that this response is greater when the immunogenetic disparity between donor and host is greater, and (3) that the mechanism governing this response involves a direct neural pathway which bypasses the hypothalamic-hypophyseal axis.

17
Geschwind N, Behan P. **Left-handedness: association with immune disease, migraine and developmental learning disorder.** *Proc Natl Acad Sci.* 1982;79:5097-100. (English)

We report an experimental study designed to test the following hypothesis derived from clinical observations: There is an elevated frequency in left-handed individuals and in their families of immune disease, migraine and developmental learning disorders. In two separate investigations the frequency of these conditions was compared in strongly left-handed subjects and in strongly right-handed controls. In each of the investigations we found markedly higher frequencies of immune disease in and in general population control subjects free of these disorders. There was a higher frequency of left-handedness in patients with migraine and myasthenia gravis than in controls. We present a brief outline of a hypothesis that may account for an increased frequency of immune disease in left-handers and in their families.

18
Grigorev VA. **Steady potential dynamics of rabbit hypothalamic structures in the early stages of the development of an immune response.** *Fiziol Zh SSSR.* 1981;67:463-7. (Russian) (no English abstract)

19
Hall NR, Lewis JK, Schimpff RD, Smith RT, Trestcot AM, Gray HE, Wenzel SE, Abraham WC, Zornetzer SF. **Effects of diencephalic and brainstem lesions on haemopoietic stem cells (abstract).** *Soc Neurosci Abstr.* 1978;4:20. (English)

A functional axis between the central nervous system and bone marrow has been postulated based upon several types of evidence. Haemopoietic cells possess receptors for certain neurotransmitter substances, nerve endings not associated with blood vessels are present in bone marrow and haemopoietic cells exhibit a light-responsive circadian rhythm. To test for the existence of a brain-bone marrow axis, C57Bl/6J and Swiss Webster mice received bilateral electrolytic lesions (300 microA anodal current for ten seconds) of the anterior hypothalamus, posterior hypothalamus, locus coeruleus or cerebellum. A standard *in vivo* technique was used to assess the number of haemopoietic stem cells. Six weeks after lesioning, the animals were exposed to a sub-lethal dose of radiation which stimulated the formation of colony forming units on the surface of the spleen (CFU-S). Only those subjects that had received locus coeruleus lesions had significantly reduced numbers of CFU-S when compared with control values. Macroautoradiography following the injection of Fe[59] revealed many of these colonies to be erythrocytic. An *in vitro* clonal assay was used to assess the number of granulocytic progenitor cells. Bone marrow cells seeded into either soft agar or methyl cellulose produced significantly reduced numbers of granulocyte macrophage colonies (GM-CFC) when the donor animals had received locus coeruleus lesions. This reduction was more pronounced in animals with bilateral lesions than in animals with unilateral lesions. Preliminary evidence suggests that this effect can be reversed by administering amphetamines. Animals with locus coeruleus lesions were also found to have lower peripheral blood white cell counts when compared with controls; however, the lesions had no effect of the differential cell count. Haemagglutinating antibody titers five days after the injection of sheep red blood cells were not affected by the locus coeruleus lesions. These data suggest an interaction between the nucleus locus coeruleus and haemopoietic stem cells in the bone marrow. The mechanism by which this interaction is able to occur is currently under investigation.

20
Hall NR, Lewis JK, Smith RT, Zornetzer SF. **Effects of locus coeruleus and anterior hypothalamic brain lesions on antibody formation in mice (abstract).** *Soc Neurosci Abstr.* 1979;5:511. (English)

Previous data have shown that electrolytic lesions of the nucleus locus coeruleus are capable of inhibiting the subsequent formation of both granulocyte-macrophage colonies in tissue culture and hemopoietic colony forming units on the spleen induced by radiation exposure. Hemopoietic stem cells arising in the bone-marrow give rise to lymphocytes under the influence of the appropriate microenvironmental factors. The possibility that lesions of the nucleus locus coeruleus might exert an inhibitory influence over the immune system as measured by antibody formation was subsequently investigated. Adult C57Bl/6J female mice received bilateral lesions induced electrolytically (300 microA for 10 seconds) in either the nucleus locus coeruleus or the anterior hypothalamus. Control animals were given nembutal anesthesia but were not manipulated surgically. All subjects were ovariectomized to eliminate differences that might have been due to cyclic fluctuations of ovarian hormones. Animals were allowed 6 weeks recovery time before being injected with antigen. Sheep red blood cells were washed in hemagglutination buffer and injected i.p. in 0.25 cc of RPMI 1640 media. Five days later, the subjects were sacrificed by decapitation and trunk blood was collected as a source of serum for measuring hemagglutinating antibody titers. Brains were removed and sectioned for histologic verification of the lesion site. Animals in both lesion groups were found to be good antibody responders. There was no statistical difference between those animals that had received lesions of the locus coeruleus and those with anterior hypothalamic lesions. Neither of the values obtained from the lesioned animals differed from the unlesioned control titer. These data suggest that the inhibitory influence of locus coeruleus lesions upon bone marrow stem cells is not manifested by a functional impairment of the immune system as assessed by using the above paradigm.

21
Jankovic BD, Isakovic K, Knezevic Z. **Ontogeny of the immuno-neuroendocrine relationship: early thymec-**

tomy of the chick embryo. *Immunol Lett.* 1979;1:7. (English) (unavailable at publication)

22
Jankovic BD, Isakovic K, Kuezeiaavic A. **Ontogeny of the immuno-neoroendocrine relationship. Changes in lymphoid tissues of chick embryos surgically decapitated at 33-38 hours of incubation.** *Dev. Comp Immunol.* 1978;2:479-91. (English)

The prosencephalen, and primordium of the hypophysis were surgically removed from chick embryos at 33-38 hours of incubation. The thymus, bursa of Fabricus, spleen, bone marrow and liver were examined cytomorphologically on day 15, 17 and 19. T marker-bearing and Bu marker-bearing lymphocytes were identified by immunofluorescence. Decapitated embryos tended to be smaller than sham-decapitated controls of the same age, and exhibited retarded development of the thymus, bursa, spleen and liver. Decapitation particularly affected the cellular composition of the bursa and spleen, induced a decrease in the number of lymphocytes, and caused a striking depletion of lymphocytes bearing Bu antigen. This experiment showed an interdependence between lymphoid (immune), nervous and endocrine centers in the chick embryo.

23
Jankovic BD, Isakovic K, Micic M, Knezevic Z. **The embryonic lympho-neuro-endocrine relationship.** *Clin Immunol Immunopathol.* 1981;18:108. (English) (unavailable at publication)

24
Jankovic BD, Jovanova K, Markovic BM. **Effect of hypothalamic stimulation on immune reactions in the rat.** *Period Biol.* 1979;81:211. (English) (unavailable at publication)

25
Keller SE, Shapiro R, Schleifer SJ, Stein M. **Hypothalamic influences on anaphylaxis** (abstract). *Psychosom Med.* 1982;44:302. (English)

Anterior hypothalamic lesions placed prior to antigen sensitization afford significant protection against lethal anaphylaxis in the guinea pig. The effects of hypothalamic lesions on anaphylaxis could be related to antigen specific and nonspecific changes in the immune system as well as to changes in tissue factors and organ responsivity. The present study was undertaken to clarify some of the mechanisms which may be involved in the protective effect of anterior hypothalamic lesions on lethal guinea pig anaphylaxis by the investigation of the effect of the placement of lesions following sensitization. Twenty-one days post-sensitization with ovalbumin, bilateral anterior hypothalamic lesions were placed stereotaxically in guinea pigs. Controls consisted of sham and non-operated animals. Seven days after the stereotaxic procedure, the lesioned, sham-operated and non-operated animals were randomly divided into four subgroups and challenged by intracardiac injections of 0.25, 0.375, 0.5 or 2.0 mg ovalbumin. Survival in the different groups was analyzed by regression of the arc sin of the proportion of surviving animals in relation to antigen dose. Anterior hypothalamic lesions were found to have no significant protective effect on lethal anaphylaxis in the animals sensitized prior to placement of lesions with each of the 4 challenge doses of ovalbumin. Furthermore, the severity of anaphylaxis in the survivors was not altered in the lesioned animals. Since anterior hypothalamic lesions placed presensitization but not postsensitization provide protection against lethal anaphylaxis, the hypothalamic effect appears to be related to immune components of the anaphylactic reaction. The findings of the present study further suggest that while the hypothalamus may influence the target organ, these effects are not sufficient to inhibit anaphylaxis.

26
Keller SE, Stein M, Camerino MS, Schleifer SJ, Sherman J. **Suppression of lymphocyte stimulation by anterior hypothalamic lesions in the guinea pig.** Cell Immunol. 1980;52:334-40. (English)

Anterior hypothalamic lesions in the guinea pig inhibited lymphocyte stimulation in whole blood cultures with the antigen tuberculin and with the mitogen phytohemagglutinin (PHA) and suppressed the delayed cutaneous hypersensitivity response to tuberculin. The lesions did not affect the stimulation of purified lymphocytes with either tuberculin or PHA. The anterior hypothalamic lesions had no effect on the absolute number of T and B lymphocytes.

27
Lambert PL, Harrell EH, Achterberg J. **Medial hypothalamic stimulation decreases the phagocytic activity of the reticuloendothelial system.** Physiol Psychol. 1981; 9:193-6. (English)

Although research has linked the CNS with changes in immunoresponsivity, the possible role of the CNSD in altering reticulodothelial activity is lacking. The present study investigated the possible relationship between hypothalamic structures and changes in responsivity of the reticuloendothelial system. Eight male albino Sprague-Dawley rats received bilateral electrode implants in the ventromedial area of the hypothalamus, and following brain stimulation, reticuloendothelial activity was assessed 3, 6, 12, 24 and 96 hours after stimulation. Brain stimulation decreased phagocytic activity of the reticuloendothelial system. Findings may increase understanding of a possible neural mechanism underlying relationships between stress and resistance to disease states.

28
Lapin V. **Pineal gland and malignanoy.** Osterr Z Onkol. 1976;3:51-60. (German)

During the last few decades, a great deal of new knowledge about morphology, physiological and biochemical activities of the pineal gland has been gained, but there is still little information available about the correlation of the pineal gland to disease, especially to neoplasias. Various studies have pointed out that the pineal gland might have an influence on the growth and genesis of malignant tumors. The aims of this paper is to review the recent as well as the previous literature concerning the possible role of this gland in neoplastic growth. This survey is not considered to exhaustively analyze all the data on this issue, but it is intended to provide an additional analysis to the previous review made up to 1953 by Kitay and Altschule.

29
Lapin V. **Pineal influences on tumor.** Prog Brain Res. 1979;52:523-33. (English) (no abstract)

30
Mathe AA, Yen SS, Sohn RJ, Kemper T. **Effect of hypothalamic lesions on anaphylactic release of PGs from guinea pig lung.** Adv Pharmacol Ther, Proc Int Congr Pharmacol, 7th, 1978. 1979. (English) (unavailable at publication)

31
Maxwell MH. **Leucocyte diurnal rhythms in normal and pinealectomised juvenile female fowls.** Res Vet Sci. 1981;31:113-5. (English)

Peripheral blood from a group of control and pinealectomised juvenile female fowls was examined to establish which leucocytes manifested a diurnal rhythm and what effect pinealectomy had on these cells. The results showed that sinificant diurnal rhythms were displayed by the heterophils, lymphocytes and monocytes ($p<0.001$) but not by the eosinophils or basophils. Comparisons made between the control and pinealectomised birds revealed that the heterophil ($p<0.01$) and monocyte ($p<0.1$) counts were higher in the operated birds whereas the lymphocytes were lower ($p<0.1$) The eosinophils and basophils were unaffected. The removal of the pineal gland did not alter the normal diurnal rhythm of the cells.

32
Nagy E, Berczi I. **Immunodeficiency in hypophysectomized rats** (abstract). Fed Proc, Fed Am Soc Exp Biol. 1979;38:1355. (English)

The response of hypophysectomized, sham-operated and non-operated female Fischer 344 and Wistar-Furth rats were compared to various antigenic stimuli. Antibody production against sheep red blood cells was virtually eliminated by hypophysectomy as measured by hemaggluntination. Treatment of the antisera with 2-mercaptoethanol (2ME) revealed that both the 2ME sensitive (IgM) and 2ME resistant (IgG) antibody classes were affected. The antibody production of hypophysectomized rats could be restored partially by the transplantation of an anterior pituitary tumor (MtT/W10). Delayed hypersensitivity response to dinitrochlorobenze and the development of adjuvant arthritis after treatment with Freund's complete adjuvant were significantly suppressed in hypophysectomized animals. Skin graft survival was also prolonged in hypophysectomized rats when compared to controls. In all the above studies sham-operated rats responded as well as did not-operated controls. The results indicate that the pituitary gland plays an important role in immune reactions.

33
Nagy E, Berczi I. **Immunodeficiency in hypophysectomized rats.** Acta Endicrinol. 1978;89:530-7. (English)

The response of hypophysectomized, sham-operated and

non-operated female Fischer 344 and Wistar-Furth rats was compared to various antigenic stimuli. Antibody production against sheep red blood cells, skin response to dinitrochlorobenzene and the development of adjuvant arthritis after treatment with Freund's complete adjuvant were all markedly suppressed in hypophysectomized animals. Sham-operated rats responded as well as did non-operated controls. Skin graft survival was also prolonged in hypophysectomized rats when compared to controls. These results indicate that the pituitary gland plays an important role in immune reactions.

34
Okouchi E. **Thymus, peripheral tissue and immunological responsiveness of the pituitary dwarf mouse.** *J Physiol Soc Japan.* 1976;38:325-35.

Snell's pituitary dwarf mice (dw) were used for studies on the relationship between hypophysis and lymphoid organs. The age-dependent changes of thymus or spleen weights of dwarf mice were compared with those of normal littermates. The suppression of growth of the thymus or spleen in dwarf mice was recognized at the fifth day of age. Although involution of the thymus varied among animals, a strong positive correlation was demonstrated between relative thymus weight and body weight in 30-40 days old dwarf mice. Lymphoid organs of dwarf mice were reconstituted by injection of growth hormone and/or thyrotoxin. Relative thymus weight significantly increased in dwarf mice when the treatment with growth hormone started at 7 days of age, but the same treatment at 3 months of age did not show any effect on the increment of relative thymus weight. On the other hand, the antibody-forming capacity against sheep erythrocytes of dwarf mice was significantly increased even when the treatment with growth hormone was started at 3 months of age. A marked increase in the number of lymphoid cells in dwarf mice was observed by treatment with thyroxin, even if treatment was started either at 7 days or 3 months of age. Similar changes were also obtained in the antibody-forming capacity.

35
Paunovic VR, Petrovic S, Jankovic BD. **Influence of early postnatal hypothalamic lesions on immune responses of adult rats.** *Period Biol.* 1976;78:50. (English) (unavailable at publication)

36
Pierpaoli W, Maestroni GJ. **Thymus-programmed pineal circadian cyclicity promotes genesis of transplantation immunity: symposium on neuroimmunomodulation.** *Proc XXVIII Int Congr.* (Budapest, 1980). 1981. (English) (unavailable at publication)

37
Quay WB, Gorray KC. **Pineal effects on metabolism and glucose homeostasis: evidence for lines of humoral mediation of pineal influences on tumor growth.** *J Neural Transm.* 1980;47:107-20. (English)

Results from animal experiments support the hypothesis that pineal gland function can influence some aspects of tissue metabolism and glucose homeostasis. Evidence of pineal effects on particular endocrine and sympatheto-adrenal

targets contributes to an understanding of indirect routes by which pineal activity can possibly affect the growth and activity of some kinds of tumors, in part through nutrient and metabolic effects in the tissue environment of the tumor cells.

38
Reilly FD, McCuskey PA, Miller ML, McCuskey RS, Meineke HA. **Innervation of the periarteriolar lymphatic sheath of the spleen.** *Tissue Cell.* 1979;11:121-6. (English)

During the course of a neurohistochemical and two independent electron microscopic studies of the mouse spleen, unmyelinated adrenergic nerves containing numerous dense core and lucent vesicles and devoid of neurolemma were observed adjacent to reticular cells and lymphocytes in the white pulp. Some of these nerves formed an intimate relationship with these cells. Since adrenergic substances have been reported to modulate the cell cycle of lymphocytes *in vitro,* these findings are suggestive of a neural influence on the cell cycle of lymphocytes *in vivo.*

39
Reilly FD, McCuskey RS, Meineke HA. **Studies on the hematopoietic microenvironment; VIII--Adrenergic and cholinergic innervation of the murine spleen.** *Anat Rec.* 1976;185:109-17. (English)

Neurohistochemical techniques were used to confirm morphologically the distribution of adrenergic and cholinergic nerves to the splenic microvasculature. The results form the basis of this report. Using these methods, adrenergic innervation was observed only in the adventitia of arteries and arterioles. No cholinergic innervation was found in this site. No adrenergic or cholinergic innervation could be demonstrated to the channels of the red pulp, venules or veins. These data provided morphological evidence that in the murine spleen only splenic arteries and arterioles are innervated; and these have only an adrenergic innervation.

40
Rella W, Lapin V. **Immunocompetence of pinealectomized and simultaneously pinealectomized and thymectomized rats.** *Oncology.* 1976;33:3-6. (English)

The cellular and antibody-mediated immune responsiveness was studied in adult rats which had the pineal and/or the thymus gland removed within 36 hours after birth. The immunological parameters measured were: skin graft rejection, haemolytic plaque formation, and haemagglutinating antibody formation in response to sheep red blood cells and the stimulation of lymphoid cells from the spleen by phytohaemagglutinin and lipopolysaccharide. The removal of the pineal gland had little effect on the degree of immunocompetence in normal or immunosuppressed animals. In some of the immunological tests an accelerated response was observed, which suggests that lymphoid cells from pinealectomized or pinealectomized-thymectomized animals proliferate more rapidly upon contact with antigen or mitogen. This accelerated cell proliferation, unlike the immunodepression of the host, could explain the enhanced growth of transplantable tumors observed in pinealectomized animals.

41

Renoux G, Biziere K, Renoux M, Guillaumin JM. **The cerebral cortex regulates immune responses in the mouse.** *C R Acad Sci (D) (Paris).* 1980;290:719-22. (French)

Ablation of the left cerebral cortex abrogates the production of thymic hormone, reduces the number of spleen T cells and impairs immunization with sheep erythrocytes. In addition, partial decortication inhibits the ability of sodium diethyldithiocarbamate (DTC) to increase the level of circulating thymic hormone, as well as the number of splenic T cells. Therefore, the cerebral cortex would display an important role to maintain body integrity and relations with the external environment, through its effects on the immune system.

42

Roszman TL, Cross RJ, Brooks WH, Markesbery WR. **Hypothalamic-immune interactions; I--The effect of hypothalamic lesions on the ability of adherent spleen cells to limit lymphocyte blastogenesis.** *Immunology.* 1982;45:737-43. (English)

Animals with electrolytic pre-optic and anterior hypothalamic (AHT) lesions show impaired mitogen-induced lymphocyte blastogenesis which is restored by removal of a population of spleen cells with macrophage-like properties. Although suppressor macrophages are detectable in normal and control rats, substantially more activity is present following AHT destruction. Abrogation of lymphocyte activation does not result from increased numbers of splenic macrophages. These data indicate that one mechanism by which neuroimmunomodulation occurs is by induction of a qualitative alteration in the function of naturally occurring suppressor macrophages.

44

Simon RH, Lovett EJ III, Tomaszek D, Lundy J. **Electrical stimulation of the midbrain mediates metastatic tumor growth.** *Science.* 1980;209:1132-3. (English)

Pulmonary metastases were counted 10 days after female rats received tail-vein injections of Walker-256 carcinosarcoma cells. Previous observations that halothane anesthesia plus hind-limb amputation increases the number of metastases were confirmed. Amputation under the analgesia of electrical stimulation of the midbrain was found to increase metastatic activity. However, the stimulus-produced analgesia alone also increased the number of metastases. Systemically-administered naloxone blocked the analgesic effect of midbrain stimulation but did not block the increase in the number of pulmonary metastases.

45

Soriano FM, Del Campo FJS, Garcia JL, Agreda VS. **Ultrastructural variations in the thymus after pinealectomy.** *Morfologia normal y patologica.* 1980;4:17-26. (Spanish) (unavailable at publication)

46

Spector NH, Koob GF, Baron S. **Hypothalamic influence upon interferon and antibody responses to Newcastle Disease Virus infection: preliminary report.** *Proc Int Union Physiol Sci.* 1977;13:711. (English) (unavailable at publication)

47

Srebro Z, Brodzicki S. **Changed activity in the hypothalamic neurosecretory centers and the pituitary gland of mice in the course of tetanus toxoid immunization.** *Folia Biol.* 1978;26:257-62. (Polish) (unavailable at publication)

48

Stein M, Schiavi RC, Camerino MS. **Influence of brain and behavior on the immune system.** *Science.* 1976;191:435-40. (English)

It has been shown experimentally that psychosocial processes influence the susceptibility to some infections, to some neoplastic processes, and to some aspects of humoral and cell-mediated immune responses. These psychosocial effects may be related to hypothalamic activity. Reviewing the mechanisms that may be involved in the role of the hypothalamus in immune responses indicates that there is no single mediating factor. Various processes may participate, including the autonomic nervous system and neuroendocrine activity. The research reviewed has been limited primarily to a consideration of the effect of hypothalamic lesions on humoral immune responses. There is some evidence indicating that hypothalamic lesions also modify cell-mediated immune responses. Further research is required to evaluate the effect of the hypothalamus on cell-mediated immunity.

49

Stein M. **Stress, brain and immune function** (abstract). *The Gerontologist.* 1982;22:203. (English)

Numerous studies have shown an association between psychosocial phenomena and pathological states in which immune processes are involved such as bacterial and viral infections, neoplastic disorders, allergy and anaphylaxis and organ transplantation. This presentation is concerned with the relationship between stress and specific measures of immune function. We have investigated in widowers the effects of bereavement on mitogen induced lymphocyte stimulation utilizing a prospective longitudinal design. The findings revealed a significant depression of lymphocyte responses to the mitogens, PHA, Con A, and PWM, during the first two months following the death of a spouse. There was a return in the lymphocyte response to prebereavement levels by 5 months following the death which persisted for the next 12 months. We have been investigating the role of the central nervous system in relation to immune processes for a number of years. The experiments have demonstrated that lesions in the anterior hypothalamus of guinea pigs suppress humoral and cell mediated responses. These findings suggest a biological basis for a link between psychosocial processes, immune function, and health and illness. Some of the biological processes which may be involved in the association between stress and immune function will be reviewed.

50

Terribile V, Caldesi-Valeri V, Lion R. **Is immunity related to the central nervous system?** *Aggressologie.* 1979;20:133-4. (English) (no abstract)

51

Uede T, Ishii Y, Matsuura A, Shimogawara I, Kikuchi K. **Immunohistochemical study of lymphocytes in rat pineal gland: selective accumulation of T lymphocytes.** *Anat Rec.* 1981;199:239-47. (English)

Morphological and immunohistochemical studies were performed to examine the existence of lymphocytes in the brain of rats. Special attention was paid to the time course of the appearance of lymphocytes in and around the pineal gland. Rabbit anti-rat T cell and anti-rat immunoglobulin sera were used for identification of T and B cells in tissue sections. Immunoperoxidase and immunofluorescence techniques were employed to identify cells reacting with anti-T and anti-immunoglobulin sera. No lymphocytes were found in the brain of rats until 20 days after birth. Small clusters of lymphocytes appeared in the pineal region by 30 days of age, after which they gradually increased in number, forming massive clusters in the pineal region by 120 days. Along with an increase in the number of lymphocytic cells, there was a gradual increase of cells reacting with anti-T cell serum. These T cells were only a minority of pineal lymphocytes in younger animals, but 90% or more cells were stained by anti-T cell serum at 120 days after birth. The remaining cells did not react with anti-immunoglobulin sera either. These findings suggest that the gradual increase of T lymphocytes in the rat pineal region is a simple reflection of the normal course of maturation of T cells, and the pineal gland in the rat may have some role in immune responses within the brain.

52

Warejcka DJ, Levy NL. **Central nervous system (CNS) control of the immune response: effect of hypothalamic lesions on PHA responsiveness in rats (abstract).** *Fed Proc, Fed Am Soc Exp Biol.* 1980;39:914. (English)

We questioned whether the immune system is under any form of CNS control. Bilateral electrocoagulative lesions were stereotaxically-placed in various nuclei of the hypothalamus (HT) in adult male Fischer rats. Control group A received burr holes only, while a second control group (B) received bilateral lesions in the thalamus or zona inserta. No difference in survival, gross neurologic function or weight was observed between the 3 groups. 14 d after surgery peripheral blood lymphocytes were tested for responsiveness to phytohemagglutinin (PHA). Spontaneous ^{3}H-thymidine uptake was the same among the 3 groups. All rats bearing bilateral HT lesions had PHA responses less than 40% of the mean response of control group A over an 8-fold PHA dose range. Animals with lesions in the anterior, dorsomedial or ventromedial nuclei consistently had responses near zero. In contrast, animals in the operated control group B had PHA responses of 83-97% of the mean control A level. Spleen cells tested 53-55 d after surgery showed identical results but less marked depression of PHA responsiveness. Preliminary results showed that the response to pokeweed mitogen was even more depressed than that to PHA in animals with HT lesions. The response to concanavalin A was only slightly depressed.

53

Williams JM, Felten DL. **Sympathetic innervation of murine thymus and spleen: a comparative histofluorescence study.** *Anat Rec.* 1981;199:531-42. (English)

Fluorescence microscopy of thymus and spleen from four strains of mice (C3H and ICR controls, AKR spontaneously leukemic and NZB autoimmune) revealed varicose noradrenergic (NE) fibers in perivascular and parenchymal regions of both organs. Thymic innervation was largely perivascular, but isolated islands and strings of free NE fibers were noted among thymic parenchymal cells. A morphological proximity between NE fibers in the thymus and mast cells was noted in all strains studied, but was exceptionally prominent in the NZB thymus. Perivascular plexuses within the splenic white pulp sent single NE fibers between the surrounding lymphocytes. Catecholamines and histamine have been shown to modulate lymphocyte development and activity *in vitro*. The present study provides morphological evidence that both NE and histamine are available to lymphocytes in thymus and spleen, and thus provides morphological evidence for neural modulation of immune activity *in vivo*.

54

Williams JM, Peterson RG, Shea PA, Schmedtje JF, Bauer DC, Felten DL. **Sympathetic innervation of murine thymus and spleen: evidence for a functional link between the nervous and immune systems.** *Br Res Bull.* 1981;6:83-94. (English)

Sympathetic innervation was demonstrated in perivascular and parenchymal regions of murine thymus and spleen. Catecholamine varicosities were associated with mast cells in these areas. The antibody response to sheep red blood cells of 7 week old mice, sympathectomized with 6-hydroxydopamine (6-OHDA) at birth, was significantly elevated compared with saline-treated controls. Alpha- methyl tyrosine (alpha-MT) and 6-OHDA treatment of mice, producing a more complete sympathectomy, showed a significantly enhanced anti-SRBC response with respect to mice treated with only alpha-MT or 6-OHDA. Catecholamine levels in thymus, spleen and adrenals of treated and control mice were measured using liquid chromatography with electrochemical detection (LCEC). The sympathetic nervous system apparently has a functional role in modulating the humoral immune response *in vivo*.

55

Wolf S. Brain, behavior and bodily disease. **Introduction: the role of the brain in bodily disease.** *Res Publ Assoc Res Nerv Ment Dis.* 1981;59:1-9. (English) (unavailable at publication)

Immunology of the nervous system

56

Belokrylov GA. **Antigenic similarity between immune response stimulators from the thymus and brain cortex.** *Biull Eskp Biol Med.* 1980;90:330-2. (Russian)

Rabbit antisera against low molecular weight polypeptides from the thymus (thymosin and thymarin), cortex (cortexin) and white matter of the brain of calves were cross-absorbed with these polypeptides and tested in the complement fixation test with these preparations and in the complement-dependent cytotoxicity test with thymic and bone marrow cells. The results showed that thymosin, thymarin and cortexin are antigenically similar, but differ in antigenic structure from polypeptide from white matter of the brain. Biological effect of polypeptides from the thymus and brain cortex is connected with thymus-dependent lymphocytes and does not depend on B-cells. Cross absorbtion revealed that antisera against polypeptides from thymus and cortex of the brain contain antibody both against common antigens and antigens specific for the appropriate preparation only. Antigenic set of polypeptide from the thymus (thymarin) corresponds more closely to thymic antigen as compared to polypeptide from the brain cortex (cortexin).

57

Brouet JC, Toben H. **Characterization of a subpopulation of human T lymphocytes reactive with an heteroantiserum to human brain.** *J Immunol.* 1976;116:1041. (English)

A rabbit antiserum to human fetal brain reacted after suitable absorptions with a subpopulation of human normal T cells. The distribution of reactive T cells varied according to the organ tested: 23% of peripheral blood lymphocytes, 5% of tonsil lymphocytes, and less than 1% of thymocytes were positive. Reactive cells did not transform after phytohemagglutinin or pokeweed stimulation but were at least weakly stimulated by allogeneic cells. T-derived neoplastic cells from one case of T acute lymphoblastic leukemia, two patients with Sezary syndrome, and from three out of five cases of T chronic lymphocytic leukemias (CCL) yielded negative results. In contrast, all the leukemic cells from two other patients with T-derived CLL were positive suggesting a proliferation of homogeneous cells arising from only a subpopulation of T lymphocytes.

58

Campbell DG, Williams AF, Bayley PM, Reid KBM. **Structural similarities between Thy 1 antigen from rat brain and immunoglobulin.** *Biochem Soc Symp.* 1980;45:45-50. (English) (no abstract)

59

Cunningham J, De Vere-Tyndall A, McCullagh P. **Recognition of histocompatibility determinants controls reactivity of auto-sensitized lymphocytes against neural tissues.** *J Exp Med.* 1980;151:1299-1304. (English)

Thoracic duct lymphocytes from rats sensitized against syngeneic spinal cord rapidly produced damage in cultures of syngeneic cerebellar cells but coexist indefinitely with allogeneic cultures. Lymphocytes from donors that have been sensitized against allogeneic spinal cord attack cultures of syngeneic and specific allogeneic cerebellum but not cells from rats of a third, unrelated strain.

60

Dalchau R, Kirkley J, Fabre JW. **Monoclonal antibody to a human brain granulocyte-T lymphocyte antigen probably homologous to the W3/13 antigen of the rat.** *Eur J Immunol.* 1980;10:745-9. (English) (unavailable at publication)

61

Fujita S, Kitamura J. **Origin of brain macrophages and the nature of the microglia.** *Prog Neuropath.* 1976;3:1-50. (English) (no abstract)

62

Golub ES. **Connections between the nervous, haematopoietic and germ-cell systems** (news and views). *Nature.* 1982;299:283. (English)

63

Horvat J, Jankovic BD, Mitrovic K. **Shared antigenicity between rat brain synaptic vesicles and B lymphocytes.** *Period Biol.* 1979;81:83. (English) (unavailable at publication)

64

Horvat J, Mostarica M, Jankovic BD. **Cross-reactivity between anti-rat nervous tissue antibodies and heterologous thymocytes.** *Period Biol.* 1976;78:108. (English) (unavailable at publication)

65
Ignatov SA, Vedernikova LV, Burbaeva GSH, Lozovskii DV. **Antigenic composition of protein fractions of the human cerebral cortex extracted by chromatography on DEAE-cellulose.** *Zh Nevropatol Psikhiatr.* 1977;77:273-8. (Russian)

In fractionating a phosphate protein extract from the human brain cortex on DEAE-cellulose 10 fractions of the basic acid proteins were received. Analyses of these fractions were conducted by the method of disc electrophoresis in polyacrilamide gel with dodecylsulphate NA and a subsequent separate straining of the densitograms of proteins and glycoproteins, precipitation in agar gel, immunoelectrophoresis and auto-immunography with the use of labeled I^{125} antibodies to rabbit gamma-globulin. In the first 2 basic fractions there were brain specific antigens with electrophoretic mobility of the $beta_2$-gamma-globulin. In the first acid fraction--2 antigens: $alpha_1$-globulin and $alpha_2$-globulin of a glycoprotein nature. In subsequent acid fractions--one antigen with a mobility of $alpha_1$-globulin. A study of the antigen activity of these fractions in a complement fixation test on cold with the serum of schizophrenic patients and disseminated sclerosis depicted differences in the activity of the basis and acid fractions.

66
Isakovic K, Terzic G, Rajcevic M, Jankovic BD. **Antigenic correlation between human brain and T and B tonsillar lymphocytes.** *Period Biol.* 1979;81:87. (English) (unavailable at publication)

67
Jankovic BD, Horvat J, Mitrovic K, Mostarica M. **Rat brain-lymphocyte antigen: characterization by rabbit antisera to rat brain tubulin and S-100 protein.** *Immunochemistry.* 1977;14:75. (English) (unavailable at publication)

68
Jankovic BD, Horvat J, Mitrovic K, Mostarica M. *In vitro* **cross-reacting antibodies from rabbit antisera to rat brain synaptic membranes and thymocytes.** *Scand J. Immunol.* 1977;6:843. (English) (unavailable at publication)

69
Jankovic BD, Horvat J, Mitrovic K. **Antigenic correlation between rat brain synaptic vesicles and rat bone marrow B lymphocytes.** *Experientia.* 1979;35:1393. (English) (unavailable at publication)

70
Jankovic BD, Savic V, Soltes S, Horvat J, Mitrovic K. **Thymocyte-neuron antigenic correlation: anti-thymocyte membrane antibodies modify bioelectrical activity of Helix pomatia neurons.** *Immunol Lett.* 1980;1:275. (English) (unavailable at publication)

71
Krakowka S, Wallace AL, Koestner A. **Shared antigenic determinants between brain and thymus-derived lymphocytes in dogs.** *Acta Neuropathol.* 1981;54:75-82. (English)

Canine anti-canine myelin, canine distemper convalescent, and control sera were tested for the presence of antilymphocyte antibodies in a complement-dependent microcytotoxicity assay. Sera were cytotoxic for CT 45-S cells, a canine origin thymic lymphoma, canine thymocytes, and phytomitogen-transformed canine peripheral blood lymphocytes. The cytotoxic effect was removed by absorption with canine white matter but not by absorption with galactocerebroside. The data suggests that the specificity of antimyelin and anti-lymphocyte antibodies is directed toward a common antigen (canine Thy-1). It is likely that, in canine distemper, these antibodies are produced following the lymphotropic phase of viral infection. The possibility that similar autoimmune phenomena observed in multiple sclerosis patients occur via an unrecognized infectious event in lymphoid tissues is raised.

72
Morimoto C, Abe T, Toguchi T, Homma M. **Characteristics and functional specificity of anti-human BAT (brain associated thymocyte antigen) serum.** *Tohoku J Exp Med.* 1980;130:321-34. (Japanese)

A rabbit antiserum to human fetal brain after multiple absorption reacted with 100% of thymocytes, 55% of peripheral blood lymphocytes and 90% of enriched T lymphocytes, but not significantly with B lymphocytes. Spontaneous SRBC rosette formation was inhibited by anti-BAT pretreatment, but EAC rosette formation remained unaffected. The anti-serum was itself highly stimulatory. However, cells treated with the antiserum and complement exhibited marked inhibition of responsiveness to Con A, little effect with PHA and no alteration with PWM. The MLC reaction was inhibited only when the responder cells were treated with the antiserum and complement. Treatment of sensitized lymphocytes with the antiserum and complement caused a dose-dependent suppression of blastogenic response to both PPD and n-DNA. No effect, however, was noted in MIF producing cells. Con A-induced suppressor function of lymphocytes was abolished by treatment with the antiserum and complement. These results indicate that the anti-BAT serum obtained by us can be utilized for the isolation of T lymphocyte subsets.

73
Mostarica M, Horvat J, Jankovic BD. **Antigenic determinants shared by rat, mouse and hamster thymocytes and brain.** *Period Biol.* 1976;78:110. (English) (unavailable at publication)

74
Mostarica M, Horvat J, Mitrovic K, Jankovic BD. **Cross-reactivity between rat brain subcellular fractions and T and B lymphocytes.** *Scand J Immunol.* 1977;6:731. (English) (unavailable at publication)

75
Shinefeld LA, Sato JL, Rosenberg NE. **Monoclonal rat anti-mouse brain antibody detects Abelson murine leukemia virus target cells in mouse bone marrow.** *Cell.* 1980;20:11-17. (English)

We report the characterization of a monoclonal antibody which detects a surface antigen expressed by the bone marrow target cell of A-MuLV. Treatment of bone marrow cells with this antibody and complement results in >95% loss of the A-MuLV-derived *in vitro* transformed foci. The surface antigen detected by this antibody is also expressed on A-MuLV-transformed lymphoid cell lines, thymocytes, and some peripheral lymphocytes. This antigen is not expressed, however, by the pluripotent hematopoietic stem cell defined by the spleen colony-forming assay. We present evidence that the antigen detected is neither a virally encoded product, nor exclusively associated with the BALB/c genome.

76

Siadak AW, Nowinski RC. **Thy-2: a murine thymocyte-brain alloantigen controlled by a gene linked to the major histocompatibility complex.** *Immunogenetics.* 1981;12:45-58. (English)

We describe a new murine cell-surface alloantigen, provisionally designated Thy-2, which is expressed primarily on thymocytes and brain tissue. Although Thy-2 is also expressed at lower levels on bone marrow spleen cells, this antigen does not appear to be present on lymph node, liver, or red blood cells. Immunoprecipitation of surface-labeled thymocyte extracts from a variety of inbred strains reveals this antigen to be a single polypeptide of 150,000 daltons. Quantitative membrane immunofluorescence demonstrates that Thy-2 is a minor cell-surface component which is present on the majority of thymocytes. Mice heterozygous at the Thy-2 locus express approximately 50 percent as much antigen as positive homozygotes. Expression of the Thy-2 alloantigen is controlled by a single semi-dominant gene located approximately 3 cM to the right of the H-2K locus on chromosome 17.

77

Ting JP, Shigekawa BL, Linthicum DS, Weiner LP, Frelinger JA. **Expression and synthesis of murine immune response-associated (Ia) antigens by brain cells.** *Proc Natl Acad Sci.* 1981;78:3170-4. (English)

This paper provides biochemical and histochemical evidence that a fraction of murine brain cells express and synthesize Ia (Immune response-associated) antigens. Both I-A and I-E subregion products are detected on frozen sections of mouse brains by immunoperoxidase staining. Most of these Ia-bearing cells are located in white matter tracts and appear to be intrafascicular oligodendrocytes. In contrast, cells in the gray matter rarely display detectable Ia antigens on their cell surfaces. Specificity of the staining was confirmed by absorption studies. Biochemical evidence for the active synthesis of Ia antigens by brain cells was obtained by immunoprecipitation of [^{3}H]leucine/tyrosine-labeled, NP-40-extracted cell lysates with monoclonal anti-Ia reagent. Both the alpha and beta subunits of Ia antigens were identified by NaDodSO$_4$ electrophoresis. By contrast, anti-mu serum failed to precipitate any product, thus eliminating contaminant B lymphocytes as a source of Ia antigens.

78

Watanabe M, Noguchi T, Tsukada Y. **Regional, cellular, and subcellular distribution of Thy-1 antigen in rat nervous tissues.** *Neurochem Res.* 1981;6:507-19. (English)

The regional, cellular, and subcellular distribution of Thy-1 antigen in rat nervous tissues was investigated with rabbit and anti-rat thymus antiserum. Thy-1 antigen was found most abundantly in the cerebrum, including the cerebral cortical layer, caudate nucleus, thalamus, and hypothalamus, and in the midbrain. It was found in lower amounts in the pons, medulla oblongata, cerebellum, and spinal cord. The content of Thy-1 antigen, however, was low in the retina, cervical sympathetic ganglion, and sciatic nerve, and there was little in the pineal body and adrenal medulla. Thy-1 antigen was present in the neuronal cell-enriched fraction, whereas the glial cell-enriched fraction lacked Thy-1 antigen. In a subcellular fractionation study, Thy-1 antigen was found to occur mainly in the synaptosomal membrane and microsomes and was low in the highly purified myelin fraction. The amount of Thy-1 antigen in the cerebral synaptosomal fraction was much higher than those in the cerebellar synaptosomal fraction. The distribution of Thy-1 antigen among the respective areas within the cerebrum was not significantly different, and it is suggested that Thy-1 antigen may be present evenly in the neuronal membranes of the cerebrum. Based on these results, Thy-1 antigen is considered to represent a useful marker of cerebral neuronal membranes, especially in the synaptic region, regardless of the kind of neurotransmitters.

Neurochemical influences on immune function

Neuroendocrine influences on immune function

Hormones

79
Abraham AD, Buga G. **^{3}H-testosterone distribution and binding in rat thymus cells in vivo.** *Molec Cellular Biochem.* 1976;13:157-63. (English)

Autoradiography and biochemical investigations showed that [^{3}H]-testosterone where injected intraperitoneally into white male rats was incorporated rapidly into thymus lymphocytes. Thymic cortex contained more silver grains than medulla, and larger lymphocytes were more labeled than medium or small lymphocytes. Cytosol fraction of thymus cells labeled *in vivo* with [^{3}H]-testosterone, contained the largest quantity of labeled hormone. A 4S cytosol fraction binds [^{3}H]-testosterone. This could be separated by Sephadex chromatography or by linear sucrose gradient centrifugation. Nuclear extract contained also a small quantity of the labeled hormone.

80
Ahlqvist J. **Endocrine influences on lymphatic organs, immune responses, inflammation and autoimmunity.** *Acta Endocrinol Suppl (KHB).* 1976;206:3-136. (English) (no abstract)

81
Aoki N, Wakisaka G, Nagata I. **Effects of thyroxine on T-cell counts and tumor rejection in mice.** *Acta Endocrinol.* 1976;81:104-9. (English)

In an attempt to study the effect of thyroxine on peripheral T-cell (thymus-derived lymphocyte) counts or immunological functions, inbred C3H/He mice (8-10) were injected subcutaneously with thyroxine for 3 months. After treatment for 3 months the mice were examined for peripheral T-cell counts, thymic incorporation of tritiated thymidine and rejection of tumour transplants. The number of T cells was counted by the indirect immunofluorescense method using anti-theta C3H serum after separation of lymphocytes on "Ficoll-Conray". It was revealed that the peripheral counts of both lymphocytes and T-cells were increased in the thyroxine-treated group as compared with the control group, as was reported in the patients with Graves' disease. Thymic incorporation of tritiated thymidine was also found to be significantly increased in the thyroxine-treated group. In addition, in order to study T-cell activity of the host, thyroxine-treated and control mice were challenged with Ehrlich carcinoma cells at several concentrations (10^2, 10^4 and 2×10^6 per mouse). It was found that rejection of tumour transplants was significantly enhanced in the T-cell rich mice. Thus, it is possible that thyroxine affects peripheral T-cell counts and enhances immunological functions of the host.

82
Beck-Nielsen H, Kuhl C, Pedersen O, Bjerre-Christensen C, Nielsen TT, Klebe JG. **Decreased insulin binding to monocytes from normal pregnant women.** *J Clin Endocrinol Metab.* 1979;49:810-4. (English)

To ascertain whether the decrease of glucose tolerance in pregnancy might be mediated by changes in insulin receptors, we have studied insulin binding to monocytes in 12 normal women during late pregnancy and 14 healthy, young, normal weight, nonpregnant female controls. The pregnant women had significantly higher fasting insulin concentrations in plasma than the controls (18 ± 3.5 vs. 8 ± 1.1 microU/ml; $p<0.01$). Fasting concentrations of glucose and ketone bodies in plasma were not significantly different in the two groups. Insulin binding to monocytes from pregnant women was about 35% lower at each insulin concentration tested compared to the nonpregnant controls ($p<0.01$ at tracer insulin concentrations). Changes in cellular insulin binding were due to changes of the receptor number per cell, whereas the receptor affinity was unaffected. Insulin binding was not significantly correlated with the fasting plasma insulin in either of the two groups ($p>0.1$). Our results suggest that the deterioration of glucose tolerance in normal late pregnancy might be explained by a decrease of insulin sensitivity caused by a reduction of the number of insulin receptors.

83
Becker B, Shier DH, Palmberg PF, Waltman SR. **HLA antigens and corticosteroid response.** *Science.* 1976;194:1427-8. (English)

Compared with normal individuals, patients with primary open-angle glaucoma have increased prevalences of HLA-B12 and B7 antigens and are more responsive to glucocorticoids. Lymphocytes from both ocular normotensive and glaucomatous individuals with the HLA-B12 antigen require significantly ($p<0.02$) lower concentrations of prednisolone to inhibit phytohemagglutinin-induced transformation.

84
Bensman A, Dardenne M, Bach JF, Valleteau deMouillac J,

Lasfargues G. **Decrease of thymic hormone serum level in Cockayne syndrome.** *Pediatr Res.* 1982;16:92-4. (English)

Previous reports concerning children with Cockayne syndrome had described decreased T cell proliferative responses and renal anomalies which could be associated with immunologic disturbances. Herein, the thymic function was evaluated by measuring the serum level of thymic hormone. This serum level was found to be undetectable or decreased in seven cases of Cockayne syndrome. Active serum concentrations varied between 0 and 1/8, whereas normal children of the same age show activity in the range between 1/16 and 1/64. In contrast, T cell function, explored by phytohemagglutinin and Concavalin A responses, and mixed lymphocyte cultures was normal. Whether or not this premature sign of immunological aging is primary or secondary to other manifestations of the syndrome is still difficult to assess.

85
Berenbaum MC, Cope WA, Bundick RV. **Synergistic effect of cortisol and prostaglandin E on the PHA response.** *Clin Exp Immunol.* 1976;26:534-41. (English)

Surgical and thermal trauma in man are followed by depressed immunological responses *in vivo* and reduced lymphocyte reactivity *in vitro*. The possibility that these are related to trauma-induced rises in tissue levels of cortisol and prostaglandins was examined by studying the effect of a wide range of concentrations of cortisol and prostaglandin E_2 (PGE)$_2$, separately and together, on the phytohaemagglutinin (PHA) response of human peripheral blood lymphocytes. These effects were plotted on two-dimensional dose:effect graphs; the shapes of the curves connecting combinations of equal effect (isoboles) showed that these agents acted with marked synergy in suppressing the response, provided they were present while the response was taking place. Synergy was also shown by using a simple equation relating the concentrations of the agents producing a given effect when used in combination to the concentrations needed to produce the same effect when used separately. Cortisol at concentrations reached in the peripheral blood after trauma in man (1.4 x 10^{-6}M) and PGE$_2$ at concentrations expected in traumatized tissues (up to 4 x 10^{-7}M) each suppressed the response only slightly. The former reduced the response to 0.7 of controls and the latter to 0.5 (means of seven subjects). When both were present together at these concentrations, the response was markedly depressed (mean, 0.06, range 0.02-0.13 of controls). However, when lymphocytes were incubated at 37°C with cortisol and PGE$_2$ for 20 hr and then washed before exposure to PHA, the response was not inhibited, even by substantially higher concentrations than the above, and was usually moderately enhanced. Therefore, these *in vitro* experiments do not explain the depressed PHA response observed in peripheral blood lymphocytes after trauma. It is possible, however, that raised cortisol and prostaglandin levels depress the reactivity of lymphocytes while they remain in the traumatized region and its lymph drainage area.

86
Besedovsky HO, Del Rey A, Sorkin E. **Antigenic competition between horse and sheep red blood cells as a hormone-dependent phenomenon.** *Clin Exp Immunol.* 1979;37:106-13. (English)

Various mechanisms for understanding antigenic competition have been proposed, such as macrophage availability, suppressor cells and their soluble products. In view of the regulatory function of some hormones on the immune system, the role of immunosuppressive adrenal corticosteroids in antigenic competition was investigated. When horse red blood cells (HRBC) were injected into rats a five-fold increase in corticosterone blood levels was measured by day 6 and a strong decrease was noted on day 11. In animals injected with HRBC and on day 6 with a second antigen (sheep red blood cells, SRBC), the corticosteroid level was high on day 11. Such high levels are immunosuppressive. To impede such increases in adrenal hormone levels, rats were adrenalectomized. Adrenalectomized or sham-operated animals receiving SRBC only showed no difference in plaque-forming cell (PFC) numbers. All sham-operated rats injected first with HRBC and 5 days later with SRBC showed the expected antigenic competition. Adrenalectomized rats also injected with both antigens sequentially had a five fold increase in number of PFC when compared with the sham-operated controls which had received both antigens. A detailed analysis of these data revealed that a proportion of adrenalectomized animals had PFC numbers within the normal range. *In vitro,* hydrocortisone enhances the response of spleen cells when only one antigen (SRBC) is present. Prior addition of the unrelated antigen (HRBC) impedes this enhancement. Thus, in a hydrocortisone-enriched culture medium, the presence of the first antigen can interfere with the immune response to the second unrelated antigen, mimicking *in vitro* a condition of antigenic competition. These findings indicate that hormones may have a role in antigenic competition.

87
Besedovsky HO, Del Rey A, Sorkin E. **Lymphokine-containing supernatants from Con A-stimulated cells increase corticosterone blood levels** (communication). *J Immunol.* 1981;126:385-7. (English) (no abstract)

88
Besedovsky HO, Sorkin E. **Hormonal control of immune processes.** *Proc 5th Int Congr Endocrinol, Excerpta Medica.* Vol. 2. V H T James (ed.). Amsterdam: Oxford U. Press, 1977. Pp. 504-13. (English)

Our knowledge of the capacity of the immune system to recognize foreign macromolecules is still largely fragmentary, despite its extraordinary growth these past twenty years. It is now appreciated that it is made up of an enormously complex and heterogeneous population of lymphocytes and their major products, the antibodies and lymphokines, accessory phagocytic cells, such as the macrophages, and effector mechanisms such as complement. This paper will concern itself with the presentation of evidence for physiological links between the immune system and the neuro-endocrine system and a network of immune-neuro-endocrine interactions will be proposed. Finally, the issue of a possible regulatory role of hormones in immune processes will be considered. Given the enormous complexity of the immune system and the endocrine system, the interactions and relationship between these major entities are hardly likely to be simple.

89
Besedovsky HO, Sorkin E. **Network of immune-neuroendocrine interactions.** *Clin Exp Immunol.* 1977;27:1-12. (English)

In order to bring the self-regulated immune system into conformity with other body systems, its functioning within the context of an immune-neuroendocrine network is proposed. This hypothesis is based on the existence of afferent-efferent pathways between immune and neuroendocrine structures. Major endocrine responses occur as a consequence of antigenic stimulation and changes in the electrical activity of the hypothalamus also take place; both of these alterations are temporally related to the immune response itself. This endocrine response has meaningful implications for immunoregulation and for immunospecificity. During ontogeny, there is also evidence for the operations of a complex network between the endocrine and immune system, a bidirectional interrelationship that may well affect each developmental stage of both functions. As sequels the functioning of the immune system and the outcome of this interrelation could be decisive in lymphoid cell homeostasis, self-tolerance, and could also have significant implications for pathology.

90
Bjune G. *In vitro* **lymphocyte responses to PHA show covariation with the menstrual cycle.** *Scand Congr Immunol.* 1979;abstract 51. (English) (unavailable at publication)

91
Blalock JE, Smith EM. **Human leukocyte interferon (HuIFN-alpha): potent endorphin-like opioid activity.** *Biochem Biophys Res Commun.* 1981;101:472-8. (English)

Human leukocyte interferon, but not fibroblast or immune interferons, bind to opiate receptors *in vitro*. When injected intracerebrally into mice, human leukocyte, but not fibroblast or immune interferon, caused potent endorphin-like opioid effects. These effects include analgesia, lack of spontaneous locomotion and catalepsy. All of these actions of human leukocyte interferon were preventable and reversible by the opiate antagonist naloxone. The findings suggest that some of the side effects of leukocyte interferon therapy may be mediated by opiate receptor binding. They also provide evidence for a regulatory circuit between the immune and neuroendocrine system. This putative circuit could be an etiologic site for certain psychopathological states.

92
Blalock JE, Smith EM. **Human leukocyte interferon: structural and biological relatedness to adrenocorticotropic hormone and endorphins.** *Proc Natl Acad Sci.* 1980;77:5972-4. (English)

Anti-alpha-corticotropin [anti-ATHalpha] (also alpha-melanotropin) and anti-gamma-endorphin antisera neutralized human leukocyte interferon activity but not fibroblast interferon activity. Human leukocyte interferon was not neutralized by anti-human luteinizing hormone (lutropin) or follicle-stimulating hormone (follitropin) antisera. Conversely, antisera to human leukocyte interferon neutralized ACTH activity. The neutralization of human leukocyte interferon by anti-

human leukocyte interferon serum was partially blocked by ACTH. These studies show strong antigenic relatedness among human leukocyte interferon, ACTH and endorphins, implying that there are underlying structural similarities. Structural relatedness is shown by pepsin cleavage of ACTH activity from human leukocyte interferon. The implications for the natural functions of human leukocyte interferon are discussed.

93
Bloom B. **Interferon and the immune system.** *Nature.* 1980;284:593-5. (English) (no abstract)

94
Carter J. **The effect of progesterone, oestradiol and HCG on cell-mediated immunity in mice.** *J Reprod Fertil.* 1976;46:211-6. (English)

During pregnancy in mice, cell-mediated immunity as measured by a contact allergic reaction to picryl chloride was diminished ($p<0.001$). Mice in which delay of implantation was maintained by progesterone, and mice with progesterone- and oestradiol-maintained pregnancies, also showed a reduction in the inflammatory response. The response of pseudopregnant mice did not differ from that of the non-pregnant controls. Young mice sensitized before complete immunological competence gave a 50% response. The response doubled in animals given a second sensitization. The extent of the response in females with delay of implantation varied inversely with the dose of progesterone. A range of oestrogen doses gave the same depression in the response when given to pseudopregnant animals. Administration of HCG to pseudopregnant mice also reduced the inflammatory response.

95
Cattaneo R, Saibene V, Margonato A, Pozza G. *In vitro* **effects of insulin on peripheral T-lymphocyte E-rosette function from normal and diabetic subjects.** *Boll Ist Sieroter.* 1977;56:139-43. (Italian)

Juvenile-onset diabetics (JOD) have a significantly low peripheral T-lymphocyte count. *In vitro* exposure of diabetic lymphocyte cultures to insulin causes a significant T-cell count increase and thereafter no significant difference is detectable among JOD, maturity-onset diabetics (MOD) and normal subjects (NS) T-cell counts. This finding supports the hypothesis that the T-lymphocyte depressed function present in JOD is a secondary phenomenon due to *in vivo* insulin deficiency. Possible mechanisms of insulin action in restoring E-rosette function are discussed.

96
Chretien PB, Lipson SD, Makuch RW, Kenady DE, Cohen MH. **Effects of thymosin *in vitro* in cancer patients and correlation with clinical course after thymosin immunotherapy.** *Ann NY Acad Sci.* 1979:332:1135-47. (English) (unavailable at publication)

97
Christie KE, Kjosen B, Solberg CO. **Influence of hydrocortisone on granulocyte function and glucose metabo-**

lism. *Acta Pathol Microbiol Scand Sect C.* 1977;85:284-88. (English) (unavailable at publication)

98
Cohn DA, Hamilton JB. **Sensitivity to androgen and immune response: immunoglobulin levels in two strains of mice, one with high and one with low target organ responses to androgen.** *RES, J Reticuloendothel Soc.* 1976;20:1-10. (English)

Mechanisms underlying the low immune responses of males compared to females have remained poorly understood; however, there is some suggestion that among males as a group, those with high target organ responses to androgen may have lower levels of certain immunoglobulins than other males. To investigate the possibility of a relationship between a high sensitivity to androgen and a low immune response, levels of immunoglobulins were determined in 2 strains of mice previously classified by seminal vesicle bioassay as high (C57L/J) and low (A/J) responders to androgen. Individual assays of plasma immunoglobulins were performed when the mice were 14 weeks old by quantitative radial immunodiffusion. Among C57L/J mice (the high androgen responder strain), males had lower values of IgM and IgG_2 than females of the same strain and lower values than A/J males (the low androgen responders). In contrast, no sex differences in levels of immunoglobulins were observed among A/J mice. Adult mice of both strains, gonadectomized within 3 days of birth, showed the same marked strain differences as intact mice but did not show increased levels of immunoglobins compared to sham operated mice. Since levels of IgM and IgG_2 C57L/J males remained low regardless of whether the mice were castrated or intact, the concentration of androgen in mature mice was clearly not responsible for their low immuglouIin levels. Instead, the results with multiple animals of each strain indicated that high sensitivity to androgen in adult males consistently correlated with low levels of IgfM and IgG_2.

99
Cooper DA, Duckett M, Petts V, Penny R. **Corticosteroid enhancement of immunoglobulin synthesis by pokeweed mitogen-stimulated human lymphocytes.** *Clin Exp Immunol.* 1979;37:145-51. (English)

The effect of the addition *in vitro* of corticosteroid on pokeweed mitogen (PWM)-induced Ig synthesis by human peripheral blood lymphocytes were studied. IgG in supernatants produced under standardized culture conditions was measured by double antibody radioimmunoassay. The addition of $10^{-6}M$ prednisolone caused a remarkable enhancement of PWM-stimulated IgG synthesis beginning at day 4 of culture and increasing at a faster rate than that in cultures with PWM alone. $10^{-6}M$ prednisolone resulted in a geometric mean enhancement of 5.6-fold of PWM-stimulated IgG synthesis in all twenty-five normal controls studied. This enhancement occurred up to 3 days after the addition of PWM. $10^{-6}M$ and $10^{-5}M$ prednisolone resulted in significantly greater enhancement of PWM-stimulated IgG synthesis than $10^{-7}M$ prednisolone. Hydrocortisone, prednisolone, methylprednisolone, betamethasone and dexamethasone at $10^{-6}M$ were all equally effective in the enhancement of PWM-induced IgG synthesis.

100
Cove-Smith JR, Kabler P, Pownall R, Knapp MS. **Circadian variation in an immune response in man.** *Brit Med J.* 1978;2:253-4. (English)

We recently showed the circadian rhythm of the immune response in the skin to challenge with oxazolone in oxazolone-sensitized rats. Others have shown that renal transplant survival in rats varies with the time of transplantation. Circadian variations have been observed in the response of human lymphocytes to mitogen stimulation, but results are conflicting and may depend on whether whole blood or isolated lymphocytes are used in the assay. There is little information about circadian variations in human immune responses *in vivo*. The response to intradermal tuberculin is a typical example of cell-mediated immunity: 70% of the cells present in the lesion at 48 hours are mononuclear cells, predominantly lymphocytes. Intradermal injection of purified protein derivative of tuberculin (PPD) to a standard depth (Heaf test) was used to study the response to challenge at different times of day.

101
Curtis JJ, Gall JH, Woodford SY, Saykaly RJ, Luke RG. **Comparison of daily and alternate-day prednisone during chronic maintenance therapy: a controlled crossover study.** *Am J Kidney Dis.* 1981;1:166-71. (English)

To determine if dose spacing of low dose chronic suppressive corticosteroid therapy would result in different effects on circulating T lymphocytes and hypothalamic-pituitary-adrenal (HPA) axis suppression, a crossover trial of two maintenance steroid regimens was performed. Twenty stable renal allograft recipients were treated for 6 mo with daily prednisone (DS) and then the same patients were abruptly converted to alternate-day prednisone (ADS) for another 6 mo. Total prednisone dosage was identical during the 6-mo study periods and only dose spacing differed. Both circulating T lymphocytes numbers and responsiveness to mitogens were less on the DS regimen. Patients gained weight on DS and lost weight on ADS. Five of the 20 patients developed infections on DS. However, HPA suppression was not different on the two regimens. These findings suggest that dose spacing alters the immunosuppressive and metabolic response to prednisone, even at low dose.

102
DiSorbo D, Rosen F, McPartland RP, Millolland RJ. **Glucocorticoid activity of various progesterone analogs: correlation between specific binding in thymus and liver and biologic activity.** *Ann NY Acad Sci.* 1977;286:355-66. (English)

When tested in an in *vitro* assay system, progesterone and various analogs of this steroid were shown to compete with [^{3}H]triamcinolone acetonide (TA) for specific glucocorticoid receptors in both rat liver and thymus. Of these analogs, the following derivatives of progesterone were potent competitors of TA binding and, when injected into adrenalectomized rats, induced regression of the thymus and marked increases in hepatic tyrosine aminotransferase activity: 11-beta-hydroxyl, 6-alpha-dimethyl, and 6-alpha-methyl-17-alpha-hydroxyl. In contrast, progesterone, 16-alpha-methyl, and 17-alpha-hydroxy progesterone competed with TA *in vitro* but failed to elicit either gluco- or antiglucocorticoid activity *in vivo*. Also, we observed that the oral contraceptive 6-alpha-methyl-17-(1-propynyl)testosterone competes very effectively with TA in a cell-free preparation of rat liver and induces an increase in hepatic tyrosine aminotransferase activity. The 11-beta-hydroxyl group has previously been thought to be essential for glucocorticoid activity. Our studies indicate that substitution of progesterone or testosterone with 6-alpha-methyl group negates the need for an 11-beta-hydroxyl substituent as a prerequisite for glucocorticoid activity.

103

Dilman VM, Anisimov VN, Ostroumova MN, Morozov VG, Khavinson VK, Azarova MA. **Study of the anti-tumor effect of polypeptide pineal extract.** *Oncology.* 1979;36:274-80. (English)

Bovine pineal polypeptide extract (PPE) exerted an anti-tumor effect on mouse-transplantable tumors: mammary cancer (RSM), squamous cell cervical carcinoma (SCC), hepatoma-22A and lympholeukemia LI0-1, and had no effect on Harding-Passey melanoma and leukemia L-1210. It was shown that PPE possessed the ability to decrease the incidence of DMBA-induced mammary adenocarcinomas in rats. The daily administration of 0.5 mg PPE prolonged the life span of rats by 25% and failed to influence spontaneous tumor development. The arguments in favor of a possible mechanism of anti-tumor action of the pineal gland are submitted. It is suggested that the anti-tumor effect of PPE may occur when the syndrome of cancrophilia is induced by tumor transplantation or chemical carcinogens.

104

Dimitriu A. **Suppression of macrophage arming by corticosteroids.** *Cell Immunol.* 1976;21:79-87. (English)

Normal mice macrophages are rendered cytotoxic by treatment with the acellular supernatant fraction of a mixed lymphocyte culture between skin graft recipient and donor spleen cells. The factor inducing this macrophage cytotoxicity is termed macrophage "arming" factor or MAF. Corticosteroids administered *in vivo* or *in vitro* depress the macrophage arming phenomenon. These hormones do not prevent MAF production by sensitized lymphocytes in the presence of donor cells, but they alter the capacity of normal macrophages to be armed. Macrophages originating from *in vivo* corticoid-treated mice present a diminished ability to become cytotoxic when incubated with MAF-rich supernatants. On the other hand, the *in vitro* treatment of normal macrophage monolayers with steroids in doses as low as 0.01-0.1 microg/ml suppresses their capacity to be armed. This effect is more intensive when macrophages are pretreated with corticosteroids before arming. These results suggest that the alteration of the macrophage arming phenomenon could be one of the corticosteroid immunosuppressive mechanisms.

105

Dumont F, Barrois R. **Electrokinetic properties and mitogen responsiveness of mouse splenic B and T lymphocytes following hydrocortisone treatment.** *Int Arch Allergy Appl Immunol.* 1977;53: 293-302. (English)

CBA mice received single intraperitoneal injection of hydrocortisone acetate (OHC) in a dose of 125 mg/kg body weight. At various times thereafter, electrophoretic mobility (EPM), surface immunoglobulin (SIg) and *in vitro* DNA synthetic reactivity to concanavalin A (Con A), phytohemagglutinin (PHA), lipopolysaccharide (LPS) and tuberculin (PPD) were investigated on splenic lymphocytes. OHC was found to deplete rapidly the spleen to a minimum of 18% of control cellularity by day 4 posttreatment. At this time, the proportions of low mobility (LM) and SIg-bearing lymphocytes (B cells) were reduced respectively to 28% (control 54%) and 20% (control 45%). The proportion of high mobility (HM) lymphocytes (T cells) was increased to 72% (control 45%). While the mean EPM of LM cells (0.71) was only slightly and transiently reduced, that of HM cells was significantly augmented (1.24) over control value (1.16). This latter finding was interpreted as indicating the selective removal by OHC of a T cell subpopulation with a mean EPM around 1.10. Changes in mitogenic responsiveness were consistent with these alterations of B and T cell compartments. Despite a marked drop in spontaneous ^{3}H-thymidine uptake, the absolute response to T cell mitogens Con A and PHA remained relatively unchanged. By contrast, the reactivity to B cell mitogens LPS and PPD was strongly depressed. Starting by day 12, regeneration and normalization of lymphocyte populations proceeded slowly and were not achieved before day 26-34.

106

Eriksson B, Hedfors E. **The effect of adrenalin, insulin and hydrocortisone on human peripheral blood lymphocytes studied by cell surface markers.** *Scand J Haematol.* 1977;18:121-8. (English)

Changes in numbers of peripheral blood lymphocytes from healthy individuals were calculated from samples collected before and after parenteral administration of adrenalin, insulin and hydrocortisone, respectively. A marked increase in circulating lymphocytes was noted in response to adrenalin and insulin. However, subpopulation analysis showed a decrease in the proportion of T-lymphocytes, estimated as cells forming rosettes with sheep red blood cells after incubation in the cold and a corresponding increase in proportion of lymphocytes having receptors for C3 (non-T-lymphocytes). In contrast, lymphocyte numbers were unaffected by hydrocortisone. The results indicate that a decreased proportion of circulating T-lymphocytes and an increase of non-T-lymphocytes may be the result of adaptive changes in response to various forms of stress and hence is to be expected in several clinical conditions.

107

Etzkorn J, Hopkins P, Gray J, Segal J, Ingar SH. **Beta-adrenergic potentiation of the increased *in vitro* accumalation of cycloleucine by rat thymocytes induced by triiodothyronine.** *J Clin Invest.* 1979;63:1172-80. (English).

We have previously demonstrated that 3,5,3'-triiodothyronine (T_3), whether administered *in vivo* or added to suspending media *in vitro*, promptly stimulates the *in vitro* accumulation of the non-metabolized amino acids, alpha-amino-isobutyric acid, and cycloleucine (CLE) by thymocytes isolated from weanling rats. In these *in vitro* interaction between catecholamines and T_3 with respect to this effect. The previously reported enhancement of CLE accumulation in thymocytes by T_3 *in vitro* (1 microM) was confirmed. When added alone in concentrations ranging between 10 nM and 0.1 mM, the adrenergic agonists, epinephrine and norepinephrine had no effect on CLE accumulation. At a concentration of 1 microM, isoproterenol, terbutaline, and phenylephrine were also without effect. However, the effect of T_3 was clearly potentiated by the concomitant addition of epinephrine, norepinephrine, and possibly isoproterenol, whereas terbutaline and phenylephrine were without effect. Neither basal nor T_3-enhanced CLE accumulation was affected by the addition alone of adrenergic blocking agents, propranolol (0.1 mM), phentolamine (10 microM), or practolol (0.1 4mM). Nevertheless, the beta$_1$- and beta$_2$-antagonist, propranol, and the beta$_1$-antagonist, practolol, blocked the increment of CLE accumulation produced by epinephrine; the alpha-antagonist, phentolamine, was without effect. The enhancement of CLE accumulation that occurred in the presence of T_3, with or without epinephrine was seen to be a result of an inhibition of CLE efflux, because T_3 alone inhibited CLE efflux, and this effect was increased when epinephrine was also present. On the other hand, neither T_3 alone nor T_3 plus epinephrine appreciably altered the rate of inward transport of CLE. As judged from studies of the ability of thymocytes to exclude trypan blue, neither T_3 alone nor T_3 plus epinephrine either enhanced or impaired viability of cells during 3 h periods of incubation. Cell water content, measured with [^{3}H]urea, was unaffected by T_3, either alone or in the presence of epinephrine. In confirmation of previous results, the stimulatory effect of T_3 on CLE accumulation was unaffected by concentrations of puromycin sufficient to inhibit protein synthesis by at least 95% and the potentiating action of epinephrine on the response to T_3 was similarly unaffected. From these findings, it is concluded that the effect of T_3 to increase CLE accumulation by thymocytes *in vitro*, thought itself independent of adrenergic mediation, is potentiated by beta$_1$-adrenergic stimulation. This interaction appears distinctly different from other thyroid hormone-catecholamine interactions, in which thyroid hormones enhance physiological responses to catecholamines. Its mechanism remains unclear, but the properties of the T_3 effect, and possibly the interaction itself, suggest that T_3 enhances CLE accumulation by an action at the level of the cell membrane.

108

Fauci AS, Pratt KR, Whalen G. **Activation of human B lymphocytes; IV--Regulatory effects of corticosteroids on the triggering signal in the plaque-forming cell response of human peripheral blood B lymphocytes to polyclonal activation.** *J Immunol.* 1977;119:598-603. (English)

In vitro hydrocortisone in physiologic and pharmacologically attainable concentrations caused a marked enhancement of the PWM-induced PFC response of normal human peripheral blood B lymphocytes. This effect was seen only when hydrocortisone was added within the first 24 hr of culture and only when hydrocortisone and PWM were present together in cultures. Only suprapharmacologic concentrations of hydrocortisone (10^{-3}M) were capable of suppressing early B cell activation. Late stages of antibody production and secre-

tion were resistant to suppression by even these extraordinarily high concentrations. Hydrocortisone did not replace the T cell requirement of PWM-induced PFC responses. A single dose of *in vivo* hydrocortisone (400 mg) to normal adult volunteers did not produced this enhancing effect when PFC responses were measured *in vitro* in the absence of hydrocortisone. The data strongly suggest that the enhancing effect of hydrocortisone was due not to elimination of naturally occurring suppressor cells, but to a modulation of the triggering signal either directly on the B cell itself or via the balance of positive and negative T cell regulation of B cell activation.

109

Fauci AS. **Mechanisms of corticosteroid action on lymphocyte subpopulations; II--Differential effects of *in vivo* hydrocortisone, prednisone and dexamethasone on *in vitro* expression of lymphocyte function.** *Clin Exp Immunol.* 1976;24:54-62. (English)

The present study was undertaken to determine what, if any, differential effects various commonly used corticosteroid preparations had on the numbers and specific functions of lymphocyte subpopulations when these agents were administered in equivalent pharmacological dosages. Normal volunteers received a single dose of either 320 mg of hydrocortisone intravenously, 80 mg of prednisone orally, or 12 mg of dexamethasone orally. There was a marked lymphocytopenia and monocytopenia maximal 4-6 hr following administration of all three corticosteroid preparations with almost identical kinetics and degree of fall in total cell numbers as well as proportions of thymus-derived and bone marrow-derived lymphocytes. Hydrocortisone and prednisone caused only a slight suppression of phytohaemagglutinin (PHA)-induced lymphocyte blastogenesis which could be reversed at supra-optimal concentrations of PHA. On the contrary, dexamethasone administration caused a marked suppression of PHA responses which was not reversed by supra-optimal PHA stimulation. In addition, hydrocortisone and prednisone administration did not suppress non-specific PHA-induced cellular cytotoxicity, while dexamethasone caused a marked suppression ($p<0.001$) of cytotoxicity. These studies show that although equivalent anti-inflammatory doses of these three corticosteroid preparations cause almost identical suppression of the numbers of circulating lymphocyte populations, they have a differential effect on certain *in vitro* functional correlates of cell-mediated immunity.

110

Fauci AS. **Mechanisms of the immunosuppressive and anti-inflammatory effects of glucocorticosteroids.** *J Immunopharmacol.* 1978-9;1:1-25. (English)

Corticosteroids have multifaceted effects on various phases of inflammatory and immunological activity. These include effects on vascular and tissue responses, effects on the movement of traffic of inflammatory or immunologically reactive cells, direct effects on functional capabilities of cells, and direct or indirect effects on various soluble factors mediating inflammation or immunologic activity. It is clear that there is a differential sensitivity of various populations and subpopulations of cells to the corticosteroid modulation of cellular kinetic patterns, cellular interactions, and functional capabilities. In general, corticosteroids have a much greater and more obvious effect on the traffic and kinetics than on the functional properties of cells involved in inflammation and immunologic activity. Hypotheses concerning the precise mechanisms of many of these effects have been proposed, but still await verification and possibly amplification.

111

Fernandes G, Halberg F, Yunis EJ, Good RA. **Circadian rhythmic plaque-forming cell response of spleens from mice immunized with SRBC.** *J Immunol.* 1976;117:962-6. (English)

Studies under controlled conditions of lighting and temperature revealed clear evidence of circadian periodicity with respect to the number of PFC present in the spleens of BALB/c mice 3 or 4 days after immunization with SRBC. Striking differences in proliferative responses of spleen lymphocytes to PHA or Con A were also observed at two different circadian times. Large proliferative responses occurred at the time when injection of antigen and/or sampling for PFC yielded a low PFC formation (early in the daily dark span) and small proliferative responses occurred at the time when antigen injection and sampling yielded high formation of PFC (early in the daily light span). These findings indicate that care should be taken to control the circadian timing of stimulation and sampling in studies of immune responses, and that rhythmically varying aspects constitute a new dimension of immunologic processes awaiting further analysis in both the circadian and weekly spectral regions.

112

Gillis B, Crabtree GR, Smith KA. **Glucocorticoid-inhibition of T cell growth factor production; I--The effect of mitogen-induced lymphocyte proliferation.** *J Immunol.* 1979;123:1624-31. (English)

Although it has been clearly established that glucocorticoids inhibit mitogen- or antigen-induced lymphocyte proliferation, the mechanism underlying these effect has remained ill-defined. Recently, it has become evident that T cell proliferation is mediated by a soluble T cell growth factor (TCGF) released by mitogen/antigen stimulated T cells. Therefore it seemed probable that the inhibitory effects of glucocorticoids were manifested either at the level of TCGF production or at the level of the activated T lymphocyte. We found that differentiated cytolytic T lymphocytes harvested from TCGF-dependent long-term culture were only mildly sensitive to inhibitory effects (25 to 30% inhibition) of glucocorticoids as measured by decreased cellular proliferation and the incorporation of tritiated thymidine. The degree of inhibition observed was most probably mediated through glucocorticoid receptors in that the half-maximal inhibitory glucocorticoid concentration correlated with half-maximal glucocorticoid receptor saturation. In contrast, we found that mitogen-induced TCGF production and T cell proliferation were completely inhibited by pharmacologic concentrations of dexamethasone (10^{-6}M). Finally, the YCGF supplementation of mitogen-stimulated cultures treated with maximal inhibitory concentrations of dexamethasone resulted in complete amelioration of glucocorticoid suppression. These results indicate that a major mechanism of glucocorticoid-mediated

immunosuppression may occur at the level of the TCGF-production cell, resulting in the control of clonal expansion of activated T cells via inhibition of TCGF production.

113

Gillis S, Crabtree GR, Smith KA. **Glucocorticoid-induced inhibition of T cell growth factor production; II--The effect on the** *in vitro* **generation of cytolytic T cells.** *J Immunol.* 1979;123:1632-8. (English)

The previous communication presented data detailing that glucocorticoid hormones exhibited slight but significant inhibitory effects on the proliferation of cytolytic T cells maintained in long-term T cell growth factor (TCGF)-dependent cultures. However, most importantly, glucocorticoids were shown to inhibit T-lymphocyte proliferation via a profound effect on TCGF production. Addition of exogenous TCGF to glucocorticoid-treated human, mouse, or rat T cell mitogen-stimulated lymphocytes restored normal levels of proliferation. These observations led us to propose that the immunosuppressive effects of glucocorticoid hormones were mediated by controlling the production of the T cell proliferation-inducing agent, TCGF. Results of experimentation detailed in this communication provide further evidence in support of this hypothesis. We found that although glucocorticoid hormones had little effect on the cytolytic reactivity of T cells harvested from TCGF-dependent culture, treatment of mixed lymphocyte cultures (MLC) with identical glucocorticoid hormone concentrations completely abrogated *in situ* TCGF production and alloantigen-directed cytolysis. The inhibitory effects of glucocorticoids in MLC could be eliminated once again simply by the delayed addition of exogenous TCGF. These observations coupled with those detailed in the previous report provide evidence that, rather than effecting lysis of potentially reactive mature lymphocytes, glucocorticoids influence the development of T cell-mediated immune reactivity by inhibiting TCGF production, which in turn serves to inhibit the clonal expansion of activated T cells.

114

Ginsberg AM, Clutter WE, Shah SD, Cryer PE. **Triiodothyronine-induced thyrotoxicosis increases mononuclear leukocyte beta-adrenergic receptor density in man.** *J Clin Invest.* 1981;67:1785-91. (English)

Beta-adrenergic receptors are increased in some tissues of experimentally thyrotoxic animals but are reported to be unchanged in mononuclear leukocytes of spontaneously thyrotoxic humans. The effects of triiodothyronine [T_3] (100 microg/d for 7 d) and placebo were examined on high-affinity mononuclear leukocyte beta-adrenergic receptors in 24 normal human subjects, using a double-blind design. Beta-adrenergic receptors were assessed by specific binding of the antagonist (-)[^{3}H]-dihydroalprenolol binding from 25 ± 3 to 57 ± 9 f[femto]mol/mg protein (p<0.001). The latter was attributable, by Scatchard analysis, to an increase in beta-adrenergic receptor density (967 ± 134 to 2250 ± 387 sites/cell, p<0.01); apparent K_d did not change. Placebo administration had no effects. Marked inter- and intraindividual variation in mononuclear leukocyte beta-adrenergic receptor density was also noted. Because this was approximately 3-fold greater than analytical variation, it is largely attributable to biologic variation. The finding of a T_3-induced increase in mononuclear leukocyte beta-adrenergic receptor density in human mononuclear leukocytes, coupled with similar findings in tissues of experimentally thyrotoxic animals, provides support for the use of mononuclear leukocytes to assess receptor status in man. There is considerable biologic variation in beta-adrenergic receptor density in man. The findings of thyroid hormone-induced increments in beta-adrenergic receptor density provide a plausible mechanism for the putative enhanced responsiveness to endogernous catecholamines of patients with thyrotoxicosis.

115
Glasser L, Heustis DW, Jones JF. **Functional capabilities of steroid-recruited neutrophils harvested for clinical transfusion.** *N Engl J Med.* 1977;297:1033-36. (English)

To determine whether steroids exert a direct inhibitory effect on neutrophil function, thus contraindicating their use to increase granulocyte yields for white-cell transfusions to infected neutropenic patients, we gave normal donors a single intravenous dose of dexamethasone (4 mg per square meter of body-surface area). Approximately two hours later the absolute neutrophil count increased from an initial value (mean ± 1 S.D.) of 3800 ± 1400 to 5700 ± 2400 per microliter. Granulocytes were then collected by discontinuous-flow centrifugation and tested. Viability (98.4 per cent), the percentage of neutrophils capable of phagocytosis (97.6), particle accumulation (12.3 candida per phagocyte), fungicidal activity (1.08 "ghost" yeast cells per phagocyte), the percentage of bacteria killed (97.7) and chemotaxis (119 per cent) did not significantly differ from observations in nontreated paired controls. The functional competence of neutrophils used for granulocyte transfusions was not altered after short-term exposure of these healthy donors to steroid medication.

116
Goldstein AL, Thurman GB, Low TLK, Rossio JL, Trivers GE. **Hormonal influences of the reticuloendothelial system: current status of the role of thymosin in the regulation and modulation of immunity.** *RES, J Reticuloendoth Soc.* 1978;23:253-66. (English)

The thymus gland controls the development and maintenance of immune balance by secreting a family of polypeptide hormones termed thymosin. These hormones, and possibly others, act on thymic-dependent lymphocytes (T cells) at several points in the maturation sequence to ensure the cells' development and function. Ongoing studies suggest that the lack of adequate production and utilization of these thymic factors causes an immune imbalance and may contribute to the etiology of many diseases. Using a partially purified preparation, thymosin fraction 5, we have established that thymosin can correct some of the immunologic deficiencies resulting from the lack of thymic function in several animal models, as well as in humans with primary and secondary immunodeficiency diseases. Several biologically active peptides present in thymosin fraction 5 contribute to its biologic activity. Several of these peptides have now been purified, and one, termed thymosin alpha$_1$, has been sequenced. It appears that these peptides act individually, sequentially or in concert to influence the development of T cell subpopulations. Thymosin

alpha$_1$ is highly acidic (pH 4.2), heat stable protein with a molecular weight (MW) of 3,108. Biologically, thymosin alpha$_1$ is from 10 to 1,000 times as active as fraction 5 in inducing maturational and functional changes in T cell subpopulations in specific *in vitro* and *in vivo* assays, e.g., erythrocyte-rosette (E-rosette) formation, surface marker induction, macrophage inhibitory factor (MIF) induction, lymphotoxin production and mitogenic activity. Clinically, over 50 children with primary immunodeficiency diseases and 150 cancer patients have now been treated with thymosin according to Phase I and Phase II protocols. No evidence of central nervous system, liver, kidney or bone marrow toxicity has been observed, and the side effects have been minimal. Eighty percent of the pediatric patients who have responded *in vitro* to thymosin have responded *in vivo* with increases in T cell numbers and function. Significant clinical improvement has been seen in over 50% of the pediatric patients who responded *in vitro*. Greater than 75% of the Phase I cancer patients who responded to thymosin *in vitro* have shown increases in numbers of T cells following thymosin treatment. Although the clinical studies with thymosin are still in the developmental stage, the positive results seen with thymosin in the reconstitution of the immune system of immunodeficient children have broad implications in dealing with many of the serious immunodeficiency diseases, cancer and autoimmune disease.

117
Goodwin JS, Messner RP, Williams RC Jr. **Inhibitors of thymus-derived cell mitogenesis: effect of mitogen dose.** *Cell Immunol.* 1979;45:303-8. (English)

The inhibitory effects of 7 compounds (hydrocortisone, histamine, interferon, isoproterenol, norepinephrine, serotonin and GABA) were tested in phytohemagglutinin (PHA)-stimulated cultures of human peripheral blood mononuclear cells as a function of PHA concentration. The cultures stimulated by suboptimal levels of PHA were much more sensitive to inhibition by the added compounds, with the curve of percentage inhibition vs. concentration of inhibitor shifted to the left by greater than 2 orders of magnitude in all cases. At the lower doses of mitogen, concentrations of hydrocortisone, histamine, interferon and isoproterenol which approach the concentrations of these or analogous compounds *in vivo* caused significant and substantial inhibition of the mitogen response.

118
Gunn T, Reece ER, Metrakos K, Colle E. **Depressed T cells following neonatal steroid treatment.** *Pediatrics.* 1981; 67:61-7. (English)

Fourty-four patients received two doses of 12.5 mg/kg of hydrocortisone or placebo on the first day of life in an attempted therapy for respiratory distress syndrome. Follow-up studies were performed on survivors at 5 years of age in ten steroid-treated and seven placebo-treated respiratory distress syndrome subjects. There were no significant differences in growth, intelligence tests, or neurologic examinations in the patients assessed. Abnormal EEGs are present in both groups. Immunologic tests showed no differences in lymphocyte counts, immunoglobulin levels, diphtheria and tetanus antibody titers, or complement components. Diminished percentages of T lymphocytes were found in steroid patients (53%) compared to control subjects (69%). There were also increased percentages of lymphocytes with C3 receptors in steroid patients (20.1%) compared to control patients (13.8%). Episodes of otitis and/or pneumonia were documented in eight of 11 steroid-treated patients between the ages of 1 and 5 years, compared to two of seven patients in the placebo group in the same time period. It is concluded that large doses of steroids on the first day of life may induce lasting immunologic abnormalities and may predispose to an increased incidence of infections.

119

Gupta P, Rapp F. **Effect of hormones on herpes simplex virus type 2-induced transformation.** *Nature.* 1977; 267:254-5. (English) (no abstract)

120

Haynes BF, Fauci AS. **The differential effect of *In vivo* hydrocortisone on the kinetics of subpopulations of human peripheral blood thymus-derived lymphocytes.** *J Clin Invest.* 1978;61:703-7. (English)

The present study was undertaken to determine the effect of *in vivo* hydrocortisone on the kinetics of subpopulations of normal human peripheral blood (PB) thymus-derived (T) cells. Normal volunteers received a single i.v. dose of hydrocortisone, and blood was taken just before, as well as 4, 24, and 48 h after hydrocortisone administration. T cells were purified from each specimen, and proportions and absolute numbers of T lymphocytes bearing receptors for the Fc portion of IgG (T_G) and for the Fc portion of IgM (T_M) were enumerated by rosetting T cells with bovine erythrocytes which had been coated with either antibovine erythrocyte IgG or IgM. 4 h after i.v. administration of hydrocortisone, T_M cells decreased from 52 ($\pm$ 5%) to 23 ($\pm$ 6%) of PB T cells (p<0.01) and the absolute number of T_M cells decreased from 1,028 ($\pm$ 171) per mm^3 to 103 ($\pm$ 23) per mm^3 (p<0.001). In contrast, relative proportion of T_G cells increased from 22 ($\pm$ 4%) to 66 ($\pm$ 7%), while the absolute numbers of T_G cells were essentially unchanged (p>0.2). *In vitro* studies involving preincubation of T cells with hydrocortisone before rosette determination of T_G or T_M cells demonstrated that the decrease in absolute numbers of T_M cells did not represent hydrocortisone interference with T_M rosette formation, nor did it represent a switch of T_M cells to T_G cells. Thus, administration of hydrocortisone to normal subjects produces a selective depletion from the circulation of T lymphocytes which possess receptors for the Fc portion of IgM (T_M cells) and of T cells which possess no detectable Fc receptor ($T_{non-M. non-G}$ cells). T_G cells are relatively resistant to the lymphopenic effect of hydrocortisone. These data clearly demonstrate that *in vitro* corticosteroids have a differential effect on the kinetics of identifiable and distinct subsets fo cells in the human T-cell class.

121

Helderman JH, Strom TB. **Specific insulin binding site on T and B lymphocytes as a marker of cell activation.** *Nature.* 1978;274:62-3. (English) (no abstract)

122

Huddlestone JR, Merigan TC Jr, Oldstone MBA. **Induction and kinetics of natural killer cells in humans following interferon therapy.** *Nature.* 1979;282:417-9. (English)

Natural killer (NK) cells are non-B, non-T lymphocytes that effect spontaneous cytolysis of both virus-infected and neoplastically transformed target cells. These NK lymphocytes have been detected in several species including man. Interferon is a primary regulator of natural killer activity. Because NK cells have been implicated in the regulation of tumor cell expression and can be induced by interferon in murine models, we have studied patients receiving large doses of interferon to determine (1) whether interferon could induce NK lymphocytes in the peripheral blood of man, and (2) whether there are characteristic kinetics for the appearance, disappearance and reactivation of NK lymphocytes following interferon therapy. We report here the activation of human NK cells by the systemic inoculation of human subjects with interferon. Five patients received interferon as therapy for non-Hodgkin's lymphoma. All showed a marked increase in NK cell activity 12-24 h after inoculation. Peak NK activity occurred 18 h after introducing interferon, and thereafter declined rapidly but remained above pre-interferon levels. Induced NK activity occurred with reintroduction of interferon but at lower levels of activity and with different kinetics.

123

Hunninghake GW, Fauci AS. **Immunologic reactivity of the lung; III--Effects of corticosteroids on alveolar macrophage cytotoxic effector cell function.** *J Immunol.* 1977;118:146-50. (English)

The effects of various *in vitro* and *in vivo* regimens of corticosteroid administration on guinea pig alveolar macrophages were studied. Corticosteroid-induced immunosuppression was assessed by the effect of drug administration on the total numbers and functional capabilities of alveolar macrophages as measured by the PHA-induced and antibody-dependent cellular cytotoxicity assays against sheep red blood cell targets. *In vivo* administration of either hydrocortisone sodium succinate (100 mg/kg/one dose) or cortisone acetate (100 mg/subcutaneously for 7 days) caused a marked increase in the numbers of alveolar macrophages recovered from the teased lung cell suspensions at 4 and 24 hr, respectively, after the last injection. Both regimens of corticosteroid administration cause similar levels of peripheral blood lymphocytopenia and monocytopenia 4 and 24 hr, respectively, after the final injection. Neither *in vitro* hydrocortisone (0, 1 and 10 microg/ml) nor hydrocortisone (100 mg/kg) *in vivo* had any effect on either the PHA-induced or antibody-dependent cellular cytotoxicity of alveolar macrophages. In marked contrast, cortisone acetate, depo-preparation which gives sustained elevations of plasma cortisol levels similar to those found for a brief period after i.v. injection of hydrocortisone caused a marked decrease in cytotoxic effector function of alveolar macrophage suspensions. In a separate experiment, the suppressed killer cell function of the alveolar macrophages from steroid-treated animals was found not to be related to an intrinsic defect in killing of bound target cells since the defect in killing could be overcome by increasing the density of antibody and PHA on the target cells.

124

Johnson HM, Smith EM, Torres BA, Blalock JE. **Regulation of the** *In vitro* **antibody response by neuroendocrine hormones.** *Proc Natl Acad Sci.* 1982;79:4171-4. (English) (unavailable at publication)

125

Kater L, Oosterom R, McClure JE, Goldstein AL. **Presence of thymosin-like factors in human thymic epithelial conditioned medium.** *Int J Immunopharmacol.* 1979; 1:273-84. (English)

The objective of the present study was to determine whether or not thymosin and conditioned medium from human thymus epithelial cultures (HTECM) contain similar fractions, capable of inducing T-cell differentiation. Therefore, we tested the ability of rabbit antisera to different thymosin fractions (thymosin fractions 4, 6 and alpha₁) of both bovine and human origin to block the stimulatory effect of HTECM on Con A and PHA response of mouse thymocytes. We also looked for reactivity of the antisera toward tissues of man, mouse and calf, and to tissue cultures of man and mouse. Anti-thymosin fraction 5 and 6, but not anti-thymosin-alpha₁, were found to inhibit the stimulatory effect of HTECM on both Con A and PHA responses. This cannot be attributed to cytostatic or cytotoxic effect of the antisera on thymocytes. No effect was seen when using antiserum to kidney fraction 5 or normal rabbit serum. In both tissue sections and tissue cultures of the different species tested, anti-thymosin reacts only with thymus epithelial cells. The reactivity is blocked by neutralizing the antisera with thymosin fraction 5 but not by kidney fraction 5. The reactivity is also strongly diminished by neutralizing the antisera with HTECM but not with supernatants of conditioned media from non-thymic tissues. The observations are highly suggestive for the presence of similar fractions in HTECM and thymosin, and that both are secreted by thymus epithelial cells.

126

Keller AJ, Irvine WJ, Jordan J, Loudon NB. **Phytohemagglutinin-induced lymphocyte transformation in oral contraceptive users.** *Obstet Gynecol.* 1977;49:83-91. (English)

Phytohemagglutinin (PHA)-induced lymphocyte transformation (PILT) was determined in 217 women taking oral contraceptives and 203 control women by means of the uptake of ³H-thymidine into DNA of lymphocytes cultures in heterologous serum. Depressed PILT responses were observed in oral contraceptive users as compared with age-matched controls, and the magnitude of depression correlated with the duration of oral contraception and was inversely related to the clinical progestagenic potency of the component steroids. An additional group of 21 women, tested within 1 year (mean 3 months) of cessation of oral contraception, showed persistent depression of PILT responses. Suppression of lymphocyte transformation in autologous as compared with homologous, normal serum suggests that serum inhibitory factors may be important. We found no evidence for a direct suppressive *in vitro* effect of synthetic estrogens and gestagens. The prevalence of autoantibodies in oral contraceptive users was similar to that in control subjects.

127

Kenny JF, Pangburn PC, Trail G. **Effect of estradiol on immune competence:** *In vivo* **and** *In vitro* **studies.** *Infect Immun.* 1976;13:448-56. (English)

The administration of a single dose of 2.5 microg of microcrystalline estradiol-17-beta from 1 day before and up until 3.5 days after the administration of 3 x 10⁵ heat-killed Escherichia coli significantly increased numbers of splenic anti-E. coli antibody-producing cells in male mice sacrificed 4 days after receiving antigen. Administration early in the proliferative phase of antibody production, i.e., 1 day before or 1 day after the antigen, appeared to increase numbers of antibody-producing cells more than when it was administered at a later time. When given 2 days before the antigen or 2 h before sacrifice no effect was observed. Spleen cells harvested from male animals injected 3 days before with 5 x 10⁶ heat-killed E. Coli were incubated for 24 h *in vitro* with estradiol in concentrations ranging from 5 pg to 20 ng/ml. With concentrations of 500 pg to 5,000 pg/ml, significant increases in antibody-producing cells were not observed after a 2-h incubation period. Uptake of tritiated thymidine was increased in thymic and spleen cells incubated for 24 h with 500 pg of estradiol per ml; a concentration of 20 ng/ml slightly (but insignificantly) decreased uptake. Findings suggest that estradiol, in concentrations that approximate physiological serum levels in females, enhances mitosis of immunocompetent cells. This phenomenon may have bearing on the better immunological responsiveness of females than males.

128

Klareskog L, Forsum U, Peterson PA. **Hormonal regulation of the expression of Ia antigens on mammary gland epithelium.** *Eur J Immunol.* 1980;10:958-63. (English)

Guinea pig and mouse mammary gland epithelial cells express Ia antigen-like molecules that react specifically with a rabbit anit-Ia antigen antiserum. The murine Ia antigen-like molecules were shown to share alloantigenic determinants with regular spleen cell Ia antigens. The expression of the mammary gland Ia antigens is under hormonal control, i.e., the Ia antigen expression is induced by pregnancy and lactation and can also be induced by the exogenous administration of lactotropic hormones.

129

Knox AJ, Von Westarp C, Row VV, Volpe R. **Demonstration of the production of human thyroid-stimulating immunoglobulins (HTSI) by Graves' lymphocytes cultured** *In vitro* **with phytohemagglutinin (PHA).** *Metab.* 1976;25:1217-33. (English)

The lymphocytes from patients with Graves' disease or from healthy subjects have been cultured *in vitro* either alone or with phytohemagglutinin (PHA). After six days the culture supernatants have been assayed for their human thyroid-stimulating activity by measuring increases in adenosine 3',5' monophosphate (cyclic AMP) in human thyroid slices with which the supernatants have been incubated. Significant levels of human thyroid stimulator activity were found in the culture supernatants in eight of nine experiments in which Graves' lymphocytes were cultured with PHA. This activity has been abolished by precipitation of the IgG from the culture supernatant with goat anti-human IgG serum. In contrast, when Graves' lymphocytes were cultured alone, or when control lymphocytes were cultured either alone or with PHA, there was no overall significant production of human thyroid-stimulating immunoglobulin (HTSI). It is concluded that Graves' lymphocytes can be stimulated by PHA to produce HTSI *in vitro*. Since PHA is known to stimulate only T lymphocytes, which do not themselves elaborate immunoglobulins as B lymphocytes do, the above observations indicate a cooperation between T and B lymphocytes in production of HTSI, at least in this system.

130
Korenman S. **Oestrogen window hypothesis of the aetiology of breast cancer.** *Lancet.* 1980;1:700-1. (English) (no abstract)

131
Korneva EA. **Neurohumoral regulation of immunological homeostasis.** *Fiziol Chel.* 1976;3:469-81. (Russian) (unavailable at publication)

132
Lee K-C. **Cortisone as a probe for cell interactions in the generation of cytotoxic T cells; I--Effect on helper cells, cytotoxic T cell precursors, and accessory cells.** *J Immunol.* 1977;119:1836-45. (English)

The effect of cortisone on the *in vitro* cell-mediated cytotoxic response was investigated with respect to the participating cell types, viz., the cytotoxic T cell precursor (CTP), the helper cell, and the accessory (A) cell. Spleen and thymus cells from cortisone-treated CBA/CaJ mice were unable to generate alloreactive cytotoxic T cells when cultured with semiallogeneic (CBA/CaJ x DBA/2JF[1]) spleen cells or allogeneic (P815) tumor cells. This immunosuppression could be reversed by the addition of 2-ME to the cultures, which suggests that the CTP and helper cells were present but unresponsive. Measurements of the CTP frequency and helper activity in cultures containing 2-ME confirmed this possibility. Thus, limiting dilution analysis of spleen and thymus cells from cortisone-treated mice showed that they contained higher frequencies of CTP than cells from normal mice. Helper cell activity, as measured by the secretion of helper factor by primed cells, was found to be higher after cortisone treatment. The possibility of a defect in A cell function in spleen cells of cortisone-treated mice was suggested by 1) the ability of irradiated peritoneal macrophages to reconstitute the response, and 2) the greatly reduced efficiency of irradiated spleen cells (adherent or nonadherent) from cortisone-treated mice to restore responsiveness to nonadherent, A cell-deficient normal spleen cells. Although cortisone may exert its immunosuppressive effect on helper cells and CTP directly, it is likely that the deficiency in A cell function is at least partially responsible for the unresponsiveness of cortisone-treated cells.

133
Lee TP, Reed CE. **Effect of steroids on the regulation of the levels of cyclic AMP in human lymphocytes.** *Biochem Biophys Res Commun* 1978;998-1004. (English)

Glucocorticosteroids and estradiol increase the cyclic AMP response of lymphocytes to isoproterenol and PGE$_1$. This response, unlike the usual steroid responses initiated by specific cytoplasmic steroid receptors, does not require the biosynthesis of macromolecules for its activity. The effect may depend partially on the inhibitory effect of steroids on cyclic nucleotide phosphodiesterase. The potentiating effect of steroids, however, is greater than that which can be achieved with theophylline, a more potent inhibitor of phosphodiesterase prepared from lymphocytes.

134
Lee TP. **Effects of histamine-sensitizing factor and cortisol on lymphocyte adenyl cyclase responses.** *J Allergy Clin Immunol.* 1977;59:79-82. (English)

Levels of cyclic adenosine monophosphate (cAMP) in lymphocytes are regulated by beta-adrenergic agonists and PGE$_1$. The effect of these agonists is potentiated by cortisol. Incubation of lymphocytes with histamine-sensitizing factor (HSF) leads to loss of response to epinephrine and PGE[1]. The response can be partially restored by cortisol. Incubation of lymphocytes with beta-adrenergic antagonists such as propranolol leads to the loss of beta-adrenergic agents but not PGE$_1$. The inhibition by propranolol is not reversed by cortisol. These results suggest that the action of HSF and bordetella pertussis vaccine is not mediated through the inhibition of beta-adrenergic receptors alone.

135
Loseva TM. **Effect of thymosin on the rosette-forming capacity of peripheral blood lymphocytes from schizophrenics and healthy subjects.** *Zh Nevropatol Psikhiatr.* 1982;82:67-70. (Russian)

It has been found that the blood of schizophrenic patients contains much more thymosin-sensitive lymphocytes than the blood of healthy subjects. Thymosin produces a regulatory effect on the changed receptor activity of the T-cells revealed in the reaction of spontaneous rosette formation. The disturbances of the T-lymphocyte membrane activity that take place in schizophrenic patients can be associated with the change of the thymus hormonal function occurring in that disease.

136
Majsky A, Jakoubkova J. **Loss of HLA antigens associated with hormonal state** (letter). *Lancet.* 1976;2:859. (English)

137
Mantzouranis E, Borel Y. **Different effects of cortisone on the humoral immune response to T-dependent and T-independent antigens.** *Cell Immunol.* 1979;43:202-8. (English)

The effect of the administration of cortisone on the murine humoral immune response to either thymus-dependent (TD) or -independent (TI) antigens was studied *in vivo*. Whereas the thymus-dependent immune response was markedly suppressed, the thymus-independent immune response was preserved. The opposing effect of steroids on these two types of immune responses appears to be due to the relative independence of thymus-dependent antigens of a radioresistant cortisone-sensitive accessory cell.

138

Mason JW, Buescher EL, Belfer ML, Artenstein MS, Mougey EH. **A prospective study of corticosteroid and catecholamine levels in relation to viral respiratory illness.** *J Hum Stress.* 1979;5:18-28. (English)

Urinary 17-OHCS, epinephrine and norepinephrine levels were studied for one week before and one week after the onset of acute, severe Adenovirus 4 respiratory illness in 12 Army recruits during Basic Combat Training. During the pre-illness period, a tendency was frequently noted for all three hormone levels to show "spiking" elevations two to four days before illness onset. There was also a tendency for 17-OHCS levels to rise on the day before fever onset. The possible relationship of these pre-illness hormonal changes to stressful experiences and, in turn, to altered host resistance to infectious illness is discussed. Following onset of respiratory illness, 17-OHCS, epinephrine and norepinephrine levels all showed about 60 percent increases over the early pre-illness period baseline value. Elevations of these hormones persisted for about four to five days, roughly in correlation with fever duration, with only slight differences in configuration and timing of curves from one hormone to the next. The problem of evaluating which of several independent variables operating concurrently during infectious illness may be responsible for stimulating the final common neuroendocrine pathways is discussed.

139

McMillan R, Longmire R, Yelenosky R. **The effects of Corticosteroids on human IgG synthesis.** *J Immunol.* 1976:116:1592-5. (English)

The effect of prolonged, high-dose corticosteroid therapy on total IgG synthesis rates by human bone marrow and splenic leukocytes was studied in patients with immune thrombocytopenia. Marrow IgG production rates begin to decrease 3 weeks after beginning therapy and reach levels approximately one-fourth of pre-treatment rates after 6 weeks. No effect of corticosteroids on splenic IgG production rates could be shown. Marrow IgG synthesis rates in these patients were on the average from 3 to 10 times greater than corresponding splenic production rates and, in addition, appeared to correlate with serum IgG levels. These data suggest that the marrow is an important contributor to the total body IgG pool; and since corticosteroids appear to suppress marrow IgG production, this may be one reason for their therapeutic usefulness in antibody-mediated diseases.

140

Melmon KL, Insel PA. **Inflammatory and immune responses: cell individuality amidst ubiquitous hormonal signals.** *Johns Hopkins Med J.* 1977;141:15-22. (English) (no abstract)

141

Mendelsohn J, Multer MM, Bernheim JL. **Inhibition of human lymphocyte stimulation by steroid hormones: cytokinetic mechanisms.** *Clin Exp Immunol.* 1977;27:127-34. (English)

The steroid hormones estradiol, progesterone and testosterone, in addition to cortisol, inhibited stimulation of human peripheral blood lymphocytes by phytohaemagglutinin (PHA) and Con A. This effect upon lymphocyte transformation was assayed by three methods: quantitation of [3H] thymidine incorporation into acid precipitable material, microscopic assessment of blastic transformation and determination of the labelling index. Addition of steroid hormones at the initiation of culture resulted in a marked inhibition in all three parameters, which was observed with lower concentrations of cortisol than the other hormones. The inhibition was not attributable to cell death and could be partially reversed by removing hormones from the incubation medium after culture for 48-72 hr. Late addition of steroid hormones, 52 hr after addition of mitogen and 18 hr prior to pulse-labelling with [3H] thymidine, also resulted in reduced [3H] thymidine incorporation, accompanied by a nearly 50% reduction in the labelling indices and only a minimal decrease in the per cent transformed cells. Inhibition of lymphocyte stimulation by steroid hormones operates by the following cytokinetic mechanisms: (1) suppressed recruitment of cells from G_O to G_1 phase of the cell cycle, as indicated by the diminished per cent blasts; (2) inhibition of progression from G_1 phase into S phase, as evidenced by the reduced ratio [labelling index/blasts]; and, in the case of estradiol and rogesterone, (3) reduced rate of DNA replication or altered intracellular [3H] thymidine specific activity, as shown by the decreased [3H]thymidine incorporation/labelling index) ratio. Late addition of steroid hormones to stimulated cultures reduced the per cent of cells in LS phase, but did not revert previously transformed cycling lymphocytes to the G_O state.

142

Merikas OS, Efstratopoulos AD, Sharp JT, Marketos SG, Merikas GE. **The effect of glucocorticosteroids on antigen-induced leukocyte migration inhibition.** *Mater Med Pol.* 1979;11:10-14. (English)

The human leukocyte migration test, which is an *in vitro* correlate of cell-mediated immunity, was employed to investigate the effect of glucocorticosteroids on streptokinase-stretodornase (SK-SD)-induced leukocyte migration inhibition. The migration of peripheral blood leukocytes from three individuals lacking delayed hypersensitivity to SK-SD was not significantly inhibited in the presence of this antigen. In contrast, the leukocytes from eleven subjects with positive skin reactions to SK-SD showed significant migration inhibition when cultured with this antigen. The SK-SD-induced significant leukocyte migration inhibition was abolished when leukocytes were cultured with SK-SD and dexamethasone or hydrocortisone simultaneously. The effect of glucocorticosteroids was dose-dependent. Glucocorticosteroids had no lympholytic effect and did not alter leukocyte migration in the absence of antigen stimulation. The effect of glucocorticosteroids was irreversible because it was observed even after preincubation of the buffy coat leukocytes with dexamethasone or hydrocortisone for 30 min followed by their complete removal from the cell cultures to which SK-SD was then added. These findings are discussed. It is suggested that glucocorticosteroids block the action of leukocyte inhibitory factor on its effector cells.

143

Mishell RI, Lucas A, Mishell BB. **The role of activated accessory cells in preventing immunosuppression by hydrocortisone.** *J Immunol.* 1977;119:118-22. (English)

The generation of humoral immunity *in vitro* by normal and antigen-primed mouse spleen cells was suppressed by *in vitro* treatment with hydrocortisone. Functions of normal and antigen-activated helper T lymphocytes and of accessory cells were inhibited by the corticosteroids. Spleen cells cultured overnight in medium containing fetal bovine serum became highly resistant to the effects of hydrocortisone. Similar resistance was found to occur when spleen cells were cultured with accessory cells that previously had been activated with bacterial lipopolysaccharide. These studies show that immunologically nonspecific processes significantly alter the effects of the steroids on specific immune responses and suggest that accessory cell products modulate T cells in ways which differ from antigen induction.

144

Moore MR, Goodrum KJ, Couch R, Berry LJ. **Factors affecting macrophage function: glucocorticoid antagonizing factor.** *RES, J Reticuloendothel Soc.* 1978;23:321. (English) (no abstract)

145

Morgan JI, Bramhall JS, Britten AZ, Perris AD. **Calcium and oestrogen interactions upon the rat thymic lymphocyte plasma membrane.** *Biochem Biophys Res Commun.* 1976;72:663-72. (English)

When isolated thymic lymphocytes are equilibrated with a carbocyanine dye the degree of fluorescence is indicative of the potential difference across the plasma membrane. Increments in extracellular calcium concentrations trigger a decrease in fluorescence intensity which represents a membrane hyperpolarisation. This hyperpolarisation cannot be reversed by subsequent chelation of the calcium. Oestradiol and natural oestrogens reduced this calcium-induced potential alteration. These same steroids also blocked the calcium-induced mitotic stimulation apparent in this same cell type.

146

Mori T, Kobayashi H, Nishimoto H, Suzuki A, Nishimura T, Mori T. **Inhibitory effect of progesterone and 20-alpha-hydroxypregn-4-en-3-one on the phytohaemagglutinin-induced transformation of human lymphocytes.** *Am J Obstet Gynecol.* 1977;127:1512-7. (English)

To examine the immunobiological implications of sex steroids during pregnancy, the effects of estrone, estradiol, estriol, testosterone, dehydroepiandrosterone, 4-androstenedione, progesterone, 17-alpha-hydroxyprogesterone, and 20-alpha-dihydroprogesterone on the response of human lymphocytes to phytohemagglutinin (PHA) stimulation were investigated. Lymphocytes of 99 blood samples from 67 normal subjects who were not taking oral contraceptives were cultured in quadruplicate or quintuplicate under PHA stimulation in the absence or presence of various concentrations of each steroid, and incorporation of ^{3}H-thymidine into lymphocytes was measured. Progesterone and 20-alpha-dihydro-

progesterone at 10^4 ng per milliliter inhibited incorporation of ^{3}H-thymidine significantly by t test. The minimum effective concentration of progesterone was estimated to be 2×10^3 ng per milliliter. No effect on incorporation was observed with the other steroids. Since the effective concentrations of progesterone match those in the human placenta throughout pregnancy, progesterone was considered to suppress maternal lymphocyte response at its site of production rather than at the systemic level.

147

Nelson AM, Conn DL. **Series on pharmacology in practice; 9-- Glucocorticoids in rheumatic disease.** *Mayo Clin Proc.* 1980;55:758-69. (English)

Glucocorticoids are potent anti-inflammatory agents that play an important role in the therapy of many patients with connective tissue diseses, including systemic lupus erythematosus, polymyalgia rheumatica, various types of vasculitis, and complications of rheumatoid arthritis. Glucocorticoids reduce the number and influence the function of lymphocytes, monocytes, and eosinophils in peripheral blood. Prolonged high doses of glucocorticoids result in decreased levels of immunoglobulins, particularly IgG. Granulocytes are increased in the peripheral blood, but their migration to sites of inflammation is diminished. Glucocorticoids inhibit release of lysosomal enzymes. Although they have no effect on the factor or factors that initiate inflammation, glucorticoids have proved to be effective in the treatment of inflammatory manifestations of disease. Among significant adverse effects of glucocorticoid therapy are osteoporosis, aseptic necrosis of bone, and steroid myopathy.

148

Panoussopoulos DG, Humphrey PA, Humphrey LJ, Meek J. **Effect of various thyroid states on immunity.** *Surg Forum.* 1976;27:138-40. (English) (no abstract)

149

Papiernik M, Bach JF. **Thymocyte subpopulations in young and adult mice; II--Study of steroid-resistant populations by means of a specific heteroantiserum.** *Eur J Immunol.* 1977;7:800-3. (English)

Mouse steroid-resistant (Sr) cells of the thymus have been studied by means of a specific heteroantiserum. This antiserum was obtained in the rabbit after immunization with Sr thymocytes followed by absorption with high density cells isolated on a Ficoll density gradient shown to include a majority of steroid-sensitive (Ss) cells. Antigens defined by this antiserum were found on Sr thymocytes and on a significant portion of spleen and lymph node cells, but not on Ss cortical thymocytes. Cells sensitive to this antiserum appear early in the thymus (by day 15 of gestation) at the same time as Ss cells. These results suggest (a) the existence of an autonomous Sr cell line, with its own antigenic markers appearing early in ontogeny (at the same time as Ss cells), and showing wide heterogeneity in density, possibly linked to variable degrees in maturation, and (b) the medullary origin of some peripheral lymphocytes in lymph node and spleen cells that share antigenic markers with Sr thymocytes.

150

Parillo JE, Fauci AS. **Mechanisms of glucocorticoid action on immune processes.** *Annu Rev Pharmacol Toxicol.* 1979;19:179-201. (English) (no abstract)

151

Pattillo RA, Shalaby MR, Hussa RO, Bahl OMP, Mattingly RF. **Effect of crude and purified hCG on lymphocyte blastogenesis.** *Obstet Gynecol.* 1976;47:557-61. (English)

Crude APL hCG completely inhibited blastogenesis induced by phytohemagglutinin, pokeweed mitogen, or concanavalin A in normal lymphocytes and lymphocytes obtained from cancer patients. Phenol in quantities comparable to its concentration in commercial lyophilized APL hCG also completely inhibited all three mitogenic responses. By contrast, similar doses of highly purified hCG had no inhibitory effect; higher concentrations produced only slight inhibition. Beta-hCG had a partial (>50%) inhibitory effect that was dose-independent and non-reproducible.

152

Pedernera E, Romano M, Aguilar MC. **Influence of early surgical bursectomy on the Leydig cells in the chick embryo testis.** *J Steroid Biochem.* 1980;12:517-9. (English)

The bursa of Fabricius is an important lymphoid organ, but functions possibly as an endocrine gland. We report here on the influence of the bursa on testis development in chick embryos. The testes of embryos at 17.5 days of development were studied. Groups of embryos were surgically bursectomized at 68 h of incubation, others were bursectomized and bursa grafted; sham-operated embryos served as controls. Determinations of weight of testes, total protein content, and of *in vitro* production of testosterone by testes under hCG stimulation were performed. The quality of interstitial cells was estimated by morphometric studies. Early bursectomy resulted in a hypertrophy of the testis. Testosterone production was increased in the bursectomized embryos. Morphometric measurements showed a hypertrophy of Leydig cells. Bursal grafting prevented hypertrophy of the testes and the increase in testosterone production. These results indicate that the bursa of Fabricius influences steroid-producing cells during testis development.

153

Peterson RD, Palmer GC. **Selected hormone sensitivities of several transplantable T-cell lymphomas.** *Immunopharmacology.* 1980;2:147-55. (English)

Ten T-cell lymphomas induced in 10 C3H mice with Gross' MuLV were established as transplantable tumor lines in syngeneic mice. The responses of these lines to cortisone, histamine, norepinephrine, and prostaglandin E_1 were assessed after varying times in passage. Distinct and distinquishing sensitivity profiles were revealed.

154

Petrov RV. **Role of hormones and mediators in the functioning of the immune system.** *Vestn Akad Med Nauk SSSR.* 1980;8:3-11. (Russian)

The mediators released by stimulated lymphocytes and collectively referred to as lymphokines, provide for mediator and effector functions of lymphocytes involved in the development of immune responses. The central organs of immunity--the thymus and bone marrow--elaborate mediators that influence the maturation and functioning of T and B lymphocytes. The active thymus fraction (ATF-6) is successfully used in the treatment of states of immune deficiency and of defects in the proliferation of lymphocytes, in particular in lymphogranulomatosis. Recently, a mediator which is elaborated in the bone marrow and which affects the effector function of B cells by stimulating antibody production, has been discovered. This mediator, which is known as SAP (stimulator of antibody producers), is devoid of species specificity and is likely to find clinical application.

155

Pierpaoli W, Kopp HG, Bianchi E. **Interdependence of thymic and neuroendocrine functions in ontogeny.** *Clin Exp Immunol.* 1976;24:501-6. (English)

The immunological blockade of the adenohypophysis of athymic nude mice bearing allogeneic skin grafts prevents the reconstitution of transplantation immunity when such animals are grafted with thymus, and the grafts are permanently accepted. Newborn and adult athymic mice have markedly diminished levels of prolactin in blood and abnormally high levels of luteotropic hormone. Implantation of the thymus normalizes blood levels of these two hormones. These findings affirm the role of the thymus in the organization of the maturing brain for endocrine functions and identify prolactin as one of the hormones which play a major role in immune differentiation in early ontogeny.

156

Pierpaoli W, Kopp HG, Mueller J, Keller M. **Interdependence between neuroendocrine programming and generation of immune recognition in ontogeny.** *Cell Immunol.* 1977;29:16-27. (English)

Sequential, chronologically, and quantitatively critical inoculation of different allogeneic hybrid cells into mice during the neonatal and perinatal period results in an indefinite prolongation of the perinatal stage during which tolerance can be readily induced. Consequently, a permanent specific tolerance to the sequentially inoculated alloantigens and a parallel alternation and retardation in the maturation of the developing endocrine system which normally controls immune differentiation are observed. The endocrine and immune parameters are altered only when the successive presentation of alloantigens is begun at birth, as this is a critical stage of development at which both the neuroendocrine (hypothalamic-pituitary) and the thymo-lymphatic systems are still highly undifferentiated. The phylogenetically and ontogenetically interlocked and independent thymo-lymphatic and neuroendocrine networks thus constitute a basic homeostatic fashion. On the basis of these considerations and the experimental findings that support them, the generation of tolerance and immunity (recognition of self and nonselfcomponents of the body) appears to be a part of the definitive brain programming for neuroendocrine and immune functions in early ontogeny. This would constitute an augmented interpretation of the concept of immune tolerance as "specific central failure of the mechanisms of reponse" originally put forth by Medawar (1956).

157
Pierpaoli W, Maestroni GJ. **Pharmacologic control of the hormonally modulated immune response; III--Prolongation of allogeneic skin graft rejection and prevention of runt disease by a combination of drugs acting on neuroendocrine functions.** *J Immunol.* 1978;120:1600-3. (English)

A recently developed pharmacologic means for suppressing acquired immunity by drugs acting on neuroendocrine regulation has been applied to transplantation immune reactions. A number of drugs have been tested singly and in combination for their capacity to suppress the immune response of mice grafted with allogeneic skin. Another model involved newborn F_1 hybrid recipients inoculated with spleen cells from donors of parental strains that had been made specifically "unresponsive" by drug and alloantigen treatment. These procedures led to the identification of a combination of four drugs that induced a remarkable delay in allograft rejection and a prolonged unresponsiveness to alloantigens. This combination of drugs also abrogated the graft-vs-host-runting syndrome in newborn hybrid recipients.

158
Pierpaoli W, Maestroni GJ. **Pharmacological control of the immune response by blockade of the early hormonal changes following antigen injection.** *Cell Immunol.* 1977;31:355-63. (English)

Antigen injection into mice induces a rapid increase in blood levels of gonadotropins. Suppression of these hormonal changes by a combination of drugs acting on the neuroendocrine regulation as well as on cell membrane receptors results in a blockade of antibody synthesis and specific "tolerance." In addition, remarkable suppression of transplantation immunity is achieved.

159
Rampen FHJ, Mulder JH. **Malignant melanoma: and androgen-dependent tumour?** *Lancet.* 1980;1:562-5. (English)

Of 688 melanoma patients registered during 1956-78, 267 developed metastatic spread of the disease. Sex differences in the course of the disease in this subset were studied. Intervals between subsequent stages of melanoma activity were longer, but not significantly so, in female than male patients. Survival times from initial distant metastases were significantly longer in women than in men. Tumour doubling time of pulmonary secondaries revealed a clear tendency to a slower growth rate in female patients. Our analysis suggests that malignant melanoma might be an androgen-dependent tumour. Therapy with anti-androgens or orchidectomy deserves consideration in male patients with metastatic melanoma.

160
Reichman ME, Villee CA. **Estradiol binding by rat thymus cytosol.** *J Steroid Biochem.* 1978;9:5637-41. (English)

Preparations of rat thymus cytosol are shown to specifically bind [^{3}H]-estradiol. Binding is stable during overnight incubations at 4°C and increases linearly with increasing protein concentration in the incubation up to at least 2.2 mg/ml. There are two components with binding activity, one of high affinity, and one of lower affinity. The high affinity component has a $K_a = 1.16 \pm 0.38 \times 10^{11} M^{-1}$ and a binding capacity of $7.32 \pm 1.65 \times 10^{-15}$ mol/mg cytosol protein. On sucrose density gradients binding appears in two regions, 6.6-7.6 S and 2.5-4 S. Binding of [^{3}H]-estradiol in the 6.6-7.6 S region is competed for by a 100-fold excess of nonradioactive estradiol while this level of nonradioactive estradiol only partially competes with [^{3}H]-estradiol in the 2.5-4 S region.

161
Renoux G, Renoux M, Gyenes L, Guillaumin JM. **A comparison of the *In vivo* T-cell recruiting capacity of DTC, serum of DTC-treated mice and two synthetic hormones.** *Internat J Immunopharmacol.* 1980;2:167. (English) (unavailable at publication)

162
Riley V, Spackman DH, Fitzmaurice MA, Santisteban G, McClanahan H, Louthan S, Dennis M, Bloom J. **Enhancement and inhibition of lymphosarcoma by fluocinolone acetonide** (abstract). *Proc Amer Assoc Cancer Res.* 1976;17:161. (English)

A modulation of the neoplastic process has been obtained by administering a potent synthetic adrenocorticoid, fluocinolone acetonide (FA). This hormone induces an involution of the thymus, spleen, and lymph nodes, enlargement of the liver, and a lymphocytopenia involving T and B cells. FA also blocks the endogenous production of corticosterone in the pituitary and adrenals. Enhancement of the growth rate of 6C3HED lymphosarcoma is produced when FA is administered during the early stages of tumor growth, and spontaneous tumor regressions are prevented or diminished. In contrast administration of FA 7 days prior to tumor implantation produces an inhibition of subsequent tumor growth. This may be an expression of a homeostatic immunological rebound following suppression of various elements of the immunological competence of the host. These contrasting effects are both dose- and time-dependent. FA and related compounds, employed in conjunction with a neoplastic system that is in tenuous equipoise with the host, provide a reliable model for examining the relationships between the RES, T cells, B cells, the pituitary-adrenocortico-thymus axis, and the cancer process.

163
Ritter M. **Embryonic mouse thymocyte development enhancing effect of corticosterone at physiological levels.** *Immunol.* 1977;33:241-6. (English)

The action of corticosterone on embryonic mouse thymus development has been studied *in vitro*. Effects of the hormone on lymphoid differentiation varied according to the dose. 0.2-1.0 microg/ml had an enhancing effect, resulting in an increasing in the proportion of Thy-1.2 positive cells as compared with control cultures. Two to fifty micrograms per millilitre had an inhibitory effect, appearing to selectively kill small lymphocytes while leaving large and medium lymphocytes intact. At higher doses these immature cells were also killed.

164

Rogers P, Matossian-Rogers A. **Selection of thymocytes with the phenotypes of mature T cells using coricosteroids.** *IRCS J jMed Sci.* 1981;9:564-78. (English)

It is well established that T cells undergo a maturational stage in the thymus before becoming fully competent lymphocytes. Consequently, most thymocytes are immunoincompetent and it is only a small percentage of medullary cells that are able to respond to antigen. One way of selecting for this immunocompetent population is to administer corticosteroids to the intact animal and previous workers have used doses ranging from 1 mg to 10 mg per mouse for this purpose. We now report investigations using monoclonal antibodies and fluorescence activated cell sorter (FACS) analysis to determine which dose in this range best selects for populations with the mature phenotype since it is now apparent that the mature thymocytes display the antigen-density characteristics of peripheral T cells.

165

Rosenberg JC, Lysz K. **Suppression of human cytotoxic lymphocytes by methylprednisolone.** *Transplantation.* 1978;25:115-20. (English)

In order to gain insight into the immunosuppressive mechanism of action of corticosteroids, an in vitro model of the cellular immune response was used to study the effect of methylprednisolone on human lymphocyte-mediated cytotoxicity. Concentrations from 0.25 to 10 microg/ml were equally effective in producing 74% suppression of lymphocyte-mediated cytotoxicity when the steroid was present during the entire period of *in vitro* sensitization. A 12.5-fold increase in effector to target cell ratio was required to achieve 30%^{51}Cr release when cytotoxic lymphocytes were generated in the presence of methylprednisolone. Lymphocyte-mediated cytotoxicity was suppressed 48% when methylprednisolone was present only during the initial 24 hr of the 7-day *in vitro* sensitization period. Methylprednisolone also effectively inhibited cytotoxicity when it was incubated with sensitized lymphocytes for 3 hr before incubating these cells with target cells. Our observations suggest that two of the major immuno-suppressive mechanisms of action of methylprednisolone are suppression of the generation of cytotoxic lymphocytes and suppression of specifically sensitized cytotoxic lymphocytes.

166

Royal College of General Practitioners' Oral Contraception Study. **Reduction in incidence of rheumatoid arthritis associated with oral contraceptives.** *Lancet.* 1978;1:569-71. (English)

Analyses of the frequency of reporting of rheumatoid arthritis have been undertaken as part of the continuing major prospective survey of oral contraceptives. The rate of reporting in oral-contraceptive users (takers) is half of the rate in non-users (controls). The rates for ex-takers and controls are not materially different. The expected rise in the rate of reporting in women over 35 is apparent in controls but suppressed in takers. In the absence of any accountable bias, it is concluded that oral contraceptives protect against the development of rheumatoid arthritis. Although the effect is small, the observation may be valuable in understanding the aetiology of the disease and the mechanism of action of oral contraceptives.

167

Saxena R K, Talwar GP. **An anterior pituitary factor stimulates thymidine incorporation in isolated thymocytes.** *Nature.* 1977;268:57-8. (English) (no abstract)

168

Schlager SI. **Relationship between cell-mediated and humoral immune attack on tumor cells; I--Drug and hormone effects on susceptibility to killing and macromolecular synthesis.** *Cell Immunol.* 1981;58:398-414. (English)

The effect of metabolic inhibitors and hormones on the susceptibility of P815 murine mastocytoma cells to antibody-C' [complement] and cell-mediated killing, and on the ability of the cells to synthesize DNA, RNA, protein, carbohydrate and lipid was tested. Pretreatment of the cells with adriamycin, actinomycin D, and puromycin increased the sensitivity of the cells to killing by rabbit anti-P815 antibody plus guinea pig C', but not by allogeneic P815 sensitized spleen cells. Mitomycin C treatment enhanced the cells' sensitivity to cell-mediated, but not antibody-C', killing. Insulin and hydrocortisone, but not epinephrine, were effective in decreasing cell susceptibility to killing by both antibody-C' and cell-mediated attack systems. The kinetics of the drug-induced-increase and the hormone-induced decrease in susceptibility of the cells to antibody-C' killing correlated with a decrease and increase, respectively, in cell ability to incorporate fatty acid into complex cellular lipid. No such correlation was found between cellular lipid synthesis and tumor cell susceptibility to cell-mediated killing. Cell ability to resist either form of immune attack was not dependent on cell ability to synthesize DNA, RNA, protein or complex carbohydrate. Apparently the susceptibility of these tumor cells to antibody-C' vs. cell-mediated killing may be linked to different metabolic properties of the cells, and may reflect differences in the mechanisms of humoral vs. cellular immune attack.

169

Shkhinek EK, Dostoevskaia LP, Biriukov VD. **Role of glucocorticoids in the development of a humoral immune response in the intact organism.** *Probl Endocrinol.* 1982;28:64-70. (Russian)

The formation of the humoral immune response in experimental rabbits to typhoid VI-antigen and to sheep red blood cells was estimated from serum hemagglutinin titres. It was found to vary but insignificantly in the animals that were immunized concurrently with the blocking of the hypothalamo-hypophysio-adrenocortical system induced by intraventricular administration of dexamethasone or during stimulation of this system due to a short-term stress. The results obtained show that relatively short-term changes in the plasma 11-HCS concentration cannot lead to significant disorders in the antibody production by the organism.

170
Shyamala G, Dickson C. **Relationship between receptor and mammary tumor virus production after stimulation of glucocorticoid.** *Nature.* 1976;262:107-12. (English)

A short exposure of primary cultures of mouse mammary tumour cells to glucocorticoids results in at least three-fold stimulation of mammary tumour virus (MTV) production. Specific interaction of glucocorticoids with the cytoplasmic and nuclear receptors can also be demonstrated. The biological potency of various steroids to stimulate MTV is related directly to the retention of the steroid-receptor complex in the nuclei. Progesterone has a high affinity for the cytoplasmic receptor, is not retained by the nuclei and does not stimulate or block the basal level of MTV production. It is however, quite effective in abolishing the glucocorticoid-mediated stimulation of MTV and thus behaves as an antagonist of glucocorticoid.

171
Siiteri PK, Febres F, Clemens LE, Chang RJ, Goudos B, Stites D. **Progesterone and maintenance of pregnancy: is progesterone nature's immunosuppressant?** *Ann NY Acad Sci.* 1977;286:384-96. (English) (no abstract)

172
Sporn MB, Todaro GJ. **Autoendocrine secretion and malignant transformation of cells.** *N Engl J Med.* 1980;303:878-80. (English) (no abstract)

173
Strom TB, Bangs JD. **Human serum-free mixed lymphocytes: the stereospecific effect of insulin and its potentiation by transferrin.** *J Immunol.* 1982;128:1555-9. (English)

We have established a serum-free human mixed lymphocyte response (MLR). Proliferative unidirectional responses are discerned using peripheral blood leukocytes obtained from unrelated individuals and family members mismatched for HLA while MLR conducted between HLA identical siblings are negative. Resting lymphocytes lack insulin and transferrin receptors; activated lymphocytes are known to express insulin and transferrin receptors. Interestingly, physiologic concentrations of insulin and transferrin synergistically potentiate DNA synthesis in serum-free allogeneic cultures. To verify that the insulin effect was due to a stereospecific interaction between insulin and classical, high-affinity insulin receptors, insulin and a series of insulin-like peptides were compared in their ability to bind to alloactivated T cells and amplify the MLR. The results demonstrate the sterospecificity of the insulin effect in the receptors in the process of lymphocyte activation.

174
Strom TB, Helderman JH. **Comparison of ligand-specific rat allosensitized lymphocyte insulin receptors as assessed in binding and functional (lymphocyte-mediated cytotoxicity) assays.** *Cell Immunol.* 1980; 53:382-8. (English)

Since rigorous proof of the existence of functional cellular hormone receptors requires that similar ligand stereospecifities for binding sites and function be demonstrable, the relative capability of insulin analogs, proinsulin, and growth hormone to compete with insulin for occupation of the insulin-binding site on alloactivated lymphocytes was determined and compared to their ability to augment alloimmune lymphocyte-mediated cytotoxicity. The potency of these agents in binding and functional assays were parallel. The results demonstrate that alloactivated lymphocytes express a stereospecific, functional insulin receptor.

175
Strom TB. **Neuroendocrine influences on immunity: immunoregulation via second messenger systems** (abstract). *The Gerontologist.* 1982;22:204. (English)

The proliferative and functional capacities of T lymphocytes are bi-directionally governed by cyclic AMP and cyclic GMP. The lymphocyte membrane possesses functionally active receptors for a variety of hormones and neurotransmitters. Activation of many of these receptors results in a change in intracellular cyclic nucleotide concentrations. Lymphocyte activation results in a preprogrammed change in the identity and concentration of these receptors. It is likely that stress, through changes in these hormones and neurotransmitters, may thus alter the immune response.

176
Stutman O, Shen FW. **Post-thymic precursor cells are sensitive to steroids and belong to the Ly 1,2,3, + subset** (abstract). *Fed Proc, Fed Am Soc Exp Biol.* 1977;36:1301. (English)

We have characterized a population of immunologically incompetent post-thymic precursor cells in the periphery which give rise to immunologically competent T cells under the influence of thymic humoral factor(s). Main features of these cells are: non-recirculating; concentrated in spleen (and marrow); rapidly dividing; decline after adult thymectomy; insensitive to ALS; adherent to nylon wool; 5.8 mm/hr migration in velocity sedimentation at 1 g; light in BSA gradients; Thy. 1^+, TL^-; immunologically incompetent (no reactivity to PHA, Con A, MLR or CML). All of these features are quite different from competent T cells. The model uses 60 day-old neonatally thymectomized CBA/H mice, injected with purified post-thymic precursors of CBA/HT6T6 origin (usually from newborn spleen or adult marrow) and grafted with CBA/HT6 thymus in diffusion chambers. Our present work indicates that the post-thymic precursor is sensitive to steroids *in vivo* (250 mg/kg of hydrocortisone, i.p.) or *in vitro*; and that appropriate Ly antisera and C' can eliminate the precursor, which types as Ly.1.1, Ly.2.1 and Ly.3.2$^+$. In both instances, pre-treatment of the precursor cells with steroids or Ly sera and C', completely abrogated the ability of such cells to restore immune functions (MLR, PHA, GvH) when injected into the thymectomized model. These experiments further support our view that the cell exported by the thymus is not necessarily a competent T cell and that further maturation in the periphery is required.

177
Swierenga SHH, MacManus JP, Braceland BM, Youdale T. **Regulation of the primary immune response in vivo by parathyroid hormone.** *J Immunol.* 1976;117:1608-11. (English)

Injection of sheep red blood cells into rats stimulates splenic DNA synthesis, then increases the proportion of plaque-forming cells, and finally raises the circulating antibody level. Removal of the parathyroid glands, which causes hypocalcemia, 24 hr before antigen injection impairs all of these responses, but is without effect after antigen injection. It is suggested that parathyroid hormone and calcium control the immune response, probably by affecting the proliferative phase of this response.

178
Talal N. **Proceedings of the Kroc Foundation Conference on sex factors, steroid hormones and the host response.** *Arthr Rheum.* 1979;22:1153-1313. (English) (no abstract)

179
Teng CS, Smith BR, Clayton B. **Thyroid stimulating antibodies to the immunoglobulins in opthalmic Graves' disease.** *Clin Endocrinol.* 1977;6:207-11. (English)

Thyroid-stimulating immunoglobulins (TSI) have been detected by receptor assay in the sera of 43% of patients with opthalmic Graves' disease. Comparison of the receptor assay studies with thyroid function tests indicated that in several patients the antibodies detected by receptor assay were biologically inactive. In other patients, thyroid function appeared to be under TSI control with hyperthyroidism prevented by autoimmune destruction of the thyroid.

180
Tischler AS, Dichter MA, Biales B, Green LA. **Neuroendocrine neoplasms and their cells of origin.** *N Engl J Med.* 1977;296:919-25. (English) (no abstract)

181
Trichopoulos D, MacMahon B, Brown J. **Socioeconomic status, urine estrogens, and breast cancer risk.** *J Natl Cancer Inst.* 1980;64:753-5. (English)

Urine estrogens were measured in 46 women students, ages 15-18, at a middle-class high school in Athens and in 40 women of the same age residing at one of three orphanages in the same city. The lower socioeconomic status (SES) of the latter group was documented by their lower mean height (by 5.2 cm) and by weight (by 5.3 kg) relative to the high school students. Both in follicular and luteal phases of the menstrual cycle, the women with lower SES had 50% higher estriol ratios (ratio of the concentration of estriol to the sum of the concentrations of estrone and estradiol). In luteal specimens the concentration of all three major estrogens was higher in the group with low SES than in the women in the other group, but the concentration of estriol was most increased. There was also an indication of less frequent anovular cycles among the women with low SES. These findings are consistent with hypotheses linking either the estriol ratio or the frequency of anovular cycles to breast cancer risk.

182
Tyan ML. **Genetic control of hydrocortisone-induced thymus atrophy.** *Immunogenetics.* 1979;8:177-81. (English) (no abstract)

183
Volpe R. **The role of autoimmunity in hypoendocrine and hyperendocrine function: with special emphasis on autoimmune thyroid disease.** *Ann Intern Med.* 1977; 87:86-99. (English)

There is considerable evidence to suggest that the organ specific autoimmune endocrinopathies are primary disorders of the lymphoid system. Although proof is not complete, the basic genetic defect in each condition may be one of immune surveillance, that is, a defect in suppressor "T" lymphocytes. Combinations of two or more of these conditions may be due to the concurrence of two or more specific defects in immune control, as well as the random appearance of the appropriate self-directed "forbidden" clones of lymphocytes. In this concept, there is no need for antigenic alteration (only antigenic availability) to initiate these disorders. Both cell-mediated and humoral immunity seem essential, with roles for immune complexes and "killer" cells as well. Antireceptor antibodies are of particular interest in Graves' disease, where they are stimulatory: other antireceptor antibodies have been found that are blocking antibodies, and others may merely bind without either stimulating or blocking.

184
Webel ML, Ritts RE Jr. **The effects of corticosteroid concentrations on lymphocyte blastogenesis.** *Cell Immunol.* 1977;32:287-92. (English)

High concentrations of methylprednisolone added for prolonged periods *in vitro* to lymphocyte cell cultures inhibited allogeneic-cell-induced or phytohemagglutinin (PHA)-induced blastogenesis in contrast to lower concentrations which were inhibitory only if added before or within several hours of blastogenic induction.

185
Weinstein Y, Lindner HR, Eckstein B. **Thymus metabolises progesterone: possible marker for T-lymphocytes.** *Nature.* 1977;266:632-3. (English) (no abstract)

186
Weinstein Y. **20-alpha-hydroxysteroid dehydrogenase: a T lymphocyte-associated enzyme.** *J Immunol.* 1977; 119:1223-9. (English)

20-alpha-Hydroxysteroid dehydrogenase (20-alpha-SDH), an enzyme which reduces progesterone to 20-alpha-dihydroprogesterone, was found to be associated with T lymphocytes. 20-alpha-SDH activity was present in spleen cells bearing theta antigen, spleen cells nonadherent to nylon wool (T lymphocyte-enriched population), and in thymocytes. Almost no enzymatic activity was found in bone marrow cells from normal mice and in spleen cells from neonatally thymectomized or athymic nude mice. T cell mitogens (PHA and Con A), but not the B cell mitogen LPS, induced high levels of enzymatic activity 48 h after addition to spleen cell cultures.

The level of 20-alpha-SDH activity in lymphocytes was age-dependent. At the age of 4 weeks, 20-alpha-SDH activity in thymocytes, spleen cells, and lymph node lymphocytes was 3 to 5 times higher than at 8 and 16 weeks. Progesterone (5.0 x 10^{-7}) was found to inhibit thymocyte proliferation after exposure to mitogens, but not 20-alpha-dihydroprogesterone (10^{-6}M). 20-alpha-SDH may protect the embryonic thymocytes against high concentrations of progesterone.

187
Weinstein Y. **Impairment of the hypothalamo-pituitary-ovarian axis of the athymic "nude" mouse.** *Mech Ageing Dev.* 1978;8:63-8. (English)

Pituitary and serum levels of LH and FSH and hypothalamic GnRH content were measured in acyclic, congenitally athymic (nu/nu) female mice. No significant differences were found between athymic and normal dioestrous mice of the same age (3 months). The serum LH level of the athymic mouse failed to increase 6 days after ovariectomy, but increased in response to injectin of GnRH. The results suggest that the athymic nude mice suffer from impairment of hypothalamic control of the pituitary.

188
Werb Z. **Biochemical actions of glucocorticoids on macrophages in culture: specific inhibition of elastase, collagenase, and plasminogen activator secretion and effects on other metabolic functions.** *J Exp Med.* 1978; 147:1695-1712. (English)

Glucocorticoids have a major role in the therapy of inflammatory and immunologically mediated diseases. The precise mechanism of the suppressive and anti-inflammatory effects of these drugs is still unknown, but the functions of the mononuclear phagocyte system are generally believed to be sensitive to glucocorticoid action. During glucocorticoid administration *in vivo*, monocytopenia occurs and monocytes fail to accumulate at inflammatory sites. In the presence of glucocorticoids, macrophages do not respond to macrophage migration inhibitory factor, and fail to become "armed" or activated. In experiments *in vivo* it is difficult to determine whether glucocorticoids are acting directly on macrophages or indirectly on lymphocytes and other cells that produce mediators of macrophage function. Macrophages may serve as a direct target for the therapeutic actions of anti-inflammatory steroids. In the accompanying paper, I establish that mononuclear phagocytes contain specific, high affinity receptors for glucocorticoids. In the present paper, I examine the action of glucocorticoids on biochemical functions of monocytes and macrophages cultured *in vitro*. Mononuclear phagocytes at all stages of maturation are sensitive to glucocorticoids. Production of monocytic and granulocytic colonies from bone marrow precursors and the secretion of elastase, collagenase, plasminogen activator, and nonspecific neutral proteinases by mature macrophages are inhibited by physiological concentrations of glucocorticoids. I have studied macrophages from glucocorticoid-sensitive (rabbit, mouse) and glucocorticoid-insensitive (human, guinea pig) species, and all show similar glucocorticoid-mediated actions, even though they differ in hormone-mediated effects on lymphocytes. Because steroid concentrations comparable to those for

saturating the high affinity glucocorticoid binding sites suppress macrophage secretion and colony formation, it is likely that these effects are mediated by specific glucocorticoid receptors.

189
Williams RM, Kraus LJ, Inbar M. et al. **Circadian bioperiodicity of natural killer cell activity in human blood (individually assessed).** *Chronobiologia.* 1979;6:172. (English) (no abstract)

190
Wyle FA, Kent JR. **Immunosuppression by sex hormones; I--The effect upon PHA- and PPD-stimulated lymphocytes.** *Clin Exp Immunol.* 1977;27:407-15. (English)

Progesterone, estradiol, testosterone, cortisol, and 11-desoxycortisol (Compound S) were added to cultures of human lymphocytes stimulated with phytohaemagglutinin (PHA) and purified protein derivative (PPD). The immunosuppressive effect of cortisol was verified and the three sex-steroid hormones were also found to inhibit lymphocyte transformation although at concentrations higher than for cortisol. Compound S, a steroid of low biological potency, also had immunosuppressive activity. At concentrations (0.01-1.0 microg/ml), progesterone, oestrogen, testosterone, and Compound S augmented the transformation response to PPD but not to PHA. Marked variation from individual to individual in the suppressive effects of all the steroids were noted. The clinical implications of immunosupppression by the sex steroid hormones are discussed.

191
Yamasaki H, Yamamoto T. **Inhibitory effect of adrenal glucocorticoids on histamine release.** *Jpn J Pharmacol.* 1963;13:223-4. (English) (unavailable at publication)

Hormone receptors on lymphocytes

192
Baxter JD, Funder JW. **Hormone receptors.** *N Engl J Med.* 1979;301:1149-61. (English) (no abstract)

193
Bhathena SJ, Schecter GP, Gazdan A, Louie J, Recant L. **Glucagon and somatostatin receptors on circulating human mononuclear leukocytes.** *62nd Annual Meeting Endocrinol Soc.* 1980; abstract no. 329. (English) (unavailable at publication)

194
Cooke T, George D, Shields R, Maynard P, Griffiths K. **Oestrogen receptors and prognosis in early breast cancer.** *Lancet.* 1979;1:995-7. (English)

In a study of the role of oestrogen-receptor analysis in early breast cancer the oestrogen-receptor content of the tumour was estimated in 286 patients undergoing mastectomy. These patients were followed for up to 39 months, and the recurrence of disease was noted in relation to the presence or absence of oestrogen receptor. Recurrence-rates were significantly higher in patients whose tumours did not contain receptors than in those whose tumours did. This same relationship was seen when women with and without axillary metastases were considered separately. The highest rates of recurrence were in women with axillary lymph-node involvement whose tumours lacked oestrogen receptors. Women without axillary-node involvement whose tumours lacked oestrogen receptors showed the same high rate of recurrence as all women with axillary-node involvement. The oestrogen-receptor content of a primary breast cancer appears to be an independent guide to early recurrence of the disease.

195
Csaba G, Sudar F, Dobozy O. **Triiodothyronine receptors in lymphocytes of newborn and adult rats.** *Horm Metab Res.* 1977;9:499-501. (English)

Cytoplasmic and nuclear incorporation of ^{125}I triiodothyronine by thymic lymphocytes has been demonstrated by electron microscopic autoadiography. Incorporation was significantly more pronounced in the newborn than in the adult age. The information emerging from the experimental observations contributes further evidence to the more precise interpretation of receptor maturation.

196
Gozes Y, Caruso J, Strom TB. **The absence of cryptic insulin receptors on resting lymphocytes.** *Diabetes.* 1981;30:314-6. (English)

Previous experiments have demonstrated that insulin receptors emerge upon stimulated lymphocytes while resting lymphocytes lack insulin receptors. The appearance of insulin receptors is totally dependent on RNA and protein synthesis. The results suggest that insulin receptors are synthesized *de novo* or that new protein is synthesized that is responsible for activation of the receptor. In this study, we investigated the possibility that cryptic membrane receptors are present before lymphocyte activation. As a precedent, hypertonic salt solutions or enzymatic digestion have been reported to uncover cryptic insulin receptors in liver and fat cell membranes. Similar treatment of lymphocytes failed to reveal cryptic, stereospecific receptor sites, although nonspecific insulin binding did increase.

197
Grossman CJ, Nathan P, Sholiton LJ. **Specific androgen receptor in the thymus of the castrate male rat** (abstract). *Biol Reprod.* 1978;18:48A. (English)

Castration in the male rat has been shown to produce enlargement of the thymus gland while androgen or estrogen treatment results in a decrease in thymic size in these animals. We have previously shown that a specific estrogen receptor was present in thymic homogenates of castrate males. This estrogen receptor was of high affinity, low capacity, specific for estrogen and estrogen-like compounds, sedimented on sucrose gradients at 8s, possessed a KA of 6.6 x 10^9M^{-1} and was present at a concentration of 0.3 pmoles/g tissue. We now wish to report the presence of a high affinity, low capacity, specific androgen receptor in thymic homogenates. Thymic tissue was removed from 1-2 day castrate young male rats and was homogenized in 0.5M Tris (pH 7.4), 1mM EDTA, .012M

thioglycerol, 10% glycerol buffer and centrifuged at 120,000 x g for 1 hr. By Scatchard plot analysis it was shown that a specific dihydrotestosterone (DHT) receptor was present in this cytosol fraction at a concentration of 0.26 ± 0.4 pmoles/g tissue and it had a KA of 3.5 ± 0.5x10^9M^{-1}. This thymic DHT receptor sedimented on 5-20% sucrose-glycerol gradients in the 8s range and was competed for a tenfold increase in unlabelled DHT but was not affected by cortisol (F). By competition analysis it was shown that the DHT receptor has a relative binding affinity (RBA) for DHT = 100%, testosterone = 38%, estradiol = 2%, progesterone = 0.5%, while cortisol had no signficant binding. Two hour incubations of thymic homogenate with a TPNH generating system using Krebs buffer revealed that C^{14} testosterone substrate could be converted in part to DHT, 5-alpha-A-dione and 3-alpha-,5-alpha-A-diol. We conclude that the thymus contains specific androgen and estrogen receptors which may play a role in the determination of thymic function.

198
Grossman CJ, Nathan P, Taylor BB, Sholiton LJ. **Rat thymic dihydrotestosterone receptor: preparation, location and physiochemical properties.** *Steroids.* 1979; 34:539-53. (English)

Castration in the male rat has been shown to produce enlargement of the thymus gland while treatment with dihydrotestosterone (DHT) results in a decrease in thymic size in these animals. To determine if these changes might be receptor-mediated, thymus tissue from castrate male rats was removed and homogenized in buffer and centrifuged to produce cytosol. By Scatchard plot analysis, it was shown that a specific DHT receptor was present at a concentration of 0.24 ± 0.02 pmoles/g tissue and it possessed a KA of 2.51 + 0.45 x 10^9M^{-1}. This thymic DHT receptor sedimented on 5-20% sucrose gradients in the 8s region. By competition analysis it was found that testosterone only partially competed (25%) for this receptor, with virtually no binding noted for estradiol, progesterone, and cortisol. The receptor was found to be localized in the reticuloepithelial matrix of the thymus and was not present in the thymic lymphocyte fraction.

199
Grossman CJ, Sholiton LJ, Blaha GC, Nathan P. **Rat thymic estrogen receptor; II--Physiological properties.** *J Steroid Biochem.* 1979;11: 1241-6. (English)

Specific, high affinity estrogen receptor has been shown to be present in the rat thymus. From *in vivo* and *in vitro* studies as well as competition assays, the receptor possesses specificity for estradiol and the estrogen-like compound diethylstilbestrol, but not for progesterone, testosterone, triamcinolone or cortisol. By sucrose gradient centrifugation studies the thymic estrogen receptor was shown to have a sedimentation value of 7-8s in low salt buffer. Castration resulted in a decrease in thymic estrogen receptor in terms of pmol/g tissue or fmol/mg soluble protein but no change in terms of pmol/mg DNA. Estradiol injection *in vivo* resulted in a rapid decrease of measurable cytoplasmic receptor by 2.5 min, which became undetectable by 20 min and returned to control values by 24 h. Autoradiographic studies show that the radioactive label is concentrated in single cells which may be of the reticulo-epithelial variety.

200

Helderman JH, Garovoy MR, Strom TB. **B-cell alloantigen matching by the lymphocyte insulin receptor assay.** *Transplant Proc.* 1981;13:1042-3. (English) (no abstract)

201

Helderman JH, Strom TB, Garovoy MR. **Rapid MLC testing by analysis of the insulin receptor on alloactivated T lymphocytes.** *J Clin Invest.* 1981;67:509-13. (English)

Responses in the mixed lymphocyte culture (MLC) are traditionally evaluated by measurement of DNA synthesis or blast transformation. However, these events occur too late in the MLC to permit prospective matching for cadaveric renal transplantation. Presentation of allogeneic cells to the T-lymphocyte within the MLC results in the emergence of an insulin receptor pharmacokinetically similar to that on other tissues such as fat, liver, and muscle. Intrafamilial MLC were studied by simultaneous assesment of DNA synthesis and insulin receptor binding. In 68 studies from seven families that provide examples of two haplotype identical matches, haplo-identical matches and total haplo- mismatches, the presence of an insulin receptor correlated in every case with a positive MLC as estimated by [^{3}H] thymidine incorporation. A quantitative relationship existed between the strength of the MLC and the amount of receptor binding. Based on analysis of cells from several families in which cross-over events were known to have occurred, the appearance of an insulin receptor always corresponded with a mismatch at the portion of histocompatibility leukocyte antigen (HLA) chromosome bearing the D region. Finally, it was demonstrated in each of 30 cultures that insulin receptor emergence occurred significantly before detectable DNA synthesis, as early as 24 h after the initiation of the MLC well within the time constraint limitations for renal preservation. Appearance of the insulin receptor on activated lymphocytes may be a more rapid measure of mixed lymphocyte responses, and should permit prospective matching for cadaveric renal transplantation.

202

Jacobs S, Cuatrecasas P. **Insulin receptor antibodies.** *Methods Enzymol.* 1981;74:471-8. (English)

Antibodies against insulin receptors occur spontaneously in some human and mouse autoimmune diseases, and have been produced in rabbits that have been immunized with purified rat insulin receptor. These antibodies have been useful in characterizing the structure, function, and regulation of insulin receptors and have also been used to purify insulin receptors. In this chapter we will describe methods for the purification of insulin receptors, for the production of anti-receptor antibodies, and for the detection of receptor antibodies in serum.

203

Jacobs S, Cuatrecasas P. **Insulin receptor: structure and function.** *Endocrinol Rev.* 1981;2:251-63. (English)

Insulin receptor has been purified by affinity chromatography and studied by affinity labeling techniques. It is composed of two types of subunits, alpha (molecular weight approximately 135,000) and beta (molecular weight approx-imately 90,000) which form a disulfide-linked heterotetramer (alpha-beta)$_2$. Both alpha and beta subunits are glycoproteins. Both are exposed on the outer surface of the membrane. Alpha is the subunit that is predominantly affinity labeled by insulin and is probably the insulin-binding subunit; however, beta may also comprise a portion of the insulin-binding site. Receptors for insulin-like growth factors have also been affinity labeled. A photoaffinity labeling derivative of basic soma-tomedin affinity labels a protein with a subunit structure very similar to the insulin receptor. In contrast, multiplication-stimulating activity is affinity cross-linked to a protein with an entirely different subunit structure. After binding to cell surface receptors, insulin, along with its receptor, is internalized by an endocytic process, which in some cells involves coated pits. The majority of internalized insulin is ultimately degraded in lysomsomes but may first go to Golgi, GERL, or other intracellular organelles. The majority of internalized receptor is recycled to the cell membrane, perhaps after mixing with a pool of intracellular receptors in the Golgi. Down-regulation may result from an increased rate of degradation of receptors or from a redistribution of receptors from the cell membrane to an intracellular pool. Several biological effects have recently been obtained by adding insulin to broken cell preparations. These include modulation of membrane protein phosphorylation, activation of pyruvate dehydrogenase and cAMP phosphodiesterase, and inhibition of Ca-ATPase. A low molecular weight, peptide-like substance that inhibits cAMP-dependent protein kinase and activates glycogen syn-thase and pyruvate dehydrogenase has been extracted from insulin-treated skeletal muscle and is released from adipocyte membranes by insulin treatment. A similar substance, which stimulates the synthesis of RNA in isolated nuclei, is produced by perfusing rat liver with insulin. It is possible that these substances are second messengers for insulin.

204

Lesniak MA, Gorden P, Roth J. **Reactivity of non-primate growth hormones and prolactins with human growth hormone receptors on cultured human lymphocytes.** *J Clin Endocrinol Metab.* 1977;44:838-99. (English)

Ovine placental lactogen is as reactive as human growth hormone with the human growth hormone receptor of cultured human (IM-9) lymphocytes, which confirms the findings of Carr and Friesen with receptors of human liver. We now also show that bovine and ovine growth hormones and ovine prolactin have reactivity for the human growth hormone receptor on IM-9 lymphocytes that is of the same order of magnitude (0.03%) as that previously reported for human placental lactogen. The binding studies predict that these non-primate hormones will have biological effects on skeletal growth in primates, either as agonists or antagonists. Previous studies have shown that when IM-9 lymphocytes are exposed to human growth hormone for 18 h at 37°C, there is a time- and concentration-dependent loss of human growth hormone receptors, and the magnitude of the loss of receptors after preincubation for 18 h at 37°C is greater than the average occupancy of receptors under steady state conditions for 90 min at 30°C. In the present study we show that human and ovine placental lactogens, ovine prolactin, and bovine and ovine growth hormones also produce this effect on the human growth hormone receptor. Since the cellular process by which a hormone induces loss of its own receptors appears to require binding of the hormone to its own receptor as well as one or more subsequent steps in hormone action, it is likely that all of the preparations that induce receptor loss will be shown to have some agonist activity of human growth hormone in promoting skeletal growth in primates. Further, these studies extend the interrelationships between primate and non-primate pituitary and placental hormones from what has been suggested previously from biological and structural studies.

205

Lesniak MA, Roth J. **Regulation of receptor concentration by homologous hormone. Effect of human growth hormone on its receptor in IM-9 lymphocytes.** *J Biol Chem.* 1976;251:3720-9. (English)

When cultured human lymphocytes of the IM-9 line were exposed to human growth hormone (hGH) at 37°C, washed for 2 hours, and incubated with $_{125}$I-hGH , the binding of $_{125}$I-hGH was reduced. The magnitude of the reduction in binding was dependent on the concentration of growth hormone present as well as the duration of the exposure. As little as 2×10^{-10}M (5.0 ng/ml), which is a low resting concentration of hormone *in vivo* and occupies about 20% of the receptors at steady state at 30°C, produced a 50% reduction in binding while 20 ng/ml, which occupies about 50% of the receptors under steady state conditions, produced an 80% loss of receptors. Further increases in growth hormone concentration produced little further effect on receptor loss. Thus, the loss of receptors at a given concentration of growth hormone (up to 20 ng/ml) in the preincubation at 37°C was greater than the occupancy produced by that concentration of growth hormone receptors under steady state conditions at 30°C. Analysis of the data indicated that the decrease in binding of ^{125}I-hGH was due to a loss of receptors per cell without any change in affinity of receptor for hormone or in cell number. The concentration of insulin receptors on these cells was affected by the insulin concentration in the medium, and the concentration of growth hormone receptors was affected by growth hormone, but neither hormone had any effect on the heterologous receptors. Exposure of the cells to cycloheximide (0.1 mM) produced a progressive but smaller loss of growth hormone receptors, and the effect of cycloheximide was additive to the receptor loss induced by growth hormone, suggesting that cycloheximide inhibited synthesis of receptors while growth hormone accelerated loss of receptors. When growth hormone was removed from the medium, receptor concentrations were restored rapidly; half of the loss was restored by 6 to 8 hours and the full complement of receptors was restored by 24 hours following removal of the hormone. If the growth hormone was removed and replaced with cycloheximide, the return of the receptors was delayed until the cycloheximide was removed. Thus restoration of the receptors appeared to require the synthesis of new proteins. These data indicate that in the IM-9 lymphocytes the concentration of growth hormone receptors is very sensitive to regulation by growth hormone and also add further support to the suggestion that hormones in general actively regulate the concentration of their own receptors.

206

Mehta RG, Fricks CM, Moon RC. **Androgen receptors in chemically-induced colon carcinogenesis.** *Cancer.* 1980; 45:1085-9. (English)

Cytoplasmic extracts (105,000 x g supernatants) prepared from the colon of 1,2-dimethylhydrazine hydrochloride (DMH) treated male BD-IX rats bound ^{3}H-5-alpha-dihydrotestosterone (DHT) with high affinity ($K_d = 3 \times 10^{-9}$M) and low capacity (n = 20 fmoles/mg protein). Unoccupied saturable binding sites were not detected in normal intact colon but were observed in colons from gonadectomized rats. DHT receptors were present in both the ascending and descending segments of the colon. The DHT binding components sedimented as 7-8S species on linear sucrose density gradients and were effectively displaced by cyproterone acetate, but not by progesterone. Forty percent of the DMH-induced colon tumors also bond DHT with high affinity and limited capacity. These results suggest that the sex steroids are involved in carcinogen-induced colon tumorigenesis, and the action is mediated by their association with sex steroid-specific receptors.

207

Neifeld JP, Lippman ME, Tonney DC. **Steroid hormone receptors in normal human lymphocytes: Induction of glucocorticoid receptor activity by phytohemagglutinin.** *J Biol Chem.* 1977;252:2972-7. (English)

The presence of specific steroid hormone receptors in human lymphocytes was investigated in unstimulated and phytohemagglutinin-stimulated glass wool column-purified peripheral blood lymphocytes. Specific steroid binding in intact cells was determined by a whole cell competitive binding assay. Non-phytohemagglutinin-stimulated lymphocytes had about 2700 specific glucocorticoid binding sites per cell; phytohemagglutinin stimulation induced a 2- to 3-fold increase in glucocorticoid receptor activity within 16 h of culture. No estrogen, androgen, or progestin binding sites were detected in either unstimulated or phytohemagglutinin-stimulated peripheral blood lymphocytes. Scatchard analysis of glucocorticoid binding was consistent with a single class of receptor sites with a dissociation constant (K_d) of about 5.5×10^{-9}M (correlation coefficient r = -0.96). Significant competition for radiolabeled dexamethasone binding was not observed with steroids lacking glucocorticoid activity. There was good agreement between relative binding affinities of various steroids to glucocorticoid receptor in lymphocytes and ability of these steroids to inhibit phytohemagglutinin-stimulated thymidine incorporation.

208

Segal J, Ingbar SH. **Specific binding sites for the triiodothyronine in the plasma membrane of rat thymocytes. Correlation with biochemical responses.** *J Clin Invest.* 1977;252:2972-7. (English) (unavailable at publication)

209

Werb Z, Foley R, Munck A. **Interaction of glucocorticoids with macrophages: identification of glucocorticoid receptors in monocytes and macrophages.** *J Exp Med.* 1978;147:1684-94. (English)

Glucocorticoid binding was measured in resident and thiogly-collate-elicited mouse peritoneal macrophages, rabbit alveolar macrophages, and human monocytes. Two assays of binding were used--an assay with intact cells in suspension or monolayers, and an assay of cytosol and nuclear forms of glucocorticoid receptors. The mononuclear phagocytes contained approx. $4-10 \times 10^3$ high affinity receptor sites per cell, with dissociation constants of approx. 2-8 nM dexamethasone. The binding to the saturable sites was specific for steroids with glucocorticoid or antiglucocorticoid activity. Cortisol, corticosterone, and progesterone competed with dexamethasone for binding, whereas estradiol, dihydrotestosterone and 11-epicortisol competed very little. Binding of dexamethasone to cytosol and nuclear forms of the receptor complex and temperature-sensitive translocation of cytosol forms to nuclear forms were shown. At 37°C the predominant form of the hormone-receptor complex was nuclear. These results demonstrate that corticosteroids interact with macrophages at physiological concentrations.

Neuropeptides

210

Anisimov VN, Morozov VG, Khavinson VK. **Increase of the life span and decrease in the tumor incidence in C3H/Sn mice as affected by thymus and epiphysis polypeptide factors.** *Dokl Akad Nauk SSSR.* 1982;263:742-5. (Russian) (unavailable at publication)

211

Bertagna SY, Nicholson WE, Sorenson GD, Pettengill OS, Mount CD, Orth DN. **Corticotropin, lipotropin, and beta-endorphin production by a human nonpituitary tumor in culture: evidence for a common precursor.** *Proc Natl Acad Sci.* 1978;75:5160-4. (English) (unavailable at publication)

212

Chang KJ, Cuatrecasas P. **Heterogeneity and properties of opiate receptors.** *Fed Proc.* 1981;40:2729-34. (English) (no abstract)

213

Chang KJ, Hazum E, Killian A, Cuatrecasas P. **Interactions of ligands with morphine and enkephalin receptors are differentially affected by guanine nucleotide.** *Mol Pharmacol.* 1981;20:1-7. (English)

The effects of cations and GTP on morphine (mu) and enkephalin (delta) receptors were examined by using binding assays of [^{3}H] naloxone to rat brain membrane preparations and [^{3}H] diprenorphine or [^{3}H] naloxone to neuroblastoma cell membranes. The potencies and Hill coefficients (n) of many opiate agonists and opioid peptides in competing with the binding of the labeled antagonist are reduced by Na$^+$ (100 mM) and GTP (0.1 mM). These effects are qualitatively similar for both subtypes of opiate receptors. However, quantitatively, the effects of GTP are much more profound for morphine receptors than for enkephalin receptors and the effects of Na$^+$ are dependent upon the type of labeled antagonist used rather than upon receptor type. Na$^+$ does not alter the affinity of opiate antagonists. GTP reduces the affinity of naloxone to morphine-binding sites by a factor of 2.5. Mg^{2+}

(5mM) increases the potency of opiate agonists and enkephalins for both receptor sites. The combination of Na$^+$, GTP, and Mg^{2+} further reduces the affinity of enkephalins and opiate agonists for enkephalin-binding sites and the affinity of Met- and Leu-enkephalin for morphine-binding sites. However, the combination of Na$^+$, GTP, and Mg^{2+} partially restores the affinity of [D-Ala^2, Leu^5]- and [D-Ala^2, D-Leu^5]enkephalin and morphine for the morphine-binding sites. These differential effects of cations and nucleotide further emphasize the differences that exist between morphine and enkephalin receptors and indicate the complex interactions of cations and nucleotides with opiate-binding sites.

214

Gilman SC, Schwartz JM, Milner RJ, Bloom FE, Feldman JD. **Beta-endorphin enhances lymphocyte proliferative responses.** *Proc Natl Acad Sci.* 1982;79:4226-30. (English)

The opioid peptides alpha- and beta-endorphin and [D-Ala^2, Met^5] enkephalin were investigated for their effect on the proliferation of resting and activated rat splenic lymphocytes *in vitro*. Beta-endorphin enhanced the proliferative response of spleen cells to the T cell mitogens concanavalin A and phytohemagglutinin. The effect of beta-endorphin was dose-dependent and occurred at peptide concentrations similar to those found in rat plasma. Alpha-endorphin and [D-Ala^2, Met^5] enkephalin did not affect the proliferative responses to any mitogen tested. Furthermore, the potentiating effect of beta-endorphin was not reversed by treatment with 10 microM naloxone. None of the peptides had any effect on resting, unstimulated spleen cells or on the response to a mixture of lipopolysaccharide and dextran sulfate, which is specifically mitogenic for B lymphocytes. The pharmacologic properties of the beta-endorphin potentiation indicate that the effect may be mediated by a nonopiate but beta-endorphin-specific mechanism. These results suggest a possible role for peripheral beta-endorphin and may provide a link between stress and disease susceptibility.

215

Hazum E, Chang KJ, Cuatrecasas P. **Cluster formation of opiate (enkephalin) receptors in neuroblastoma cells: differences between agonists and antagonists and possible relationships to biological functions.** *Proc Natl Acad Sci.* 1980;77:3038-41. (English)

Neuroblastoma cells were used to study the surface distribution and organization of opiate (enkephalin) receptors and the possible relevance of changes in these variables to biological functions. Opiate receptors readily form clusters that are visible by image-intensifier fluorescent microscopy and are localized on both the cell body and processes. These clusters do not become internalized even during prolonged incubation periods. The receptors appear to pre-exist largely in a diffuse state, with only a very small number pre-existing as clusters. The clusters are induced within 1 hour and they are stable for prolonged (7-9hr) periods, even after removal of the receptor-bound ligand. Agonists and antagonists are both equally capable of inducing receptor clustering. However, the clusters induced by agonists are different from those induced by antagonists; the former can be dispersed by treatment with dithiothreitol. This dispersion requires removal of the receptor-bound agonist, indicating that the hormone protects or stabilizes disulfide bonds which are critical for maintenance of the clustered state. Pretreatment of cells with sulfhydryl-blocking reagents (iodoacetate, iodoacetamide, and N-ethylmaleimide) prevents cluster formation but does not alter the ability of agonists to inhibit adenylate cyclase [ATP pyrophosphate-lyase (cyclizing), EC 4.6.1.1] activity. Neither the number nor the affinity of binding sites is altered by pretreatment with opiates. These studies suggest that at least the acute, immediate biological effects of opiates and enkephalins occur prior to and are independent of the formation of gross receptor clusters. The possible relationship of cluster formation to the actions of opiates remains to be determined.

216

Hazum E, Chang KJ, Cuatrecasas P. **Role of disulphide and sulphydryl groups in clustering of enkephalin receptors in neuroblastoma cells.** *Nature.* 1979;282:626-8. (English)

Image intensified fluorescence microscopy has been very useful in visualising the patterns and mobility of receptors for epidermal growth factor (EGF), insulin and alpha$_2$-macroglobulin in intact cells. Recently we have synthesised a bioactive derivative of enkephalin, Tyr-D-Ala-Gly-Phe-Leu-Lys-rhodamine, and used it for the microscopic visualisation and localisation of opiate (enkephalin) receptors in neuroblastoma cells. In contrast to the case of polypeptide hormones, where fluorescently labelled receptors are initially distributed uniformly and quickly form patches which are subsequently internalized, the enkephalin-labelled receptor patches in neuroblastoma cells appear only slowly and are not internalised. Sulphydryl groups are involved in the binding of opiates to brain membranes and may affect differentially the binding of agonists and antagonists. Also, sulphydryl and disulphide groups are involved in the binding sites of adrenergic, cholinergic and muscarinic receptors. These observations prompted us to examine the effects of disulphide and sulphydryl reagents on the clustering of opiate (enkephalin) receptors in N4TG1 neuroblastoma cells. We report here that in these cells there are reactive sulphydryl and disulphide groups which are essential for cluster formation (but not binding), and that a sulphydryl-disulphide exchange reaction may be involved in this process. In addition, the sulphydryl reagents seem to dissociate the two steps of binding and cluster formation, and thus provide a tool for studying the pharmacological importance of receptor clustering.

217

Hazum E, Chang KJ, Cuatrecasas P. **Specific nonopiate receptors for beta-endorphin.** *Science.* 1979;205:1033-5. (English)

Iodinated beta H$_2$-D-alanineendorphin exhibits specific binding to cultured human lymphocytes. The binding is inhibited by low concentrations of beta-endorphin and its D-analine derivative, but is not affected by opiate agonists and antagonists, or by enkephalin analogs, beta-lipotropin, adrenocorticotrophic hormone, or alpha-melanocyte-stimulating hormone; this suggests the existence of a specific, non-opiate binding site (receptor) for beta-endorphin. The carboxy-terminal region of beta-endorphin is essential for this binding

activity, since alpha-endorphin is not active. Beta-endorphin may be a circulating hormone with peripheral physiological effects that are not primarily mediated through interactions with opiate or enkephalin receptors.

218

Hinterberger W, Cerny C, Kinast H, Pointer H, Trag KH. **Somatostatin reduces the release of colony-stimulating activity (CSA) from PHA-activated mouse spleen lymphocytes.** *Experientia.* 1977;34:860-2. (German)

PHA-activated lymphocytes release colony-stimulating activity (CSA) for macrophage-granulocyte precursor cells (colony forming units, CFU$_c$) in the culture medium. Somatostatin, known to interfere with ribosomal protein synthesis, was demonstrated to reduce the release of CSA from PHA-treated mouse spleen lymphocytes.

219

Lazarus LH, Perrin MH, Brown MR, Rivier JE. **Mast cell binding of neurotensin; II--Molecular conformation of neurotensin involved in the stereospecific binding to mast cell receptor sites.** *J Biol Chem.* 1977;252:7180-3. (English)

Systematic substitution of the natural L-amino acids in neurotensin by their D isomers reveals that the COOH-terminal portion of this tridecapeptide is required for binding to mast cell receptors: D-amino acid replacements from Pro[10] through Leu[13] substantially decrease that binding. Either blockage of the COOH-terminal carboxyl group as with N-methylamidation, or formation of a cyclic structure by the inclusion of a disulfide bond, a Cys[2,13], markedly reduces the specific binding to mast cell receptor sites. Modifications in the NH$_2$-terminal portion of neurotensin do not affect the binding to mast cells. However, D-Arg[8] and D-Arg[9] substitutions increase binding by factors of 5- to 6-fold. The hydroxyl group at position 3 or 11 is not essential for binding since Phe[3] or Phe[11] is equivalent to Tyr[3] or Tyr[11]. The COOH-terminal penta- and hexapeptides are able to displace approximately 70% ^{125}I-neurotensin relative to the intact peptide. Of 18 other biologically active peptides tested, only xenopsin, a naturally occurring COOH-terminal analog of neurotensin, and bradykinin effectively compete in the binding assay to an extent of 60 and 100%, respectively. Histamine, diphenhydramine, and noradrenaline are ineffective in this regard.

220

Miller GC, Murgo AJ, Plotnikoff NP. **The influence of leucine and methionine enkephalin on immune mechanisms.** *Int J Immunopharmacol.* 1982;4:366-7. (English)

Leucine (leu) and methionine (met) enkephalin (enk) at concentrations ranging from 10^{-2} to 10^{-20} mg/ml influence neutrophil chemiluminescence and the activity of T lymphocytes as measured by "active" T cell rosettes, but have no significant influence on phytohemagglutinin, pokeweed and concanavalin A stimulated lymphocyte transformation on cells from healthy controls and cancer patients. The observed responses were increased, decreased or of no significant effect depending on the enkephalin, its concentration and the individual subject. The observed decreased responses for chemiluminescence and "active" T cell rosette percentages were similar for the control and cancer group; however, the observed increased activity for chemiluminescence was only demonstrated in cells from the cancer patients while increased percentages of "active" T cell rosettes were apparent in both groups.

221

Moody TW, Pert CB, Gazdar AF, Carney DN, Minna JD. **High levels of intracellular bombesin characterize human small-cell lung carcinoma.** *Science.* 1981;214:1246-8. (English)

"Small cells" or "oat cells" characterize a virulent form of lung cancer and share many biochemical properties with peptide-secreting neurones. The neuropeptide bombesin is present in all small-cell lines examined, but not in other lung cancer cell lines, suggesting that bombesinergic precursor cells in lung may give rise to this disease.

222

Pierpaoli W, Maestroni GJ. **Pharmacologic control of the hormonally modulated immune response; II--Blockade of antibody production by a combination of drugs acting on neuroendocrine function--its prevention by gonadotropins and corticotropin.** *Immunol.* 1978;34:419-30. (English)

Injection of a combination of three drugs, 5-hydroxy-tryptophan, the alpha-blocker phentolamine and the neuroleptic drug haloperidol into mice before or together with sheep red blood cells (SRBC) induces a complete and long-lasting inhibition of antibody production to SRBC and leads to specific unresponsiveness. The mice unresponsive to SRBC respond normally to another antigen. Treatment with a combination of luteotropic (LH), follicle stimulating (FSH) and corticotropic hormone (ACTH) before administration of drugs and antigen prevents the immune blockade. Injection of SRBC induces an early elevation of LH in blood. This effect is prevented by previous administration of the three drugs in combination. The hormonal response to a second injection of the same antigen of mice previously made "unresponsive" is different from that of immunized animals. The suppression of these hormonal changes which follow antigen injection by drugs acting on neuroendocrine regulation and cell membrane adrenergic receptors represents a step forward in efforts aimed at a pharmacological control of acquired immunity.

223

Plotnikoff NP, Miller GC, Murgo AJ. **Enkephalins-endorphins: immunomodulators in mice.** *Int J Immunopharmacol.* 1982;4:366-7. (English)

Continuing studies in BDF_1 mice inoculated with concentrations of L1210 leukemia cells ranging from 1 x 10^2 to 1 x 10^4 with varying treatment concentrations of leucine (leu) and methionine (met) enkephalin (enk) indicate that the enkephalins can alter the rate of mortality when compared to untreated controls. The *in vivo* studies appear to correlate to *in vitro* findings in which phytohemagglutinin-stimulated lymphocyte transformation is also affected by leu-enk and met-enk. Other enkephalins-endorphins studied include beta-endorphin as well as the synthetic enkephalin derivative FK33,438. The

enkephalin-endorphin antagonist naloxone also modifies the rate of mortality of mice inoculated with the L1210 leukemia cells. These studies suggest that the enkephalins are endogenous immunomodulators.

224

Plotnikoff NP. **The central nervous system control of the immune system. Enkephalins: antitumor activities** (abstract). *Ann Mtg Am Coll Neuropsychopharmacol.* San Diego, Dec. 1981. P. 67. (English)

225

Poupland A, Bottazzo GF, Doniach D, Roitt IV. **Binding of human immunoglobulins in pituitary adrenocorticotropin hormone cells.** *Nature.* 1976;261:142-4. (English) (no abstract)

226

Pullan PT, Clement-Jones V, Corder R, Lowry PJ, Rees GM, Rees LH, Besser GM, Macedo MM, Galvao-Teles A. **Ectopic production of methionine enkephalin and beta-endorphin.** *Brit Med J.* 1980;280:758-9. (English)

Immunoreactive methionine enkephalin and beta-endorphin were sought by serial dilution of tissue extracts and assay of chromatographic fractions in non-endocrine tumour tissue from three patients with the ectopic adrenocorticotropin syndrome associated with carcinoid tumours and in normal lung tissue and thymic tissue from a patient with myasthenia gravis. In all cases serial dilution of extracts showed parallelism to standard radioimmunoassay curves. The two peptides were found in high concentration in the three tumours but were undetectable in the control tissues. In a single case tested, the methionine enkephalin concentration in a vein draining the tumour was twice that in a peripheral vein. In view of their profound effects on behaviour in animals and potent analgesic activity in animals and man the ectopic secretion of methionine enkephalin and beta-endorphin may modify the clinical features of a wide variety of tumours and produce some of the diverse clinical syndromes associated with malignancy.

227

Roberts NJ Jr. **ACTH production by leukocytes** (letter). *N Engl J Med.* 1982;306:1296. (English)

228

Smith EM, Blalock JE. **Human lymphocyte production of corticotropin and endorphin-like substances: association with leukocyte interferon.** *Proc Natl Acad Sci.* 1981;78:7530-4. (English)

Human leukocyte interferon (HIFN-alpha) preparations contain immunologically and biologically recognizable endorphin and corticotrophin-like (ACTH-like) activities. The ACTH bioactivity was demonstrable only after pepsin or acid treatment. Highly purified HIFN-alpha was composed of two molecular species of interferon (18,500 and 23,000 daltons). Endorphin activity was associated with both of these molecules. Pepsin treatment of the 23,000-dalton but not the 18,500-dalton HIFN-alpha generated ACTH activity. In acid, the 23,000-dalton HIFN-alpha broke down into the

18,500-dalton form and ACTH (4500 daltons). The ACTH derived from HIFN-alpha by pepsin digestion comigrated with a purified ACTH standard in NADODSO$_4$/polacrylamide gel electrophoresis. HIFN-alpha-producing lymphocytes showed positive immunofluorescence after staining with highly specific antisera to ACTH alpha- and gamma-endorphin. Essentially 100% of the human peripheral lymphocytes were capable of producing both ACTH and gamma-endorphin-related substances, presumably associated with HIFN-alpha. These results strongly suggest a circuit between the immune and neuroendocrine systems which involves neuroendocrine hormone-like substances, some of which are associated with HIFN-alpha.

229
Snyder SH, Childers SR. **Opiate receptors and opioid peptides.** *Annu Rev Neurosci.* 1979;2:35-64. (English) (no abstract)

230
Theoharides TC, Douglas WW. **Somatostatin induces histamine secretion from rat peritoneal mast cells.** *Endocrinology.* 1978;102:1637-40. (English)

Cyclic somatostatin strongly stimulated secretion of histamine from rat peritoneal mast cells. The energy, temperature and calcium dependence of this effect indicate that the action of somatostatin on the mast cells is similar to that of the classic mast cell secretagogue compound 48/80 and is to induce exocytosis.

231
Wagner H, Hengst K, Zierden E, Gerlach U. **Investigations of the antiproliferative effect of somatostatin in man and rats.** *Clin Exp Metab.* 1979;27:1381-6. (English)

Growth-hormone-release-inhibiting hormone (SRIF; somatostatin) is a potent inhibitor of the secretion of several hormones on the pituitary and the pancreas. Recently, we have shown that somatostatin inhibits endotoxin-induced leukocytosis in man. The present studies were carried out to investigate further effects of somatostatin on the hemopoietic system as well as on mesenchymal cells in man and rats.

232
Wybran J, Appelboom T, Famacy J-P, Govaerts A. **Suggestive evidence for receptors for morphine and methionine-enkephalin on normal human blood T-lymphocytes.** *J Immunol.* 1979;123:1068-70. (English)

This study reports the *in vitro* influence of morphine, dextromoramide, levomoramide, and methionine-enkephalin upon normal human T blood lymphocytes by using the active and total rosette tests. Morphine and dextromoramide inhibited the percentage of active T rosettes. This effect was completely reversed in the presence of naloxone, their specific antagonist. The specificity was further demonstrated by the absence of the effect of levomoramide, the inactive enantiomere, upon the rosette system. Methionine-enkephalin increased the percentage of active T rosettes. This effect was specifically inhibited by naloxone. These observations suggest that normal human blood T lymphocytes bear surface receptor-like structures for morphine, dextromoramide, and methionine-enkephalin. Such findings may provide a link between the central nervous system and the immune system.

233
Zozulia AA, Patsakova EK, Kost NV. **Reaction between endogenous opiates and human peripheral blood lymphocytes.** *Zh Nevropatol Psikhiatr.* 1982;82:60-3. (Russian)

The radioreceptor method and determination of the content of cAMP in lymphocytes were used to study the interplay of met-enkephalin with human peripheral blood lymphocytes. The characteristics of specific binding of endogenous opiate with the cells, as well as a decrease in the activity of lymphocyte adenylate cyclase observed under the effect of met-enkephalin proved the presence of a specific interplay between the physiological concentrations of the opiate with lymphocytes. It is suggested that it is determined by the existence of two parallel mechanisms: a process having some features in common with the receptor binding and limited transport of the opiate inside the cell.

234
Zozulia AA, Patsakova EK, Kost NV. **Reaction between methionine enkephalin and human lymphocytes.** Vestn *Akad Med Nauk SSSR.* 1982;1:28-32. (Russian)

The interaction of methionine enkephalin with lymphocytes of human peripheral blood was studied by the radioreceptor method and by determining the activity of adenylate cyclase (from the level of cAMP in lymphocytes). ^{3}H-methenkephalin was found to be specifically bound by the cells and the adenylate cylcase activity was shown to be reduced by the action of this endogenous opiate. It is suggested that the interaction of methenkephalin with the cells under study is due to the existence of two mechanisms, one of which has properties of receptor interaction and the other involves limited transport of the opiate into the interior of the cells.

Neuropharmacologic influences on immune function

Neurotransmitters

235
Askenase PW, Bursztajn S, Gershon MD, Gershon RK. **T cell-dependent mast cell degranulation and release of serotonin in murine delayed-type hypersensitivity.** *J Exp Med.* 1980;152:1358-74. (English)

We have previously suggested that the release of serotonin (5-hydroxytryptamine) (5-HT) by local tissue mast cells is required for the elicitation of delayed-type hypersensitivity (DTH) in mice. In the current study, light microscopic radioautographs from animals treated with [^{3}]5-HT indicated that local mast cells released 5-HT between 6 and 18 h during the evolution of DTH. Ultrastructural examination of mast cells revealed surface activation, indicated by extension of surface filopodia, and degranulation by fusion and exocytosis. Light and electron microscopic studies of the endothelium of postcapillary venules at sites of DTH revealed the development of gaps between adjacent cells. The development of gaps permitted extravasation of tracers that was abolished by depletion or antagonism of 5-HT. Thus mast cells degranulated and released 5-HT in DTH, and this 5-HT acted on local vessels. Recipients of nonadherent, non-immunoglobulin-bearing sensitized lymphocytes also demonstrated similar mast cell degranulation and the formation of endothelial gaps. This indicated that mast cell degranulation and 5-HT release in murine DTH were probably T cell dependent.

236
Askenase PW, Schwartz A, Siegel JN, Gershon RK. **Role of histamine in the regulation of cell-mediated immunity.** *Int Arch Allergy Appl Immunol.* 1981;66:225-33. (English) (no abstract)

237
Barnes P, FitzGerald G, Brown M, Dollery C. **Nocturnal asthma and changes in circulating epinephrine, histamine and cortisol.** *N Engl J Med.* 1980;303:263-7. (English) (no abstract)

238
Borresen T, Palmgren N, Christensen NJ. **Absence of catecholamines in malignant tumors.** *Eur J Cancer.* 1980;16:123-5. (English)

Noradrenaline and adrenaline concentrations were measured in tissue specimens of malignant and non-malignant tumors as well as in adjacent normal tissue. Tissue specimens were obtained immediately after surgical excision. Noradrenaline and adrenaline were nearly absent from all malignant tumors examined. In specimens from 7 tumors from 6 different organs mean noradrenaline concentration averaged 1.7% of normal values. Several cases of leiomyoma of uterus examined similarly contained very small amounts of noradrenaline while other benign lesions such as serous cystadenoma of the ovary, hyperplasia of the prostate gland and fibroadenoma of the breast contained approximately normal amounts of noradrenaline. The very low noradrenaline concentrations in malignant and in some non-malignant tumors indicate, in all probability, lack of sympathetic innervation.

239
Crary B, Borysenko M, Borysenko J, Benson H. **Release of granular lymphocytes into peripheral blood after epinephrine administration in humans: correlation with T_G lymphocytes and suppression of mitogen-responsiveness** (abstract). *Fed Proc, Fed Am Soc Exp Biol.* 1982; 41:591. (English)

A single subcutaneous injection of 0.2 mg epinephrine causes a transient lymphocytosis in peripheral blood. Wright-Giemsa stained slides reveal that within 15 min after injection, granular lymphocytes increase 4-fold, while non-granular lymphocytes increase 2-fold; levels of both cell types return to baseline by 2 hrs. Rosette assays reveal that numbers of T_G lymphocytes fluctuate in parallel with granular lymphocytes (correlation coefficient, r = 0.97). The proliferative response to pokeweed mitogen and phytohemagglutinin by mononuclear cells (MNC) is greatly suppressed for up to one hour after

epinephrine. The degree of suppression is highly correlated with the percentage of T_G cells present. Removal of adherent monocytes does not abrogate suppression. MNC from epinephrine-treated subjects are able to suppress the mitogen-induced proliferation of untreated allogeneic lymphocytes. Treatment of normal MNC for 2 hr or 18 hr *in vitro* with various concentrations of epinephrine has no effect on subsequent proliferation in response to mitogens. These data support previous studies by others indicating that T_G lymphocytes are granular lymphocytes and further suggest that epinephrine causes a transient alteration of immune homeostasis by inducing the release of activated suppressor cells into the peripheral circulation.

240
Crary B, Borysenko M, Sutherland DC, Kutz I, Borysenko J, Benson H. **Decrease in mitogen responsiveness of mononuclear cells from peripheral blood after epinephrine administration in humans.** *J Immunol.* 1983;130:694-7. (English)

A single subcutaneous injection of 0.2 mg epinephrine into healthy human subjects caused a transient lymphocytosis in peripheral blood. Mononuclear cells (MNC), isolated at various times after epinephrine administration, were cultured in the presence of mitogens. The blastogenic responses to pokeweed mitogen (PWM) and phytohemagglutinin (PHA) were significantly reduced for up to 60 min post-epinephrine ($p<0.05$); the response to concanavalin A (Con A) was reduced in the 15 min samples only. All responses returned to pre-injection levels by 120 min post-injection. Removal of adherent monocytes from MNC isolates prior to culture did not restore normal mitogen responsiveness. When MNC were cultured in the absence of mitogens there was no difference in survival between pre- and post-epinephrine samples. Incubation of untreated MNC for 2 hr or 18 hr *in vitro* with various concentrations of epinephrine (10^{-5} to 10^{-1} mg/ml) had no effect upon the subsequent blastogenic response to mitogens. Other workers have reported that epinephrine administration causes alterations in the composition of the circulating lymphocyte pool. Taken together, these data suggest that the reduction in mitogen responsivenesss after epinephrine is the result of changes in the distribution of lymphocyte subclasses in peripheral blood.

241
Depelchin A, Letesson JJ. **Adrenaline influence on the immune response; II--Its effects through action on the suppressor T-cells.** *Immunol Lett.* 1981;3:207-13. (English)

Experiments were carried out to specify the adrenaline target among the immunocompetent cells. Adrenaline administered for some hours exerted opposite effects on the natural PFC and RFC: the first were enhanced and the second significantly reduced. These paradoxical results were intrepreted as a consequence of the inhibition of the suppressor T-cells in the resting status. Adrenaline appeared to act on the sensitive cells through beta- rather than through alpha-receptors. Further experiments on the adrenaline influence on the syngeneic barrier phenomenon and on the cellular balance at its termination seemed to indicate that adrenaline was directly inhibitory for the T_S but not for their precursors. These results are discussed in the light of the cellular networks regulating the immune response.

242

Depelchin A, Letesson JJ. **Adrenaline influence on the immune response; I--Accelerating or suppressor effects according to the time of application.** *Immunol Lett.* 1981;3:199-205. (English)

The intervention of adrenaline in the immunoregulation was investigated through the modification of the anti-SRBC PFC response of mice after its i.p. administration (4 micrograms) at various intervals before SRBC antigen. When the interval was less than 24 h, adrenaline accelerated the immune kinetics. This modification was apparent on both direct and indirect PFC, as well as on naive and immune mice. However, mice treated from 2 days showed a suppression of the response. The adrenaline effect subsisted on the adoptive response of spleen cells drug-treated either *in vivo* or *in vitro*. The mitogenic response after *in vitro* PHA or LPS stimulation of spleen cells from adrenaline-treated mice indicated that the T-cells were the drug target. The physiological role of the adrenaline and immunological influences of acute stress are discussed in the paper.

243

Devoino LV, Eliseeva LS, Eremina O, Idova GV, Cheido MA. **5-hydroxytryptophan effect on the development of the immune response: IgM and IgG antibodies and rosette formation in primary and secondary responses.** *Eur J Immunol.* 1976;5:394-9. (English)

In animals immunized with bovine serum albumin, 5-hydroxytryptophan prolonged the latent period of the IgM and IgG primary responses, decreased response intensity, delayed the response peak and suppressed IgG immunological memory. In 5-hydroxytryptophan-treated mice, the number of rosette-forming cells (RFC) in the lymph node and spleen decreased during the primary and secondary responses. This effect was due to the decreased number of IgG RFC and to the later involvement of IgM RFC in the immune response. The absence of the secondary response was related to unprimed IgG memory cells. 5-hydroxytryptophan does not inhibit the primary and secondary responses after the connections between the hypothalamus and pituitary have been disrupted. The participation of the N raphe-hypothalamic-pituitary system in immuno-regulation and the putative mechanism underlying serotonin effect on the immune response are discussed.

244

Devoino LV, Morozova NB. **Nonspecific suppressor cells in the inhibiting action of serotonin on immunogenesis.** *Dokl Akad Nauk SSSR.* 1981;256:506-9. (Russian) (unavailable at publication)

245

Devoino LV, Morozova NB. **Participation of suppressor cells in the depressing action of serotonin on immunogenesis.** *Zh Mikrobiol Epidemiol Immunobiol.* 1979;5:60-4. (Russian)
The transfer of 20 x 10^6 T and B cells of lymphoid organs from donors immunized with sheep erythrocytes and having elevated serotonin level to recipients immunized with SRBC decreased the intensity of immune response (rosette formation and direct plaque formation). The elevation of serotonin level in the donors induced the appearance of T and B suppressors in the thymus and the bone marrow respectively and increased the population of T and B suppressors in the spleen and, to a lesser extent, in lymph nodes.

246

Eliseeva LS, Stefanovich LE. **Specific binding of serotonin by blood leukocytes and peritoneal cells in the mouse.** *Biokhimiia.* 1982;47:810-3. (Russian)

It was shown that blood leukocytes and peritoneal cells of mice specifically bind serotonin (5-hydroxytryptamine) in amounts which exceed manifold its binding by the cells of thymus, lymphatic nodes, spleen, Peyer's patches and bone marrow. The nature of this binding suggests that peritoneal cells and blood leukocytes contain cell populations (apart from those already known) capable of binding and trapping of serotonin.

247

Engel EK, Trotter JL, MacFarlin DE, McIntosh CL. **Thymic epithelial cell contains acetylcholine receptor** (letter). *Lancet.* 1977;1:1310-1. (English)

248

Fedorova NV, Golikov PP, Ershova NV, Golikov AP, Syromiatnikova ED. **Changes in the indices of blast transformation reactions of the peripheral blood lymphocytes and in the level of 11-hydrocorticosteroids, serotonin and histamine in acute myocardial infarct.** *Klin Med.* 1982;60:43-5. (Russian) (unavailable at publication)

249

Foon KA, Wahl SM, Oppenheim JJ, Rosenstreich DL. **Serotonin-induced production of a monocyte chemotactic factor by human peripheral blood leukocytes.** *J Immunol.* 1976;117:1545-52. (English)

Serotonin and histamine are released during the early phase of inflammatory reactions. To determine if these vasoactive amines might play a role in the cell-mediated phase of inflammation, studies were undertaken to assess their influence on some immunologic functions of human peripheral blood leukocytes (PBL). PBL were cultured with serotonin or histamine, and assayed for a proliferative response and their cell-free supernatants were assayed for the presence of a mediator with chemotactic activity for monocytes. When serotonin was cultured with PBL factors chemotactic for monocytes as well as polymorphonuclear leukocytes were produced in the absence of a proliferative response. Production of the factor chemotactic for monocytes was specifically blocked by methysergide, a serotonin antagonist and nonspecifically blocked by cycloheximide which interferes with leukocyte protein synthesis. Some decarboxylated precursors of serotonin also induced the monocyte chemotactic factor. This serotonin-induced chemotactic factor was demonstrated to be a product of mononuclear cells, and the majority of chemotactic activity was physicochemically similar to the previously characterized lymphocyte-derived chemotactic factor, suggesting that this factor is a lymphocyte product. In contrast to serotonin, histamine did not stimulate the production of monocyte chemotactic factor, nor did it induce proliferation. However, when 10^{-5}M histamine was added to a substimulatory concentration of serotonin (10^{-5}M), chemotactic activity comparable to or greater than the peak activity of serotonin alone was measured. This synergistic effect between serotonin and histamine suggests that the combination of these two amines may contribute to the induction of monocyte exudation in inflammatory reactions.

250
Fujiwara H. **Effect of chemical mediators (histamine, bradykinin, serotonin and acetylcholine) on antigen- or mitogen-induced lymphocyte activation (author's translation)** *Arerugi.* 1982;31:29-37. (Japanese) (no English abstract)

251
Ganguly P, Fossett NG. **Induction of serotonin secretion by cross-linking of surface receptors of a derivative of wheat germ agglutinin on human platelets.** *Biochem Biophys Res Commun.* 1981;99:176-82. (English)

A nonagglutinating derivative of wheat germ agglutinin has been prepared that binds to platelets and precipitates an antibody to the lectin. Platelets treated with this inactive derivative released serotonin when exposed to bivalent F(ab)$_2$, but not monovalent Fab, fragments of the lectin antibody. Bridging of platelet-bound Fab by an antibody again induced secretion. The F(ab)$_2$ or Fab fragments plus IgG, without the derivative, did not induce secretion. This secretion was not affected by indomethacin showing a direct activation of platelets. Platelets treated with Con A followed by F(ab)$_2$ to Con A did not secrete. In addition, lentil lectin failed to release platelet serotonin. The receptors of the lectin derivative are mobile on the platelet surface and their redistribution may lead to secretion.

252
Gerritsen SM, Akkerman JW, Nijmeijer B, Sixma JJ, Witkop CJ, White J. **The Hermansky-Pudlak syndrome: evidence for a lowered 5-hydroxytryptamine content in platelets of heterozygotes.** *Scand J Haematol.* 1977; 18:249-56. (English)

A Dutch kindred with the Hermansky-Pudlak syndrome (HPS) is described. We show for the first time evidence of a lowered platelet 5-hydroxytryptamine content in obligate heterozygotes. Platelet ATP and ADP levels and ATP/ADP ratio were normal in these patients. Platelet aggregation with the ADP, collagen and adrenaline was within the normal range. In contrast to the homozygous HPS patients the heterozygotes are normally pigmented and none has diaphanous irides, nystagmus or a bleeding tendency. All homozygous HPS patients have the typical triad of oculocutaneous albinism, pigmented macrophages in the bone marrow and a bleeding disorder, based on a platelet dysfunction. The platelets showed the typical characteristics of a storage pool deficiency. Their platelet factor 3 availability was decreased and the aggregation patterns showed an absent second wave with ADP, adrenaline and absent collagen aggregation. Platelet ADP levels were strongly decreased in all homozygous HPS patients, whereas ATP was lowered only in 3 out of 6 HPS patients. The 5-hydroxytryptamine content of their platelets was very low (15-20% of normal).

253
Gordon MA, Cohen JJ, Wilson IB. **Muscarinic cholinergic receptors in murine lymphocytes: demonstration by direct binding.** *Proc Natl Acad Sci.* 1978;75:2902-4. (English)

Using [^{3}H]quinuclidinyl benzilate as a specific cholinergic muscarinic ligand, it has been demonstrated that lymphocytes have muscarinic binding sites. There are approximately 200 sites per cell and the dissociation constant for quinuclidinyl benzilate is approximately 1×10^{-9}M. Quinuclidinyl benzilate receptor binding is blocked by atropine and oxotremorine.

254
Grabczewska E, Ryzewski J, Krzystyniak K. **Studies on cyclic AMP-cyclic GMP cooperation and on the influence of acetylcholine, adrenaline and thiols in lymphocyte reactivity.** *Arch Immunol Ther Exp.* 1978;26:357-9. (Polish)

In rat lymph node lymphocytes, maximal stimulation of the response after suboptimal doses of PHA (1/2 of the optimal dose), measured by the incorporation of ^{3}H-thymidine, after 10^{-6}M acetylcholine and after 10 min interval between PHA and acetylcholine application was obtained. In these experiments inhibition of acetylcholine action by its muscarinic antagonists was not observed. It was shown that exogenous cAMP as well as other factors which increase cAMP level in lymphocytes had opposite effects to those which could be caused by increasing cGMP. Acetylcholine in optimal concentration (10^{-6}M) as well as thiols, did not increase the level of endogeneous cAMP in rat lymphocytes.

255
Gruchow HW. **Catecholamine activity and infectious disease episodes.** *J Hum Stress.* 1979;5:11-17. (English)

The profile of 3-hydroxy-4-methoxy mandelic acid (VMA) excretion was studied in relation to reported acute infectious disease episodes. Daily VMA excretion levels and symptom reports were analyzed for a group of 47 volunteers over a four-week period. Results showed a tendency for elevated VMA levels to occur with greater frequency within three days prior to the onset of symptoms. These findings are interpreted as suggesting that elevated levels of catecholamine activity may increase susceptibility to disease by interfering with the immune response, and in the presence of an agent lead to an infectious disease episode.

256
Gushchin GV, Shkhinek EK. **Participation of cholinergic mechanisms in the regulation of immunological processes.** *Farmakol Toksikol.* 1979;42:635-9. (Russian)

Chronic administration of cholinomimetic (arecolin, pilocarpin, nicotin) and cholinolytic (benzohexonium, pedifen) drugs produces changes of different directions in the number of rosette-forming cells in the spleens of CBA mice immunized with sheep red blood cells. The analysis performed does not allow the effect of the drugs on immunologic processes to be accounted for by an immediate action on lymphoid cells or by an action of the function of the pituitary-adrenal system.

257

Herman JJ, Brenner JK, Colten HR. **Inhibition of histaminase release from human granulocytes by production of histaminase activity.** *Science.* 1977;2206:77-8. (English)

Imidazoleacetic acid, a product of the action of histaminase (E.C. 1.4.3.6) on histamine, inhibits specific release of histaminase from human peripheral blood granulocytes with an inhibition constant between 5×10^{-9}M and 1×10^{-8}M. Hence modulation of enzyme release is indirectly mediated by the activity of the enzyme.

258

Idova GV, Cheido MA. **Formation of an IgM and an IgG immune response depending on the redistribution of T- and B-subpopulations under the action of serotonin.** *Zh Mikrobiol Epidemiol Immunobiol.* 1979;7:54-9. (Russian)

The syngeneic transfer of spleen cells or spleen and lymph node cells from donors with an elevated serotonin level stimulated, in comparison with the control animals, immune response in the recipients subjected to sublethal irradiation, which was manifested by an increase in the number of plaque-forming and rosette-forming cells. After the combined transfer of spleen cells and bone marrow cells from similar animals a decrease in the number of plaque-forming and rosette-forming cells was observed, while after the transfer of spleen and thymus cells the intensity of immune response remained unchanged. Serotonin was supposed to induce the redistribution of T and B cells in the non-immunized animals, so that suppressor cells migrated from the spleen and the lymph nodes to the bone marrow.

259

Igari T, Takeda M, Obara K, Ono S. **Catecholamine metabolism in patients with rheumatoid arthritis.** *Tohoku J Exp Med.* 1977;122:9-20. (Japanese)

The amount of urinary catecholamine of healthy subjects and patients with rheumatoid arthritis, particularly before and after synovectomy, was studied. (1) The urinary catecholamine of patients with rheumatoid arthritis showed a lower value than that of healthy subjects. The greater the amount of intraarticularly injected steroids was and the more severe the stage and class of rheumatoid arthritis were, the lower the level of adrenaline was and the more reduced the activity of phenylethanolamine-N-methyltransferase was. (2) The level of urinary noradrenaline in patients with rheumatoid arthritis was lower than that of healthy subjects, but there was no relationship between the level of noradrenaline and the amount of intraarticularly injected steroids. Considering that noradrenaline tended to approach the normal level as the stage or class of rheumatoid arthritis was more severe, the level of urinary noradrenaline in patients with rheumatoid arthritis seems to reflect the existence of a certain compensa-

tory system in the enzyme system of catecholamine metabolism rather than the influence of the adrenal cortex system. (3) The urinary catecholamine was decreased after synovectomy; especially, noradrenaline level was remarkably decreased. These results suggest that catecholamine plays an important role in the appearance of pain or other clinical signs in rheumatoid arthritis.

260

Jones WO, Rothwell TLW, Adams DB. **Studies on the role of histamine and 5-hydroxytryptamine in immunity against the nematode *Trichostrongylis colubriformis*.** *Int Arch Allergy Appl Immunol.* 1978;57:48-56. (English)

A temporal relationship was established between the onset of expulsion of the parasitic nematode *Trichostrongylus colubriformis* from the intestine of both vaccinated and adoptively immunized guinea pigs with a sudden increase in small intestinal mucosal histamine to two or three times preinfection levels. However, in guinea pigs whose capacity to expel *T. colubriformis* was inhibited by treatment with anti-lymphocyte serum, mucosal histamine remained at preinfection levels. The results support previous findings which suggest an important role for histamine in the effector mechanism of the immune response of guinea pigs against *T. colubriformis*.

261

Kasprisin DO, Pang EJ. **The effect of epinephrine on granulocyte adhesion.** *Experientia.* 1978;34:119-20. (English)

Preincubation of blood from normal human volunteers with epinephrine significantly decreased the granulocytes' ability to adhere to nylon fibres. Possible significance for the *in vivo* correlation is discussed.

262

Khamidov D KH, Nishanbaev KN, Michnik SE. **Electron cytochemical determination of adenylate cyclase in bone marrow cells under the action of adrenaline epinephrine.** *Probl Gematol Pereliv Krovi.* 1979;24:46-7. (Russian)

The electron-cytochemical method was used to show unequal activity of adenylate cyclase on plasmatic membranes of rat bone marrow cells at various levels of differentiation. In mature granulocytes, lymphocytes, monocytes and erythrocytes dense granules are distributed through the whole plasmatic membrane, while in juvenile cells (promyelocytes, myeloblasts, erythroblasts, lymphoblasts) poor activity of adenylate cyclase is observed. The sensitivity of cells to adrenaline [epinephrine] increases with the progress of the cellular differentiation.

263

Kirtland HH, Mohler DN, Horwitz DA. **Methyldopa inhibition of suppressor- lymphocyte function: a proposed cause of autoimmune hemolytic anemia.** *N Engl J Med.* 1980;302:825-32. (English)

To test the hypothesis that methyldopa induces red-cell autoantibodies by inhibiting the activity of suppressor lymphocytes, we studied its effect on several immune functions.

Methyldopa inhibited T-lymphocyte suppression of IgG production by peripheral-blood mononuclear cells stimulated by pokeweed mitogens. This effect occurred in isolated T cells incubated with methyldopa and in T cells obtained from patients taking methyldopa. In addition, the drug caused a 30 to 80 per cent reduction in the proliferative response of peripheral-blood mononuclear cells to mitogens *in vitro*, and this reduction primarily involved the activation of T lymphocytes. Methyldopa also caused a persistent elevation of intracellular lymphocyte cyclic AMP *in vitro* and *in vivo*. We postulate that methyldopa alters the immune system by causing a persistent increase in lymphocyte cyclic AMP, which inhibits suppressor T-cell function. These effects may lead to unregulated autoantibody production by B cells in some patients.

264

Krall JF, Connelly M, Tuck ML. *In vitro* desensitization of human lymphocytes by epinephrine. *Biochem Pharmacol.* 1982;31:117-9. (English)

Exposure of target tissues to beta-adrenergic catecholamines causes both an increase in cAMP synthesis and a time-dependent loss of sensitivity to further stimulation by these same hormones. In man, this agonist-specific desensitization is a target tissue property *in vivo* as well as *in vitro*, but the mechanism by which it occurs is poorly understood. Beta-adrenergic catecholamine desensitization was initally believed to be the consequence of agonist-induced loss of functional cell surface beta-adrenergic receptors, but more recent evidence of substantive decreases in sensitivity with little or no change in receptor number indicates a more complex mechanism or mechanisms distal to the interaction between hormone and receptor. In general, the rate at which desensitization occurs appears to be hormone and/or cell specific with a time course of days or hours in some cases and minutes in others. Presumably, desensitization protects hormone-sensitive tissues from "over-stimulation," so that rate of progression might be expected to proceed as a function of the seriousness of the consequences of over-stimulation. Using an accessible human target tissue, we found that desensitization of lymphocytes isolated from human subjects undergoing isoproterenol infusion proceeded with rapid time course. Desensitization *in situ* proceeded without detectable changes in beta-adrenergic receptor concentration, and similar losses of sensitivity could be induced in the lymphocytes *in vitro*. These results suggested that human tissues have a mechanism for rapidly reducing their sensitivity on exposure to beta-adrenergic catecholamines, and we sought to determine how acute this response might be.

265

Kraus LJ. **Augmentation of human natural killer cell activity by catecholamines** (abstract). *The Gerontologist.* 1982;22:204. (English)

Recent research in both man and animals indicates the important contribution of neural and endocrine influences to the maintenance of balanced immune function. Previous studies have shown stress related changes in the composition of mononuclear cell subsets. Both epinephrine and norepinephrine have been shown to influence immune response. The percentage of large granular T_G lymphocytes is reportedly increased in response to stress. These T_G lymphocytes are the effectors of natural killer cell activity (NKCA). NKCA is a parameter of cell mediated immune function believed to play a major role in host defense against viral infection and immune surveillance of neoplastic growth. We have found a marked augmentation of NKCA following *in vivo* administration of epinephrine or norepinephrine in normal human subjects. Decreased sensitivity of target tissues to the actions of hormones and other regulatory substances is a primary characteristic of aging. Desensitization may occur as a consequence of exposure to elevated levels of these substances. Age-associated elevation of catecholamine levels has been demonstrated. Such changes may have profound effects on aspects of immunity and may thus be implicated in age-associated changes in immunity.

266

Kudintseva TZ. **Concentration of catecholamines, their precursors, vanilmandelic acid and monoamine oxidase in patients with rheumatism in the active phase.** *Vrach Delo.* 1977;7:33-5. (Russian) (unavailable at publication)

267

Le Fur G, Phan T, Canton T, Tur C, Uzan A. **Evidence for a coupling between dopaminergic receptors and phospholipid methylation in mouse B lymphocytes.** *Life Sci.* 1981;29:2737-49. (English) (unavailable at publication)

268

MacGregor RR. **Granulocyte adherence changes induced by hemodialysis, endotoxin, epinephrine, and glucocorticoids.** *Ann Intern Med.* 1977;86:35-9. (English)

Granulocyte adherence was studied in several situations of altered granulocyte kinetics. During the transient granulocytopenia of hemodialysis, adherence increased to 481.7% of baseline by 15 min and was normal by 60 min. One hour after endotoxin administration, adherence was 160.5% of control as granulocyte counts fell to 21.4%; conversely, the 24-h postdose granulocytosis was associated with a 43.0% decrease in adherence. Epinephrine produced a 25.8% decrease in adherence, with demargination granulocytosis 146.1% of control period. Alternate-day prednisone administration inhibited adherence by 38.9% on the "on" day, concomitant with prolonged granulocyte intravascular half-life, but adherence returned to normal on the "off" day when intravascular half-life is normal. In each situation, a plasma factor not present in serum was responsible for the modified adherence; if these factors produce the same adherence changes *in vivo*, they may be responsible for the alterations noted in granulocyte kinetics.

269

Marone G, Lichtenstein LM. **Adenosine-adenosine deaminase modulation of histamine release.** *J Allergy Clin Immunol.* 1978;61:131. (English)

Adenosine (but not adenine) inhibits antigen or anti-IgE-induced histamine release from human basophils in a dose-dependent fashion; inhibition begins at about 10^{-7}M and peaks at 10^{-4}M. Adenosine inhibits in the first stage of histamine release but is without activity in the second stage. The same or slightly lower concentrations of adenosine increased the cAMP level of mixed leukocytes; $10^{-6}M$ caused an increase of about 75%; while the peak level, $10^{-5}M$, lead to a 300% increase. The increase in cAMP levels begins within 1 min, peaks at 8 to 15 min, and returns to baseline by 45 to 60 min. Inhibition of histamine release is also observed with an adenosine deaminase (ADA) inhibitor, EHNA, in the presence of serum. The inhibition is dose-dependent with respect to both sera in the range of 1% to 20%, and EHNA concentration (10^{-7} to $10^{-6}M$) and is presumably due to the serum adenosine level since dialyzed serum is ineffective. EHNA, by itself, failed to inhibit histamine release at the range of concentrations which are effective in the presence of serum. Decreased levels of ADA have been noted in about one half the cases of severe combined immune deficiency (SCID). Since the adenosine-ADA system controls histamine release and since histamine has marked and usually inhibitory effects on lymphocyte function, we suggest that the present observations may help elucidate the mechanism of the lymphocyte dysfunction observed in SCID.

270

Martin TW, Lagunoff D. **Inhibition of mast cell histamine secretion by N-substituted derivatives of phosphatidylserine.** *Science.* 1979;204:631-3. (English)

The structural basis for the highly specific action of phosphatidylserine in enhancing mast cell histamine secretion induced by concanavalin A was investigated by studying the activities of three N-substituted derivatives: N-acetyl phosphatidylserine, N-1-dimethylaminonaphthaline-5-sulfonyl phosphatidylserine, and N-4-nitrobenzo-2-oxa-1,3-diazole phosphatidylserine. None of the derivatives was capable of activating concanavalin A-induced histamine secretion at concentrations two or three times that required for maximal activation by phosphatidylserine. Instead, the derivatives were found to inhibit the secretory response of mast cells to the calcium ionophore A23187 as well as to concanavalin A. The inhibition was noncytotoxic, partially reversible by washing, and associated with binding of N-substituted phosphatidylserine to the mast cell.

271

Maslinski W, Grabczewska E, Ryzewski J. **Acetylcholine receptors of rat lymphocytes.** *Biochim Biophys Acta.* 1980;633:269-73. (English)

The conditions of the binding of acetylcholine have been studied in lymphocytes isolated from rat peripheral lymph nodes. Acetylcholine appeared to penetrate the lymphocyte membrane. We have confirmed the presence of muscarinic receptors, which, however, are not involved in transport of acetylcholine through the membrane. The receptors of the nicotine type on lymphocytes are demonstrated by the decrease of acetylcholine binding in the presence of a specific antagonist, tubocurarine. These nicotinic receptors may be involved in acetylcholine transport into the cells.

272

Mato M, Ookawara S, Uchiyama Y. **The effects of L-DOPA, serotonin, reserpine and chlorpromazine on the daily rhythm of fluorescent intensity in leucocytes and blood platelets.** *Acta Histochem (Jena).* 1976;57:198-204. (English)

1) The rhythmic fluctuation of fluorescent intensity of leucocytes and platelets of rats was modified by administration of some drugs such as L-DOPA, serotonin, reserpine and chlorpromazine. Timing of administration was determined to get clearcut results. The different results were expected by the administration of drugs at the other time of day. 2) The administration of L-DOPA enhanced the fluorescent intensity of leucocytes and platelets and the tincture of them tended strongly to be green at 4 to 10 h after the treatment. The administration of serotonin suppressed the fluorescent intensity of leucocytes temporarily, but inversely enhanced the intensity of platelets significantly. Reserpine and chlorpromazine had a similar suppressive effect on the fluorescent intensity of leucocytes and platelets within 30 h after the treatment. Compared with them, the influence of reserpine was stronger than that of chlorpromazine. 3) In fact these drugs made a marked influence on the rhythmic fluctuation of fluorescent intensity in leucocytes and platelets, but the physiological rhythmicity remained in the ground of modified fluctuation of rats which were treated by those drugs. In a previous report (Mato *et al.*, 1975), a fluorescent material was demonstrated in leucocytes and platelets using a modification of the Falck-Hillarp technic (Falck *et al.*, 1962), and the dominant component of the fluorescent material was ascertained to be serotonin. Further, the fluorescent intensity of rat's leucocytes and platelets fluctuated representing a bimodal daily rhythm. In this paper, the authors' attention was focused to elucidate the effects of some drugs on the rhythmicity and the concentration of fluorescent material in leucocytes and platelets. The present study will afford valuable information concerning the leucocytes as a kind of store house of biogenic monoamines.

273

Miles K, Quint'ans J, Chelmicka-Schorr E, Arnason BG. **The sympathetic nervous system modulates antibody response to thymus-independent antigens.** *J Neuroimmunol.* 1981;1:101-5. (English)

Sympathetic nerve endings were destroyed with 6-hydroxydopamine (6-OHDA) and the response to thymus-dependent and -independent antigens compared in 6-OHDA-treated and control mice. A significantly enhanced plaque-forming cell response to 2 thymus-independent antigens was observed in the 6-OHDA-treated mice; in contrast, the response to a thymus-dependent antigen was normal. The findings point to a selective modulation of antibody response by the sympathetic nervous system.

274

Monroe EW, Jones EH. **Urticaria: an updated review.** *Arch Dermatol.* 1977;113:80-90. (English)

Urticaria can result from many different stimuli, and numerous factors, both immunologic and nonimmunologic, are involved in its pathogenesis. Most commonly considered of immunologic mechanisms is the type I hypersensitivity state mediated by IgE. Another immunologic mechanism involves the activation of the complement cascade, which produces anaphylatoxins that can release histamine. Immunologic, nonimmunologic, genetic, and modulating factors converge on mast cells and basophils to release mediators capable of producing urticarial lesions. In addition to the clinical and laboratory diagnosis and treatment regimens, we review such mediators as histamine, kinins, serotonin, slow-reacting substance of anaphylaxis, prostaglandins, acetylcholine, fibrin degradation products, and anaphylatoxins that increase vascular permeability and can thereby produce wheals. Special consideration is given to histamine and the basophils, including the modulating role of intracellular levels of cyclic adenosine monophosphate.

275

Moore A, Weksler BB, Nachman RL. **Platelet FcIgG receptor: increased expression in female platelets.** *Thromb Res.* 1981;21:469-74. (English)

Platelet serotonin release, stimulated by heat-aggregated IgG was compared using washed platelets from normal female and normal male donors. There was significantly more serotonin released from female platelets at each concentration of aggregated IgG tested than from male platelets. Thrombin-induced platelet release of serotonin was identical in both sexes. These results suggest that female platelets bear increased FcIgG receptors or that they are more sensitive to FcIgG receptor-induced platelet stimulation. This finding may be of importance in the pathogenesis of certain immune-complex-associated diseases which predominantly affect the female population.

276

Motulsky HJ, Insel PA. **Adrenergic receptors in man.** *N Engl J Med.* 1982;307:18-29. (English)

The catecholamines norephinephrine and epinephrine are key regulators of many physiologic events in human beings; norephinephrine acts primarily as a neurotransmitter released from sympathetic-nerve terminals, and epinephrine functions as a circulating hormone released from the adrenal medulla. These catecholamines initiate target-cell responses by binding to specific recognition sites, the adrenergic receptors. That receptors are the initial decoders of extracellular messages is a concept that has guided research on hormone and neurotransmitter action for many years. Most recently (since 1975), investigators have directly probed these receptors by using radioactively labeled hormone and drug derivatives, termed radioligands. These radioligand-binding techniques have been used to characterize and quantitate adrenergic receptors and to examine their regulation in many animal tissues and cultured cells. In addition, clinical investigators have applied radioligand-binding methods to study alpha- and beta-adrenergic receptors in human tissues--the topic of this review. This is a review of work published through the end of 1981, and discusses general concepts of radioligand-binding studies, properties of adrenergic receptors from various human tissues, physiologic alterations of adrenergic receptors, and changes of adrenergic receptors in disease states.

277

Osband M, Gallison D, Miller B, Agarawel RP, McCaffrey R. **Concanavalin A activation of suppressor cells medi-** ated by histamine and blocked by cimetidine (abstract). *Clin Res.* 1980;28:356A. (English)

Human peripheral blood lymphocytes (PBL) are activated to become suppressor cells by overnight incubation with Concanavalin A (Con A). This activation by Con A has become the standard method for the evaluation of suppressor cell function in patients. Incubation of PBL with histamine also activates suppressor cells. This activation is blocked by cimetidine, an H_2 antagonist, but not by diphenhydramine, a H_1 antihistamine. We report now that incubation of PBL with Con A causes histamine release into the supernatant medium, and that the inclusion of cimetidine or histaminase in the culture prevents Con A activation of suppressor cells. PBL were incubated for 24 hours in medium only or medium containing Con A (6 microg/ml), cimetidine (10^{-3}M) or histaminase (1 unit/ml), in various combinations. The cells were washed, added to autologous carried lymphocytes and the entire cell mixture stimulated by allogeneic lymphocytes for 7 days in a one-way MLC. Cells incubated in Con A alone suppressed the MLC 59%. Cells incubated in Con A + cimetidine suppressed only 6%, and those incubated in Con A + histaminase suppressed only 1%. This blocking of the Con A activation by cimetidine or histaminase implies the presence of histamine. This was further supported by the result that the incubation of PBL with Con A causes release of histamine into the supernatant medium, peaking after 4 hours, at 10^{-5}M, a concentration high enough to activate directly suppressor cells. We conclude that the Con A activation of suppressor cells is mediated by histamine release and actually measures the resultant histamine activation of suppressor cells.

278

Paegelow I, Lange P. **Pharmacological studies on lymphocytes; 1--Effects of 5-hydroxytryptamine, bradykinin, and lymphokines on the migration of lymphocytes in vitro.** *Agents Actions (Suppl).* 1982;10:255-65. (English)

The migration of lymphocytes from several sources and several species was assessed in modified Boyden chambers. The migratory ability of resident thymocytes from cats, guinea pigs and rats is generally comparable. In rats a non-adherent T-cell population from lymph nodes and from the ductus thoracicus showed higher spontaneous mobility than thymocytes. The migration of all tested lymphocytes was significantly stimulated by 5-HT and bradykinin in a dose-dependent manner. Lymphokine preparations with a MIF-activity less than 0.8 increased the migration of lymphocytes, too. It could be suggested that 5-HT and bradykinin together with lymphokines play a role in the movement of lymphocytes.

279

Peterson CS, Herlin T, Esmann V. **Effects of catecholamines and glucagon on glycogen metabolism in human polymorphonuclear leukocytes.** *Biochim Biophys Acta.* 1978;542:77-87. (English)

Addition of 10 microM of the alpha-adrenergic agonist phenylephrine to polymorphonuclear leukocytes suspended in glucose-free Krebs-Ringer bicarbonate buffer (pH 6.7) activated phosphorylase, inactivated glycogen synthase R maximally within 30 s and resulted in glycogen breakdown. Phenylephrine increased ^{45}Ca efflux relative to control of ^{45}Ca prelabelled cells, but did not affect cyclic adenosine 3',5'-monophosphate (cAMP) concentration. The effects of phenylephrine were blocked by 20 microM phentolamine and were absent in cells incubated at pH 7.4. The same unexplained dependency of extracellular pH was observed with 2.5 nM-microM glucagon, which activated phosphorylase and inactivated synthase-R, but in addition caused a 30 s burst in cAMP formation. 25 nM glucagon also increased ^{45}Ca efflux. The activation of phosphorylase by phenylephrine and possibly also by glucagon are thought to be mediated by an increased concentration of cytosolic Ca^{2+}-activating phosphorylase kinase. The effects of 5 microM epinephrine were independent of extracellular pH 6.7 and 7.4 and resulted in a sustained increase in cAMP, an activation of phosphorylase and inactivation of synthase-R within 15 s, and in glycogenolysis. The effects of both compounds were blocked by 10 microM propanolol, whereas 10 microM phentolamine had no effect on the epinephrine action. The efflux of ^{45}Ca was not affected by either isoproterenol or epinephrine. The beta-adrenergic activation of phosphorylase is consistent with the assumption of a covalent modification of phosphorylase kinase by the cAMP dependent protein kinase. Phosphorylation of synthase-R to synthase-D can thus occur independently of increase in cAMP, but the evidence is inconclusive with respect to the cAMP-dependent protein kinase also being in this phosphorylation.

280

Reed CE, Busse WW, Lee TP. **Adrenergic mechanisms and the adenyl cyclase system in atopic dermatitis.** *J Invest Dermatol.* 1976;67:333-8. (English)

Patients with atopic dermatitis have abnormal autonomic responses of the arterioles, pilomotor smooth muscle, and sweat glands. Their lesions have been reported to contain increased amounts of the neurohumors, acetylcholine and norepinephrine, as well as increased activity of acetylcholinesterase and catechol-o-methyltransferase. *In vitro* studies of epidermis show that beta-adrenergic agonists fail to evoke the normal inhibition of mitosis of basal cells of patients with atopic dermatitis. Epidermis removed not only from the lesions, but also from normal-appearing skin, responded abnormally. The increase in intracellular levels of cAMP after exposure to catecholamines was similar in normal and atopic epidermis. Lymphocytes and PMN leukocytes isolated from patients with atopic dermatitis show a decreased physiologic response (glycogenolysis and inhibition of lysosome enzyme release) and a decreased rise in intracellular levels of cAMP upon incubation with beta-agonists, but a normal response to PGE_1. Cortisol increases the response of lymphocyte adenyl cyclase to both agonists and, in the case of the patients with atopic disease, more than overcomes the depressed response to beta agonists. Because the leukocytes respond normally to PGE_1 and because others have reported normal activities of skin and adenyl cyclase, phosphodiesterase, and protein kinases, we conclude that the step responsible for the diminished beta adrenergic response lies antecedent to the catalytic site of adenyl cyclase.

281

Richman DP, Arnason BG. **Nicotinic acetylcholine receptor: evidence for a functionally distinct receptor on human lymphocytes.** *Proc Natl Acad Sci.* 1979;76:4632-5. (English)

The presence of three distinct cholinergic receptors on human lymphocytes was suggested by the effects of carbamoylcholine on lymphocyte proliferation *in vitro*. The cells responded to both 0.1 nM and 1 microM carbamoylcholine by increased proliferation which was blocked by the muscarinic antagonist atropine. This effect occurred in both mitogen-stimulated cells (maximum effect at 24 hr) and nonstimulated cells (maximum effect at 72 hr). In contrast, 1^{-10}nM carbamoylcholine produced diminished *in vitro* proliferation, an effect which was blocked by the nicotinic antagonists alpha-bungarotoxin and d-tubocurarine.

282

Ring J, O'Connor P. **In vitro histamine and serotonin release in atopic dermatitis.** *Int Arch Allergy Appl Immunol.* 1979;58:322-30. (English)

6 patients suffering from severe atopic dermatitis with high serum IgE were investigated. 3 of the patients had elevated plasma histamine levels (1.5-2.0 ng/ml). Compared to 9 nonatopic normal volunteers, the patient showed increased *in vitro* histamine release from peripheral leukocytes after stimulation with iothalamate and methacholine: while there was no significant histamine release at a methacholine concentration of $10^{-4}M$ in normals, 4 of the patients with atopic dermatitis showed measurable histamine release under these conditions *in vitro*. The uptake of radio-labeled serotonin by platelets *in vitro* was decreased in two of the patients. There was no significant difference in serotonin release induced *in vitro* by different concentrations of thrombin, epinephrine and methacholine; 2 patients showed an increased platelet release reaction after iodipamide stimulation. It is concluded that a general tendency to release vasoactive mediators, even after "nonimmunologic" stimulation, might play a role in the pathogenesis of atopic dermatitis.

283

Rocklin RE, Greineder DK, Melmon KL. **Histamine-induced suppressor factor (HSF): further studies on the nature of the stimulus and the cell which produces it.** *Cell Immunol.* 1979;44:404-15. (English)

Guinea pig lymphocytes are stimulated by histamine to produce a soluble factor with immunosuppressive properties. This factor, termed histamine-induced suppressor factor or HSF, abrogates the production of migration inhibitory factor (MIF) and proliferative response to specific antigen. In the present study we have determined the lymphocyte subpopulation which elaborates HSF, the lymphoid tissue source, the kinetics of its generation in relation to immunization, and the nature of the histamine receptor involved in modification of the release of HSF. HSF activity could be detected in populations of cells from spleen and lymph nodes prior to active immunization of the donor, but not in cells from the donor's blood or thymus. Following immunization with *ortho*-chloro benzoyl-bovine gamma-globulin in complete Freund's adjuvant (CFA), more HSF activity was detected in cells from the donor's spleen and lymph nodes. The peak response was seen 2 weeks postimmunization when significant amounts of HSF also were made by cells from the blood and thymus. Concentrations of T-cell-enriched and B-cell-enriched pupulations were tested for their ability to make HSF. We found that T-cell-enriched, but not B-cell-enriched populations, made significant amounts of HSF. Cells from the lymph nodes of immunized donors were chromatographed over affinity columns made of insolubilizaed conjugates of histamine with albumin. The nonretained cells were unable to generate HSF, whereas HSF activity was detected in the cells that were retained by the columns. This finding strongly suggests that the HSF-producing cells have receptors for histamine. Cells from CFA-immune lymph nodes were incubated with H_1 (2-methyl histamine) and H_2 (4-methyl histamine) agonists to determine their relative potency and, therefore, the nature of the histamine receptors on these cells that were modifying HSF release. Although both agonists could induce generation of HSF when high concetnrations (10^{-3}M) were used, only the H_2 agonist stimulated production or release of HSF at lower concentrations (10^{-5}M). These HSF-producing cells appear to be selectively sensitive to H_2 agonists and likely have a predominance of H_2 receptors. Allergic mediators other than histamine were studied to determine their ability to allow elaboration of HSF-like activity from CFA-immune lymph node cells. Serotonin (10^{-3}M), slow-reacting substance of anaphylaxis (100 units/ml), eosinophil chemotactic factor (tetrapeptide; 10^{-5}M), and prostaglandin E_1 (10^{-4}M) were unable to induce HSF-like activity in lymph node cells from donors immunized with CFA. Furthermore, other agents which raise intracellular levels of cyclic adenosine 3',5'-monophosphate (cyclic AMP) such as isoproterenol and cholera toxin, as well as the dibutyryl form of cyclic AMP itself, were also unable to generate HSF-like activity. Thus, histamine is unique among the allergic mediators in stimulating elaboration of the suppressive substance. These findings also suggest that the ability of histamine to stimulate HSF may not reside in the conventional pathway linked to cAMP accumulation, but rather to an as yet undefined pathway of cell activation. A model is presented which further implicated histamine as a modulator of cellular immune reactions.

284

Rocklin RE. **Role of histamine as a modulator of cellular-immune function.** *Monogr Allergy.* 1979;14:134-7. (English)

The effects of histamine on vascular permeability and smooth muscle are well known. It is only recently, however, that we have begun to appreciate its role as a modulator of leukocyte function in general and lymphocyte function in particular. In previous studies reported in a guinea pig model, histamine was shown to suppress *in vivo* delayed hypersensitivity and *in vitro* lymphocyte proliferation and the production of macrophage migration inhibitory factor (MIF). An analysis of the mechanism of suppression by histamine *in vitro* revealed that the drug did not affect macrophage responses to MIF or antigen presentation to lymphocytes. Instead it was found that lymphocytes chromatographed on histamine affinity columns produced MIF and proliferated in the presence of histamine. The latter observation suggested the possibility that the histamine-responsive cells had a regulatory function

and subsequently led to the finding that lymphocytes stimulated by histamine elaborated a soluble suppressor factor termed histamine-induced suppressor factor (HSF). In the present studies, which were carried out in collaboration with Drs. Kenneth L. Melmon and Dirk Greineder, we have investigated the cell source of the suppressor factor, the kinetics of its production in relation to immunization, the lymphocyte subpopulation which elaborates the factor and the nature of the stimuli. These questions were examined using either the guinea pig model, or more recently, an assay to detect HSF production by human cells. The method for producing and assaying HSF involves a two-step procedure. In the first step, lymphocytes from a variety of sources are isolated and cultured *in vitro* without or with varying concentrations of histamine for 18 h. The cell-free supernatants from these cultures are obtained and dialyzed to remove the histamine. The supernatants are then used to resuspend fresh indicator cells which are assayed for MIF production or proliferation. The effect of the histamine-induced supernatant (compared to its control supernatant) on either MIF or proliferation gives an indication of the amount of suppressor factor in that supernatant.

285

Roskowski W, Plaut M, Lichtenstein LM. **Selective display of histamine receptors on lymphocytes.** *Science.* 1977; 195:683-5. (English)

Histamine, acting on histamine 2 receptors, increases intracellular cyclic adenosine monophosphate (AMP) and thus modulates the immunologic functions of lymphocytes. Lymphocyte cyclic AMP levels were used to follow the development of histamine receptors. The B lymphocytes have no functional histamine receptors. As T lymphocytes "mature" in immunologic function--from thymocytes to cortisone-resistant thymocytes to splenic T lymphocytes--their response of these subpopulations of lymphocytes to isoproterenol is the inverse of the histamine response. It is suggested that the changing display of histamine receptors plays an important part in the control of immunologic responses.

286

Rothschild AM. **Plasma kallikrein-generating activity evoked by rat peritoneal fluid mast cells following treatment with epinephrine, 8-bromo-cyclic GMP or compound 48-80.** *Biochem Pharmacol.* 1981;30:481-8. (English)

Acting in a dose-dependent fashion, l-epinephrine (E) caused rat peritoneal fluid cells to rapidly deplete rat plasma kininogen *in vitro*; 48-bromo-(cGMP) (8-Br-cGMP) behaved similarly; $N_6{}^2$l0-dibutryl-(cAMP) (di BU-cAMP) inhibited this effect of E or 8-Br-cGMP. After fractionation of peritoneal-fluid cells by differential centrifugation, this kininogen-depleting activity was observed only in mast cells; eosinophils, lymphocytes, and monocytes were inactive. E-treated mast cells were able to hydrolyze the trypsin substrates N-p-toluenesulfonyl-arginine-methyl-ester (TAME) or N-benzoyl-arginine-ethyl-ester and to generate the capacity to hydrolyze these substrates in rat plasma; because this activity accompanied kininogen depletion, it was attributed to plasma kininogenase (plasma kallikrein). DFP inhibited the mast cell esterase activity toward TAME but did not prevent activated cells from depleting plasma kininogen. Thus, mast cell-bound arginginase ester esterase may not have been necessary for the activation of plasma kininogenase. Mast cell heparin, exposed following E or 8-Br-cGMP treatment, may have been the activator of plasma kallikrein. Unlike DFP, Trasylol [polyvalent bovine proteinase inhibitor (BPTI)] inhibited both mast cell esterase and kininogen-depleting activity. This inhibitor may have acted on mast cells both as a heparin antagonist and as a non-specific esterase inhibitor. Compound 48/80 (p-methoxyphenethyl methylamine formaldehyde product), at concentrations causing 40% release of mast cell histamine, failed to cause mast cells to exhibit the ability to activate plasma kallikrein. At high concentrations it activated the kininogen-depleting action of mast cells, but to a lesser degree than did E or 8-Br-cGMP. These compounds did not release histamine. The ability to activate plasma kininogenase apparently was present in non-histamine-releasing mast cells.

287

Schleimer R. **Regulatory roles of histamine in the immune system.** *Proc West Pharmacol Soc.* 1978;21:145-50. (English) (no abstract)

288

Schmutzler W. **Pharmacological aspects of immune reactions.** *Allergol Immunopathol (Madr).* 1978;6:345-60. (English)

"Immunopharmacology" evolved as a field of research in its own right when it was appreciated that pharmacological methods can contribute to the understanding of immune mechanisms on the one hand or can be used to influence or even control immune reactions at all stages and levels. The best studied subjects of immunopharmacology are release and effects of the chemical mediator substance which are responsible for the reactions of effector cells, thus causing the clinical symptoms in allergic or inflammatory diseases. In type I allergic (anaphylactic) reactions the primary target cells are tissue mast cells or basophil granulocytes which discharge their granular contents upon interaction of immunoglobulin E fixed to their surface with the specific antigen or--in the anaphylactoid reaction--upon stimulation with an appropriate chemical substance (so-called histamine-liberator). In both cases the stimulus leads to an influx or intracellular shift from one compartment to another of calcium ions, which in turn trigger membrane fusion and degranulation. This process can vary from a physiological secretion (in the case of IgE antigen-interaction) to pathological cytolysis (in the case of high concentrations of activated complement components or other chemical histamine releasers). As long as it is secretory, it is subject to vegetative and hormonal modulation and regulation, mainly by catecholamines and other substances which increase cellular cAMP levels or inhibit calcium fluxes. Although cholinergic stimuli under certain circumstances induce mast cell degranulation and histamine release, no definite role has yet been established for cholinergic mechanisms in type I allergies. Type II (cytotoxic) and type III (immune complex-mediated) allergies share the complement requirement. As far as mast cells and basophils are involved in such reactions their sensitivity towards pharmacological modulators is comparable to reactions induced by chemical histamine releasers. Otherwise, these types of allergic reac-

tions are dominated by phenomena of general inflammation. In those, mainly cytotoxic effects of lipases and hydrolases are involved. Cyclic AMP-active agents have therefore quite limited modulating effects and steroid hormones are more effective in inhibiting the acute lesions of type II and III allergies. Only during the last decade the involvement of chemical mediators in type IV (cellular immunity) allergic reactions has been appreciated. 26 different factors (called lymphokines) have been discovered and classified as mediators of cellular immune reactions. However, rather little is yet known about their chemical nature and about the influence of drugs on their production and action.

289

Schwartz A, Askenase PW, Gershon RK. **Histamine inhibition of the in vitro induction of cytotoxic T-cell responses.** *Immunopharmacology.* 1980;2:179-90. (English)

Addition of 10^{-3} to 10^{-6} M histamine (H) to mixed leukocyte cultures (MLCs) inhibited primary *in vitro* induction of cytotoxic T lymphocytes specific for either allogeneic or trinitrophenol modified syngeneic target cells. The use of specific H agonists implicated H_2 but not H_1 receptor triggering in the mediation of these effects. Unlike *in vivo*-induced allogeneic CTLs, the addition of H to assay culture failed to influence the effector function of *in vitro*-induced CTLs of either specificity. Kinetic studies showed that this difference might be due to loss of functional H receptors after the initiation of the *in vitro* MLC, and   demonstrated that H interferes with an early event in the generation of CTLs. These data indicate that H receptors are not merely markers for CTL precursors, but that they are functional receptors, and suggest that H may play an important role in regulating both the generation and effector function of CTLs *in vivo*.

290

Schwartz A, Sutton SL, Askenase PW, Gershon RK. **Histamine inhibition of concanavalin A-induced suppressor T-cell activation.** *Cell Immunol.* 1981;60:426-39. (English) (unavailable at publication)

291

Shapiro HM, Strom TB. **Electrophysiology of T lymphocyte cholinergic receptors.** *Proc Natl Acad Sci.* 1980; 77:4317-21. (English)

The presence of functional muscarinic-cholinergic receptors on at least some T-lymphocytes is suggested by the existence of saturable, high-affinity, specific muscarinic binding in T cell-enriched, but not in B cell-enriched, cell suspensions and by observed cholinergic effects on lymphocytes, (e.g., increased lytic capacity of cytotoxic lymphocytes preincubated with muscarinic agents). In this study, we used flow cytometry and a fluorescent probe of membrane potential, the cyanine dye 3,3'-dihexyloxacarbocyanine iodine, to examine the effects of cholinergic agonists and antagonists on the membrane potentials of lymphocytes in T cell-enriched and B cell-enriched suspensions. Acetylcholine (ACCHO) and carbamoylcholine (CBMCHO) depolarized the membranes of T cells, but not of B cells; the maximal depolarization was produced by 10 nM ACCHO or by 1 nM CBMCHO. Depolarization following exposure to these concentrations of agonists was maximal by

5-8 min; T cell membrane potentials returned to control values by 13-15 min. Less marked depolarization was produced by 100 nM ACCHO ad 10 nM CBMCHO; 100 pM CBMCHO was only slightly less effective than 1 nM CBMCHO, and the depolarization persisted 12 min after exposure. Depolarization induced by 1 nM ACCHO was abolished when ACCHO was combined with 10 nM atropine but not when ACCHO was combined with 1 nM atropine or 200 nM D-tubocurarine. The time course of the membrane potential response and its dependence on the relative concentrations of ACCHO and specific cholinergic blocking agents correlate well with both binding studies and biological effects. Our results provide evidence that T lymphocytes have functional muscarinic receptors; the flow cytometric method should be generally applicable to studies of the electrophysiology and pharmacology of receptor-ligand interactions.

292

Shaskan EG. **Evidence in humans and mice for a dopamine-modulation of cell-mediated immunity. In:** *Proceedings, 7th meeting of the International Society for Neurochemistry, Jerusalem, Isr.* 1979:577. (English)

There exist numerous reports in the literature in which it is suggested that individuals who are genetically low for platelet monoamine oxidase activity (MAO) are predisposed to psychiatric disorders, including schizophrenia, manic-depressive illness, and alcoholism. Is there any selective advantage to low MAO? Or, does high MAO predispose to any illnesses? Through fully prospective, epidemiologic studies of two infectious viral diseases, infectious mononucleosis (IM) and dengue fever (DF), preliminary results suggest that genetically high MAO predisposes to clinical IM in those individuals acquiring the Epstein-Barr Virus (EBV), but MAO does not appear to be a host factor predisposing to DF, following infection by a Dengue virus. EBV infection is combated by a predominantly humoral immune response. Accordingly, the above epidemiologic studies in humans have stimulated pharmacological studies in mice in order to better define a possible brain biogenic amine to CMI response, while Dengue virus infection is combated by a predominantly humoral immune response. Accordingly, the above epidemiologic studies in humans have stimulated pharmacological studies in mice in order to better define a possible brain biogenic amine to CMI system axis. A delayed-type hypersensitivity reaction in C57Bl/6J mice was used, sensitizing and challenging with dinitrochlorobenzene. By varying the sequence of haloperidol injections (0.5 mg/kg) in relation to the afferent and efferent arms of the immune response, these treatments produced either an immunopotentiation or an immunosuppression. All of the above results are consistent with a brain dopamine-CMI system axis.

293

Shelhamer JH, Marom Z, Kaliner M. **Immunologic and neuropharmacologic stimulation of mucous glycoprotein release from human airways in vitro.** *J Clin Invest.* 1980;66:1400-8. (English)

Human bronchial airways obtained after surgical resection were maintained in tissue culture for 24-48 h. Incorporation of [^{3}H] or [^{14}C]-glucosamine, [^{14}C] threonine or Na$_2$[^{35}S]O$_4$

to the culture media resulted in biosynthesis of 2 radiolabeled glycoproteins--one filtering in the exclusion volume of Sepharose 2B, and the other filtering with a MW of approx. 400,000. Both fractions had similar elution patterns from DEAE-cellulose anion exchange chromatography. [^{3}H]Glucosamine was incorporated equally into the 2 fractions. The effects of anaphylaxis, histamine and several neurohormones on the release of [^{3}H]glucosamine-labeled glycoproteins were analyzed, making no attempt to separate the 2 glycoprotein fractions. Mast cell degranulation apparently increases mucous release from cultured airways. Supernatant fluids from anaphylaxed peripheral human lung that contained 200-400 ng/ml histamine and 400-1000 U/ml slow-reacting substance of anaphylaxis (SRS-A) increased release by $40 \pm 18\%$. The addition of antigen to IgE sensitized airways led to the release of $26 \pm 7\%$ of the total histamine and a $36 \pm 14\%$ increase in mucous release. Reversed anaphylaxis with anti-IgE antibodies induced a $36 \pm 6\%$ release of histamine from the airways and an increase in the release of mucous glycoproteins of $25 \pm 9\%$. Exogenous histamine added to airways increased mucous glycoprotein release, an effect prevented by cimetidine, an H-2 antagonist. Selective histamine H-2, but not H-1 agonists increased mucous glycoprotein release, suggesting the possibility that anaphylaxis of airways results in increased mucous glycoprotein release partly through histamine H-2 stimulation. A cholinomimetic agonist, methacholine, increased mucous release; this response was prevented by atropine which alone had no effect. No response to beta-adrenergic stimulation with either isoproterenol or epinephrine was noted. However, alpha-adrenergic stimulation with norepinephrine combined with propranolol or phenylephrine alone resulted in dose-related increases in glycoprotein release. Both alpha-adrenergic and cholinergic stimulation of human tissues induce the formation of cGMP, and 8-bromo-cGMP added to the airways led to increased mucous secretion. Neurohormones capable of stimulating cGMP formation in human airways may lead to increased mucous glycoprotein release.

294

Sheppard JR, Gormus R, Moldow CF. **Catecholamine hormone receptors are reduced on chronic lymphocytic leukaemic lymphocytes.** *Nature.* 1977;269:693-5. (English) (no abstract)

295

Singh U, Owen JJT. **Studies on the maturation of thymus stem cells. The effects of catecholamines, histamine and peptide hormones on the expression of T cell alloantigens.** *Eur J Immunol.* 1976;6:59-62. (English)

Studies have been performed in order to investigate the effects of catecholamines, histamine, peptide hormones and various other agents known to increase cellular adenosine 3',5'-cyclic monophosphate (cAMP) levels, on the expression of Thy-1 and TL antigens on 14-day fetal thymic stem cells. It has been shown that the proportions of Thy-1 and TL positive cells, as detected by dye exclusion cytoxicity tests, can be significantly increased by some of these agents and that these effects may be inhibited by beta-adrenergic and H$_G$ antagonists. The value of these tests as a means for studying normal thymic stem cell maturation and for investigating T cell deficiency is discussed.

296

Singh U. **Effect of catecholamines on lymphopoiesis in fetal mouse thymic explants.** *J Anat.* 1979;279-92. (English)

Fetal thymic explants (14 days of gestation) from BALB/c mice were grown in organ culture for up to 12 days and the pattern of lymphopoiesis was monitored by [124]IUdR incorporation and cell yields of such lobes in the presence of adrenergic agents. It was observed that, after 3 days of cultures, phenylephrine stimulated lymphopoiesis in thymic explants, whereas some inhibition was observed with isoproterenol. These observations were confirmed by autoradiography. It was also observed that cells obtained from phenylephrine-treated cultures had greater mitogen reactivity than either control (untreated) isoproterenol-treated cultures. The possible role of cyclic nucleotides as intracellular mediators of thymocyte maturation is discussed.

297

Sokol WN, Beall GN, Kruger SR. **Specificity studies of leukocytic catecholamine receptors.** *Int J Clin Pharmacol Biopharm.* 1978;16:173-6. (English)

Using tritium-labeled dl(±)epinephrine, we have extended previous studies demonstrating binding of epinephrine to human leukocytes. We have now further assessed the biological significance of this catecholamine binding by comparing the specificity of binding by human leukocytes with the ability of these compounds to inhibit epinephrine-stimulated adenyl cyclase. Binding is specific for catechols, but does not distinguish between physiologically active and inactive stereoisomers, nor between alpha- and beta-adrenergic agonists. Although 2.5 x 10-4M l(-)DOPA, dopamine, d(+)epinephrine and serotonin failed to stimulate leukocytic 4adenyl cyclase and prevented adenyl cyclase stimulation by 2.5 x 10 $^{-4}$M l(-)epinephrine, the inhibition of adenyl cyclase by d(+)epinephrine is noncompetitive. This catechol- binding site is clearly not the beta-adrenergic receptor. Its physiological significance, if any, remains to be elucidated.

298

Stepien H, Kunert-Radek J, Karasek E, Pawlikowski M. **Dopamine increases cyclic AMP concentration in the rat spleen lymphocytes *in vitro.*** Biochem Biophys Res Commun. 1981;101:1057-63. (English)

The effect of dopamine on the cyclic AMP concentration in the rat spleen lymphocytes has been investigated *in vitro.* It has been shown that dopamine in concentration above 10^{-6}M induces a significant increase of cyclic AMP level. The maximal stimulatory effect was observed after 10 minutes of the lymphocytes incubation with dopamine. These data suggest that the dopamine receptor in lymphocyte belongs to D-1 category.

299

Strom TB, Lane MA, George K. **The parallel, time-dependent, bimodal change in lymphocyte cholinergic binding activity and cholinergic influence upon lymphocyte-mediated cytotoxicity after lymphocyte activation.** *J Immunol.* 1981;127:705-10. (English)

The potent muscarinic cholinergic antagonist 3-quinuclidinyl benzilate has been used to detect muscarinic acetylcholine receptors on rodent and human lymphocytes. Binding to B lymphocytes was minimal and was not saturable or ligand-specific. Half-maximal binding of (^{3}H)-quinuclidinyl benzilate to T lymphocytes occurred at concentrations comparable to those described in other systems, and was displaceable at physiologic concentrations by muscarinic but not nicotinic agonists and antagonists. Binding to T lymphocytes was both saturable and specific, and was found to rapidly increase significantly after mitogen activation. Activation of T lymphocytes or Lyt 1[+] subset produces an early increase and later fall in muscarinic binding, and the ability of cholinergic agonists to augment the effector function of cytotoxic T lymphocytes harvested from alloimmune rat spleen is directly related to the magnitude of muscarinic binding.

300

Szentwanyi A, Heim O, Schultze P. **Changes in adrenoreceptor densities in membranes of lung tissue and lymphocytes from patients with atopic disease.** *Ann NY Acad Sci.* 1979;332: 295. (English) (unavailable at publication)

301

Timoshenko LV, Markitaniuk SV. **Desensitizing effect of skin grafts in pregnant women with Rh-conflict (according to the data of catecholamine and serotonin metabolism).** *Akush Ginekol (Mosk).* 1980;4:29-32. (Russian)

A total of 19 grafts of a cutaneous flap taken in 13 women with Rh-conflict pregnancy were used for desensitization. Investigations of catecholamines and serotonin carried out before and 2 weeks after transplantation of the cutaneous flap revealed activation of the biosynthesis of DOPA, dopamine, noradrenaline, and adrenaline, a decrease of the serotonin level and excretion with the urine of normetanephrine, metanephrine and dioxyamygdalic acid, as well as a rise in the 5-oxidol acetic and vanilyl amygdalic acid content in the urine. These changes correlated well with the clinical effect of the graft in these pregnant women and are considered as a positive test of desensitizing therapy.

302

Tutton PJM, Barkla DH. **A comparison of cell proliferation in normal and neoplastic intestinal epithelia following either biogenic amine depletion or monoamine oxidase inhibition.** *Virchows Arch B Cell Path.* 1976;21:161-8. (English)

Epithelial cell proliferation was studied in the jejunum and in the colon of normal rats, in the colon of dimethylhydrazine-treated rats and in dimethylhydrazine-induced adenocarcinoma of the colon using a stathmokinetic technique. Estimates of cell proliferation rates in these four tissues were then repeated in animals which had been depleted of biogenic amines by treatment with reserpine and in animals whose monoamine oxidase was inhibited with treatment with nialamide. In amine-depleted animals cell proliferation essentially ceased in all four tissues examined. Inhibition of monoamine oxidase did not significantly influence cell proliferation in non-malignant tissues but accelerated cell division in colonic tumors.

303

Vetoshkin AV, Fomenko AM, Zozulia AA. **Lymphocyte serotonin receptors: a radioreceptor study.** *Biull Eksp Biol Med.* 1982;94:52-3. (Russian)

The radioreceptor method was used to find high affinity, saturable and partially reversible specific binding of ^{3}H-5HT with a gross membrane fraction of human peripheral blood lymphocytes. The Sketchard analysis demonstrated the presence of two types of the binding sites with equilibrium dissociation constants 2 nM and 66 nM. These characteristics are similar to those of ^{3}H-5HT binding with the brain receptors. The results obtained suggest the existence on human lymphocytes of two types of serotonin receptors.

304

Yu DT, Clements PJ. **Human lymphocyte subpopulations: effect of epinephrine.** *Clin Exp Immunol.* 1976; 25:472-9. (English)

The effect of administration of 0.2 mg of epinephrine (Parke-Davis) on circulatory lymphocytes was investigated in fifteen normal subjects. Blood samples were taken prior to, and 10 and 20 min after, subcutaneous injections. Thymus-derived (T) cells were assayed by sheep red blood cell rosettes, bone marrow-derived (B) cells by their complement receptors and immunofluorescent detection of FC receptors plus surface immunoglobulins. Their percentages prior to injections were 72.2 ± 1.4, 13.8 ± 1.1, and 20.3 ± 1.3. Ten minutes after injections the absolute concentrations of these cells increased to 164 ± 14%, 326 ± 57%, and 272 ± 45% respectively of the values prior to injection (averages ± standard errors). Further, when cells with receptors for both sheep red blood cells and complement were assayed by simultaneous rosette technique, they increased from 2.5 ± 0.4% to 10.5 ± 1.3% of the lymphocytes. Such changes were also observed in three subjects who had undergone splenectomy more than 2 years previously, but not in four subjects receiving injections of saline instead of epinephrine.

305

Zhikharev SS, Mineev VN. **Detection of disorders in lymphocyte adrenoreactivity in bronchial asthma.** *Lab Delo.* 1981;5:297-300. (Russian) (unavailable at publication)

Autonomic agents

306

Aarons RD, Nies AS, Gal J, Hegstrand LR, Molinoff PB. **Elevation of beta-adrenergic receptor density in human lymphocytes after propanolol administration.** *J Clin Invest.* 1980;65:949-57. (English)

Abrupt withdrawal after the chronic administration of propranolol has resulted in clinical syndromes that suggest adrenergic hypersensitivity. The effect of propranolol administration and withdrawal on beta-adrenergic receptors was studied in human lymphocyte membranes. Receptor density was quantitated by direct binding assays with the radioligand [125$_I$]iodohydroxybenzylpindolol. Administration of propranolol (160 mg/d) for 8 d resulted in trough plasma levels of approx. 35 ng/ml. By day 5 of propranolol administration the density of beta-adrenergic receptors had increased 43 ± 4% (p$<$0.01) above pretreatment levels. Abrupt withdrawal of propranolol was followed by the disappearance of propranolol from the plasma within 24 h. The density of beta-adrenergic receptors did not return to pretreatment level for several days. Physiologic supersensitivity of beta-adrenergic receptor-mediated responses was suggested by the appearance of significant increases in the orthostatic change in heart rate (p$<$0.05) and the orthostatic change in the heart rate-systolic blood pressure product (p$<$0.01) during the first 48 h after propranolol withdrawal. These data show that propranolol administration leads to an increase in the density of beta-adrenergic receptors in human tissue. The results are consistent with the hypothesis that some of the untoward effects observed after abrupt discontinuation of propranolol are caused by beta-receptor-mediated adrenergic hypersensitivity.

307

Anderton BH, Axford JS, Cohn P, Marshall NS, Shen L, Sprake S. **Inhibition of lymphocyte capping and transformation by propanolol and related compounds.** *Br J Pharmacol.* 1981;72,69-74. (English)

1) The effects of propranolol on phytohaemagglutinin (PHA)-induced transformation of murine T lymphocytes and capping of anti-IgG on the surface of murine B lymphocytes have been examined. 2) A 50% inhibition of transformation was observed with 10^{-5} M propranolol, whereas a higher concentration of the order of 10^{-3} M propranolol was required to inhibit capping by 50%. The (+) and (-) isomers of propranolol proved equipotent in these respects, and the relative potencies of selected analogues of propanolol (alprenolol, oxprenolol, metoprolol, practolol, and sotalol) coincided with their potencies as membrane stabilizers; however, lymphocyte transformation was consistently more sensitive than capping. 3) Similar effects were also seen with quinidine, chlorpromazine and lignocaine, and it was concluded that the inhibition of both lymphocyte functions was due to the membrane stabilizing actions of propranolol.

308

Bishopric NJ, Cohen HJ, Lefkowitz RJ. **Beta-adrenergic receptors in lymphocyte subpopulations.** *J Allergy Clin Immunol.* 1980;65:29-33. (English)

To further evaluate the potential utility of lymphocyte beta-adrenergic receptor assays in the study of receptor alterations in human disease, we studied highly purified populations of B and T lymphocytes in peripheral blood to see if differences existed in the concentration or affinity of beta-adrenergic receptors and catecholamine-responsive cAMP levels. The mean number of receptors present in particulate fractions of B cells did not differ significantly from the number found in T cells. Similarly, no significant difference in the dissociation constant for (-)[6H]dihydroalprenolol was found. Cyclic adenosine monophosphate (cAMP) accumulation in whole lymphocytes as measured by radioimmunoassay was comparable, although a tendency toward lower basal and stimulated levels in the T cells was evident. The data suggest that differences observed in concentrations of beta-adrenergic receptors or catecholamine-responsive cAMP accumulation in lymphocytes from patients with varying illnesses are not likely to be due to differences in the proportions of circulating B and T lymphocytes.

309

Boxer LA, Allen JM, Baehner RL. **Diminished polymorphonuclear leukocyte adherence function dependent on release of cyclic AMP by endothelial cells after stimulation of beta-receptors by epinephrine.** *J Clin Invest.* 1980;66:268-74. (English)

To investigate the biochemical and cellular basis for the rise in polymorphonuclear leukocyte (PMN) count during epinephrine administration, PMN from (human) subjects receiving epinephrine were studied for their capacity to adhere to nylon wool fibers and endothelial cell monolayers. After administration of epinephrine, the PMN count increased by 80% at 5 min, and isolated PMN adherence to nylon fibers fell from a base line of 44 ± 2 to $18 \pm 3\%$. When subjects were infused with the beta-antagonist propanolol before receiving epinephrine, the PMN count failed to rise and PMN adherence was normal. Exposure of PMN endothelial cell monolayers exposed to 0.1 microM epinephrine led to diminished PMN adherence that could be blocked by 10 microM propanolol but not by 10 microM phentolamine. Sera obtained from subjects 5 min after receiving epinephrine or from supernates derived from endothelial cell monolayers exposed to 90 nM epinephrine inhibited PMN adherence to nylon fibers. Addition of anti-cyclic AMP antisera but not anti-cyclic GMP antisera to the postepinephrine sera or to the postepinephrine supernate derived from the endothelial cell monolayers abolished their inhibitory effect of PMN adherence to nylon fibers. Direct exposure of PMN to epinephrine failed to affect their adherent properties. Because it was previously shown that endothelial cells contain beta-receptors and respond to catecholamines by raising their intracellular concentrations of cyclic (c)AMP, and that PMN adherence is attenuated by cAMP, it would appear that diminished PMN adherence after epinephrine administration is mediated through endothelial cell beta-receptor activity, which in turn impairs PMN margination *in vivo* and could account for the rise in circulating PMN.

310

Brodde O-E, Engel G, Hoyer D, Bock KD, Weber F. **The beta-adrenergic receptor in human lymphocytes: subclassification by the use of a new radio-ligand, ($\pm$)-[125]Iodocyanopindolol.** *Life Sci.* 1981;29:2189-98. (English)

($\pm$)-[125]Iodocyanopindolol (ICYP), a new radio-ligand with high affinity and specificity to beta-adrenoceptors was used to identify and characterize beta-adrenergic receptors in human lymphocytes. Binding of ICYP was saturable with 1.56 ± 0.2 fmol ICYP specifically bound/10^6 cells at maximal occupancy of the sites and of high affinity ($K_d = 57 \pm 7.1$ pM, n=4). In contrast to [125]iodohydroxybenzylpindolol, ICYP-binding was not affected by phentolamine (up to 10^{-4}M) or serotonin (up to 10^{-5}M). Analysis of inhibition of ICYP-binding via a pseudo-Scatchard-plot ("Hofstee-plot") by beta$_1$-selective (practolol, metoprolol) and beta$_2$-selective (IPS 339, zinterol) adrenergic drugs resulted in linear plots suggesting the existence of a homogeneous population of beta-adrenergic receptors in human lymphocytes. From the resulting K_d-values for practolol (16.8 microM), metoprolol (4.11 microM), zinterol (0.08 microM) and IPS 339 (0.002 microM) it is concluded that the beta-adrenergic receptor present in human lymphocytes is of the beta$_2$-subtype. According to its low non-specific binding and its high specificity to beta-adrenergic receptors ICYP appears to be an ideal ligand for long-term studies on the regulation of beta-adrenergic receptors of human lymphocytes.

311

Busse WW, Anderson CL, Hanson PG, Folts JD. **The effect of exercise on the granulocyte response to isoproterenol in the trained athlete and unconditioned individual.** *J Allergy Clin Immunol.* 1980;65:358-64. (English)

Many factors will influence the tissue response to catecholamine stimulation. Isolated human granulocytes (PMN) release the lysosomal enzyme beta-glucuronidase following incubation with complement-activated zymosan particles. Isoproterenol, histamine and prostaglandin E$_1$ (PGE$_1$) inhibit this PMN release of beta-glucuronidase. The effect of exercise on this *in vitro* granulocyte response was studied in 2 groups: 6 highly conditioned marathon runners and 7 unconditioned subjects (n=7). A 13 km run did not produce leukocytosis in the highly conditioned marathon runners and the granulocyte response to isoproterenol was unchanged in cells obtained immediately following the run. The 7 unconditioned subjects exercised to a maximal response on the treadmill. Following exercise there was an increase in plasma catecholamines, a significant leukocytosis and granulocytes from the immediate postexercise period responded less well to isoproterenol.

312

Busse WW, Lee TP. **Decreased adrenergic responses in lymphocytes and granulocytes in atopic eczema.** *J Allergy Clin Immunol.* 1976;58:586-96. (English)

The physiologic and cyclic adenosine monophosphate (cAMP) response to beta adrenergic stimulation in lymphocytes and granulocytes was examined in atopic eczema. These cells were isolated by Ficoll-Hypaque gradient from 10 patients with atopic eczema, and their responses were compared to 10 normal subjects. In eczema, basal concentrations of cAMP were normal in both lymphocytes and granulocytes. Lymphocyte cAMP response in eczema was decreased both to epinephrine (10^{-5} M) and to isoproterenol (10^{-5} M) but normal to prostaglandin E$_1$ (PGE$_1$). It was also noted that the glycogenolysis response to isoproterenol was significantly less at 10^{-5} M in eczema, but the fall in glycogen was normal with PGE (10^{-5} M and 10^{-7} M). The inhibition of lysosomal enzyme release from granulocytes after zymosan stimulation was significantly less (p<0.01) in eczema with all concentrations of isoproterenol tested. There was also a decrease in cyclic AMP and response to isoproterenol in the polymorphonuclear leukocytes. PGE$_1$ inhibited lysosomal enzyme release and stimulated cAMP normally. In eczema, both lymphocytes and polymorphonuclear leukocytes have a decreased beta-adrenergic response.

313

Colucci WS, Alexander RW, Williams GH, Rude RE, Holman BL, Konstam MA, Wynne J, Mudge GH Jr, Braunwald

E. **Decreased lymphocyte beta-adrenergic receptor density in patients with heart failure and tolerance to the beta-adrenergic agonist pirbuterol.** *N Engl J Med.* 1981; 305:185-90. (English)

We compared the initial and long-term effects of the beta-adrenergic agonist pirbuterol in 12 patients with chronic congestive heart failure. The drug's initial effect was a 35 per cent increase in cardiac index, but there was no significant change in heart rate or mean arterial pressure. After one month of therapy, the mean cardiac index and ejection fraction had returned to base-line values, and no clinical effect was evident in most patients. This apparent tolerance was not accompanied by changes in heart rate, blood pressure or body weight, and it occurred in the presence of therapeutic drug levels during long-term therapy. The density of beta-adrenergic receptors on lymphocytes from patients treated with pirbuterol was significantly depressed as compared with that of patients with heart failure of comparable severity but not treated with pirbuterol. We conclude that tolerance to the hemodynamic and clinical effects of pirbuterol develops during long-term administration. This tolerance may be related to a decrease in myocardial or vascular beta-adrenergic receptors or both.

314
Conolly ME, Greenacre JK. **The lymphocyte beta-adrenoreceptor in normal subjects and patients with bronchial asthma; the effect of different forms of treatment on receptor function.** *J Clin Invest.* 1976;58:1307-16. (English)

Beta-adrenoceptor function has been compared in lymphocytes of normal subjects, asthmatic patients taking large does of beta-adrenergic bronchodilators, and comparable asthmatics treated exclusively with nonadrenergic medication. The effect of prolonged administration of beta-adrenoceptor agonists on receptor function in normal subjects has also been examined. Beta-receptor response in each situation was quantitated by changes in levels of cyclic AMP, measured by protein-binding assay. Dose response curves to isoproterenol (10 nM-0.1 mM) have been constructed for each group. Maximal increase in cyclic AMP in lymphocytes from normal subjects ($393.2 \pm 44.0\%$) and in asthmatics on nonadrenergic preparations (408.3 ± 46.7) was significantly greater ($p<0.001$) than in asthmatics taking large doses of beta-sympathomimetics ($67.5 \pm 24.2\%$). Depression of the cyclic AMP response appeared to correlate with the degree of exposure to beta-adrenergic agonists but not with the prevailing severity of the patient's asthma. Withdrawal of beta-adrenergic drugs was followed by a reversion of the cyclic AMP response to normal values, which suggests that the depression was drug-induced rather than an inherent feature of the disease. This interpretation was confirmed by the finding that prolonged exposure of normal subjects to high doses of a beta-adrenergic agonist caused a marked and significant ($p<0.001$) reduction in the cyclic AMP response, very similar to that seen in asthmatics on large doses of adrenergic bronchodilators. A possible link between drug-induced changes in the cyclic AMP response and the rise in the United Kingdom asthma death rate in the 1960's is discussed.

315
Conolly ME. **Cyclic nucleotides, beta receptors, and bronchial asthma.** *Adv Cyclic Nucleotide Res.* 1980;12:151-9. (English) (no abstract)

316
Davies AO, Lefkowitz RJ. **Corticosteroid-induced differential regulation of beta-adrenergic receptors in circulating human polymorphonuclear leukocytes and mononuclear leukocytes.** *J Clin Endocrinol Metab.* 1980; 51:599-605. (English)

A method of reproducibly measuring human leukocyte beta-adrenergic receptor density and affinity has been developed and applied to the study of receptor regulation in man. The method has the advantages of using a membrane preparation which binds highly specifically and employing techniques such as using low concentrations of [^{3}H]dihydroalprenolol, analyzing the data by computer modelling techniques, and providing data from both granulocytes and lymphocytes in the same individual to minimize measurement errors. Using this methodology, human beta-adrenergic receptor regulation is examined. Cortisone acetate was found to induce an acute rise in granulocyte beta-adrenergic receptor density and adenylate cyclase activity and an acute fall in lymphocyte beta-adrenergic density. This potentially differential regulation of a single receptor subtype in two lines of leukocytes has important implications for the study of receptor regulation in man using leukocyte models.

317
Del Rey A, Besedovsky HO, Sorkin E, De Prada M, Bondiolotti GP. **Sympathetic immunoregulation: difference between high- and low-responder animals.** *Am J Physiol.* 1982;242:R303. (English)

A quantitative relationship is reported between the magnitude of the immune response of rats to SRBC and diminution of splenic noradrenaline (NA). A decrease in concentration and content of NA in the spleen on day 3 after immunization was evident in both high and low responder animals, whereas a diminished concentration of NA persisted only in the high responders. This continuing NA diminution in high responder animals is associated with increase in spleen weight, probably attributable to blood accumulation. These findings are consonant with the concept that the sympathetic nervous system is involved in immunoregulation.

318
Dulis BH, Wilson IB. **The beta-adrenergic receptor of live human polymorphonuclear leukocytes.** *J Biol Chem.* 1980;255:1043-8. (English)

The beta-adrenergic receptor of human polymorphonuclear leukocytes was identified on whole live cells using the high-affinity antagonist [^{3}H]dihydroalprenolol ([^{3}H]DHA). For these studies, it was necessary to inhibit nonspecific retention of permeable amines, including [^{3}H]DHA and propranolol, by these cells. The lysosomotropic agent, chloroquine, effectively decreased nonreceptor uptake without affecting receptor binding. In the presence of chloroquine, agonist potency in competing for [^{3}H]DHA binding was of the order isoproterenol>epinephrine>norepinephrine, and the (-)isomer of isoproterenol is at least 10 times as potent a competitor as is the (+)isomer. Saturation was observed at low ligand concentrations, and equilibrium and kinetic techniques gave $K_d = 0.4$ to 0.5 nM, with approximately 1800 sites/cell. Specific binding is a linear function of cell concentration over a 5-fold range. Antagonist concentrations displacing specific [^{3}H]DHA binding correlate well with concentrations which block agonist effects on lysosomal enzyme release. Close agreement was seen between constants for binding competition and for inhibition of enzyme release for the agonists isoproterenol and epinephrine. Using these live cells, the effects of colchicine on adrenergic binding parameters were investigated. Values for K_d or K_i and nH for the antagonists, (+)-propranolol and [^{3}H]DHA, as well as the number of sites per cell, are unchanged by preincubation with colchicine. K_i values for agonist competition for [^{3}H]DHA binding sites are reduced 4- to 6-fold, and nH is increased to unity. The order of agonist affinity is unchanged by the presence of colchicine. Another inhibitor of microtubule polymerization, vinblastine, causes comparable changes in agonist binding parameters, while the inactive isomer of colchicine, lumicolchicine, has no effect. The possible role of microtubules in regulating equilibrium agonist affinity was discussed.

319

Eskra JD, Stevens JS, Carty TJ. **Beta$_2$-adrenergic receptors in thymocytes (abstract).** *Fed Proc, Fed Am Soc Exp Biol.* 1978;37:687. (English)

The nature of murine thymocyte beta-adrenergic receptor subtype (beta$_1$ or beta$_2$) was investigated. The specificity of beta-agonist action on thymocytes in suspension was measured by the accumulation of cellular cAMP in the presence of the phosphodiesterase inhibitor, Ro 20-1724 [4-(3-butoxy-4-methoxybenzyl)-2-imidazolidinone]. The potency ranking of 4 standard beta-agonists is: isoproterenol (EC$_{50}$, 0.01 microM) > epinephrine (EC$_{50}$, 0.1 microM) > norepinephrine (EC$_{50}$, 5 microM). Preferential activity of the (-)-stereoisomer is observed. Salbutamol and solterenol, selective beta$_2$-agonists, stimulate increases in cAMP levels at low concentration. Butoxamine, a specific beta$_2$-antagonist, causes competitive inhibition of the isoproterenol response, while practolol, a specific beta$_1$-blocker is less effective. Based on this evidence, it is concluded that murine thymocytes have beta$_2$-adrenergic receptors coupled to adenyl cyclase.

320

Ferreia GG, Massuda-Brascher HK, Javierre MQ, Sassine WA, Lima AO. **Rosette formation by human T and B lymphocytes in the presence of adrenergic and cholinergic drugs.** *Experientia.* 1976;32:1594-6. (English)

It was shown that adrenergic drugs, which increase the intracellular levels of cAMP, inhibit the rosette formation by T-lymphocytes, but stimulate the rosettes produced by B-lymphocytes. Cholinergic drugs, which increase the levels of cGMP, on the contrary, stimulate the formation of rosettes by T-lymphocytes but inhibit those produced by B-lymphocytes.

321

Fraser CM, Venter JC, Kaliner M. **Autonomic abnormalities and autoantibodies to beta-adrenergic receptors.** *N Engl J Med.* 1981;305:1165-70. (English)

We identified autoantibodies to beta$_2$-adrenergic receptors in the plasma of three apparently normal subjects, four patients with allergic asthma, one subject who was "preallergic" (at risk of allergy), and one patient with cystic fibrosis. Although these antibodies appeared to be heterogeneous, they shared the ability to affect binding of [^{125}I]protein A to calf-lung membranes, to inhibit beta-adrenergic ligand binding to calf-lung beta-adrenergic receptors, and to precipitate solubilized calf-lung beta-adrenergic receptors in an indirect immunoprecipitation assay. The presence of autoantibodies to beta-adrenergic receptors in these subjects correlates with abnormal autonomic responsiveness characterized by alpha-adrenergic and cholinergic hypersensitivity and beta-adrenergic hyposensitivity. These findings suggest that autoantibodies to beta-adrenergic receptors may play a part in the development of autonomic abnormalities.

322

Fraser J, Nadeau J, Robertson D, Wood AJJ. **Regulation of human leukocyte beta-receptors by endogenous catecholamines: relationship of leukocyte beta-receptor density to the cardiac sensitivity to isoproterenol.** *J Clin Invest.* 1981;67:1777-84. (English)

High levels of beta-receptor agonist down-regulate beta-receptor density on circulating leukocytes in man; factors controlling receptor density under physiological conditions were not previously defined. To determine whether beta-receptor density is normally down-regulated by circulating, physiological levels of catecholamines the relationship between receptor density and catecholamine levels was examined. Urinary epinephrine and norepinephrine were significantly reciprocally correlated to lymphocyte receptor density. A similar relationship existed between beta-receptor density and supine plasma epinephrine, norepinephrine, upright epinephrine and norepinephrine levels. Change in Na$^+$ intake from 10 to 400 meq/day caused a 52% increase in lymphocyte and a 48% increase in polymorphonuclear beta-receptor density. The changes in receptor density were accompanied by an increase in the sensitivity to isoproterenol measured as a fall in the dose of isoproterenol required to raise the heart rate by 25 beats/min. Beta-receptor density on lymphocyte and polymorphonuclear cells was significantly correlated to the cardiac sensitivity to isoproterenol. Propranolol administration resulted in an increase in the density of beta-receptors on lymphocyte and polymorphonuclear cells that correlated with the subject's pretreatment catecholamine levels. Physiological levels of catecholamines normally down-regulate beta-receptors in man and blockade of this down-regulation by propranolol apparently allows receptor density to increase.

323

Fugner A. **Inhibition of antigen-induced histamine release by beta adrenergic stimulants in vivo.** *Int Arch Allergy Appl Immunol.* 1977;54:78-87. (English)

IgE-mediated histamine release was studied using the method of passive peritoneal anaphylaxis (PPA) in the rat. Some beta-adrenergic stimulants markedly inhibited this reaction *in vivo*, the order of potency (ED_{50} microg/kg i.v.) of agents tested being fenoterol, salbutamol and isoproterenol. Higher activity against the simultaneously measured dye extravasation suggested a dual effect of the drugs on both the cellular (inhibition of histamine release) and the vascular level. The order of potency in modifying vascular injury was, however, reversed, isoproterenol and not fenoterol being relatively more active here, as could be shown by further experiments. Inhibition of histamine release is discussed with respect to (a) methodical requirements and (b) the suggestion that beta$_2$-receptor stimulants (fenoterol, salbutamol) are more selective than isoproterenol.

324

Galant SP, Allred SJ. **Demonstration of beta$_2$-adrenergic receptors of high coupling efficiency in human neutrophil sonicates.** *J Lab Clin Med.* 1980;96:15-23. (English)

Using highly purified (>95%) neutrophil (PMN [polymorphonuclear leukocyte]) sonicates, beta-adrenergic (beta$_1$/beta$_2$) pattern of adenylate cyclase activation after agonist stimulation and the coupling characteristics of the beta-adrenergic receptor to the adenylate cyclase enzyme were studied. Adenylate cyclase was highly responsive to agonist activation, with peak isoproterenol (100 microM) stimulation causing the generation of 119 ± 9.5 (mean $\pm$ SEM [SE of mean]) pmol/mg per min cyclic[c]AMP (224% above basal levels) compared to 171.7 ± 8.6 following NaF (10mM) stimulation. The agonist pattern of adenylate cyclase activation suggested the presence of beta$_2$-adrenergic receptors, as isoproterenol with a K_{act} [activation constant] of 0.7 microM was more potent than epinephrine (K_{act} = 90 microM). Butoxamine (beta$_2$-antagonist) was approx. 25 times more potent than practolol (beta$_1$-antagonist), with $K_{d's}$ of 0.75 and 17.5 microM respectively. Receptor coupling efficiency was determined by measuring isoproterenol binding and adenylate cyclase activation with the same PMN sonicates and incubation conditions for each assay. The apparent K_d for isoproterenol binding was 2.82 ± 0.53 microM, the K_{act} was 0.47 ± 0.05 microM and the mean K_d/K_{act} ratio was 6.5. Using sucrose gradient-purified PMN sonicates, isoproterenol required the guanine nucleotides GTP or Gpp(NH)p [5'-guanylyl-imidodiphosphate] to activate adenylate cyclase. The GTP effect on adenylate cyclase responsiveness to isoproterenol was associated with a 10-fold decrease in the isoproterenol binding affinity. Apparently the human PMN has beta$_2$-adrenergic receptors which are highly coupled to the adenylate cyclase enzyme. PMN sonicates provide a suitable model for the study of beta$_2$-adrenergic receptors and the mechanism of hormone-induced adenylate cyclase activation in man.

325

Galant SP, Duriseti L, Underwood S, Insel PA. **Decreased beta-adrenergic receptors in polymorphonuclear leukocytes after adrenergic therapy.** *N Engl J Med.* 1978; 299:933-6. (English) (no abstract)

326

Galant SP, Lundak RL, Eaton L. **Enhancement of early human E rosette formation by cholinergic stimuli.** *J Immunol.* 1976;117:48-51. (English)

The effects of the cholinergic stimuli carbamylcholine (carbachol) and dibutyrol cyclic guanosine monophosphate (DBcGMP) were determined on both "early" and "total" E rosette formation. Ficoll-Hypaque-separated lymphocytes were preincubated with either carbachol or DBcGMP over a 10^{-3} to 10^{-13}M dose range. Both agents significantly enhanced "early", but not "total" E rosette formation. Peak enhancement above control values ocurred at 10^{-7}M (72%) and 10^{-9}M (69%) for carbachol and 10^{-5}M (70%) and 10^{-7}M (70%) for DBcGMP. Kinetic studies showed a rapid onset of enhancement (2.5 min) for carbachol, whereas DBcGMP required 15 min for significant enhancement to occur. The muscurinic nature of carbachol enhancement of E rosettes was demonstrated. Atropine at 10^{-7}M completely abolished the carbachol effect while showing little inhibition of the DBcGMP effect on rosette formation. These studies indicate that the cholinergic stimuli carbachol and DBcGMP significantly enhance the "early" E rosette former in man. Human T lymphocytes appear to have functional cholinergic receptors that can be blocked by the muscarinic antagonist atropine. The role of the cyclic nucleotides and their stimulants on the immune system is incompletely understood, but it would appear that they are extremely important in the differentiation and function of the T lymphocyte. E rosette formation may be a useful model in man for studying the effects of the cyclic nucleotides on the human T lymphocyte.

327

Galant SP, Underwood S, Duriseti L, Insel PA. **Characterization of high-affinity beta$_2$-adrenergic receptor binding of (-)[^{3}H]dihydroalprenolol to human polymorphonuclear cell particulates.** *J Lab Clin Med.* 1978;92:613-8. (English)

Human PMNs have well-described responses to beta-adrenergic catecholamines; these include elevation of cellular levels of cyclic AMP and inhibition of the release of lysosomal contents. Using the radioactive beta-adrenergic antagonist (-)-[^{3}H]DHA in direct ligand-binding studies, we have identified and characterized beta-adrenergic receptors on particulate preparations of PMNs. These particulates bind DHA rapidly ($t_{1/2}$<1 min) and reversibly ($t_{1/2}$= 8 to 9 min). DHA binding is saturable and of high affinity (dissociation constant= 1 to 5 nM) and low capacity (870 ± 128 receptors/cell, mean $\pm$ SD) to a single class of binding sites. Competition for DHA binding sites by both beta-adrenergic agonists and antagonists is stereoselective [(-)-isomers more potent than (+)-isomers]. The rank order of potency of adrenergic agents in such competition studies indicates that these receptors are of the beta$_2$ type. Since PMNs can be obtained in high purity with relative ease, the combined use of pharmacologic and ligand-binding sites in PMNs provide a useful system for studying beta-adrenergic receptors and their function in human subjects.

328

Grabczewska E, Krzystyniak K, Ryzewski J. **Cholinergic stimulation of lymphocytes *in vitro*.** *Bull Acad Sci Biol.* 1979;27:883-7. (English)

The authors found that the stimulators--acetylcholine and PHA--mutually interfere in affecting the incorporation of

[³H]thymidine in cultures of rat lymphocytes from peripheral lymph nodes. A positive effect of acetylcholine was obtained only when the lymphocytes had previously been subjected to suboptimal doses of PHA. Proliferation was inhibited whenever the sequence of the stimulators was changed or the lymphocytes were stimulated with an optimal dose of PHA. The effect of muscarinic antagonists of acetylcholine was opposite to that caused by acetylcholine itself. Changes in cAMP and cGMP levels in lymphocytes treated with acetylcholine and PHA were determined.

329
Grieco MH, Siegel I, Goel Z. **Modulation of human T lymphocyte rosette formation by autonomic agonists and cyclic nucleotides.** *J Allergy Clin Immunol.* 1976; 58:149-59. (English)

Early rosette formation by T lymphocytes appear to be modulated by cyclic nucleotides. Dibutyryl cyclic 3',5' adenosine monophosphate (cyclic AMP) 10^{-2} M inhibited E rosette formation up to 83%, while 10^{-6} M 8-bromo-cyclic guanosine monophosphate (cyclic GMP) increased rosette formation maximally to 67.4% with less pronounced effect at increased concentrations. T lymphocyte receptors for beta- adrenergic, alpha-adrenergic, and muscarinic cholinergic agonists appear to influence rosette formation. Isoproterenol 10^{-2} M induced 67.3% inhibition, while phenylephrine 10^{-5} M and carbamylcholine 10^{-4} M were associated with enhanced rosette formation of 67.2% and 57.8%, respectively. Selective blockade with propranolol, phentolamine, and atropine indicated the presence of separate receptor sites. The lack of effect of histamine at concentrations of 10^{-3} M and above suggests the absence of specific receptors on peripheral human lymphocytes.

330
Hall NR, McClure JE, Hu S-K, Tick NT, Seales CM, Goldstein AL. **Effects of chemical sympathectomy upon thymus-dependent immune responses (abstract).** *Soc Neurosc Abstr.* 1980;6:68. (English)

Several immunologic parameters were measured in C57Bl/6J male mice following treatment with 100 mg/kg i.p. of 6-hydroxydopamine (6-OHDA). Twenty-four hours after drug treatment, a single i.p. injection of sheep red blood cells (SRBC) was given to the primary (1°) immune response subjects (n=8). Secondary (2°) immune response animals (n=8) received a second SRBC injection 21 days after the first sensitization. The immune system was evaluated 5 days after the final antigen injection. A single cell suspension of spleen cells was dispensed in triplicate onto agarose-coated slides for the plaque forming cell assay (PFC). An enzymatic assay was used to measure thymocyte levels of terminal deoxynucleotidyl transferase (TdT) and a radioimmunoassay was used to measure serum levels of thymosin alpha₁. No significant differences between body, thymus and spleen weights were measured between the 6-OHDA versus the saline treated control group in either the 1° or 2° immune response. Antibody production as measured by PFC and hemagglutination assays was significantly reduced in the drug treated animals after 1° and 2° exposure to the SRBC's. The response to LPS was also reduced, but 6-OHDA increased the spleen cell response to Con A, PHA-P and PWM. These increased

measures were observed only in the 1° immune response group. Thymocyte TdT levels were significantly elevated by 6-OHDA treatment in the 1° response group but were not different from control values in the 2° response mice. Preliminary measurement of thymosin alpha₁ revealed a significant increase in levels of this peptide hormone in the serum of drug treated animals in both the 1° and 2° response groups. These data suggest involvement of the autonomic nervous system in modulating the immune response to thymus-dependent antigens. The possibility that the endocrine thymus performs an important function in a central nervous system-immune system axis is currently being investigated.

331
Harden TK, Cotton CU, Waldo GL, Lutton JK, Perkins JP. **Catecholamine-induced alteration in sedimentation behavior of membrane-bound beta-adrenergic receptors.** *Science.* 1980;210:441-3. (English)

Incubation of astrocytoma cells with catecholamines results in decrease in catecholamine-stimulated adenylate cyclase activity and a concomitant alteration in the sedimentation properties of particulate beta-adrenergic receptors. The altered receptors exhibit agonist binding properties similar to those of receptors that are "uncoupled" from adenylate cyclase.

332
Ito M, Sless F, Parrott DM. **Evidence for control of complement receptor rosette-forming cells by alpha- and beta-adrenergic agents.** *Nature.* 1977;89:266:633-5. (English) (no abstract)

333
Johnson DL, Gordon MA. **Effect of chronic beta-adrenergic therapy on the human lymphocyte response to concanavalin A.** *Res Commun Chem Pathol Pharmacol.* 1981;32:377-80. (English)

Lymphocytes isolated from cystic fibrosis patients chronically treated with beta-adrenergic agonists respond significantly differently to epinephrine modulation of mitogen challenge than cystic fibrosis patients not receiving beta-adrenergic therapy and than normal human volunteers. Those patients on chronic beta-adrenergic therapy are insensitive to the modulating effects of l-epinephrine. This observation is discussed in terms of adrenergic receptor alteration and/or different cystic fibrosis disease states.

334
Kasahara K, Tanaka S, Hamashima Y. **Suppression of the primary immune response by chemical sympathectomy.** *Res Commun Chem Pathol Pharmcol.* 1977; 16:687-94. (English)

The effects of general sympathectomy with 6-hydroxydopamine (6-OHDA) on antibody production to sheep red blood cells (SRBC) were studied in mice. Intraperitoneal administration of 6-OHDA in a dose of 1 to 300 mg/kg resulted in a significant decrease in hemagglutinin titer and number of direct plaque-forming cells which were observed only in the early period of the primary immune response. Following treatment with 6-OHDA 10 mg/kg i.p., the noradrenaline content in murine spleen was significantly reduced from 63 to 42% of control value between 2 and 10 days after injection indicating that chemical sympathectomy supresses the primary immune response.

335

Koslov VK, Arkhangel'skaia SL, Vasil'eva EF. **Beta-adrenoreceptors on the surface membranes of lymphocytes and macrophages.** *Biull Eksp Biol Med.* 1978; 85:723-5. (Russian)

In experiments *in vivo* and *in vitro* on sensitized and intact guinea pigs and Wistar rats, the effect of beta-adrenergic stimulants (adrenaline and isoproterenol) and a beta-adrenergic blocker (propranalol) on lymphocytolysis and the reaction of macrophage adherence inhibition was studied. Adrenaline and isoproterenol were shown to inhibit the antigen interaction with both sensitized and intact cells. Restoring the sensitivity of cells to the antigen, propranalol destroys the defensive action of adrenaline and isoproterenol.

336

Krall JF, Connelly M, Tuck ML. **Acute regulation of beta-adrenergic catecholamine sensitivity in human lymphocytes.** *J Pharmacol Exp Ther.* 1980;214:554-60. (English)

Human lymphocytes were used to examine acute regulation of adenylate cyclase by beta-adrenergic catecholamines in man. Hormone sensitivity was evaluated with respect to the requirements for agonist-induced desensitization of lymphocyte cAMP production. Lymphocytes from control or agonist-treated subjects were isolated by centrifugation of Ficoll-Hypaque gradients. cAMP was measured by competitive protein-binding assay. Beta-adrenergic receptors on intact lymphocytes were quantitated by Scatchard analysis of specific binding of the beta- adrenergic antagonist (-)[^{3}H]dihydroalprenolol. Binding sites displayed high affinity ($K_d < 1.5$ nM) and stereospecificity characteristic of beta-adrenergic receptors characterized previously by using membrane fragments. Studies examining cells exposed to isoproterenol *in vitro*, were compared with cells from *in vivo* studies obtained from subjects during isoproterenol infusion. cAMP generation by human lymphocytes *in vitro* was rapidly increased by 1 microM isoproterenol (3.2 ± 0.4 to 6.6 ± 0.6 pmol of cAMP/10^6 cells). Cells incubated with 1 microM isoproterenol for 30 min *in vitro* rapidly lost responsiveness to rechallenge with the agonist. Over an isoproterenol concentration range 0.1-100 microM, agonist-dependent desensitization of adenylate cyclase was accompanied by a parallel reduction in beta-adrenergic receptor number. In contrast, cells incubated with very low (0.01 nM) concentrations of isoproterenol demonstrated rapid desensitization of cAMP production independent of changes in beta-adrenergic receptor number. Lymphocytes from subjects receiving isoproterenol infusion showed desensitization of agonist-dependent cAMP production without significant reduction in beta- adrenergic receptor number. Additional time course studies revealed that the desensitized state persisted *in vitro* and *in vivo* for several hours after removal of the agonist. Catecholamine agonists are capable of inducing rapid prolonged reductions in sensitivity of lymphocyte cAMP production *in vitro* and *in vivo*. Over a wide dose range acute decreases in cAMP production

in vitro are mediated by a reduction in beta-adrenergic receptor number. Exogenous hormone-induced refractoriness *in vivo*, and at low agonist doses *in vitro*, may not be associated with similar changes in receptor number. This may reflect higher agonist concentrations achievable *in vitro* or indicate that mechanisms independent of receptor changes contribute to desensitization of beta-adrenergic-mediated adenylate cyclase in man.

337

Minakuchi K, Ogawa K, Ban M, Satake T. **Decreased generation of cyclic AMP in lymphocytes by beta-adrenergic stimulation in heart failure.** *Jpn Heart J.* 1981;22:585-92. (English)

Peripheral blood lymphocytes from 31 normal subjects and 29 patients with heart diseases were stimulated by isoproterenol, and cyclic AMP level in lymphocytes was assayed. Simultaneously plasma norepinephrine concentration at rest was measured. In normal subjects the generation of cyclic AMP after the stimulation decreased with age. The response of lymphocytes in patients of NYHA classes III and IV was significantly smaller than in the normal, age-matched control. Plasma norepinephrine concentration of patients of classes II, III, and IV rose significantly above normal. In congestive heart failure, a significant correlation between plasma norepinephrine concentration and increase of lymphocyte cyclic AMP was demonstrated. From these results it was suggested that beta-adrenergic receptors in congestive heart failure were desensitized.

338

Morris HG, Rusnak SA, Selner JC, Barnes J. **Diminished leukocyte cyclic AMP responses to adrenergic stimulation after therapeutic administration of beta-adrenergic agonists.** *Chest.* 1978;73:973-4. (English) (no abstract)

339

Morris HG, Rusnak SA, Selner JC, Barzens K, Barnes J. **Adrenergic desensitization in leukocytes of normal and asthmatic subjects.** *J Cyclic Nucleotide Res.* 1977;3:439-46. (English)

Cyclic AMP was measured in leukocytes of normal asthmatic subjects before and after one week of treatment with equal amounts of ephedrine. During the control and placebo periods, the measurements of cyclic AMP in leukocytes of asthmatic subjects were similar to those of normal individuals. After one week of treatment with ephedrine, both groups exhibited suppression of the leukocyte cyclic AMP response to adrenergic stimulation *in vitro*; however, the suppression of response was significantly greater in asthmatic subjects (p<.01). Subcutaneous administration of epinephrine was followed by further suppression of the leukocyte cyclic AMP response to *in vitro* stimulation which was similar in both groups during all treatment periods. The results indicate that *in vivo* exposure to adrenergic medications is followed by desensitization of the leukocyte responses to subsequent adrenergic stimulation *in vitro*. After administration of small doses of medication, the severity and/or duration of desensitization is significantly greater in asthmatic leukocytes.

340

Mue S, Ohmi T, Tamura G, Ishihara T, Fujimoto S, Takishima T. **The effect of sympathomimetic drugs on immediate skin reactions and metabolic responses in asthmatic patients.** *Ann Allergy.* 1979;43:302-9. (English)

The varied effects of intradermal injection of isoproterenol and propranolol on the immediate skin reaction were studied in relation to the metabolic responses to the i.v. injection of epinephrine. In asthmatic patients whose skin reaction was not suppressed with $10^{-7}M$ isoproterenol, the hypoglycemic response after the injection of epinephrine was significantly reduced.

341

Patterson R, Suszko IM, Metzger WJ, Roberts M. *In vitro* **production of IgE by human peripheral blood lymphocytes: effect of cholera toxin and beta-adrenergic stimulation.** *J Immunol.* 1976;117:97-101. (English)

Peripheral blood lymphocytes from two human donors with elevated serum IgE concentrations were maintained in short-term tissue culture preparations. Repeated culture preparations demonstrated that IgE was produced *in vitro* in amounts that could be measured by the double antibody radioimmunoassay technique. The amount of IgE produced by replicate cultures of cells from a single bleeding of the donor was similar when the cultures were simultaneously prepared. In contrast, IgE production by the same donor's lymphocytes varied when the culture preparations were initiated from separate bleedings. The results of simultaneous cultures of a single bleeding were sufficiently consistent to provide a means of testing the effect of pharmacologic agents on the *in vitro* production of IgE. Cholera toxin effected a marked reduction in production of IgE by lymphocytes of both cell donors. Isoproterenol showed marked inhibition of IgE production at 10^3M but cell viability studies suggested that this may have been due to decreased cell viability. At lower, nontoxic concentrations of isoproterenol (10^4M-10^6M) slight but definite inhibition of *in vitro* IgE production was evident. This inhibition was more pronounced subsequent to the first 24 hr of exposure of the cells to isoproterenol.

342

Pochet R, Delespesse G, Gausset PW, Collet H. **Distribution of beta- adrenergic receptors on human lymphocyte sub-populations.** *Clin Exp Immunol.* 1979;38:578-84. (English)

A technique is described allowing the quantification and the characterization of specific beta-adrenergic receptors in intact living human lymphocytes. ^{125}I-Iodohydroxybenzylpindolol (HYP), a potent beta-adrenergic antagonist, was used to label specific binding sites on unfractionated lymphoid cells and on purified subpopulations of T (thymus-derived) (F_1 and F_2) and B (bone marrow-derived) cells. F_1 and F_2 were obtained by filtration through nylon wool column as previously described; they differ in their response to mitogens and in their interactions with adherent cells and B cells. ^{125}I-HYP binding to unfractionated lymphocytes was a saturable, stereospecific and rapid process with a K_d of 2.5 $10^{-10}M$ and a binding capacity of 400-600 sites/cell. Bindings on unfractionated

lymphocytes, purified B cells and T cells of the F_2 fraction were similar. No detectable binding was noted on T cells from the F_1 fraction. Enriched T cells obtained by a rosetting technique displayed 200 receptors/cell. (These findings have relevance to the influence of catecholamines on immune functions.)

343

Ponassi A, Burzzi P, Parodi GB, Sacchetti C, Morra L. **Influence of the spleen on blood distribution of leukocytes producing colony-stimulating activity in man.** *Blut.* 1981;42:41-6. (German)

The colony-stimulating activity (CSA) produced by the blood leukocytes was studied before and after epinephrine administration in 10 normal, 15 splenomegalic and 7 splenectomized subjects through a double layer agar culture system. A significant increase of mean values of the CSA/ml produced by blood monocytes was observed after epinephrine administration in the groups of normal and splenomegalic subjects. In the group of splenectomized subjects the baseline mean values of CSA/ml of blood was higher than those observed in the other groups, but it showed no increase after epinephrine infusion. The CSA produced by 10^6 blood leukocytes was similar in all 3 groups of subjects and was not similarly modified by epinephrine administration. The leukocytes producing CSA are distributed within 2 rapidly exchangeable blood compartments, the spleen representing an important section of the marginal compartment of blood monocytes.

344

Scorza-Smeraldi R, Smeraldi E, Fabio G, Bellodi L, Sacchetti E, Rugarli C. **Interference between anti-HLA antibodies and adrenergic receptor-binding drugs.** *Tissue Antigens.* 1977;9:163-6. (English) (no abstract)

345

Singh U, Millson DS, Smith PA, Owen JJT. **Identification of beta-adrenoreceptors during thymocyte ontogeny in mice.** *Eur J Immunol.* 1979;9:31-5. (English)

Thymocytes have been studied at various stages during ontogeny in relation to their responsiveness to beta-adreno-receptor agonists and ability to bind L-[propyl-2,3,-^{3}H]dihydroalprenolol ([^{3}H]DHA), a specific radioligand of the beta-adrenoreceptor. Specific [^{3}H]DHA binding and activity of an isoproterenol-sensitive adenylate cyclase were compared and correlated between (14 to 20 day) fetal mouse thymocytes and young adult thymocytes. Preliminary experiments show that [^{3}H]DHA binding to thymocytes demonstrated the kinetics, affinity and sterospecificity expected of binding to adenylate cyclase-coupled beta-adrenoreceptors. Similarly, isoproterenol was shown to selectively increase intracellular adenosine 3',5'-cyclic monophosphate (cAMP) levels and was antagonized by propranolol (a beta-adrenoreceptor antagonist), but not by phentolamine (an alpha-adrenoreceptor antagonist), nor by lignocaine (a local anesthetic). The rises in fetal thymocyte cAMP levels found after stimulation with isoproterenol were of greater magnitude than in adult thymocytes. The number of [^{3}H]DHA-binding sites in both fetal and adult thymocytes was the same (B_{max} = 50 fmol/2×10^6 cells). However, the affinity of the binding sites for [^{3}H]DHA was less for the adult cells than the fetal cells (with K_D values of 8.0 and 22 nM, respectively); this was in the embryonic cells.

347

Tohmeh JF, Cryer PE. **Biphasic adrenergic modulation of beta-adrenergic receptors in man: agonist-induced early increment and late decrement in beta-adrenergic receptor number.** *J Clin Invest.* 1980;65:836-40. (English)

Beta-adrenergic receptors in mononuclear leukocyte preparations were assessed with (-)[^{3}H]-dihydroalprenolol binding studies during the infusion of adrenergic agonists into normal human subjects. During the infusion of isoproterenol into 7 subjects, mean ($\pm$ SE) (-)[^{3}H]-dihydroalprenolol binding increased from 25 ± 3 f[femto]mol/mg protein to 47 ± 8 fmol/mg protein (p<0.02) at 0.5 h and 40 ± 3 fmol/mg protein (p<0.01) at 1 h and decreased to 12 ± 1 fmol/mg protein (p<0.01) at 4-6 h. During the infusion of epinephrine into 3 subjects mean (-)[^{3}H]dihydroalprenolol binding increased from 32 ± 3 to 63 ± 3 fmol/mg protein (p<0.01) at 0.5-1 h. By Scatchard plot analysis, the changes were attributable to changes in the number of available binding sites rather than changes in binding affinity. The observed changes in the number of (-)[^{3}H]dihydroalprenolol binding sites were not paralleled by changes in total mononuclear cell counts or in T [thymus-derived] lymphocyte, B [bone marrow-derived] lymphocyte and monocyte distributions. Adrenergic agonists may modulate the number of available beta-adrenergic receptors on circulating mononuclear cells in a biphasic manner with an early increment and a late decrement, in man. The finding that the increase in pulse rate in response to a pulse infusion of isoproterenol was significantly greater after 0.5-1 h of agonist infusion suggests that the observed early agonist-induced increment in beta-adrenergic receptor number on circulating cells is paralleled by increments in extra-vascular beta-adrenergic receptor sensitivity.

348

Tuck ML, Fittingoff D, Connelly M, Krall JF. **Beta-adrenergic catecholamine regulation of lymphocyte sensitivity heterologous desensitization to prostaglandin E$_2$ by isoproterenol.** *J Clin Endocrinol Metab.* 1980; 51:1-6. (English)

Human lymphocytes isolated from peripheral blood increased c[cyclic] AMP production up to 2.5-fold in a dose-dependent manner in the presence of the beta-adrenergic catecholamine agonist isoproterenol and up to 5-fold in the presence of prostaglandin E$_2$ (PGE$_2$). Cells maximally stimulated by PGE$_2$ failed to show further increases in cAMP production when isoproterenol was also added, suggesting that the same cells were sensitive to both agonists. When incubated with isoproterenol for up to 430 min and then washed free of the agonist before restimulation with fresh isoproterenol or PGE$_2$, cells showed a time-dependent loss of sensitivity to both agonists. Isoproterenol-dependent desensitization to PGE$_2$ was both less extensive and more slowly developing than desensitization to isoproterenol, and proceeded in the presence of indomethacin and in indomethacin-pretreated cells. Both desensitizaion to PGE$_2$ and cAMP production demonstrated similar isoproterenol dose dependency with a half-maximal concentration of 0.1 microM, but neither 8-

bromo-cAMP nor 8-bromo cGMP had the desensitizing effects of isoproterenol. Evidence of similar heterologous desensitization to PGE$_2$ by isoproterenol was sought *in vivo* by infusing subjects with the beta-adrenergic catecholamine. Lymphocytes isolated during the course infusion showed a loss of sensitivity to both isoproterenol and PGE$_2$ over a 60 min period. Lymphocytes from asthmatic eceiving chronic beta-adrenergic catecholamine therapy (80 mg metaproterenol/day) also showed reduced sensitivity to both isoproterenol and PGE$_2$ compared to cells from normal subjects. Beta-adrenergic catecholamines apparently have heterologous desensitizing effects in human tissues, at least with respect to PGE$_2$. Heterologous desensitization is a property of acute regulation of beta-adrenergic catecholamine and PGE$_2$ target cell function and occurs *in vivo* as well as *in vitro*. Some therapeutic effects of beta-adrenergic catecholamine administration may be attributed to desensitization to more than one agonist.

349

Vardanian IK, Golubeva NN, Seslavina LS, Sitkovski MV. **Interaction of noradrenaline and alpha-adrenoblockers with lymphoid cells.** *Fiziol Zh.* 1979;25:627-33. (Russian)

An attempt is made to find out the effect of norepinephrine and alpha-adrenoblocking agents on the lymphocyte surface membranes and realization of a transmembrane signal at the metabolic and functional level of the immunocompetent cells. It is shown that unidirectional inhibitory effect of the above drugs provokes different changes in metabolism, which results in various functional changes of immunocompetent cells.

350

Welscher HD, Cruchaud A. **Conditions for maximal synthesis of cyclic-AMP by mouse macrophages in response to beta-adrenergic stimulation.** *Eur J Immunol.* 1978;8:180-4. (English)

The synthesis of cyclic AMP by mouse peritoneal macrophages in response to stimulation by isoproterenol was studied as a function of drug concentration, incubation time and cell density. Cyclic AMP levels of macrophages increased 3 to 3.5 times over the control level 20 sec after the addition of 10^{-3}M isoproterenol. Under these conditions the dose response could be followed down to an isoproterenol concentration of 10^{-6} to 10^{-7} M. When cell suspensions were inactivated as early as 1 sec after the addition of the drug, the increase in cyclic AMP was much greater (153 vs. 25 pmol/10^7 cells). Macrophage suspensions of high cell density were less responsive than those of low cell density. In the absence of any inhibitor of phosphodiesterase, the stimulatory effect of isoproterenol was always of short duration. The maximal effect of beta-adrenergic stimulation probably occurs in less than 1 sec at a cell density less than 2×10^6 cells/ml. The beta-blocking drug Visken abolished the observed effects.

351

Williams LT, Snyderman R, Lefkowitz RJ. **Identification of beta-adrenergic receptors in human lymphocytes by (-)[^{3}H]alprenolol binding.** *J Clin Invest.* 1976;57:149-55. (English)

Human lymphocytes are known to possess a catecholamine-responsive adenylate cyclase which has typical beta-adrenergic specificity. To identify directly and to quantitate these beta-adrenergic receptors in human lymphocytes, (-)[³H]alprenolol, a potent beta-adrenergic antagonist, was used to label binding sites in homogenates of human mononuclear leukocytes. Binding of (-)[³H]alprenolol to these sites demonstrated the kinetics, affinity and stereospecificity expected of binding to adenylate cyclase-coupled beta-adrenergic receptors. Binding was rapid ($t_{1/2}$<30 s) and rapidly reversible ($t_{1/2}$<3 min) at 37°C. Binding was a saturable process with 75 ± 12 fmol (-)[³H]alprenolol bound/mg protein (mean $\pm$ SEM) at saturation, corresponding to about 2,000 sites per cell. Half-maximal saturation occurred at 10 nM (-)[³H]alprenolol, which provides an estimate of the dissociation constant of (-)[³H]alprenolol for the beta-adrenergic receptor. The beta-adrenergic antagonist, (-)propranolol, potently competed for the binding sites, causing half-maximal inhibition of binding at 9 nM. Beta-adrenergic agonists also competed for the binding sites. The order of potency was (-)isoproterenol > (-)epinephrine > (-)norepinephrine which agreed with the order of potency of these agents in stimulating leukocyte adenylate cyclase. Dissociation constants computed from binding experiments were virtually identical to those obtained from adenylate cyclase activation studies. Marked stereospecificity was observed for both binding and activation of adenylate cyclase. (-)Stereoisomers of beta-adrenergic agonists and antagonists were 9- to 300-fold more potent than their corresponding (+)stereoisomers. Structurally related compounds devoid of beta-adrenergic activity such as dopamine, dihydroxymandeliic acid, normetanephrine, pyrocatechol and phentolamine did not effectively compete for the binding sites. (-)[³H]alprenolol binding to human mononuclear leukocyte preparations was almost entirely accounted for by binding to small lymphocytes, the predominant cell type in the preparations. No binding was detectable to human erythrocytes. These results demonstrate the feasibility of using direct binding methods to study beta-adrenergic receptors in a human tissue. They also provide an experimental approach to the study of states of altered sensitivity to catecholamines at the receptor level in man.

352

Williams RS, Guthrow CE, Lefkowitz RJ. **Beta-adrenergic receptors of human lymphocytes are unaltered by hyperthyroidism.** *J Clin Endocrinol Metab.* 1979;48:503-5. (English)

Lymphocytes from 12 patients with untreated hyperthyroidism were compared to lymphocytes from age- and sex-matched euthyroid control subjects to test the hypothesis that alterations in beta-adrenergic response mechanisms occur in human hyperthyroidism. The binding of (-)[³H]dihydroalprenolol, a compound previously shown in these cells to label binding sites having the characteristics of beta-adrenergic receptors, was assayed and no significant difference was found between the two groups. In addition, the accumulation of cAMP in response to isoproterenol was determined by RIA and, again, no difference was found.

353

Winchurch RA, Mardiney MR Jr. **The effects of adrener-gic agonists and blockers on antigen-induced DNA synthesis in vitro.** *Biomedicine.* 1977;26:36-42. (English)

The effects of both alpha- and beta-adrenergic agonists and blockers on antigen-stimulated DNA synthesis in human lymphocyte cultures were studied. Results show that antigen-induced responses were enhanced by the presence of the beta blockers, propranolol and dichloroisoproterenol, and that this effect appeared to be specific blocking of the lymphocyte beta receptor since D(+)propranolol, a compound devoid of such activity, has no effect. Similarly, an alpha-adrenergic agonist such as norepinephrine enhanced lymphocyte responsiveness.

Psychotropic agents

354

A-Wahid F, Meisheri KD, Isom GE. **Suppression of morphine physical dependence and tolerance by immune activation.** *Proc West Pharmacol Soc.* 1979;22:483-8. (English)

Numerous studies indicate chronic responses to opiates may involve, in part, an immune component and that alteration of the immune system changes opiate responses. Kornetsky & Kiplinger demonstrated that serum from tolerant animals can alter the antinociceptive action of morphine in the serum recipients. Berkowitz & Spector produced active immunization which altered the disposition of the narcotic and the pharmacological response was reduced. Suppression or stimulation of the immune system alters physical dependence and tolerance development to morphine. Cosenza and Kohler demonstrated that the immunoglobulin receptor for an antigen is potentially antigenic. Antibodies directed against the immunoglobulin receptor suppress specifically immune responses to that antigen and antireceptor antibodies will suppress immune responses *in vivo*. In the present study, this antireceptor antibody technique was used to alter physical dependence and tolerance to opiates in laboratory animals. Rabbit antimorphine serum was used as an antigen in the active immunization of laboratory animals. Theoretically this immunological technique may induce formation of antimorphine receptor antibodies and alter the function of the endogenous opiate receptor.

355

Baker GA, Santalo R, Blumenstein J. **Effect of psychotropic agents upon the blastogenic response of human T-lymphocytes.** *Biol Psychiat.* 1977;12:159-69. (English)

Antischizophrenic agents, phenothiazine and nonphenothiazine, inhibit the transformation of the T-lymphocyte *in vitro*. This inhibition occurs only in the early event and is neither competitive with dopamine, nor appears to involve Na^+/K^+ adenosine triphosphatase. RNA synthesis is more sensitive to the inhibitory effect than DNA or protein synthesis. This leads to the conclusion that chlorpromazine may act by inhibiting the synthesis of newly formed RNA, and subsequently, transformation, rather than by alteration of the cell membrane.

356

Balitskii KP. **Increase in the antitumor protection of the** body by pharmacological correction of the neurohumoral status. *Vopr Onkol.* 1982;28:50-4. (Russian) (unavailable at publication)

357
Barker W, Rodenheaver GT, Edgerton MT, Edlich RF. **Damage to tissue defenses by a topical anesthetic agent.** *Ann Emerg Med.* 1982;11:307-10. (English)

The purpose of this study was to determine the effect of a topical application of a solution containing 0.5% tetracaine, 1:2000 epinephrine, and 11.9% cocaine on the wound's ability to resist infection. In this experimental study, this solution potentiated the development of wound infection. This effect can be explained by its vasoconstrictive action limiting access of the cellular defenses to the bacteria on the wound surface.

358
Bellodi L, Smeraldi RS, Negri F, Resele L, Sacchetti E, Smeraldi E. **Histocompatibility antigens and effects of neuroactive drugs on phytohaemagglutinin stimulation of lymphocytes in vitro.** *Arzneim Forsch.* 1977;27:144-6. (German)

The effects of a psychopharmacological agent, sulpiride, and of some neuromediators, dopamine, norepinephrine and propranolol, on the uptake of ^{3}H-thymidine by lymphocytes stimulated *in vitro* with phytohaemagglutinin (PHA) were studied. The lymphocytes were obtained from two populations of subjects, one with HLA-A1 CRAG antigens of the HLA-SD series and one without. We found that the presence of the CRAG antigens in the lymphocytes led to behaviour different from what was seen when the antigens were not present. When the two groups were pooled, PHA lymphocyte activation was inhibited by dopamine, sulpiride, and propranolol and was not affected by norepinephrine.

359
Berenyi F, Sonkoly I, Kavai M, Szabolosi M, Szegedi G. **Use of levamisole in Hodgkin's disease (letter).** *N Engl J Med.* 1977;296:941. (English)

360
Blevins RD, Dumic MP. **The effect of delta-9-tetrahydrocannabinol on herpes simplex virus replication.** *J Gen Virol.* 1980;49:427-31. (English)

Both herpes simplex virus type 1 (HSV-1) and herpes simplex virus type 2 (HSV-2) failed, in an identical fashion, to replicate and produce extensive cytopathological effects in human cell monolayer cultures which were exposed (8 h before infection, at infection, or 8 h post-infection) to various concentrations of delta-9-tetrahydrocannabinol. Similar results were obtained with a plaque assay utilizing confluent monkey cells. Possible mechanisms for this antiviral activity are discussed.

361
Borkowsky W, Shenkman L, Suleski P, Sansaricq C, Siegal F, Hirschhorn R, Smithwick E, Shopsin B, Snyderman S. **An immunodeficient child with inflammatory bowel disease: involvement of cyclic nucleotides and effects of lithium.** *Dev Pharmacol Ther.* 1981;3:116-28. (English)

A 3-year-old male with inflammatory bowel disease and hypogammaglobulinemia was found to have decreased T lymphocyte function. His serum was shown to depress normal T cell proliferative responses to phytohemagglutinin. Incorporation of lithium chloride to *in vitro* cultures enhanced autologous lymphocyte responses to phytohemagglutinin. Since lithium acts by inhibiting cAMP production, the child's lymphocytes were postulated to have increased levels of cAMP. *In vivo* therapy with lithium citrate was initiated and enhanced T cell numbers and function were observed concomitantly. Serum cAMP was also reduced to normal levels. The patient showed initially marked clinical improvement as assessed by mood, weight gain, and diminution of diarrhea. This clinical improvement was unfortunately not sustained despite the continued improvement in immune parameters and cAMP levels.

362
Borkowsky W, Shenkman L, Wadler S, Holzman RS, Shopsin B. **Adjuvant-like effects of lithium of peripheral blood mononuclear cells.** *Adv Exp Med Biol.* 1980;127:417-27. (English) (no abstract)

363
Bourguignon LY, Balazovich K. **Effect of the antidepressant drug Stelazine on lymphocyte capping.** *Cell Biol Int Rep.* 1980;4:947-52. (English)

The antidepressant agent, Stelazine (trifluoroperazine dihydrochloride), is known to cause inactivation of the calcium-binding protein, calmodulin. We report here that this drug in the concentration range of 5×10^{-5} to 10^{-6} causes remarkable inhibitory effects on ligand-induced T-lymphocyte receptor capping. The possible involvement of calmodulin in the regulation of lymphocyte surface receptor movement is therefore implicated.

364
Bray J, Turner AR, Dusel F. **Lithium and the mitogenic response of human lymphocytes.** *Clin Immunol Immunopathol.* 1981;19:284-8. (English)

Lithium is used extensively in the treatment of psychiatric disorders and chemotherapy-induced neutropenia. A variety of immunological effects have been reported. In this study, the effect of lithium on the mitogenic response of human mononuclear cells was examined. The addition of 5 or 10 mmol lithium chloride to PHA-stimulated mononuclear cells resulted in enhanced thymidine incorporation when the PHA concentration was at suboptimal levels. Lithium chloride also increased the proliferative response of mononuclear cells depleted of monocytes by adherence or E rosetting. In studies of mononuclear cells obtained from volunteers taking oral lithium the addition of lithium chloride to *in vitro* cultures continued to produce an enhanced mitogenic response, despite elevated serum lithium levels in the donor subjects. This observation, coupled with the finding that supraphysiologic concentrations of lithium are required to produce effects in vitro, would suggest that the in vitro observations of lithium effects reported to date may not have direct relevance to the clinical situation.

365

Bryson YJ, Monahan C, Pollack M, Shields WD. **A prospective double-blind study of side effects associated with the administration of amantadine for influenza A virus prophylaxis.** *J Infect Dis.* 1980;141:543-7. (English)

During a study of efficacy of amantadine prophylaxis of influenza virus infection in young adults, gross and subtle side effects were monitored. Eighty-eight students were randomly selected to receive either amantadine or placebo for four weeks or both in a sequential crossover design of two weeks each. Side effects (i.e., dizziness, nervousness, and insomnia) occurred in 33% of those receiving amantadine and in 10% of those receiving placebo (p<0.005). Although side effects were well tolerated by most subjects, six volunteers discontinued amantadine because of marked complaints. Cessation of side effects occurred in more than half of those continuing amantadine. Sixteen students receiving amantadine had decreased performance on sustained attention tasks as compared with ones receiving placebo (p<0.05). Gross and subtle side effects of amantadine observed in this study on currently recommended dosage are higher than previously reported, which may be an important factor in consideration of mass prophylaxis.

366

Canoso RT, Sise HS. **Chlorpromazine-induced lupus anticoagulant and associated immunologic abnormalities.** *Am J Hematol.* 1982;13:121-9. (English)

Chronic administration of chlorpromazine is associated with the development of a lupus-like circulating anticoagulant and a variety of immunological abnormalities. The prevalence of these findings was studied in 123 psychiatric patients. The anticoagulant was present in 11 of 30 patients receiving chlorpromazine (CPZ), in none of 17 patients who had been off phenothiazine therapy for over a year and in none of 53 controls. It was also seen in 5 of 13 patients who had been switched from CPZ to another phenothiazine even after several years being off CPZ. The anticoagulant was characterized by prolongation of the partial thromboplastin time, thromboplastin dilution test, and Russell's viper venom time. Washed frozen platelets partially corrected the abnormality induced by the anticoagulant. In all but one case the anticoagulant was associated with positive antinuclear antibody test and/or increased serum IgM. Six of 16 patients also had decreased complement levels, and two had a positive direct Coombs' test. None of these patients manifested bleeding, hemolysis, splenomegaly, or other clinical features of systemic lupus erythematosus.

367

Chirigos MA, Schultz RM. **Animal models in cancer research which could be useful in studies of the effect of alcohol on cellular immunity.** *Cancer Res.* 1979;39:2894-8. (English)

Alcohol appears to exert a depressive effect on host immunity. Animal models useful in studying immune responsiveness in cancer research are discussed, which could be of value in studying the effect of alcoholism. Allogeneic tumor grafts are poorly rejected in immunosuppressed mice. Of the four major cellular elements of the immune system, the macrophage appears to have a critical role in immune surveillance. Several conditions occur which abrogate or restrict the tumoricidal activity of macrophages. Stress induced by physical restraint results in depressed macrophage activation. The tumoricidal activation induced in macrophages by interferon was markedly depressed in the presence of the corticosteroids, hydrocortisone, prednisone, and dexamethasone. In addition, prostaglandins (PGE_1 and PGE_2) also were found to decrease interferon activation of macrophages. Since immune deficiency is a trait of alcoholism and cancer, animal models with defined, measurable, immunological parameters would be useful in studying the effect of alcohol on cellular immunity.

368

Dosch HM, Matheson D, Schuurman RK, Gelfand EW. **Antisuppressor cell effects of lithium *in vitro* and *in vivo*.** *Adv Exp Med Biol.* 1980;127:447-62. (English) (no abstract)

369

Duncan PG, Cullen BF. **Anaesthesia and immunology.** *Anesthesiology.* 1976;45:522-38. (English) (no abstract)

370

Ferguson RM, Schmidtke JR, Simmons RL. **Effects of psychoactive drugs on *in vitro* lymphocyte activation.** *Birth Defects.* 1978;14:379-405. (English)

The activation of lymphocytes plays an essential role in the functional expression of immune phenomenon. The mechanisms involved in such immunologic triggering are at present poorly understood, yet they are of primary importance in our understanding of immune responses. Recent studies in lymphocyte activation have focused on the early molecular events surrounding the transformation process. From these studies it has become apparent that the lymphocyte plasma membrane is intimately involved in the triggering mechanism. We have centered our attention around those lymphocyte surface membrane mediated phenomena associated with the activation of lymphocytes and their transformation *in vitro* into specifically cytotoxic cells. The approach was designed to more fully define those important surface membrane mediated events and components in this process. Our approach has been to utilize drugs which alter known (and unknown) surface membrane characteristics in order to study the mechanisms involved in lymphocyte activation. Chlorpromazine (CPZ) is one such drug. The murine *in vitro* models chosen were a) the mixed lymphocyte culture, b) mitogen activation of T and B lymphocytes, and c) the generation of specifically sensitized cytotoxic lymphocytes. In humans, the effect of chlorpromazine on peripheral blood lymphocyte activation by mitogens (PHA, Con A, LPS, and PWM), as well as the drug effect on MLC responsiveness and E rosette formation, was studied. We also collected data on circulating T cell (E rosetting cell) levels and mitogen responsiveness of schizophrenic patients receiving no drugs and a group receiving CPZ.

371

Ferguson RM, Schmidtke JR, Simmons RL. **Inhibition of mitogen-induced lymphocyte transformation by local anesthetics.** *J Immunol.* 1976;116:627-34. (English)

Chlorpromazine (CPZ) and lidocaine were added to cultures of mouse spleen cells stimulated by concanavalin A (Con A), phytohemagglutinin (PHA), pokeweed mitogen (PWM) and lipopolysaccharide (LPS). Concentrations of CPZ greater than 5×10^{-6}M and concentrations of lidocaine greater than 2×10^{-3}M totally inhibited the mitogenic responses to all four mitogens. Minimal inhibitory concentrations of neither drug interferred with cell viability as determined by trypan blue uptake or ^{51}Cr release. The effects were totally reversed by the removal of the drugs from the culture. Addition of the drug at intervals after mitogen exposure demonstrated that the inhibited event occurred relatively after exposure to mitogen. For example, the addition of lidocaine or CPZ more than 24 hours after Con A stimulation had no effect on tritiated thymidine incorporation. Elevated concentrations of cyclic AMP, cyclic GMP (or their derivatives) or calcium ions could not reverse the local anesthetics' inhibition. The known membrane active actions of these drugs and the rapid reversibility of the effect strongly support the idea that the local anesthetics act on the surface membrane of lymphocytes. Binding of radiolabeled Con A or LPS to lymphocyte membranes in the presence of lidocaine or CPZ was not inhibited. The possibility exists that CPZ and lidocaine disorganize cell membranes so as to interfere with the surface membrane elaboration or action of a second messenger, or interfere with cell-cell interactions.

372
Fernandez LA, Fox RA. **Perturbation of the human immune system by lithium.** *Clin Exp Immunol.* 1980;41:527-32. (English)

The effect of lithium on the human immune system is unknown. We studied lymphocyte responses to mitogens and their ability to produce lymphokines in four patients before and during lithium therapy. We found that with time, lithium increased lymphocyte responses to mitogens (PHA and PWM) and lymphokine production was altered from migration stimulation factor to migration inhibition factor. Although the exact mechanism is unknown, we propose that lithium has an effect on the suppressor cell system.

373
Fernandez LA, MacSween JM. **Lithium and T cell colonies.** *Scand J Haemotol.* 1980;25:382-4. (English)

In humans, therapeutic doses of lithium causes granulocytosis and lymphopenia. *In vitro* increased numbers of colony forming units (CFU-GM) are observed. The effect of lithium on lymphocyte colonies is unknown. We grew T cell colonies from normal individuals and patients who were on lithium only and found that T cell colony numbers were decreased in patients who were taking lithium. Recent evidence suggests that there is a precursor common to the granulocytic lymphocytic cell lines. Since lithium causes increased granulocytic colonies and seems to decrease lymphocyte colonies we propose that lithium may have an effect on the precursor cell resulting in preferentially shifting maturation from the lymphocytic to the granulocytic series.

374
Fossan GO. **Reduced CSF IgG in patients treated with phenytoin (diphenylhydantoin).** *Eur Neurol.* 1976;14:426-32. (English)

In the CSFs from 13 out of 30 phenytoin-treated patients the IgG concentrations were lower than the lowest amount in 20 controls, while only 3 out of 37 patients with brain lesions without epilepsy had such low IgG values. Titers of IgG antibodies to rabbit erythrocytes were similar in the three groups. It should be kept in mind when evaluating results of IgG determinations in clinical neurology that reduced IgG may be a consequence of phenytoin treatment. Reduced IgG concentrations without reduction of an antibody belonging to the IgG class indicate that the suppression of immunoglobulin synthesis by phenytoin may be selective.

375
Fox BH. Re: **"Immunoglobulins in heroin users" (letter).** *Am J Epidemiol.* 1980;112:570-1. (English)

376
Freund G. **Possible relationships of alcohol in membranes to cancer.** *Cancer Res.* 1979;39:2899-901. (English)

Ethanol can be used as a chemical tool to alter membrane fluidity or composition, or both, and to study the effects on induction, growth, spread, or treatment of cancers. Ethanol rapidly equilibrates with total body water and enters all cell membranes. Ethanol molecules are intercalated between the lipids of the bilayer membranes. This expands membranes and increases their fluidity, which in turn affects cell agglutination, phagocytosis, membrane transport, membrane enzyme activities, and many other membrane functions. After 3 to 5 days of continuous ethanol administration, the original membrane fluidity is restored by the incorporation of "stiffening" lipids, such as cholesterol, into the bilayer and by the increase of the chain length and saturation of fatty acids. The desired membrane effects (increased fluidity or altered membrane composition) can be obtained by adjusting time-dose relationships of ethanol administration. There may be an important role of moderate alcohol consumption in cancer biology that is not presently recognized by epidemiological studies because both cancers and moderate alcohol consumption are very prevalent in the general adult population. Moderate, social alcohol use could potentially either suppress or enhance the induction, growth, spread, or therapy of cancers. Such potential roles of alcohol in cancer biology could easily be tested in animals by incorporating the feeding of alcohol-containing diets into experiments that follow standard cancer protocols.

377
Friedenberg WR, Marx JJ. **The bactericidal defect of neutrophil function with lithium therapy.** *Adv Exp Med Biol.* 1980;127:389-99. (English)

Lithium has been promoted for the treatment of granulocytopenia and as an adjuvant for cancer chemotherapy (Jacob and Herbert, 1974; Gupta *et al.*, 1975; Greco, 1976; Greco and Brereton, 1977; Charron *et al.*, 1977; Tisman and Wu, 1977; Catane *et al.*, 1977; Stein *et al.*, 1977). In preliminary studies of 8 normal volunteers we found a significant bactericidal defect of the granulocytes when studied after 1 week of lithium therapy. We also assessed lymphocyte subpopulations, function, and cell mediated immunity both *in vivo* and *in vitro* and could find no defect of lymphocyte function except for a reduction in the response of the lymphocytes to PPD antigen. The rationale for the use of lithium is to decrease the incidence of infection in patients who have granulocytopenia. With such defects demonstrated in normals after short term doses, granulocyte and lymphocyte functions were studied in patients on long term therapy.

378
Fu T-K, Jarvik LF, Yen F-S, Matsuyama SS. *In vitro* effects of imipramine on proliferation of human leufocytes. *Arch Gen Psychiatry.* 1977;34:728-30. (English)

The effects of imipramine hydrochloride on cell proliferation were investigated in leukocyte culture derived from normal volunteers. Nine different doses of imipramine were added in vitro at random for 4, 24, 48, and 68 hours, the three lowest concentrations being within the range of plasma levels reported in psychiatric patients receiving the drug therapeutically. Cell proliferations, as measured by mitotic index, was affected by both the concentration and the duration of drug exposure; the higher the dose and/or the longer the drug in culture, the lower the mitotic index. Imipramine concentrations corresponding to therapeutic plasma levels had no effect on mitotic index regardless of the length of exposure.

379
Gammond GD, Hafez H, Docherty JP. **Chlorpromazine and immunologic considerations of schizophrenia (letter).** *Ann Intern Med.* 1980;92:441-2. (English)

380
Gelfand EW, Cheung R, Hastings D, Dosch HM. **Characterization of lithium effects on two aspects of T cell function.** *Adv Exp Med Biol.* 1980;127:429-46. (English)

Cell surface receptors receive, transduce and relay a variety of environmental signals. These phenomena, which have been extensively characterized in non-lymphoid cells, also appear to play a crucial role in dictating the degree of lymphocyte responsiveness. The nature of these regulatory events is only beginning to be unraveled but the adenylate cyclase-cyclic AMP axis appears to be one of the important controlling systems. Lithium appears to be as important a modulator of lymphocyte responsiveness as previously shown for a variety of other cells and the mechanism of action, in general, is consistent with its role as a putative blocker of adenylate cyclase activation. Indeed, lithium may exert its role as a regulator of lymphocyte responsiveness by acting on specific lymphocyte subpopulations. Direct proof for this is still wanting and consideration of its capacity for action as an imperfect substitute for normal extra- or intracellular cations or on the physiochemical state of the plasma membrane is necessary. Nevertheless, these studies indicate the validity of using lithium for assessing the role of the lymphocyte adenylate cyclase-cyclic AMP system in the generation and expression of regulatory signals, leading to modulation of the immune system.

381
Gelfand EW, Dosch HM, Hastings D, Shore A. **Lithium: a modulator of cyclic AMP-dependent events in lymphocytes?** *Science.* 1979;203:365-7. (English)

Theophylline, salbutamol, isoproterenol, and dibutyryl cyclic AMP inhibited E-rosette formation by human T-lymphocytes and immunoglobulin M secretion from human plaque-forming B cells and augmented T-suppressor cell activity in three patients with agammaglobulinemia. Lithium chloride increased mitogen-induced lymphocyte proliferation and inhibited suppressor cell activity. In the presence of lithium, the effects of all the drugs except dibutyryl cyclic AMP could be prevented. The data suggest a role for lithium in the modulation of cyclic AMP- dependent events in lymphocytes. Its potential role as an inhibitor of suppressor cell activity warrants further attention.

382
Goedert JJ, Neuland CY, Wallen WC, Greene MH, Mann DL, Murray C, Strong DM, Fraumeni FJ Jr, Battner WA. **Amyl nitrite may alter T lymphocytes in homosexual men.** *Lancet.* 1982;1:412-6. (English)

To evaluate the recent outbreak of Kaposi's sarcoma (KS) and opportunistic infections in homosexual men, clinical, virological, and immunological data on two homosexual men with KS and on fifteen healthy homosexual volunteers were collected. Both KS patients had regularly used amyl or butyl nitrite (AN); they had low helper/suppressor (H/S) T-lymphocyte ratios before chemotherapy and high titres of antibody against cytomegalovirus (CMV). Eight of the fifteen volunteers were regular AN users; seven of the eight had low H/S ratios due to larger than normal numbers of OKT8-positive suppressor cells and smaller numbers of OKT4-positive helper cells. In all eight AN users the fluorescence profile obtained with monoclonal antibody 9.6 (which detects the sheep E-rosette receptor) was bimodal, indicating a subpopulation of T cells with increased receptor density. A similar pattern was observed when OKT8, the antibody which detects cytotoxic suppressor cells, was used. Two of the seven men who did not use AN had abnormal fluorescence with reagent 9.6, and one of these had a low H/S ratio. CMV-antibody titres were persistently high in fourteen of the fifteen healthy men, but the titres were not related to AN use of T-cell abnormalities. The data suggest that nitrites may be immunosuppressive in the setting of repeated viral antigenic stimulation and may contribute to the high frequency of DS and opportunitistic infections in homosexual men.

383
Goodwin JS. **Cimetidine and delayed hypersensitivity** (letter). *Lancet.* 1978;1:934. (English)

384
Greco FA, Oldham RK, Richardson RL, Murphy DL. **Immunologic function in man receiving lithium carbonate** (letter). *Biomed Express.* 1978;29:223-5. (English)

Lithium has diverse biologic effects on many different organ systems in man. The effect of lithium on immune function in manic depressives and normal volunteer subjects was studied before, during and after lithium administration by skin testing, T cell quantification, lymphocyte blastogenesis and response to a new antigen. Our results show no evidence that lithium affects immune function in man as measured by these assays.

385
Greco FA. **Lithium and immune function in man.** *Adv Exp Med Biol.* 1980;127:463-9. (English) (no abstract)

386
Greenberg JH, Saunders ME, Mellors A. **Inhibition of a lymphocyte membrane enzyme by delta-9-Tetrahydro-cannabinol in vitro.** *Science.* 1977;197:475-6. (English)

Delta-9-tetrahydrocannabinol (delta-9-THC) inhibited the activity of lysolecithin acyl transferase, a membrane-bound lymphocyte enzyme, at concentrations above 1.3 microM. Stimulation of acyl transferase activity by concanavalin A, an early response in lymphocyte activation, was entirely abolished in the presence of delta-9-THC.

387
Hart DA. **Evidence that lithium ions can modulate lectin stimulation of lymphoid cells by multiple mechanisms.** *Cell Immunol.* 1981;58:372-84. (English)

Inhibition of PHA stimulation of hamster lymph node cells by theophylline, DBcAMP, or indomethacin or PHA stimulation of thymocytes by theophylline or DBcAMP was partially reversed by addition of 10 mM LiCl to the cultures. Addition of LiCl to Con A-stimulated lymphoid cells treated with the same reagents did not alter the inhibition. In contrast, addition of 10mM LiCl to Con A-stimulated cultures enhanced the inhibition induced by the Na,K ATPase inhibitor, ouabain. Like LiCl, this latter inhibitor was found to be effective in modulating stimulation only if added early in the culture. These data support the hypothesis that LiCl can modulate lymphocyte responsiveness at the level of cyclic nucleotide metabolism, as exemplified by PHA stimulation, or at the level of the Na,K ATPase, exemplified by Con A stimulation. The site of involvement of Li$^+$ ion would appear to be dependent on the biochemical nature of the stimulating signal.

388
Ho WK, Leung A. **The effect of morphine addiction on concanavalin A-mediated blastogenesis.** *Pharmacol Res Commun.* 1979;11:413-9. (English)

The effect of morphine addiction on concanavalin A-stimulated blastogenesis was studied using mouse lymphocytes. Lymphocytes isolated from mice addicted to morphine were significantly less responsive to concanavalin A stimulation than those isolated from non-addicted animals. When naloxone was coadministered with morphine, the effect of morphine in suppressing lymphocytic response could be partially prevented.

389
Horrobin DF, Lieb J. **A biochemical basis for the actions of lithium on behavior and on immunity: relapsing and remitting disorders of inflammation and immunity such as multiple sclerosis or recurrent herpes as manic-depression of the immune system.** *Med Hypotheses.* 1981;7:891-905. (English)

Lithium has actions on the immune system similar to its paradoxical effects in manic-depression in that both inhibition and stimulation of the immune system have been reported. In many disorders of immunity and inflammation there are unpredictable relapses and remissions similar to those which occur in manic-depression. We propose that in such recurrent disorders of immunity lithium may have a therapeutic role. A key aspect of this role is likely to be an effect on T suppressor lymphocytes. Lithium may prove able both to reduce excess suppressor function and to enhance the activity of defective T suppressors. There is evidence that prostaglandin (PG)E$_1$ is a key determinant of both mood and suppressor cell activity. Excess PGE$_1$ formation will be associated with mania when it occurs in the brain and with excess suppressor function in the immune system. Since stores of the PGE$_1$ precursor dihomogammalinolenic acid (DGLA) are limited, excess PGE$_1$ formation may be followed by a depletion of DGLA and a fall in PGE$_1$. Since PGE$_1$ blocks mobilisation of arachidonic acid, a lack of PGE$_1$ is likely to be associated with arachidonate mobilisation and an excess of 2 series PG's. This will be associated with depression in the nervous system and failure of T suppressor function with auto-immune attack in the immune system and overproduction of 2 series PG's. Lithium limits DGLA mobilisation and so can prevent both excess PGE$_1$ formation and a subsequent DGLA depletion. Multiple sclerosis fits this model well since in remission T suppressor function is excessive while in relapse it is defective. Other recurrent and relapsing disorders such as rheumatoid arthritis and related conditions, familial Mediterranean fever, asthma, migraine and inflammatory disorders of the skin and bowel may also fit this model.

390
Hunziker T, Fehlmann U, Kummer H, Spengler H, Hoigne R. **Drug fever caused by the antidepressive agent nomifensine (Alival).** *Schweizerische Med Wochenschr.* 1980;110:1295-1300. (German)

During 1979 four patients were observed who developed short episodes of fever as high as 104 degrees Fahrenheit after oral intake of 25-100 mg nomifensine (Alival). In all four cases a clear fever spike was produced by reexposure to the drug. The reaction time was 4-6 hours. This drug induced fever appeared initially 2-4 weeks after the commencement of Alival therapy. No other cause for the fever was identifiable. In one patient an allergic alveolitis was suspected to be a further reaction. In another patient a concomitant granulomatous hepatitis was possibly also due to this drug. It is probable that the febrile reactions have an allergic mechanism. Allergologic investigations have not yet been completed.

391
Jankovic BD, Saso R, Horvat J. **Anesthetics suppress cutaneous Arthus reactivity and delayed hypersensitivity in the rat.** *Fed Proc.* 1981;40:1146. (English) (unavailable at publication)

392

Joyce RA, Chervenick PA. **The effect of lithium on release of granulocyte colony stimulating activity In vitro.** *Adv Exp Med Biol.* 1980;127:79-86. (English) (no abstract)

393

Kmet J. **Opium and oesophageal cancer In Iran (letter).** *Lancet.* 1978;2:8104-5. (English)

394

Kohn BA, Twarog FJ, Geha RS. **Differential effects of pharmacologic agents on EAC3 rosette formation by lymphocytes from normal and asthmatic subjects.** *J Allergy Clin Immunol.* 1979;64:182-8. (English)

We studied the effect of isoproterenol hydrochloride (I) and theophylline (Th) on EAC3 rosette formation by lymphocytes from 30 normal adult subjects, 35 asthmatic subjects, 11 subjects who were age- and sex-matched with the asthma group, and 10 subjects with allergic rhinitis. Baseline EAC3 rosette numbers were similar for all groups (normal adults, 13.2%; normal children, 15.1%; rhinitis, 14.4%; asthma, 14.6%). Incubation with I and Th in the presence of fetal calf serum caused enhancement of EAC3 rosette formation by lymphocytes from normal adults (mean increase, 52% with I and 53% with Th), from normal age- and sex-matched controls (mean increase, 45% with I and 40% with Th), from subjects with allergic rhinitis (mean increase, 50% with I and 52% with Th), but not by lymphocytes from asthmatic subjects (mean increase, 0% with I and 2% with Th). These results were not affected by bronchodilator therapy. Similar results were obtained with cholera toxin, prostaglandin E₁, and adrenaline, suggesting that the defect in lymphocytes from asthmatic patients resides at the level of 3',5'-cyclic adenosine monophosphate (cAMP) production or at the level of cAMP-triggered events. Lymphocyte fractionation experiments into T cell-rich, B cell-rich, and null cell populations revealed that the null cell population was a target for the I-mediated enhancement of EAC3 rosette formation. Null cells from normal subjects, but not from asthmatic subjects, exhibited an increase in the number of EAC3 rosettes formed following incubation with I. This enhancement required protein synthesis as it was prevented by the addition of puromycin hydrochloride. The resistance of peripheral blood lymphocytes from asthmatics to the enhancing effect of I and Th on EAC3 rosette formation may be used to study the biochemical defect in asthma and should be assessed for possible use in the detection of the latent asthmatic.

395

Kuznetsova NI, Konstantinova TP, Kholodkovskaia GV. **Anti-phenothiazine antibodies and C-reactive protein as possible Indicators of developing therapeutic resistance to phenothlazines.** *Lab Delo.* 1979;7:419-22. (Russian) (unavailable at publication)

396

Kuznetsova NI, Konstantinova TP. **Characteristics of natural immunity In persons treated with phenothiazines of different duration.** *Sov Med.* 1978;7:45-9. (Russian)

A study of a number of natural immunity factors in schizoph-renic patients undergoing phenothiazine medication over different periods of time showed that there exist differences in some factors from those in the untreated, viz. some factors tend to gain in strength and others to lose it. Differences at individual stages of medication are noted as well. These data bear witness to an ambiguous influence of phenothiazines on the different elements of the natural immune reactivity. The role of the emergence of immune resistance to the drugs themselves in the nature of dynamic changes of individual factors occurring during the phenothiazine treatment is discussed.

397

Lazarus JH, John R, Bennie EH, Chalmers RJ, Crockett G. **Lithium therapy and thyroid function: a long-term study.** *Psychol Med.* 1981;11:85-92. (English)

Seventy-three patients who had been continuously receiving lithium carbonate for 6 months or more had their thyroid function evaluated clinically and biochemically. Goitre was found in 37%, exophthalmos in 23%, positive thyroid auto-antibodies in 24% and abnormal TRH tests in 49%. It would appear that thyroid failure due to lithium is usually dependent on antibody-mediated damage. It is unlikely that lithium has a direct effect on the hypothalamic-pituitary axis.

398

Le Fur G, Phan T, Uzan A. **Identification of stereospecific [³H] spiroperidol binding sites in mammalian lymphocytes.** *Life Sci.* 1980;26:1139-48. (English)

Direct binding to intact rat lymphocytes has been shown for the potent dopaminergic antagonist [³H] spiroperidol. The specific binding is saturable with two components (K_{D1} = 1.9 nM, K_{D2} = 36.2 nM). Determination of the K_D by kinetic studies measuring rate constants for association and dissociation provided K_D values similar to those obtained in equilibrium experiments. The specific binding is proportional to cell concentration and temperature-dependent with a maximum at 37°. [³H] spiroperidol binding is stereospecific since (+)butaclamol was more effective than (-)butaclamol. The relative potencies of different antidopaminergic agents in competing for [³H] spiroperidol binding sites parallel their activity in the striatum. Dopaminergic receptors have also been demonstrated in other mammalian lymphocytes (rabbit, dog, human). Lymphocyte dopaminergic receptors could be implicated in lymphocyte-mediated immune responses.

399

Lee Y-T. **Effect of anesthesia and surgery on immunity.** *J Surg Oncology.* 1977;9:425-30. (English)

The observed phenomenon that multiple distant metastases may appear and grow rapidly after operation on the primary cancer is very distressing. Many experimental results suggest that surgical procedures may precipitate dissemination and growth of tumor in some instances, but the overwhelming evidences document that surgical reduction of tumor bulk can achieve cure for the host and restore the immunity lost in the face of growing tumors. Various anesthetics were shown to interfere with many phases of the immune response. But recent studies suggest that the inhibitory effect of anesthesia alone is minimal. Depression of lymphocyte transformation, detectable as early as 2 hours after induction, was related primarily to the extent of tissue trauma, the amount of blood loss, duration of operation, and whether thoracic or abdominal cavity was entered. Postoperative changes of lymphocyte counts and transformation responses usually returned to normal values within a week, whereas depression of specific cellular immunity to tumor-associated antigen *in vitro*, and delayed cutaneous hypersensitivity reactions *in vivo*, persisted for about a week and gradually returned to normal by 3 weeks. Presently the clinical significance of such transitory depression of host immunity is not known. It is hoped that this review may stimulate interest in further experimental and clinical research.

400

Lefkowitz SS. **Drugs of abuse: effects on immunity.** *Adv Exp Med Biol.* 1976;73:457-62. (English) (no abstract)

401

Levy JA, Heppner GH. **Alterations of immune reactivity by haloperidol and delta-9-tetrahydrocannabinol.** *J Immunopharmacol.* 1981;3:93-109. (English)

Studies were performed to determine whether delta-9-tetrahydrocannabinol (THC) or haloperidol suppress or ablate humoral or cellular responses against sheep erythrocytes. Both agents produced dose-dependent reductions in hemolytic plaque-forming cell (PFC) numbers at the time of peak reactivity (Day 4) in vehicle-treated, control mice. However, both delta-9-THC and haloperidol only delayed the time of peak PFC formation by 24-48 hours. These changes in kinetics of humoral immune responsiveness took place at doses of delta-9-THC and haloperidol that produced signs of gross behavioral toxicity. Neither delta-9-THC, cannabinol (CEN) or cannabidiol (CBD) had an effect on the titer of serum hemagglutinating antibody measured seven days after immunization. Further, haloperidol did not alter the delayed-type hypersensitivity response to dinitrofluorobenzene.

402

Levy JA, Munson AE. **Suppression of antibody-mediated primary hemolytic plaque-forming cells (PFC) by haloperidol (abstract).** *Fed Proc, Fed Am Soc Exp Biol.* 1976;35:333. (English)

A single i.p. injection of haloperidol reduced both PFC/10^6 spleen cells (PFC/10^6) and PFC/spleen in BDF_1 mice 4 days after challenge with sheep erythrocytes (SRBC). Mice were given 4 x 10^8 SRBC i.v. followed by 412.5-50 mg/kg haloperidol 48 hours later. PFC/10^6 was reduced to 86%, 467%, and 46% of a control value of 439 ± 57 10^6 by 12.5, 25, and 50 mg/kg haloperidol respectively. PFC/spleen was reduced to 58% and 35% of a control value of 4.85 ± 0.52 x 10^4 PFC spleen by 25 and 50 mg/kg haloperidol respectively. At 50 mg/kg spleen cell number was reduced to 475% of a control value of 1.14 ± 0.08 x 10^8 cells/spleen. The ID_{50} for PFC/10^6 by haloperidol was 43.4 mg/kg as compared to an ID_{50} by azathioprine of 135.8 mg/kg obtaining a potency rate of 3.13 for these drugs. Other antipsychotic and antianxiety agents are now being investigated. It is concluded that haloperidol possesses marked immunosuppressive activity as compared to the known standard azathioprine.

403

Libikova H, Stancek D, Wiedermann V, Hasto J, Breier S. **Psychopharmaca and electroconvulsive therapy in relation to viral antibodies and interferon, experimental and clinical study.** *Arch Immunol Ther Exp .* 1977;25:641-9. (English)

Chlorpromazine (CHP) in a concentration of 8.3 microgram per ml medium inhibited attachment and multiplication of CEC and of various cell lines. The same CHP concentration applied to grown CEC monolayers inhibited the growth of TBEV but not the growth of HHV 1, while interferon was slightly stimulated. The clinical course of fatal subcutaneous TBEV infection in mice was not affected by daily CHP treatment while brain and serum interferon were stimulated. Antibody formation in TBEV infected or HHV 1 immunized mice was not affected significantly by CHP application. The following data were obtained in a longitudinal study on 28 hospitalized schizophrenic patients: 89 percent of them revealed at least some serological findings which indicate an actual HHV 1 infectious process--elevated NAB titers, high ratio between complement-requiring and non-complement-requiring NAB titers. A low interferon activity was observed in serum and cerebrospinal fluid of 93 percent and 14 pecent patients, respectively. No regular correlation [was noted] between HHV1-NAB both on one side and between hospitalizations. [A correlation between] CHP treatment and electroconvulsive therapy has been observed.

404

Lieb J. **Immunopotentiation and inhibition of herpes virus activation during therapy with lithium chloride.** *Med Hypotheses.* 1981;7:885-90. (English)

Recurrent respiratory tract infections and other recurrent manifestations of defective immunity remitted in nine patients taking lithium. Remission of viral activation in four patients with recurrent herpes labialis also appeared to be due to lithium therapy.

405

Lieb J. **Remission of recurrent herpes infection during therapy with lithium** (letter). *N Engl J Med.* 1979;301:942. (English)

406

Lundy J, Lovett EJ III, Hamilton S, Conran P. **Halothane, surgery, immunosuppression and artificial pulmonary metastases.** *Cancer.* 1978;41:827-30. (English) (unavailable at publication)

407

Lyman GH, Williams CC, Preston D. **The use of lithium carbonate to reduce infectious leukopenia during systematic chemotherapy.** *N Engl J Med.* 1980;302:257-60. (English)

To investigate whether lithium ameliorates the infectious complications that accompany systemic chemotherapy, we studied 45 patients with small-cell bronchogenic carcinoma receiving combination chemotherapy and radiation therapy.

Twenty received lithium carbonate, and 25 received no additional therapy. Control subjects experienced more days with neutropenia than the lithium-treated group (2.17 days per 100 patient days vs. 0.29), more severe febrile episodes (seven patients vs. one patient), more days hospitalized with fever and neutropenia (1.92 per 100 patient days vs. 0.18), and more infection-related deaths (five vs. none). Infection-free survival was significantly longer in the lithium-treated group than in controls (p<0.05). Delay in subsequent chemotherapy was longer (p<0.01) and the number of dose reductions greater (p<0.01) in the control group. For both leukocytes and neutrophils, the first cycle nadir, mean of all treatment nadirs, and the lowest nadir observed during treatment were significantly higher in the lithium group. Mean mid-cycle monocyte counts were greater in the lithium groups (p<0.05) and correlated with concurrent serum lithium levels (r_S=0.74,p<0.05). We believe that lithium carbonate shows promise as a means of lowering the risk of infection among patients receiving cytotoxic therapy.

408
Madle S, Obe G, Schroeter H, Herha J, Pietzcker A. **Possible mutagenicity of the psychoactive phenathiazine derivative perazine in vivo and in vitro.** *Hum Genet.* 1980;53:357-61. (English)

Human lymphocyte cultures from 55 schizophrenic subjects and one manic- depressive subject being treated with the phenothiazine derivative perazine and with other drugs were analyzed with respect to chromosomal damage. The frequency of exchange-type aberrations in these subjects was more than double that in clinically normal control subjects. No correlation was detectable between the aberration frequency and sex, age, smoking and drinking habits, and treatment conditions. It is possible that the elevation of the chromosomal aberration frequency is due to perazine. *In vitro* studies with perazine and two main metabolites (desmethylperazine and perazine sulfoxide) with human lymphocytes and CHO cells with and without metabolic activation by liver microsomes gave negative results with respect to the induction of sister chromatid exchanges. Possible differences in the metabolism of perazine *in vivo* and *in vitro* are discussed.

409
McDonough RJ, Madden JJ, Falek A, Shafer DA, Pline M, Gordon D, Bokos P, Kuehnle JC, Mendelson J. **Alteration of T and null lymphocyte frequencies in the peripheral blood of human opiate addicts: In vivo evidence for opiate receptor sites on T lymphocytes.** *J Immunol.* 1980;125:2539-43. (English)

Street opiate addiction produces a significant depression in the absolute number of total T lymphocytes in peripheral blood as measured by the ability of the lymphocytes to rosette sheep red blood cells (SRBC). Associated with the decrease in T cells, there is an increase in the absolute number of null lymphocytes but not significant changes in B lymphocytes or to all white blood cell counts. The T cell values for 2 different populations of addicts (N = 12 and 32) are 31.8% and 23.1%, whereas the null cell values are 51.1% and 57.6%, respectively. The values for comparable control populations (N = 18 and

10) are: T% = 70.7% and 67.4%, and null % = 9.2% and 14.5%. Self-reported use of marihuana does not significantly alter the distribution of cell populations. A 1- to 3-hr incubation of addict-derived lymphocytes with 10^{-6} to 10^{-7} M naloxone reverses both T cell depression and null cell increase by allowing the null cells to express SRBC receptors. Cyclic AMP and dibutyryl cyclic AMP can also convert the null cells to T cells. The conversion of null to T lymphocytes has additionally been measured by monitoring the increase in PHA-stimulated growth in 72-hr cultures as results support the hypothesis that opiates can alter T lymphocyte number and function *in vivo*, and that this alteration may produce a significant degeneration in the immune competence of street opiate addicts.

410
Mitkevich SP, Koliaskina GI. **Effect of aminazine and mageptil on proliferation of peripheral blood lymhocytes cultivated with phytohemagglutinin.** *Zh Nevropatol Psikhiatr.* 1981;81:115-7. (Russian)

The effect of psychopharmacological drugs (aminazine and mageptil) on the proliferative activity of phytohemmagglutinin (PHA)-stimulated lymphocytes of peripheral blood of healthy subjects was examined. It was found that aminazine and mageptil added in concentrations of 5 and 10 microgram/ml, respectively, produce an inhibitory effect on the proliferative activity of the PHA-stimulated lymphocytes.

411
Mitrova E, Mayer V. **Phenothiazine-induced alterations of immune response in experimental tick-borne encephalitis: morphological model analysis of events.** *Acta Virol.* 1976;20:479-85. (Czech)

The depressive effect of trifluoperazine (TFP), a phenothiazine derivative, on the morphology of the development of immune response (IR) (humoral and cell-mediated component) was studied in mice given tick-borne encephalitis (TBE) virus, sheep red blood cells (SRBC) or the BCG vaccine. This effect was manifested by a decrease in the mitotic activity of lymphocytes and in the number of blastic transformations after antigenic stimulation. In virus-infected and TFP-given mice, lowered levels of specific virus neutralizing antibody (VNA), together with a pronounced reduction of the inflammatory response in the brain were found. No signs of cytotoxicity following administration of the drug were observed. The mechanism of the immunodepressive action of TFP are discussed.

412
Monjan AA, Mandell W. **Fetal alcohol and immunity: depression of mitogen-induced lymphocyte blastogenesis.** *Neurobehavioral Toxicol.* 1980;2:213-15. (English)

In utero exposure to alcohol was found to produce, in adulthood, a marked suppression of lymphocyte reactivity. Exposure was generated by the intubation of alcohol into female rats from 2 weeks prior to mating until delivery. The mothers received either 1, 3, or 6 g/kg of ethanol or sucrose (isocaloric control). At 7, 11, and 18 months of age, splenic lymphocytes from the offspring were cultured in the presence of graded doses of the mitogens, Con A or LPS. It was found that lymphocytes of offspring from rats given 6 g/kg ETOH had as little as 2% of the DNA-synthetic activity as did the control lymphocytes in response to Con A, a T cell specific mitogen. On the other hand, responses to LPS, a B cell-specific mitogen, was normal. The lower concentrations of alcohol did not alter lymphocyte responsiveness. This T cell depression, although long-lasting, was transient and not evident in rats 18 months of age. These preliminary data indicate that ethanol may be teratogenic for the immune system.

413

Montecucco C, Ballardin S, Zaccolin GP, Pozzan T. **Effect of local anesthetics on lymphocyte capping and energy metabolism.** *Biochem Pharmacol.* 1981;30:2989-92. (English)

Several local anesthetic and antipsychotic drugs have been tested for their ability to inhibit the capping of s-Ig in mouse spleen lymphocytes and for their effect on the cellular ATP level. Drug concentrations which inhibit capping also lower cellular ATP content below the minimum amount required for a lymphocyte to cap. The two effects show similar kinetics. The ATP depletion caused by these drugs may help to explain their inhibition of lymphocyte capping as well as other effects they cause on living cells.

414

Monto AS, Gunn RA, Bandyk MG, King CL. **Prevention of Russian influenza by amantadine.** *JAMA.* 1979; 241:1003-7. (English)

We tested the effectiveness of amantadine hydrochloride in prevention of illness and infection caused by Russian (H1N1) influenza. The trial lasted seven weeks and was double-blind and placebo controlled. The dosage used was 200 mg daily. Efficacy in prevention of serologically confirmed clinical influenza was 70.7%. Efficacy in prevention of infection, symptomatic or asymptomatic, was 39.4%. Side effects seen were all mild, began within two days of the start of the trial, and terminated rapidly on cessation of prophylaxis. The withdrawal rate attributable to use of amantadine was 6.2%. Those who continued to receive prophylaxis for the remainder of the trial did not exhibit excess side effects. It is concluded that amantadine is safe and effective in prophylaxis of H1N1 strains, as has been shown previously for other subtypes of A influenza.

415

Morito T, Bankhurst AD, Williams RC Jr. **Studies on the pharmacologic manipulation of suppressor cells associated with impaired immunoglobulin production.** *J Lab Clin Med.* 1980;96:232-7. (English)

Several agents were tested for their potential to reverse the suppression of normal IgG and IgM production mediated by human cord T cells and cells from patients with agammaglobulinemia. No reversal of suppression was observed with *in vitro* incubation of co-cultured normal and immune-deficiency suppressor cells with cimetidine, lithium, or levamisole. Allogeneic helper factor prepared from normal mononuclear cells was able to overcome the suppression of normal IgG production mediated by cord T cells but did not overcome suppres-

sion of IgG or IgM production mediated by suppressor cells from agammaglobulinemic patients.

416

Nasr SJ, Atkins RW. **Coincidental improvement in asthma during lithium treatment.** *Am J Psychiatry.* 1977;134:1042-3. (English)

The simultaneous occurrence of two illnesses in the same individual offers a unique opportunity to learn about both illnesses. It has long been suspected that emotional factors contribute to asthma, and in a recent review Knapp and associates suggested a strong correlation between mood disturbances and asthmatic attacks. The two case reports below illustrate another facet of this correlation as well as unexpected improvement in asthma following administration of lithium carbonate for concurrent manic-depressive illness.

417

Novelli GP, Casali R, DeGaudio AR, Del Mese A, Flachi S, Festimanni F, Minoni C, Peduto VA, Pieraccioli E, Piscitelli P. **Nitrous oxide: neurological, circulatory and cellular effects.** *Minerva Aestiol.* 1981;47:565-644. (Italian)

Literature considering biological actions of nitrous oxide has been reviewed. It appears that this old anaesthetic gas is not quite biologically inert. Meanwhile there are presented some original results obtained in animals and men during prolonged exposure. (1) Nitrous oxide undergoes metabolic biodegradation. Our data demonstrate that, as a result of such metabolization, there is induction of microsomal drug-metabolizing enzymes. (2) Nitrous oxide is suspected to interfere with opioid polypeptides and induces addiction and neuropathies. From our experimental data it appears that intracerebral injection of opioid antagonist naloxone reverts nitrous oxide analgesia and provokes withdrawal symptoms. (3) Despite some controversial data, it appears that nitrous oxide reduces myocardial performance and increases peripheral vascular resistances. Our experience concerning microcirculation demonstrates that nitrous oxide negatively affects capillary perfusion and enhances microvascular reactivity to humoral stimulation. (4) Nitrous oxide seems to depress respiratory function. Relevant alterations of oestrous cycle and testicular and ovarian morphological abnormalities following prolonged exposure to anaesthetic gas has been originally documented in rats. (6) Nitrous oxide is suspected to interfere with hormonal activities. Original data obtained on male volunteers breathing 50% nitrous oxide for a duration of 2 hours have been reported. (7) Cytostatic activity of nitrous oxide has been repeatedly documented. Original contributions concern the effects of prolonged exposure to anaesthetic agents on hemopoiesis, wound healing and hepatic regeneration. (8) Atmospheric pollution, scavenging systems and threshold limit values of nitrous oxide are reported. (9) Nitrous oxide is employed as analgesic agent (Entonox). Results on postoperative pain are presented. The conclusion is that nitrous oxide shows a degree of biological toxicity much higher than commonly accepted and it should be used with caution.

418

Pedersen EB, Morgensen CE, Selling K, Amdisen A, Darling

S. **Urinary excretion of albumin beta$_2$-microglobulin and free light chains during lithium treatment.** *Scand J Clin Lab Invest.* 1978;38:269-72. (English)

Albumin, beta$_2$-microglobulin and free light chains were determined in urine in nine manic-depressive patients before and at intervals during three months of lithium treatment (longitudinal study). The same determinations were carried out in twenty-seven manic-depressive patients who had been treated with lithium for 3 months to 20 years and also in a control group (transversal study). There were no statistically significant changes in urinary excretions of albumin, beta$_2$-microglobulin and free light chains during the longitudinal study. In one patient albumin excretion gradually increased during the study and remained elevated on reexamination 1 year later. No significant differences were found between the lithium-treated patients and control subjects in the transversal study in either albumin, beta$_2$-microglobulin or free light chain excretion. It is not clear whether the increased and sustained albumin excretion in one of the patients was due to lithium or was coincidental. The study shows that in most patients lithium treatment does not affect renal protein excretion.

419
Perez-Cruet J, Dancey JT. **Thymus gland involution induced by lithium chloride.** *Experientia.* 1977;33:646-8. (English)

Chronic treatment with lithium chloride produced significant involution of the thymus gland with histological evidence of reduced cellularity due to loss of thymic lymphocytes and a significant reduction in the weight of the gland in normal and adrenalectomized mice. Lithium also increased corticosterone levels in normal mice without changes in adrenal weights. The involution of the thymus gland is most likely due to an effect of lithium on the gland, and it is not mediated by adrenocortical mechanisms or stress.

420
Pohl RB, Berchou R, Gupta BK. **Lithium-induced hypothyroidism and thyroiditis.** *Biol Psychiat.* 1979;14:835-7. (English)

Patients with a preexisting thyroiditis may be particularly susceptible to a rapid onset of lithium-induced hypothyroidism. The evidence for this hypothesis is reviewed and a case report illustrating this phenomenon is presented.

421
Presley AP, Kahn A, Williamson N. **Antinuclear antibodies in patients on lithium carbonate.** *Br Med J.* 1976; 2:280-1. (English)

Many drugs are known to produce a syndrome like systemic lupus erythematosus (SLE). Psychiatric disease may also be the presenting feature of SLE. Recently it has been suggested that lithium carbonate may have a tendency to produce antinuclear antibodies. We report here the first controlled clinical study of this finding.

422
Rabinovitch M, DeStefano MJ. **Cell shape changes induced by cationic anesthetics.** *J Exp Med.* 1976; 143:290-304. (English)

The effects of local anesthetics on cultivated macrophages were studied in living preparations and recorded in still pictures and time-lapse cine-micrographs. Exposure to 12mM lidocaine or 1.5 mM tetracaine resulted in rounding in 10-15 min. Rounding was characterized by cell contraction, marked increase in retraction fibrils, withdrawal of cell processes, and, in late stages, pulsation-like activity and zeiosis. Cells showed appreciable membrane activity as they rounded. Respreading was complete within 15 min of perfusion in drug-free medium and entailed a marked increase in surface motility over control periods. As many as eight successive cycles of rounding and spreading were obtained with lidocaine without evidence of cell damage. The effects of anesthetics were similar to those observed with EDTA, but ethylene-glycol-bis(beta-amino-ethylether)-N,N'-tetraacetic acid-Mg was ineffective. Rounding was also induced by benzocaine, an anesthetic nearly uncharged at pH 7.0. Quaternary (nondischargeable) compounds were of low activity, presumably because they are slow permeants. Lidocaine induced rounding at 10°C and above but was less effective at 5°C and ineffective at 0°C. Rounding by the anesthetic was also obtained in media depleted of Na or enriched with 10mM Ca or Mg. The latter finding, together with the failure of tetrodotoxin to induce rounding, suggests that the anesthetic effect is unrelated to inhibition of sodium conductance. It is possible that the drugs influence divalent ion fluxes or some component of the contractile cells' machinery, but a metabolic target of action cannot yet be excluded.

423
Rem J, Brandt MR, Kehlet H. **Prevention of postoperative lymphopenia and granulocytosis by epidural analgesia.** *Lancet.* 1980;1:283-4. (English)

Blood leukocyte counts, cortisol and glucose were measured in 12 healthy premenopausal women undergoing elective abdominal hysterectomy during general anesthesia (6 women) or epidural analgesia (T4 to S5) (6 women). Surgery during general anesthesia caused significant lymphopenia 6 and 9 h after skin incision and significantly increased granulocyte counts 6, 9 and 24 h after skin incision. Epidural analgesia prevented lymphopenia and reduced granulocytosis to about 40% of that seen in the group receiving general anesthesia. Normal increase in plasma glucose and cortisol during and after surgery was abolished by epidural analgesia. Neurogenic stimuli from the surgical area, probably through their influence on adrenal hormones (cortisol and adrenaline [epinephrine]), are apparently the main mediators of postoperative lymphopenia and are partly responsible for postoperative granulocytosis. Inhibition of the endocrine-metabolic response to surgery may prevent postoperative immunodepression.

424
Renoux G, Renoux M. **Immunopotentiation and anabolism induced by sodium diethyldithiocarbamate.** *J Immunopharmacol.* 1979;1:247-67. (English)

Sodium diethyldithiocarbamate, DTC, enhances over a large range of doses macrophage listericidal capacity and T cell activities in terms of increased IgG-antibody forming spleen cells and delayed hypersensitivity levels. Such immunopotentiation is not associated with splenomegalia or increase in lymphocyte counts. Immunopotentiation requires a preexisting link between carbon disulfide and diethylamine, since both moieties were inactive if administered alone or on separate body sites. DTC demonstrates also an anabolic effect on mice emaciated by administering a *B. melitensis* cell-wall fraction. The role of DTC on hormonal production is discussed in relation to hormone-mediated action of T cell induction.

425

Ricci P, Bándini G, Franchi P, Motta MR, Visani G, Calamandrei G. **Haematological effects of lithium carbonate: a study in 56 psychiatric patients.** *Haematologica.* 1981; 66:627-33. (Italian)

Haematological effects of lithium carbonate (LC) were investigated in 56 adult psychiatric out-patients. Results were compared with a control group of 60 healthy adults. Patients on LC had a statistically significant increase in the leukocyte count (7,600 ± 1,640/microl vs. 6,200 ± 1,600/microl; p<0.001) which was largely due to a rise in neutrophilic polymorphonucleocytes (PMNs) (4,840 ± 1,460/microl vs. 3,650 ± 1,150/microl; p<0.001). Also monocytes and eosinophils were significantly increased. Platelet counts, lymphocyte counts and haemoglobin levels did not differ in patients and control subjects. Patients were divided into three subgroups, according to the daily dose of LC they received, i.e., 1200 mg, 900 mg and 600 mg, respectively. PMN, lymphocyte and platelet counts were analyzed in this context. PMN count was positively related to the LC dose; with 600 mg, no statistical difference was observed between patients and control subjects, while 900 mg and 1200 mg were associated with increasingly higher PMN counts. A slight, not significant reduction of the lymphocyte count was observed only in those patients receiving 1200 mg LC per day. Platelet count did not vary with the drug dose.

426

Runge LA, Pinals RS, Tomar RH. **Treatment of rheumatoid arthritis with levamisole: long-term results and immune changes.** *Ann Rheum Dis.* 1979;38:122-7. (English)

We treated 29 rheumatoid arthritis patients with levamisole. On the basis of a 25% improvement in any 3 of 6 measurements 95% of the patients had a favorable response within 20 weeks. However, 64% of the patients discontinued levamisole by 40 to 60 weeks because of rash or secondary treatment failures. Delayed skin reactivity to streptokinase-streptodornase increased significantly in the entire treatment group, but there was an inverse correlation between skin test enhancement and clinical response. There was no overall change in lymphocyte response to phytohaemagglutinin (PHA) after 4 and 16 weeks of treatment, but seven patients with enhanced lymphocyte responsiveness to PHA experienced an earlier clinical response to levamisole. Treatment with levamisole frequently results in clinical improvement in rheumatoid arthritis, but this is not clearly related to a stimu-

latory effect on cell-mediated immunity. Its long-term usefulness may be limited by a high incidence of relapse and rash.

427

Shaskan EG, Lovett EJ III. **Effects of haloperidol, a dopamine receptor antagonist, on a delayed-type hypersensitivity reaction to 1-chloro, 2,4-dinitrobenzene in mice.** *Res Commun Psychol Psychiat Behav.* 1980;5:241-54. (English)

The effects of subcutaneous injections of haloperidol into C57BL/6 female mice were evaluated on the immune response to a contact allergen, DNCB. Evidence from an *in vivo*, cell-mediated immune response to DNCB suggests that haloperidol does not alter the immune response through effector mechanisms (efferent arm of response), but rather it possesses immunomodulatory properties in relation to recognition and processing of *de novo* antigen (afferent arm of response). These conclusions are made, following deliberate scheduling of drug injections in relation to time of sensitization and challenge by DNCB. While saline-vehicle injections alone, or even handling, can depress this immune response, the magnitude and paradoxical effects from haloperidol suggest that dopamine receptors are modulating this DTH response. The experiments do not distinguish between central (brain) and peripheral (lymphocytes, tissues) sites through which this highly specific dopamine-receptor antagonist may be acting. However, baseline levels of immunocompetency appear to dictate magnitudes of response to haloperidol and some dopamine-receptor agonists.

428

Shaskan EG, Lovett EJ III. **Effects of psychotropic drugs on delayed hypersensitivity reactions in mice: relevant sites of action.** In: *Proc of the 3rd World Congr of Biol Psychiatry.* C Perris, G Struwe, B Jansson (eds.). Amsterdam: Elsevier Biomedical Press, 1981. Pp. 73-84. (English)

Observations that phenothiazine drugs alter cellular immune responses (Mitrova and Mayer, 1976; Ferguson, et al., 1978) suggests involvement of dopamine receptors as non-specific immunomodulators. Theoretically, dopamine receptors modulating immune function could be directly associated with tissues and/or cells of the immune system (e.g., thymus, spleen, lymphocytes, macrophages). In fact, there is recent evidence for the existence of dopamine receptors on lymphocytes (LeFur, et al., 1980) although specific binding may be restricted to receptor antagonists (Shaskan, unpublished observations). Alternatively, immunorelevant dopamine-containing pathways might be within central nervous system structures (Hall and Goldstein, 1981). For instance, central dopamine receptors, presumably in the tubero-infundibular pathway, appear to regulate blood eosinophilia in the rat (Podolec, et al, 1979). Furthermore, chronic treatent of mice with the immediate precursor to dopamine, oral L-Dopa, prolongs mean life span presumably through reduction of intervening diseases (Cotzias, et al., 1974; Cotzias, et al 1977). Elucidation of some mechanisms for these phenomena is facilitated by studying *in vivo* and *in vitro* cellular responses in which intervening steps are well-defined. A delayed-type hypersensitivity (DTH) response represents an ideal experimental system. The "specificity" of this response is considered to result from antigen stimulation of a specific population of thymus-derived lymphocytes (T-cells), and culminates in blast transformation into either a subpopulation of cells capable of a specific immune response against the antigen or a clone of memory cells capable of more rapid response to the antigen in the future (Roitt, 1974). Other cells which mediate DTH *in vivo* include macrophages which process the antigen for initial presentation to T-cells (afferent arm) of the immune response, and function at cutaneous effector sites presumably under direction of T-cells through intercellular messengers or lymphokines (Roitt, 1974). Simply, a DTH reaction may be divided into two phases (Crowle, 1981): 1) afferent arm--the recognition and processing of *de novo* antigen (comprising the first 24-48 hours) and clonal proliferation of effector and memory lymphocytes and 2) efferent arm--the inflammatory, cellular reaction which is specific to the site of reintroduction of the antigen and which is maximum at 24-48 hours. Nonspecific immuno-modulators of DTH could act anywhere along this continuum. Within this context, ligands highly specific for dopamine receptors are evaluated in mice.

429
Shenkman L, Borkowsky W, Shopsin B. **Lithium as an immunological adjuvant.** *Med Hypotheses.* 1980;6:1-6. (English)

Lithium, an adenylate cyclase inhibitor, stimulates a variety of *in vitro* indices of immune function, including proliferation of lymphocytes in response to mitogens, rosette formation by T-cells and phagocytosis by macrophages. Lithium enhances these immunologic responses at concentrations comparable to those achieved in patients receiving lithium for treatment of manic-depressive disorders. Lithium may prove to have important therapeutic applications as an immune adjuvant, particularly in immune deficiency states associated with excessive cAMP production.

430
Shenkman L, Wadler S, Borkowsky W, Shopsin B. **Adjuvant effects of lithium chloride on human mononuclear cells in suppressor-enriched and suppressor-depleted systems.** *Immunopharmacology.* 1981;3:1-8. (English)

Lithium enhances several *in vitro* indices of immune function, including thymidine uptake by mitogen-stimulated human mononuclear cells. To further characterize the mechanism of action of lithium and to determine whether it acts by abrogating suppressor cell activity or by enhancing helper cell function, we have compared the effects of lithium on the mitogenic response of normal, suppressor-depleted and suppressor-enriched mononuclear cell preparations. In normal cultures, lithium enhanced thymidine uptake in response to concanavalin A (Con A) and phytohemagglutinin (PHA). In the suppressor-depleted cultures, thymidine uptake after Con A stimulation was significantly higher than in normal cultures, and was further enhanced by lithium. In the suppressor-enriched system, response to PHA was significantly lower than in normal cultures, and addition of lithium reversed the observed suppression. These results indicate that lithium may be enhancing thymidine uptake in response to mitogen at least in part by abrogating suppressor cell activity. The observed increase in thymidine incorporation in the suppressor-depleted cultures suggests that lithium may also have a direct stimulatory effect on helper cell activity.

431
Sierakowski S, Hryszko S, Bernacka K. **Effect of lithium chloride on lymphocyte transformation.** *Pol Tyg Lek.* 1981;36:63-4. (Polish) (unavailable at publication)

432
Silverman AY, Darnell BJ, Montiel MM, Smith CG, Asch RH. **Response of rhesus monkey lymphocytes to short-term administration of THC.** *Life Sci.* 1982;30:107-15. (English)

Four rhesus monkeys were subjected to daily administration of 2.5 mg of tetrahydrocannabinol (THC)/kg body wt, after establishing the norms for complete blood count, T- and B-cell concentrations, and the dose response of thymidine incorporation after PHA stimulation. THC was administered daily for 3 weeks, the treatment was stopped and then the animals were allowed to recover for 4 weeks. Cellular responses, incorporation studies and fibrinogen levels were determined during the treatment and recovery phases. Compared to the 4 vehicle-treated animals, the THC-treated animals experienced significant augmentation of both their total white cell and their neutrophil counts during the recovery phase which returned to normal levels during the recovery phase. There was no alteration in total lymphocyte count or T- or B-cell concentrations. Fibrinogen levels of the THC-treated animals during the treatment phase were also evaluated compared to controls, and the levels diminished to the same values as the vehicle-treated animals during recovery phase. Possible mechanisms for the response of rhesus monkeys to short-term administration of THC are discussed.

433
Skinner GR, Harley C, Buchan A, Harper L, Gallimore P. **The effect of lithium chloride on the replication of herpes simplex virus.** *Med Microbiol Immunol (Berl).* 1980;168:139-148. (English)

Lithium chloride inhibited the replication of type 1 and type 2 Herpes simplex virus at concentrations which permitted host cell replication. Virus polypeptide and antigen synthesis were unaffected while DNA synthesis was inhibited. The replication of two other DNA viruses, pseudorabies and vaccinia virus, was inhibited but there was no inhibition of two RNA viruses, namely EMC and influenza virus.

434
Skoven I, Thormann J. **Lithium compound treatment and psoriasis.** *Arch Dermatol.* 1979;115:1185-7. (English)

Observations were made of 12 cases of psoriasis that developed and three cases of psoriasis that became exacerbated during treatment with lithium compounds. Only two patients had a family history of psoriasis, and results of a search for increased frequencies of the histocompatibility antigens seen in psoriasis vulgaris were negative. The clinical features were identical to severe psoriasis vulgaris and the diagnosis was confirmed by histologic examination performed in six cases. However, the skin changes disappeared or returned to pretreatment level after withdrawal of lithium compounds. A positive provocation test result was obtained in two cases, the secondary latency time being shorter than the primary. We suggest that the psoriasis was induced or exacerbated by lithium compounds.

435

Smeraldi E, Scorza-Smeraldi R, Fabio G, Negri F. **Interference between anti-HLA antibodies and chlorpromazine metabolites.** *Psychopharmacol (Berl).* 1980;67:87-9. (English)

The interference of chlorpromazine (CPZ) and several preincubated CPZ metabolites on the lymphocyte absorption of antibodies directed against HLA-A1 and other nonrelated HLA specificities were investigated. Both CPZ and metabolites 7-OH-, Nor$_1$- and Nor$_2$-CPZ were found to interfere with the specific absorption of anti-HLA-A1 antibodies. The meaning of such a result is discussed.

436

Stamm T, Lubach D. **Undesirable side effects on the skin caused by lithium therapy: case report and references** (author's translation). *Psychiatr Prax.* 1981;8:152-4. (German)

This is a report about a 54 year old woman, who was treated with lithium carbonate because of a manic-depressive illness. As a side-effect of this medication she developed a relapsing hidradenitis suppurativa. After interruption of this therapy the illness of the skin improved, but relapsed when the therapy with lithium was started again. In this case report we give a survey about side-effects of lithium concerning the skin.

437

Stefanis C. **Biological aspects of cannabis use.** *Natl Inst Drug Abuse Res Monogr Ser.* 1978;19:149-78. (English)

In this paper the results of a multidisciplinary long-term and controlled study on chronic cannabis use are critically reviewed. The first part of the study consisted of: (A) standardization of methods and identification of the experimental sample of chronic cannabis users and matched controls; (B) comparison of the two groups on a number of variables following administration of a battery of medical, psychiatric, neurophysiologic, and psychologic tests; (C) acute cannabis inhalation experiments during which the effect of cannabis preparations of various strengths and of THC-delta-9 were studied in relation to behavioral, psychologic, neurophysiologic, and psychophysiologic responses; (D) identification of possible withdrawal symptoms during a 3-day abstinence period and reintroduction of hashish use. The second part of the study consisted of: (A) a controlled histochemical and electron-microscopic investigation of blood cells and sperm, aimed at revealing changes produced by cannabis at the molecular level, particularly in the cell-nuclear area; (B) a biochemical investigation of changes in biogenic amines and substances related to their metabolism and function during cannabis pre-smoking and post-smoking periods. Our findings from the first part of the study failed to distinguish users from nonusers on most of the investigated parameters. However, they provided useful information on a variety of controversial issues and revealed methodological limitations which should guide future research. Our findings from the second part of the study, although still preliminary, clearly indicate that cannabis use affects cell nuclear metabolism and produces changes on the molecular level potentially significant for man's biologic functioning. Furthermore, findings from this part of this study failed to distinguish users from nonusers on most of the investigated parameters. However, they provided

useful information on a variety of controversial issues and research. Our findings from the second part of the study, although still preliminary, clearly indicate that cannabis use affects cell-nuclear metabolism and produces changes on the molecular level potentially significant for man's biologic functioning. Furthermore findings from this part of this study indicated that cannabis' acute effects in man are correlated with changes in metabolism directly related to biogenic amine biosynthesis and function. It is concluded that despite advances in recent years, cannabis research has still a long way to go before providing the definitive answers to the very important questions arising from its habitual use by man.

438

Tsokos G, Mandyla H, Xanthou M, Papamichail M. **Chlorpromazine and lidocaine inhibit antibody-dependent cell-mediated cytotoxicity but not erythrocyte and antibody rosette formation.** *Int Arch Allergy Appl Immunol.* 1980;61:344-6. (English)

Pretreatment of human peripheral blood mononuclear cells with chlorpromazine and lidocaine reduces their ability to induce lysis of antibody-coated target cells. This effect of local anesthetics was not due to a reduction of binding of antibody-coated red cells to the mononuclear cells, but it was rather probably due to the inhibition of the Fc receptor on the cell membrane.

439

Turner AR, Allalunis MJ. **Oral lithium carbonate increases colony stimulating activity production from human mononuclear cells.** *Adv Exp Med Biol.* 1980;127:127-36. (English) (no abstract)

440

Uzan A, Phan T, Le Fur G. **Selective labelling of murine B lymphocytes by [^{3}H] spiroperidol.** *J Pharm Pharmacol.* 1981;33:102-3. (English) (no abstract)

441

Verma DS, Spitzer G, Gutterman JU, Beran M, Zander AR, McCredie KB. **Human leukocyte interferon-mediated granulopoietic differentiation arrest and is abrogation by lithium carbonate.** *Am J Hematol.* 1982;12:39-46. (English)

Interferon has been show to inhibit erythropoietic and granulopoietic differentiation. Since lithium carbonate (Li) elevates granulocyte levels in a variety of neutropenic disorders, we investigated the effect of Li on human leukocyte interferon (HLIF)-mediated inhibition of granulopoietic differentiation. Using an agar culture technique for cloning granulocyte-macrophage progenitor cells (GM-CFC), we demonstrated that Li blocks HLIF-induced granulopoietic differentiation arrest in a dose-dependent manner. Results of removal of T lymphocytes from marrow cells suggest that this Li effect is not mediated through marrow T lymphocytes.

442

Verrill HL, Pickard N, Gruemer HD. **Mechanisms of cellular enzyme release; I--Alteration in membrane fluidity and permeability.** *Clin Chem.* 1977;23:2219-25. (English)

Above-normal plasma enzyme activities resulting from increased release of intracellular macromolecules are an important diagnostic feature of Duchenne muscular dystrophy. These and other biochemical and histological characteristics of this disease are faithfully duplicated when imipramine and serotonin are administered to the rat. Imipramine, but not serotonin alone, causes release of enzymes from rat diaphragms and human lymphocytes and release of hemoglobin from erythrocytes *in vitro*. Quabain causes neither. Imipramine-induced enzyme release is decreased by adding ATP to the specimen *in vitro* or in hypertonic solution. Imipramine inhibits the capping phenomenon (an aggregation of antigen/antibody complexes of the membrane) of human B lymphocytes labeled with fluorescein-conjugated antihuman immunoglobulins. Serotonin alone has no such effect, but, administered together with imipramine, it potentiates the inhibition of capping by imipramine.

443

Walton B. **Anaesthesia, surgery and immunology.** *Anaesthesia.* 1978;33:322-48. (English) (no abstract)

444

Weetman AP, McGregor AM, Lazarus JH, Smith BR, Hall R. **The enhancement of immunoglobulin synthesis by human lymphocytes with lithium.** *Clin Immunol Immunopathol.* 1982;22:400-7. (English) (unavailable at publication)

445

Wessels JM. **Haematological effects of lithium: a review.** *Aggressologie.* 1982;23:105-9. (English)

Lithium in physiological concentrations causes peripheral granulocytosis. It enhances the production of colony stimulating activity and stimulates the proliferation of stem cells. In clinical practice lithium seems to be most effective in Felty's syndrome and when used in combination with cytostatic therapy. There are some indications that lithium stimulates immune reactions. It is proven that this drug augments the aggregability of thrombocytes. Striking evidence is presented that inhibition of adenylate cyclase plays a key role in the effect of lithium of the aggregability of thrombocytes.

446

Whalley LJ, Roberts DF, Wentzel J, Watson KC. **Antinuclear antibodies and histocompatibility antigens in patients on long-term lithium therapy.** *J Affective Disord.* 1981;3:123-30. (English)

A survey of antinuclear factor, histocompatibility antigens, red blood cell groups and red blood cell isoenzyme variants is reported in 54 patients on long-term lithium therapy. Eleven patients with detectable antinuclear factor could not be distinguished from 43 patients without antinuclear factor using age, sex, diagnosis, previous medication, time on lithium or usual dose of lithium. The presence of antinuclear factor was not associated with any particular genetic marker.

447

Wunderlich V, Fey F, Sydow G. **Antiviral effect of haloperidol on Rauscher murine leukemia virus.** *Arch Geschwulstforsch.* 1980;50:758-62. (German)

The neuroleptic drug haloperidol (Hal) shows, when administered in multiple intraperitoneal or intravenous injections beginning at 5 hours post inoculation of Rauscher leukemia virus to male NMRI mice, a marked activity in inhibiting virus-induced splenomegaly and prolonging mean survival time. Evidence is presented that a direct action of the drug is involved in its inhibitory effect.

448

Yoda K, Yokono S, Miyazaki M. **Anaphylactic shock during spinal anesthesia.** *Jpn J Anesthesiol.* 1980;29:941-45. (Japanese)

Anaphylactic shock during spinal anesthesia is encountered in very low incidence, however it is critical. Cases (3) of anaphylactic cardiovascular collapse during spinal anesthesia were studied. The cases had 11 points in common. To prevent anaphylactic shock, general anesthesia is preferable to spinal anesthesia in patients with asthma and other allergic factors. Skin test to local anesthetics should be performed. Epinephrine or ephedrine should be given before spinal anesthesia to avoid the release of chemical mediators of anaphylaxis.

449

Zarrabi MH, Zucker S, Miller F, Derman RM, Romano GS, Hartnett JA, Varma AO. **Immunologic and coagulation disorders in chlorpromazine-treated patients.** *Ann Intern Med.* 1979;91:194-9. (English)

The prevalence of immunologic and coagulation disorders in 75 schizophrenic patients treated with chlorpromazine or other antipsychotic drugs was evaluated. Four groups were studied: Group A, chlorpromazine treatment for more than 2 1/2 years; Group B, chlorpromazine and other antipsychotic drug treatment for more than 2 1/2 years; Group C, chlorpromazine treatment for less than 2 1/2 years; Group D, no chlorpromazine, but other antipsychotic drug treatment. Significant evaluation of serum IgM and prolongation of partial thromboplastin time were noted in patients who had long-term chlorpromazine treatment. The latter was caused by a circulating inhibitor resembling that seen with systemic lupus erythematosus. There was significant correlation between the IgM level versus chlorpromazine dose or duration of treatment and the partial thromboplastin time versus chlorpromazine dose or duration of treatment. In Groups A and B, 63% had positive antinuclear antibody test ($\geq$ 1:80), 40% had antibodies to native DNA, and 58% had antibodies to nucleoprotein. These antibodies were negative in the other groups. The percentages of T lymphocytes were below normal in 13 of 41 patients treated with chlorpromazine. Twenty of 42 patients in Groups A and B, and none of 28 in Groups C and D had splenomegaly. This study indicates that most patients on long-term chlorpromazine treatment develop one or more immunologic abnormalities.

450

Zucker S, Zarrabi MH, Romano GS, Miller F. **IgM inhibitors of the contact activation phase of coagulation in chlorpromazine-treated patients.** *Br J Haematol.* 1978; 40:447-57. (English)

In this report we have described three patients with chronic schizophrenia on long-term chlorpromazine therapy who developed asymptomatic IgM inhibitors of the intrinsic phase of blood coagulation. The anticoagulant resulted in decreased measurements of all of the plasma clotting factors in the intrinsic pathway (factors VIII, IX, XI, XII, Fletcher Factor and Fitzgerald Factor). Using crude coagulation reagents, the serum of these patients interfered with the clot promoting activity of contact product. To determine the relationship between drug therapy and these IgM inhibitors, we have studied nine additional schizophrenic patients on long-term chlorpromazine therapy. All nine chlorpromazine-treated patients had significantly increased levels of serum IgM and asymptomatic inhibitors of coagulation. We conclude that long-term high-dose chlorpromazine treatment of schizophrenic patients results in an increased concentration of IgM which has inhibitory activity in the contact phase of blood coagulation.

Other agents

451
Antonaci S. et al. *In vitro* modulation of cell-mediated immunity by prostaglandin E$_2$; I--Enhancing-inhibitory effects on antibody-dependent cellular cytotoxicity. *Prostaglandins, Leukotrienes and Med.* 1982;9:285-93. (English) (unavailable at publication)

452
Askenase PW. Role of basophils, mast cells, and vasoamines in hypersensitivity reactions with a delayed time course. *Prog Allergy.* 1977;23:199-320. (English) (no abstract)

453
Atkinson JP, Sullivan TJ, Kelly JP, Parker CW. Stimulation by alcohols of cyclic AMP metabolism in human leukocytes: possible role of cyclic AMP in the anti-inflammatory effects of ethanol. *J Clin Invest.* 1977;60:284-94. (English)

In this study ethanol and certain other short-chain aryl (benzyl and phenethyl) and aliphatic (methyl, propyl, butyl, and amyl) alcohols produced up to 10-fold increases in cyclic AMP (cAMP) concentrations in purified human peripheral blood lymphocytes. Ethanol concentrations as low as 80 mg/dl produced significant elevations in lymphocyte cAMP. Significant but less marked augmentation of cAMP in response to alcohols was observed in human platelets, human granulocytes, and rabbit alveolar macrophages. The mechanism of the alcohol-induced cAMP accumulation is probably secondary to membrane perturbation and consequent activation of adenylate cyclase, because ethanol directly stimulated this enzyme in lymphocyte membrane preparations but had no effect on lymphocyte phosphodiesterase activity. Lysosomal enzyme release, by phagocytosing human leukocytes, and aminoisobutyric acid transport in mitogen-stimulated human lymphocytes were shown to be inhibited by ethanol and other alcohols at concentrations which also elevate cAMP. In general, the magnitude of the inhibition of these inflammatory processes correlated with the ability of the alcohol to elevate cAMP concentrations. Lectin- and antithymocyte globulin-induced lymphocyte

454
Ben-Zvi A, Russel A, Shneyour A, Trainin N. Changes in intra cellular cyclic AMP levels of human peripheral blood lymphocytes in bronchial asthma. *Ann Allergy.* 1979;43:223-4. (English)

Peripheral blood lymphocytes of asthmatic patients in the acute stage manifested low basal levels of cyclic(c)AMP (which have been implicated with acquisition of immuno-competence). These levels were higher in lymphocytes of patients in remission than in controls. Trypsin treatment of lymphocytes increased cAMP content to almost the same level in both groups of patients. Presence of an additional activation site of the receptor in theophylline- and catecholamines-treated patients was suggested.

455
Benotzen K, Palit J. Modulation of human leucocyte migration inhibitory factor (MIF) by 3', 5' cyclic AMP, 3' 5'-cyclic GMP and agents known to influence intracellular cyclic nucleotide metabolism. *Acta Pathol Microbiol Scand C.* 1977;85:317-23. (English) (unavailable at publication)

456
Berenbaum MC, Purves EC, Allison IE. Intercellular immunological controls and modulation of cyclic AMP levels: some doubts. *Immunology.* 1976;30:815-23. (English)

We have re-examined two sets of observations put forward to support the hypothesis that rises in cAMP levels induced by vasoactive amines and prostaglandins are involved in the intercellular control of immunological and inflammatory processes. (1) This hypothesis is said to be supported by the fact that cholera toxin, which raises cAMP levels in lymphoid tissue *in vivo*, is immunosuppressive. However, we found that cholera toxin inhibited antibody production only if given in doses causing gross destruction of lymphoid tissue. This sort of evidence, therefore, cannot be used to support a hypothesis about homoeostasis under physiological conditions. (2) The hypothesis is also said to be supported by the claim that vasoactive amines, prostaglandins, cholera toxin and methyl xanthines, which raise cAMP cell levels *in vitro*, also inhibit the formation of haemolytic plaques by spleen cells from mice immunized with sheep red cells. However, we were unable to confirm this claim, except when the experimental conditions were such that cells were killed or other artefacts operated.

457
Bidart JM, Assicot M, Bohuon C. Catechol-O-methyl transferase activity in human mononuclear cells. *Res Commun Chem Pathol Pharmacol.* 1981;34:47-54. (English)

Catechol-O-methyl transferase activity (COMT) activity was investigated in human peripheral mononuclear cells and in human lymphoblastoid cell lines. In any case, we have detected enzymatic activity in the membrane fraction of the cells. K_m was found to be 4-9 x 10^{-6} M and the enzyme was inhibited by tropolone and the lack of magnesium. The eventual association of COMT with adrenergic receptor-adenylate cyclase system in mononuclear cells is discussed.

458

Boss GR, Erbe RW. **Decreased rates of methionine synthesis by methylene tetrahydrofolate reductase-deficient fibroblasts and lymphoblasts.** *J Clin Invest.* 1981; 67:1659-64. (English)

Methionine synthesis from homocysteine was measured in intact human fibroblasts and lymphoblasts using a ^{14}C formate label. Seven fibroblast lines and two lymphoblast lines derived from patients with 5,10-methylene tetrahydrofolate reductase deficiency had rates of methionine synthesis that were from 4 to 43% of normal. When the patients were divided by clinical status into mildly (two patients), moderately (two patients), and severely (three patients) affected, methionine biosynthesis expressed as a percent of control values was 43 and 33%, 11 and 10%, and 7, 6, and 4%, respectively, in fibroblasts. Similar data for the two lymphoblast lines were 36 and 26% for a mildly and moderately affected patient, respectively. These data are to be contrasted with the measurement of residual enzyme activity in cell extracts which agrees less precisely with the clinical status of the patients. In the presence of normal methionine synthetase activity, the rate of synthesis of methionine from homocysteine is a function of the activity of the enzyme 5,10-methylene tetrahydrofolate reductase, and measurement of the methionine biosynthetic capacity of cells deficient in this enzyme accurately reflects the clinical status of the patient from whom the cells were derived.

459

Bursztajn S, Askenase PW, Gershon RK, Gershon MD. **Role of vasoactive amines during early stages of delayed-type hypersensitivity skin reactions.** *Fed Proc.* 1978;37:590. (English)

Delayed-type hypersensitivity (DTH) in immunized mice (0.2 ml of SRBC containing 10^5 cells) induced by injecting an antigen (SRBC) was studied by light and electron microscopy during early stages of the reaction. Mast cells which are known to contain vasoactive amines at first undergo filopodia activation and 12 h later show granule alteration. The release of vasoactive amines is a gradual process and extrusion of granules was not observed. Autoradiography of immunized challenged mice injected with ^3H-5-hydroxytryptamine (1mCi/mM) show no grain accumulation over degranulated mast cells. The release of vasoactive amines causes separation of endothelial cells of postcapillary venules which results in diapedisis of blood cells. These endothelial separations are further elucidated ultrastructurally by employing colloidal carbon (100mg/kg) and by fluorescent microscopy using fluorosceinated dextrans (100mg/100gm) where the topology of the entire vasculature was delineated in a whole mount preparation. Monoamine-depleting drugs, reserpine (5mg/kg) or cyproheptadine (5mg/kg) prevented blood vessel leaks as evidenced by the tracer particles being confined to the lumen of the venous blood vessels. Alterations in the basement membrane are also described. We suggest that vasoamines may be directly involved in production of lesions seen in DTH reactions.

460

Coffey RG, Hadden EM, Hadden JW. **Evidence for cyclic GMP and calcium mediation of lymphocyte activation by mitogens.** *J Immunol.* 1977;119:1387-94. (English)

The results of 47 experiments indicate that the lectin mitogens, PHA and Con A, increase cyclic GMP (cGMP) levels in human peripheral blood lymphocytes and their incubation medium 2- to 9-fold within 10 min of stimulation. At concentrations supraoptimal for the induction of proliferation, Con A, but not PHA, induces progressive increases in cAMP and lesser increases in cGMP. Succinylated Con A (S-Con A) does not exhibit inhibition of proliferation up to concentrations of 250 microg/ml and correspondingly does not produce the cAMP increases observed with native Con A. PHA and both forms of Con A induce modest increases in cGMP in the absence of calcium and no increases in the presence of EDTA. After preexposure to Con A in the absence of calcium, the addition of calcium produces increases in cGMP. The data are consistent with the interpretation that mitogen-induced increases in lymphocyte cGMP are totally Ca^{2+}-dependent, yet only in part dependent on extracellular Ca^{2+}. The interpretation is confirmed with a divalent cation ionophore A23187, which was shown to induce lymphocyte proliferation in close association with Ca^{2+}-dependent increases in cGMP and at higher concentrations to inhibit the mitogenic effects in association with Mg^{2+}-dependent increases in cAMP. Dose-response curves for each agent showed that this capacity to increase cGMP levels was correlated with the optimal mitogenic concentration as determined by assay of DNA synthesis. The data are consistent with the postulate that cGMP participates in the positive aspects of mitogen action and that cAMP participates in the inhibitory aspects. It is concluded that coparticipation of cGMP and Ca^{2+} as essential mediators of the mitogenic signal is a sound hypothesis.

461

Cotzias CG, Tang LC. **An adenylate cyclase of brain reflects propensity for breast cnacer in mice.** *Science.* 1977;197:1094-6. (English)

High propensity for breast cancer in mice was associated with low dopamine-stimulated adenylate cyclase activity in the brain, low spontaneous motorization, and low motor responses to injections of the catecholamine precursor, L-dopa.

462

Dmitrenko NP, Komissarenko SV, Goroshnikova TV. **Adenylate cyclase from rat thymus and spleen lymphocytes.** *Biokhimiia.* 1980;45:1810-8. (Russian)

It was found that adenylate cyclase from spleen lymphocytes is more active as compared to that from thymocytes, but is less sensitive to the activating effect of epinephrine and NAF. Adenylate cyclase from different subcellular fractions of thymocytes has different sensitivity to NAF. In the microsomal and mitochondrial fractions the enzyme is inhibited by NAF 7- and 2-fold, while in cell lysate and nuclear-cellular fractions it is activated 3- and 9-fold, respectively. In the presence of NAF, adenosine, AMP, PPI and methylene diphosphonic acid inhibit the enzyme activity both in thymus and spleen lymphocytes. Creatine and CRP also significantly decrease the enzyme activity. N_4^+ and Concanavalin A have no effect and phytohemagglutinin stimulates the enzyme from both sources.

463

Gallin JI, Sandler JA, Clyman RI, Manganiello VC, Vaughan M. **Agents that increase cyclic AMP inhibit accumulation of cGMP and depress human monocyte locomotion.** *J Immunol.* 1978;120:492-6. (English)

Ascorbic acid and serotonin increased the 3',5'-guanosine monophosphate (cGMP) content and enhanced the chemotactic responsiveness of mononuclear cells from human peripheral blood. The ionophore A23187, PGE_1 and polystyrene beads increased the 3',5'-adenosine monophosphate (cAMP) content of mononuclear cells and had no effect on basal cGMP content. A23187, PGE_1 and beads caused significant increases in cAMP content in preparations of adherent cells (chiefly monocytes); PGE_1 and beads also increased cAMP content in the nonadherent cells (chiefly lymphocytes). A23187 and PGE_1 each inhibited mononuclear cell locomotion. The chemically unrelated agents, A23187, beads, and PGE_1, that raised cAMP of monocytes inhibited the accumulation of cGMP in response to serotonin and ascorbic acid. PGE_1 at a concentration that caused 349% increase in cAMP inhibited the effect of serotonin on cGMP accumulation and the amplification of chemotaxis by serotonin only 37% and 40%, respectively. In contrast A23187, which increased monocyte cAMP by only 71%, inhibited the effect of serotonin on cGMP accumulation and locomotion by 85% and 79%, respectively. Although there is no clear quantitative relationship between the increase in cAMP content and the degree of inhibition of cGMP accumulation, it is possible that the elevation of cAMP in monocytes interferes with their capacity to accumulate cGMP in response to serotonin and ascorbic acid, perhaps by increasing cGMP degradation and/or inhibiting synthesis. In any case cyclic nucleotide modulation of monocyte locomotion appears to be more closely related to intracellular cGMP content than to cAMP content.

464

Goldberg SJ, O'Shaughnessy MV, Stewart RB. **The relationship between adenosine 3',5'-cyclic monophosphate (cAMP) and interferon activity in mouse cells.** *J Gen Virol.* 1980;48:377-81. (English)

Three mouse cell lines (L, 3T3, and SV 3T3) were studied with respect to the elevation of cellular cAMP levels following interferon treatment and the effect of stimulators of cAMP levels on the antiviral activity of interferon. Interferon treatment resulted in increased cAMP levels in L and 3T3 cells but not in SV 3T3. The antiviral activity of interferon in cells treated with epinephrine and 1-methyl-3-isobutyl xanthine (stimulators of cAMP levels) was potentiated in L cells, but not in 3T3 cells and was lost in SV 3T3 cells.

465

Gurtoo HL, Parker NB, Paigen B, Havens MB, Minowada J, Freedman HJ. **Induction inhibition and some enzymological properties of aryl hydrocarbon hydroxylase in fresh-mitogen activated human lymphocytes.** *Cancer Res.* 1979;39:4620-9. (English)
Aryl hydrocarbon hydroxylase (AHH) induction may be correlated with carcinogenesis. Basal and/or polycyclic aromatic hydrocarbon (PAH)- induced AHH in mitogen-activated cultured lymphocytes obtained from healthy donors was studied for the specificity of induction and inhibition and for other enzymological proprties. Of the 24 chemicals tested, 2,3,7,8-tetrachlorodibenzo-p-dioxin, dibenz(a,h)anthracene, benz(a)anthracene 3-methylcholanthrene, beta-naphthoflavone, cholecalciferol and DL-isoproterenol were good inducers (inducibility ratio > 2.0). Other chemicals which produced effects ranging from inhibition to mild induction included 4-bromoflavone, alpha-naphthoflavone, chrysene, p,p-1,1,1-trichloro-2,2-bis (p-chlorophenyl) ethane, 7,12-dimethyl-benzanthracene, pyrene, D,L-norepinephrine, benzo(e)pyrene, lindane, n-octylamine, testosterone, 2,5-diphenyloxazole, 17-beta-estradiol, metyrapone and phenobarbital, 2,3,7,8-Tetrachlorodibenzo-p-dioxin was the most potent inducer, followed by dibenz(a,h)-anthracene benz(a) anthracene > 3-methylcholanthrene. The data suggested that the latter 4 inducers could be used interchangeably as they appear to activate the common, genetically determined factors involved in the induction of AHH. The order of potency among the inhibitors was alpha-naphthoflavone > beta-naphthoflavone, followed by 2-diethylaminoethyl-2,2-diphenylvalerate, metyrapone, 1,1,1- trichloropropene oxide and cyclohexene oxide. Depending on the concentration used, the latter 4 inhibitors produced moderate inhibition to moderate stimulation. The inhibition pattern for the basal and PAH induced AHH was indistinguishable. The half-life of the enzyme during cell culture and the K_m values of the AHH in uninduced and PAH-induced cells were also similar. 2,3,7,8-tetrachlorodibenzo-p-dioxin dibenz(a,h)anthracene, benz(a)anthracene and 3-methylcholanthrene seem to have a common mechanism of action, differing only in the degree of induction of AHH produced. Basal and induced AHH are qualitatively similar and differ only quantitatively in comparable uninduced and PAH-induced cells.

466

Hanifin JM. **Atopic dermatitis.** *J Am Acad Dermatol.* 1982;6:1-13. (English)

Atopic dermatitis is a chronically relapsing inflammatory skin disease with altered immune and pharmacologic responses. Elevated serum IgE probably reflects defective immune regulation. Various other cellular immune defects rise and fall with exacerbations and remissions of skin inflammation. Increased responsiveness to cholinergic and alpha-adrenergic agents may relate to abnormalities of cyclic nucleotide regulation. Recent observations of abnormal cyclic adenosine monophosphate (cAMP)-phosphodiesterase activity in atopic dermatitis may provide new insights into the pathogenesis and treatment of the disease.

467

Higgins TJ, David JR. **Effects of isoproterenol and aminophylline on cyclic AMP levels of guinea pig macrophages.** *Cell Immunol.* 1976;27:1-10. (English)

The levels of cyclic AMP in guinea pig peritoneal macrophages can be significantly elevated by both isoproterenol and aminophylline. The response by the macrophages to each of these agents is dose-related and is manifested by 5 min of incubation with levels returning to basal within 2 min. It is demonstrated that at times when the macrophage no longer manifests increased intracellular levels of cyclic AMP, the stimulating agent is still present in the culture medium. Furthermore, the addition of fresh isoproterenol to previously stimulated cultures does not produce a second elevation of intracellular cyclic AMP. While some of the excess intracellular cyclic AMP is excreted from the cell, there was no increasing accumulation of cyclic AMP in the culture medium with time. It is concluded from these results that after the initial response the macrophage is refractory to the stimulating agent.

468
Kalmar L, Gergely P, Nekam K, Lang I, Petranyi G. **Spontaneous rosette formation** *in vitro* **under the effect of agents affecting the cyclic nucleotide system of circulating lymphocytes of normal subjects.** *Acta Med Acad Sci Hung.* 1978;35:21-8. (Hungarian)

Aminophylline was found to affect the early and total rosette-forming capacity of human thymus-dependent lymphocytes. This may be connected with an increase in the intracellular cyclic adenosine 3',5'-monophosphate level. Acetylcholine increases the proportion of early spontaneous rosettes, a phenomenon suggestive of a shift within the lymphocyte population toward a subpopulation of higher activity. The effect of acetylcholine is possibly mediated by an increase in the intracellular cyclic guanosine 3',5'-monophosphate level. Aminophylline affects only the early rosette-forming capacity of thymus-derived lymphocytes. Levamisole has no influence on either early or total rosette-forming capacity of normal lymphocytes. The results are suggestive of definite relationships between the functional state, activity and cyclic nucleotide system of thymus-dependent lymphocytes.

469
Kalmar L, Gergely P, Petranyi G. **Dissociation of the mitogenic and rosette-forming effects of PHA to stimulators of cyclic AMP levels.** *Acta Med Acad Sci Hung.* 1978;35:147-51. (Hungarian)

The mitogenic and the spontaneous E-rosette stimulating effects of phytohaemagglutinin (PHA) were studied by examining their responses to an elevation of intracellular cAMP induced by pretreatment with aminophylline, adrenaline or PGE₁ or by adding exogenous cAMP. Elevation of the intracellular cAMP levels of lymphocytes was found to be inhibitory to the mitogenic effect of PHA, while leaving the increased early and stable spontaneous rosette formation unaffected. It also failed to depress the PHA-induced slight increase in the proportion of total spontaneous E-rosette-forming lymphocytes. The responses of the two PHA effects under study to the elevation of the cAMP level are thus dissociated, suggesting that the two effects represent two different manifestations of lymphocyte activation, though these manifestations may not be independent of each other. It has been confirmed that PHA produces a shift primarily within the T-cell population toward the active and the stable E-rosette-forming subpopulation, while the increase in the total E-rosette-forming lymphocyte population is but slight. This may possibly involve the activation of the T-derived "null" cells unable to bind sheep red blood cells without PHA treatment.

470
Kalmar L, Lang I, Gergely P, Fekete B, Petranyi G. **Effect of changes in cyclic nucleotide levels on human antibody-dependent cellular cytotoxicity.** *Acta Med Acad Sci Hung.* 1978;35:35-42. (Hungarian)

The effect of agents influencing intracellular cyclic nucleotide levels and that of exogenous cAMP was studied on the cytotoxicity of normal human peripheral blood mononuclear cells on antibody-coated human and chicken erythrocytes. Elevation of the cAMP level resulted in a marked decrease in cytotoxicity. While these effects were basically similar in the allogeneic and the xenogeneic test systems, they were more expressed in the allogeneic system.

471
Kuehl FA, Jr, Egan RW. **Prostaglandins, arachidonic acid and inflammation.** *Science.* 1980;210:978-84. (English)

The enzymatic oxidation of arachidonic acid has been shown to yield potent pathological agents by two major pathways. Those of the prostaglandin (PG) pathway, particularly PGE₂, have been implicated as inflammatory mediators for many years. The discovery and biological activities of thromboxane A₂ and prostacyclin as well as a destructive oxygen-centered radical as additional products of this biosynthetic pathway now require these to be considered as potential inflammatory mediators. Like PGE₂, their biosynthesis is prevented by nonsteroidal anti-inflammatory agents. More recently, the alternative metabolic route, the lipoxygenase pathway, has been shown to yield a new class of arachidonic acid oxygenation products, called the leukotrienes, which also appear to be important inflammatory mediators. Unlike the prostaglandins, some of which play important roles as biological regulators, the actions of the lipoxygenase products appear to be exclusively of a pathological level.

472
Lee TP, Busse WW, Reed CE. **Effect of beta-adrenergic agonist, prostaglandins, and cortisol on lymphocyte levels of cyclic adenosine monophosphate and glycogen: abnormal lymphocytic metabolism in asthma.** *J Allergy Clin Immunol.* 1977;59:408-13. (English)

Decreased beta-adrenergic regulation of cyclic adenosine monophosphate (cAMP) in lymphocytes has been described in asthma. We investigated adrenergic stimulation of glycogenolysis and responses to prostaglandin E₁ (PGE₁). Lymphocytes from 24 normal and 24 mild asthmatic subjects who had no drugs for at least 2 weeks were separated on Ficoll-Hypaque and incubated in Medium 199 with Hepes buffer. Beta-adrenergic stimulation of cAMP and glycogenolysis was reduced in the asthmatics (p<0.05). PGE₁ produced less of a rise in cAMP in asthmatics than in normals, but the difference was not significant (p>0.05) and glycogenolysis was normal. Cortisol added *in vitro* potentiates the effect of isoproterenol and PGE₁—but in the presence of cortisol the response of the asthmatic cells to isoproterenol is still lower than that of normal cells. This observation would support that "beta-adrenergic blockade" is the major defect of asthmatic cells. The conclusion is further supported by the observation that the degree of the blockade is associated with a pathologic condition.

473

Machado JA, Antunes LJ, Silva EN. **"E" Rosette formation in "active" T lymphocytes: phenomenon modulated by intracellular level of cyclic AMP and GMP** (author's transl.) *Rev Bras Pesqui Med Biol.* 1977;10:241-6. (Portuguese)

The rosette formation involving the binding of sheep red blood cells (SRBC) with active T lymphocytes was activated when the lymphocytes were incubated with levamisole, acetylcholine or carbamylcholine. Similar activation was seen when substances of glucose metabolism (lactate, fumarate or succinate) or adenosine triphosphate (ATP) were added to the incubation medium. The lymphocytes' incubation with aminophyline, isoproterenol or 2,4-dinitrophenol (DNP) inhibited the rosette formation. The inhibition promoted by aminophyline was reversed by levamisole, acetylcholine or carbamylcholine, but not when lactate or ATP was used. When the rosette formation inhibition was caused by DNP, the reversion was only possible by ATP and no effect occurred if guanil cyclase activators were added to the incubation medium.

474

Makino S, Ikemori K, Kashima T, Fukuda T. **Comparison of cyclic adenosine monophosphate response of lymphocytes in normal and asthmatic subjects to norepinephrine and salbutamol.** *J Allergy Clin Immunol.* 1977; 59:348-52. (English)

Reduced response of beta-adrenergic receptors, especially beta$_2$-receptors, has been suggested as a contributing factor in the etiology of asthma. Cyclic adenosine monophosphate (AMP) production in lymphocytes after exposure to 10^{-3} M salbutamol, predominantly a beta$_2$-receptor stimulant, was significantly less in asthmatic subjects than in normal subjects, while there was no significant difference in cyclic AMP response to 10^{-3} M norepinephrine, predominantly a beta$_2$-receptor stimulant. Both drugs evoked the maximum response at 10^{-3} M. The cyclic AMP response to salbutamol of 5 asthmatic subjects being treated with steroids was diminished significantly compared with that of 7 patients not treated with steroids; however, the response to norepinephrine was similar in both groups. The degree of abnormality in the beta$_2$-receptor response seems to be related to the severity of the asthma.

475

Masaracchia RA, Walsh DA. **Protein phosphotransferase activities and cyclic nucleotide action in proliferating lymphocytes.** *Cancer Res.* 1976;36:3227-37. (English)

Cyclic nucleotide levels, protein phosphotransferase activities, and cyclic nucleotide-binding proteins have been determined and partially characterized in the mouse lymphosarcoma P1798. This system is used as a model to understand the function of these activities in a rapidly proliferating cell. Adenosine 3',5' monophosphate (cAMP) concentrations are 5-fold higher in the lymphosarcoma cells than in thymocytes. In both the thymocytes and malignant tissue, cAMP concentrations are increased by physiological concentrations of epinephrine and prostaglandin. The guanosine 3',5'-monophosphate (cGMP) level in the lymphosarcoma is 0.1 pmol/10^6) cells and is not modified by acetylcholine, prosta-

glandin F$_2$alpha, or concanavalin A. Four protein phosphotransferase activities have been identified in the lymphosarcoma. These are the cAMP-dependent protein kinase type I and II isozymes and a "histone kinase" and a "phosvitin kinase"; neither of the latter two is regulated by cyclic nucleotides. Characterization of these enzymes was based on fractionation by De[52] chromatography, substrate specificity, interaction with the protein inhibitor of cAMP-dependent protein kinases, and sucrose gradient sedimentation rates. Both the cAMP-dependent protein phosphotransferase activity and the phosvitin phosphotransferase activity are 2-to 4-fold elevated in the lymphosarcoma cells in comparison to thymocytes. cAMP binding is associated with both the type I and II isozymes and with a fraction tentatively designated as the regulatory subunit of these enzymes. cGMP also binds to this latter fraction and to the partially purified fraction containing the type I cAMP-dependent enzyme. The histone phosphotransferase activity of this fraction is also stimulated by cGMP, but studies of the number of binding sites and of absorption to cAMP and cGMP affinity resins indicated that this fraction contains more than one species of cyclic nucleotide-binding protein.

476

Mendelsohn J, Nordberg J. **Adenylate cyclase in thymus-derived and bone marrow-derived lymphocytes from normal donors and patients with chronic lymphocytic leukemia.** *J Clin Invest.* 1979;63:1124-32. (English)

Lymphocytes were purified from peripheral blood of normal donors and patients with chronic lymphocytic leukemia (CLL) by Ficoll-Hypaque centrifugation. Adenylate cyclase activity, expressed as picomoles [^{32}P]cyclic AMP generated per milligram protein per minute, was 57 ± 4 in normals and 26 ± 4 in CLL patients. Enzyme activity, expressed as picomoles [^{32}P]cyclic AMP generated per 10^6 lymphocytes per minute, was 2.09 ± 0.19 for normal lymphocytes and 1.10 ± 0.16 for CLL lymphocytes. The differences between normal and CLL peripheral lymphocytes are highly significant ($p<0.001$) with either method of calculating activity. Cyclic AMP levels (picomoles per 10^6 lymphocytes) also differed significantly: 1.38 ± 0.29 for normals and 0.45 ± 0.08 for CLL lymphocytes. Adenylate cyclase was assayed in lymphocytes enriched for bone marrow-derived (B) cells by removing E-rosetted thymus-derived (T) cells, and enriched for T cells by harvesting E-rosetted lymphocytes or by removing B cells with nylon wool absorption. Solutions to simultaneous equations gave the following calculated enzyme activities for pure B- and T-cell subpopulations (in picomoles [^{32}P]cyclic AMP generated per milligram mg protein per minute): normal B, 196 ± 22; normal T, 30 ± 10; CLL B, 34 ± 6; CLL T, 19 ± 4. Thus, normal B-lymphocyte adenylate cyclase exceeds normal T-lymphocyte activity by more than sixfold, whereas in the case of CLL the enzyme activity in B lymphocytes is markedly reduced to levels comparable to T lymphocytes.

477

Morgan JI, Hall AK, Perris AD. **The ionic dependence and steroid blockade of cyclic nucleotide-induced mitogenesis in isolated rat thymic lymphocytes.** *J Cyclic Nucleotide Res.* 1977;3:303-14. (English)

The cyclic nucleotides adenosine 3',5'-monophosphate (cyclic AMP) and guanosine 3',5'-monophosphate (cyclic GMP) and their dibutyryl derivatives are all mitogenic in isolated thymic lymphocyte cultures. These compounds elicit this response over two distinct concentration ranges. Thus cyclic AMP is maximally effective at 10^{-7} and 10^{-13}M. Cyclic GMP is likewise maximally effective at 10^{-6} and 5×10^{-11}M. The dibutyryl derivatives also exerted their mitogenic effect over these restricted concentration ranges. The mitotic response to the higher concentrations of nucleotides is inhibited either by the presence of testosterone (0.1 microg/ml) or by the omission of magnesium ions from the medium. Estradiol addition (0.1 microg/ml) or the absence of calcium prevents the mitogenic actions of the lower cyclic nucleotide concentrations. The cyclic nucleotide analogues cyclic 2'-deoxyadenosine 3',5'-monophosphate and cyclic adenosine 2',3'-monophosphate exhibit a similar biphasic mitogenic action with ionic dependency and steroid blockade but at higher concentrations than the naturally occurring cyclic nucleotides. A number of other related nucleotides were inactive. The cyclic nucleotide phosphodiesterase inhibitor Ro 20-1724 is also mitogenic over the concentration range 10^{-5}M to 10^{-8}M a response which can be blocked by testosterone addition or magnesium omission.

478
Morris HG, Rusnak SA, Barzens K. **Leukocyte cyclic adenosine monophosphate in asthmatic children: effects of adrenergic therapy.** *Clin Pharmacol Therap.* 1977;22:352-7. (English)

Blood specimens for measurement of leukocyte cyclic adenosine monophosphate (AMP) were obtained at weekly intervals from asthmatic children who were participating in a double-blind, crossover study to compare the effects of two adrenergic agents and a placebo. When patients were treated with the placebo, the basal measurements and the cyclic AMP responses of leukocytes to *in vitro* stimulation with epinephrine (10^{-4}M) were similar to those of normal subjects but within one week after initiation of treatment with an adrenergic bronchodialator, leukocyte cyclic AMP responses to adrenergic stimulation *in vitro* decreased and remained low during the remainder of the treatment period. Within one week after discontinuation of adrenergic therapy, leukocyte cyclic AMP responses returned to the control level. Our results indicate that the alterations in leukocyte cyclic AMP metabolism which have been observed previously in asthmatic patients may result from medications used for treatment of asthma.

479
Morris RJ, Gower S, Pfeiffer SE. **Thy-1 cell surface antigen on cloned cell lines of the rat and mouse: stimulation by cAMP and by butyrate.** *Br Res.* 1980;183:145-59. (English)

The level of the Thy-1 cell surface antigen on a number of established rat and mouse nerve cell lines can be stimulated by N_6,O_2'-dibutyryl adenosine 3',5'-cyclic monophosphoric acid (Bt_2cAMP), in some cases up to the antigen level found in whole brain. On rat cell line BN1010-3, stimulation is also produced by phosphodiesterase inhibitors, adenosine 3',5'-cyclic monophosphoric acid (cAMP) and its 8-bromo deriva-

tive, and L-isoproterenol. Hence, antigen elevation appears to occur via cAMP-related metabolism. It is not a consequence of morphological changes brought about by cAMP elevation in these cells, and is apparently independent of the inhibition of cell division by the nucleotide. Elevations of intracellular cAMP levels for at least one hour are needed to produce Thy-1 stimulation, after which an enhanced level of Thy-1 is observable after about 12 h. Continuous stimulation is required to maintain elevated antigen levels, for upon removal of the stimulating agent, the level of Thy-1 returns to the original unstimulated value within 48 h. Potent stimulation of the antigen level is also obtained with butyrate at 1-2 mM, which appears to be acting by a cAMP-independent mechanism.

480
Ohara J, Kishimoto T, Yamamura Y. *In vitro* **immune response of human peripheral lymphocytes; III--Effect of anti-mu or anti-gamma antibody on PWM-induced increase of cyclic nucleotides in human B lymphocytes.** *J Immunol.* 1978;121:2058-96. (English)

Stimulation of human peripheral blood lymphocytes (PBL) with pokeweed mitogen (PWM)-induced consistent increases of intracellular levels of cyclic AMP and cyclic GMP within 15 min. Increases of cyclic AMP were observed in both B and T lymphocyte populations, but increase of cyclic GMP was observed only in the B lymphocyte population. The addition of anti-mu antibody to B cells abolished PWM-induced increase of cyclic GMP without any effect on cyclic AMP response. Anti-gamma antibody did not show any inhibitory or stimulatory effect on PWM-induced increase of cyclic GMP or cyclic AMP. Pretreatment of B cells with anti-mu antibody at 37°C for 1 hr inhibited PWM-induced increase of cyclic GMP, whereas pretreatment with anti-mu antibody at 4° did not show any inhibitory effect on PWM-induced increase of cyclic GMP. The effect of anti-mu pretreatment was reversible and pretreated cells were recovered from the inhibitory effect of anti-mu antibody after 36 hr culture.

481
Pankaskie MC, Abdel-Monem MM, Raina A, Wang T, Foker JE. **Inhibitors of polyamine biosynthesis; 9--Effects of S-adenyosyl-L-methionine analogues on mammalian aminopropyltransferases in vitro and polyamine biosynthesis in transformed lymphocytes.** *J Med Chem.* 1981;24:549-53. (English)

Seven analogues of S-adenosyl-L-methionine were studied as inhibitors or substrates for mammalian spermidine and spermine synthases. One of these, S-(5'-deoxy-5'-adenosyl)-(±)1-methyl- 3-(methylthio)propylamine (5), showed a unique spectrum of activities on the polyamine biosynthesis enzymes. It was an inhibitor of S-adenosyl-L-methionine decarboxylase from rat liver and spermine synthase from bovine brain and rat ventral prostrate. This compound was a substrate for the spermidine synthases from bovine brain and rat ventral prostrate but not a substrate for the spermine synthases from these same sources. At concentrations of 0.2 mM and higher, compound 5 blocked the increase in polyamine levels and in [3H]thymidine incorporation induced by Concanavalin A in cultured mouse lymphocytes. At approximately a 0.5 mM concentration of 5, the cellular polyamine levels and the rate of thymidine incorporation were similar to those of the unstimulated lymphocytes. Lower concentrations of 5 (0.02-0.1 mM) produced a dose-dependent increase in thymidine incorporation. A dose-dependent decrease in the cellular polyamine levels was observed in the range of 0.05-0.5 mM of the inhibitor. These results suggest that the effects of 5 on transformed lymphocytes are complex and may not be solely due to the inhibition of polyamine biosynthesis of this compound.

482

Parker CW, Kennedy S, Eisen AZ. **Leukocyte and lymphocyte cyclic AMP responses in atopic eczema.** *J Invest Dermatol.* 1977;68:302-6. (English)

Lymphocytes from subjects with mild and severe atopic eczema were compared with normal control subjects in regard to their cAMP (3',5'-cyclic adenosine monophosphate) responses to a variety of stimulatory agents. Individuals in the severe eczema group were shown to have a significant diminution in their unstimulated lymphocyte cAMP levels and absolute cAMP responses to 0.5 mM theophylline, 0.5 mM theophylline + 1 microM epinephrine, 10 mM isoproterenol, 1 mM isoproterenol, 10 mM salbutamol, and 3 microM PGE_1. Individuals with mild eczema had a reduced response to 0.5 mM theophylline. The severe eczema groups also differed in a number of these responses from a group of 5 subjects with severe psoriasis. Mixed leukocyte cAMP responses to 10 mM isoproterenol also were examined and found to be diminished in individuals with eczema.

483

Polgar P, Vera JC, Rutenburg AM. **An altered response to cyclic AMP stimulating hormones in intact human leukemic lymphocytes.** *Proc Soc Exp Biol Med.* 1977;154:493-5. (English)

Adenylate cyclase, in particulate preparations from lymphocytes of patients with chronic lymphatic leukemia (CCL), has previously been shown by us to possess a lowered basal activity and a diminished response to prostaglandin (PG) E_1, E_2, F_{-2G}alpha. Reports of cyclic AMP and PG participation in cell division and maturation and modulation of certain functions in lymphocytes suggested that the observed reduction in adenylate cyclase activity and response to stimulation may prove important in the abnormal behavior of leukemic lymphocytes. In this report, we demonstrate observations with intact human lymphocytes, normal and malignant, which indicate further that the response of adenylate cyclase to extracellular effectors has been altered in leukemic lymphocytes.

484

Ring J, Mathison DA, O'Connor R. **In vitro cyclic nucleotide responsiveness of leukocytes and platelets in patients suffering from atopic dermatitis.** *Int Arch Allergy Appl Immunol.* 1981;65:1-7. (English)

Peripheral blood leukocytes from patients with severe atopic dermatitis (serum IgE levels between 1560-28,000 U/ml) showed a significantly weaker increase in intracellular cAMP after stimulation with epinephrine (10^{-5} to 10^{-3} M) than leukocytes from normals. At the same time, stimulation with methylcholine (10^{-10} to 10^{-4} M) induced a significantly higher increase in intracellular levels of cGMP in the atopic group compared to normals. The immunomodulating agent levamisole induced a slight increase in cAMP and cGMP response both in leukocytes from atopic patients and in normals. Platelet cAMP concentrations were lowered by epinephrine stimulation both in atopics and controls. There was no effect of methylcholine upon platelet cyclic nucleotide levels in the dose range examined. Abnormal cyclic nucleotide responsiveness, not only as beta-adrenergic blockade but also as cholinergic hyperreactivity, may play a role in the pathogenesis of atopic dermatitis.

485

Ryzewski J, Roszkowski-Sliz W, Krzystyniak K. **The action of thiols on lymphocyte membranes.** *Immunology.* 1976;31:145-9. (English)

Short-term incubation with cysteine in concentrations not altering cell viability increased the amount of -SH groups on the surface of rat lymphocytes. Maximal effect was achieved in 10 min using 2 mm cysteine, which concentration also induced immediate total loss of response to adrenaline, as measured by intracellular cyclic AMP level. Neither of these effects was observed after incubation of lymphocytes with glutathione or dithiothreitol.

486

Santoro MG, Benedetto A, Carruba G, Garaci E, Jaffe BM. **Prostaglandin A compounds as antiviral agents.** *Science.* 1980;209:1032-4. (English)

Prostaglandin of the A series strongly inhibit the production of Sendai virus in Africa green monkey kidney cells and are able to prevent the establishment of persistent infection ("carrier" state). This action is specific for prostaglandin A and is not due to alteration in the host cell metabolism or in the virus infectivity. The possibility that this effect is mediated by interferon is discussed.

487

Scheid MP, Goldstein G, Boyse EA. **The generation and regulation of lymphocyte populations: evidence from differentiative induction systems in vitro.** *J Exp Med.* 1978;147:1727-43. (English)

Results with a dual assay, for the induction of Thy-1$^+$ T cells and of CR$^+$ B cells from marker-negative precursors, confirm that thymopoietin is at present the only known selective inducer of prothymocytes. In contrast, various inducers, including ubiquitin, are active in both assays. Pharmacological evidence indicates that there are different cellular receptors for ubiquitin and thymopoietin. Prothymocytes and pro-CR$^+$ B cells compose two distinct populations in bone marrow and spleen; their distribution in density gradients is different, and elimination of either population enriches the other proportionately. There are not noteworthy differences between induction of these two populations in regard to (a) kinetics (b) dependence on temperature and protein synthesis, (c) activation by cAMP, and (d) inhibition by cGMP. The opposite inductive effects of cAMP and cGMP were corroborated by the use of pharmacological agents that raise or lower the levels of intracellular cyclic nucleotides. In contrast, a third induction assay, which monitors acquisition of the PC$^+$ surface phenotype, indicates that this differentiative step, the last known for B cells, is initiated by cGMP and inhibited by cAMP. Induction of PC is also inhibited by thymopoietin, signifying that the inductive selectivity of thymopoietin is not due to restriction of its receptors to the T lineage cells. Rather it seems that receptors for thymopoietin occur also on PC-inducible and other B cells, although in this case geared biochemically to inhibition rather than expression of the succeeding gene program. This suggests a role for thymopoietin in the coordinated interregulation of lymphocyte classes, in addition to its better-known function as the thymic inducer of prothymocytes. Present data conform to a general scheme in which the cyclic nucleotides cAMP and cGMP, and agents that affect intracellular levels of these mediators, influence reciprocally the early and late (functional) phases of lymphocyte differentiation as a whole, while thymopoietin influences reciprocally the differentiation of the B and T classes of lymphocyte.

488
Schwartz A, Askenase PW, Gershon RK. **The effect of locally injected vasoactive amines on the elicitation of delayed-type hypersensitivity.** J Immunol. 1977;118:159-65. (English)

In previous work monoamine depletion due to treatment with reserpine was shown to decrease the elicitability of DTH responses in mice. In addition, treatment with monoamine oxidase inhibitors prevented the reserpine-induced decrease. These findings led to the suggestion that serotonin-induced increased vascular permeability is necessary to the development of DTH reactions, perhaps by allowing bone marrow-derived macrophage precursor cells, which are obligate components of DTH responses, to migrate through specialized venules into the site of the reaction. We have compared classical drug tachyphylaxis (temporary inhibition of the effects of a drug by prior treatment with agonists) to serotonin in vessels of mouse feet with local inhibition of DTH after serotonin pretreatment of mice. During the tachyphylactic period, DTH responses are depressed. This suggests that serotonin-induced tachyphylaxis of local endothelial receptors can be responsible for DTH inhibition. In contrast, local injection of histamine has no effect on DTH and this drug is a much less potent inducer of tachyphylaxis to serotonin-mediated vasoactive reactions. On the other hand, histamine can inhibit in vitro T cell reactions, which are not affected by serotonin. These data help to further the concept that serotonin plays an important role in the regulation of DTH in mice and that it probably does so by acting on vascular endothelium.

489
Seegmiller JE, Watanabe T, Shreier MH, Waldmann TA. **Immunological aspects of purine metabolism.** Adv Exp Med Biol. 1977;76A:412-33. (English)

The development of our knowledge of the immune system has been reviewed and evidence presented of the need for a rapid rate of purine synthesis de novo for the proliferative events in this process. The mechanism of the inhibition of the immune system in a model of ADA deficiency has been studied intensively and considerable indirect evidence obtained of adenosine toxicity as a possible mediator of a reversible inhibition of proliferation of T-cells and to a slightly lesser extent B-cells. A secondary inhibition of ADA by inosine accumulation in PNP deficiency is proposed as a unifying hypothesis in which a somewhat lesser adenosine toxicity would inhibit proliferation only of T-cells. The correction of the immune response by addition of ADA both in vitro and in vivo provides strong evidence in favor of this view. In HPRT deficiency no evidence was found of a gross impairment of the immune system; however, the HPRT enzyme is required for inhibition of the immune response by 6MP in a variety of systems using different mitogenic stimuli.

490
Shaskan EG, Peszke MA, Niederman JC, Kasl SV. **Monoamine oxidase activity (MAOA) as a screen for host-resistance to infectious disease.** Fed Proc. 1978;37:878. (English)

Cotzias and co-workers (1974) reported an increased mean life-span of mice treated chronically with oral L-DOPA, ascribing this effect to the reduction of intervening diseases. This effect is probably mediated by brain dopamine (DA) neurons, presumably via the immune system. In epidemiological studies in man, brain DA functioning may be assessed by evaluating blood platelet MAOA. The following evidence supports the assumption that platelet MAOA correlates with the physiological disposition of brain DA: 1) platelet MAO is genetically stable; 2) platelet MAOA correlates with brain MAOA, increasing with age in humans (Robinson et al., 1971); 3) platelet MAOA correlates with brain DA, following treatment with MAO inhibitors specific for the physiological "B-form"(Birkmayer et al., 1977); 4) growth hormone release, following oral L-DOPA is inversely related to platelet MAOA (Sacchar and Coppen, 1975). Our results from a fully prospective, as well as retrospective, study of infectious mononucleosis (IM) in first year cadets at the U.S. Coast Guard Academy support the notion that increased functioning of brain DA-containing neuron systems (i.e., "low" platelet MAOA) confers increased host-resistance to individuals infected by Epstein-Barr virus.

491
Singh U. **In vitro lymphopoiesis in foetal thymic organ cultures: effect of various agents.** Clin Exp Immunol. 1980;41:150-5. (English)

In this study 14-day-old foetal BALB/c mouse thymic lobes were removed and grown as organ culture in vitro for up to 6 days. The cultures were treated with agents which are known to alter the intracellular levels of cyclic nucleotides. The proliferative response of the lobes was judged by histological examination, ^{125}I-UdR uptake and cell yields of the lobes at various time intervals. The results indicate that agents which raise cyclic GMP levels stimulate the proliferative response of the lobes as judged by the various parameters used and that the response was largely restricted to the lymphoid cells. It has been suggested that most probably cyclic GMP is the positive signal for thymic lymphopoiesis perhaps not only *in vitro* but also *in vivo*.

492
Snider DE Jr, Parker CW. **Adenylate cyclase activity in lymphocyte subcellular fractions: characterization of non-nuclear adenylate cyclase.** *Biochem J.* 1977;162:473-82. (English)

Human peripheral lymphocytes were broken in a Dounce homogenizer and subcellular fractions enriched in plasma membranes or microsomal particles and mitochondria were isolated by centrifugation through a discontinuous sucrose gradient. Various agents that promote cyclic AMP accumulation in intact lymphocytes were compared in their ability to stimulate adenylate cyclase activity in the individual fractions. Plasma-membrane-rich fractions that were essentially free of other subcellular particles as judged by electron microscopy and marker enzyme measurements responded to fluoride, but weakly or not at all to prostaglandin E_1 and other prostaglandins. Microsomal and mitochondrial-rich fractions responded markedly to both prostaglandin E_1 and fluoride. In some, but not all, experiments phytohaemagglutinin produced a modest increase in enzyme activity in plasma-membrane-rich fractions. Catecholamines, histamine, parathyrin, glucagon and corticotropin produced little or no response. In the absence of theophylline, adenosine (1-10 microM) stimulated basal enzyme activity, although at higher concentrations the responses to prostaglandin E_1 and fluoride were inhibited. GTP (1-100 microM) and GMP (5-1000 microM) respectively inhibited or stimulated the response to fluoride, whereas the converse was true with prostaglandin E_1

493
Stephens CG, Snyderman R. **Cyclic nucleotides regulate the morphologic alterations required for chemotaxis in monocytes.** *J Immunol.* 1982;128:1192-7. (English)

The initial morphologic response of human monocytes to chemoattractants is a change in shape from round to a triangular "motile" configuration (polarization). At doses chemotactic *in vitro*, chemoattractants induced rapid ($t_{1/2}$ = 45 sec), sustained (greater than 40 min) polarization of monocytes in suspension. Extracellular Ca^{++} was not required for polarization induced by chemoattractants, but in the absence of Ca^{++} kinetics were slowed ($t_{1/2}$ = 6.5 min). Phenylephrine, carboamycholine, serotonin, and ascorbate also caused rapid polarization of monocytes. Unlike chemoattractants, polarization by the pharmacologic agents was unsustained (less than 15 min), absolutely required extracellular Ca^{++}, and affected about 50% of the cells responsive to chemoattractants. Based on relative sensitivities to alpha$_1$- and alpha$_2$-adrenergic agonists and antagonists, polarization caused by adrenergic agents was mediated by alpha$_2$-receptors. Muscarinic and alpha$_2$-adrenergic agonists, serotonin, and ascorbate enhanced the rate and number of monocytes polarizing to suboptimal doses of chemoattractants. Thus, the initial morphologic changes induced by chemoattractants appear to utilize an activation pathway shared with a variety of agents that enhance cGMP levels and inhibit adenylate cyclase. In contrast, theophylline, histamine, and isoproterenol, all agents

that activate adenylate cyclase and elevate cAMP levels, inhibited monocyte polarization to chemoattractants. As in PMN, pharmacologic agents that increase cAMP levels inhibited monocyte chemotaxis *in vitro*, whereas those that inhibit adenylate cyclase and increase cGMP enhanced monocyte chemotactic responses. Thus, the initial morphologic response of monocytes to chemoattractants as well as the processes required for sustained directional motility are modulated by cyclic nucleotides.

494
Stolc V. **Control of adenylate cyclase EC-4.6.1.1 by divalent cations and agonists: analysis of interactions by the Hill equation.** *Biochim Biophys Acta.* 1979;569:267-76. (English)

The analysis by the Hill equation of the results of adenylate cyclase (ATP pyrophosphate-lyase (cyclizing), EC 4.6.1.1) activation in human granulocytes resulted in the following findings: the adenylate cyclase agonists have no effect on guanyl nucleotide and divalent cation activation or inhibition of the adenylate cyclase activity since the Hill coefficients for Gpp(NH)p, Mg^{2+} and Ca^{2+} were not affected by ($\pm$)-isoproterenol, histamine or prostaglandin E_1. The fact that the Hill coefficient for 5 adenylate cyclase agonists (prostaglandin E_1, ($\pm$)-isoproterenol, histamine, (-)adrenaline [epinephrine] and ($\pm$)-noradrenaline [norepinephrine]) was approximately 0.5 or less rules out the possibility that there is a cooperation among the catalytic subunits of the adenylate cyclase. The inhibitory action of Ca^{2+} on the adenylate cyclase activity can be attributed to a competition between Ca^{2+} and Mg^{2+} by Ca^{2+} that results in a replacement of Mg^{2+} by Ca^{2+} at the intercellular Mg^{2+} binding site. The Hill coefficient for Mg^{2+} was 1.8, 2.1 and 1.7 at 0, 0.1, and 0.5 mM Ca^{2+} but decreased significantly to 1.1 at 1 mM Ca^{2+}. The exposure of whole cells to Mg^{2+}, Ca^{2+}, prostaglandin E_1 and ionophore A23187 has indicated a diverse action of divalent cations on the cyclic [c]AMP formation. Ca^{2+} and Mg^{2+} may potentiate the prostaglandin E_1 stimulatory effect on cAMP production, Ca^{2+} at the extracellular and Mg^{2+} at the intracellular site of the adenylate cyclase complex. In contrast, prostaglandin E_1-stimulated cAMP formation was inhibited when Ca^{2+} and Mg^{2+} acted at the reverse sites.

495
Strom TB, Carpenter CB. **Cyclic nucleotides in immunosuppression-neuroendocrine pharmacologic manipulation and *in vivo* immunoregulation of immunity acting via second messenger systems.** *Transplantation Proc.* 1980;12:304-10. (English) (no abstract)

496
Strom TB, Lundin AP, Carpenter CB. **The role of cyclic nucleotides in lymphocyte activation and function.** *Prog Clin Immunol.* 1977;3:115-53. (English) (no abstract)

497
Sullivan TJ, Parker CW. **Possible role of arachidonic acid and its metabolites in mediator release from rat mast cells.** *J Immunol.* 1979;122:431-6. (English)

The role of arachidonic acid (AA) metabolism in the release

of inflammatory mediators from rat mast cells was studied. Eicosa-5,8,11,14-tetraynoic acid (ETYA), an acetylenic analog of AA, was found to inhibit histamine release induced by anti-IgE, concanavalin A (Con A), or the ionophore A-23187 with ID_{50} values of 65,50, and 17 microM, respectively. Mediator release was not affected by aspirin or indomethacin in concentrations up to 60 microM. Addition of free AA (0.1 to 100 microM) to unstimulated mast cells did not initiate noncytotoxic mediator release. Preincubation of mast cells did not initiate noncytotoxic mediator release. Preincubation of mast cells with 1 to 10 microM AA inhibited subsequent release induced by anti-IgE or Con A (up to 38%). This inhibition of release was blocked if aspirin (10 microM) or indomethacin (10 microM) was present, suggesting that AA inhibition was mediated by cyclo-oxygenase products. When AA was added after secretion was initiated by anti-IgE or Con A, a modest potentiation of release was noted. These studies suggest that AA metabolism by enzyme systems other than cyclo-oxigenase is an integral part of the mast cell secretory process. Availability of free AA, however, does not appear to be a sufficient condition to initiate secretion by otherwise unstimulated cells. Activation of mast cells by secretory signals appears to lead to altered AA metabolism which in turn appears to be involved in the secretion of inflammatory mediators.

498

Sullivan TJ, Parker KL, Kulczycki A Jr, Parker CW. **Modulation of cyclic AMP in purified rat mast cells; III--Studies on the effects of concanavalin A and anti-IgE on cyclic AMP during histamine release.** *J Immunol.* 1976;117:713-6. (English)

Changes in rat mast cell cyclic adenosine 3',5' monophosphate (cAMP) concentrations during stimulation of histamine release by concanavalin A (Con A) and anti-IgE were studied. Con A caused an increase in cAMP with a mean peak level at 20 sec of 232% of control range (range 164% to 365%). Con A-stimulated cells demonstrated falls toward control levels after 20 sec, but generally remained above control for at least 5 min. By 10 min cAMP had returned to control values. The Con A effect on cAMP occurred in the absence of phosphatidyl serine but was markedly inhibited by a 5 mM alpha-methyl-D-mannose. Anti-IgE induced a less marked increase in cAMP (157% of control, range 110% to 540% of control) which reached a peak at 20 sec. Two monospecific goat anti-rat myeloma IgE antisera induced similar changes in cAMP whereas normal goat IgG had no effect. These peak values were followed by a rapid decrease in cAMP. Within 2 min the cAMP content of anti-IgE stimulated cells had fallen to levels well below control and remained below control levels from 45 sec to over 15 min. Histamine release in both systems began after the peak cAMP levels, during the period of rapid destruction of cAMP.

499

Trung PH. **Chemotaxis of human leukocytes, part 2: effects of lectins, colchicine, cytochalasin B, cyclic nucleotides and immunostimulatory products.** *Biomedicine.* 1979;30:12124. (English)

Drugs or products acting as chemo-modulators were assayed for their effect on the chemotactic activity of human normal neutrophils by a method of direct microscopic observation. Lectins (PHA[phytohemagglutin]P and Con [concanavalin] A) had an inhibitory effect at the level of 10 microg/ml. Colchicine and cytochalasin B had also an inhibitory effect at the level of 0.25 times. 10.6 M/ml and 0.20 microg/ml. For the cyclic [c] nucleotides: dibutyryl cAMP and products such as norepinephrine and aminophylline that raise the cellular level of cAMP had an inhibitory effect, whereas cGMP and carbamylcholine had a stimulatory effect. Imidazole and levamisole, caused some enhancement of chemotaxis, but it was not significant. Lectins by binding to cell surface receptors which assume the recognition of chemotactic gradient in the environment, colchicine and cytochalasin B by interfering with the cytoskeletal elements (microtubules and microfilaments) and cyclic nucleotides affected metabolic activity during cell motility. The integrity of 1 of these 3 sequences was necessary for the normal activity of chemotaxis. Animal and human models (i.e., mutant mouse bg/bg and Chediak-Higashi syndrome) gave some clue of their interrelation.

500

Wang T, Sheppard JR, Foker JE. **Rise and fall of cyclic AMP required for onset of lymphocyte DNA synthesis.** *Science.* 1978;201:155-7. (English)

The adenosine 3',5'-monophosphate (cyclic AMP) levels of mouse lymphocytes rose and fell sharply 10 hours after stimulation with concanavalin A. Treatment of the cells with indomethacin reversibly prevented the increase in cyclic AMP and the subsequent onset of DNA synthesis. When the heightened cyclic AMP before S phase was maintained by either inhibiting phosphodiesterase or by adding the 8-bromo derivative of cyclic AMP, DNA synthesis was also blocked. Both the increase and decrease in cyclic AMP appear to be required for progression of lymphocytes into the S phase of growth.

501

Weinstein Y, Melmon KL. **Control of immune responses by cyclic AMP and lymphocytes that adhere to histamine columns.** *Immunol Commun.* 1976;5:401-16. (English)

Mixed lymphocytes from human peripheral blood, murine spleens, lymph nodes or thymus glands have pharmacologically specific receptors for histamine, beta-mimetic catecholamines and prostaglandins. When these cells are exposed to the panoply of drugs mentioned above, their intracellular cyclic AMP concentrations increase. The biologic consequences of such an increase were at first elusive. Now we know that the immune potential of some murine spleen cells may be modulated and the release of lysosomal enzymes and histamine from human leukocytes may be inhibited. This paper concentrates on the effects that manipulation of cells with amine receptors has on their immune function. Recent studies have revealed that a subpopulation of splenic suppressor T cells responds to increases in its cyclic AMP content by reversing its suppressive effects on the humoral antibody response. When these T cells are removed from the murine cell population by their differential adherence to insolubulized conjugates of histamine with albumin, the remainder of the cells are more responsive to sheep cell antigen, as tested by transferring the spleen cells together with the antigen into lethally irradiated recipient animals. The suppressor T cells that adhere to the insolubilized conjugates of histamine-albumin (called histamine-rabbit serum albumin-Sepharose, or HRS) are Ia positive, they appear to have receptors for histamine, beta-adrenergic amines and prostaglandins of the E series, and when stimulated by these agents their *in vivo* and *in vitro* suppressor actions are reversed. The reversal seems quantitatively dependent on cyclic AMP accumulation. Receptors for the amines and prostaglandins are found on the T cell precursors of cell-mediated immunity. They develop on some T effector cells in selected models of allogeneic target cell lysis. The receptors also appear to develop on selected B cells once these cells become committed to antibody production. The distribution of receptors on all leukocytes has not been adequately studied nor has their full potential in the immune response been studied in detail.

502

Welscher HD, Cruchaud A. **The influence of various particles and 3',5'-cyclic adenosine monophosphate on release of lysosomal enzymes by mouse macrophages.** *RES, J Reticuloendothel Soc.* 1976;20:405-20. (English)

Mouse peritoneal macrophages cultured with particulate material released beta-glucoronidase, beta-galactosidase and cathepsin D in a comparable manner. This release was measurable after less than 5 min incubation and showed a 3- to 10-fold increase over control levels after 60 to 180 min. The degree of release depended upon the concentration and the chemical nature of the particles. At the concentrations used, zymosan had a more powerful effect than IgM-coated heat-aggregated human IgG which in turn was more potent than uncoated IgG. The phagocytosis of sheep erythrocytes was also determined. Although both lysosomal enzyme release and phagocytosis were reduced by either dibutyryl-cyclic AMP, theophylline or isoproterenol, intact phagocytosis was found not to be an essential prerequisite for enzyme release. Indeed, blockade of phagocytosis by cytochalasin B considerably increased the release of lysosomal enzymes. The total amount of all enzymes tested remained unchanged up to 180 min of incubation. The cellular level of cyclic AMP in macrophages was 63 ± 6 pmoles per 10^7 cells. This level appeared to be the same in resting and phagocytizing cells. Also, both isoproterenol and theophylline caused only a moderate and transient increase in cyclic AMP at the very beginning of incubation. Beta-adrenergic blockade suppressed the effect of isoproterenol.

503

Wisloff F, Christoffersen T. **Role of cyclic nucleotides in human lymphocyte-mediated antibody-dependent cytotoxicity.** *Int Arch Allergy Appl Immunol.* 1977;53:42-9. (English)

Experiments were carried out in order to throw light on the role of cyclic AMP and cyclic GMP in the modulation of the expression of antibody-dependent cytotoxicity mediated by human peripheral blood lymphocytes *in vitro*. Chicken erythrocytes were used as target cells. Support for an inhibitory role of cyclic AMP was derived from the marked suppression

of cytotoxicity by dibutyryl cyclic AMP. Cyclic AMP itself had little effect. Isoproterenol, prostaglandin E_1 and prostaglandin E_2 increased cyclic AMP concentrations and strongly inhibited the cytotoxic effect of the lymphocytes. Histamine showed very slight elevation of the cyclic AMP level and suppression of the cytotoxicity. Theophylline did not increase the cyclic AMP concentration, but potentiated the effects of isoproterenol and prostaglandin E_1 on the cyclic AMP levels, and significantly inhibited cytotoxicity. No clear effects were seen when cyclic GMP, dibutyryl GMP, acetylcholine or carbacholine were added to the cells. The results indicate that in this system cyclic AMP inhibits cytotoxicity, while no evidence for a role of cyclic GMP has been obtained.

504

Zhikharev SS, Mineev VN. **Features of cyclic nucleotide metabolism in leukocytes of patients with bronchial asthma.** *Ter Arkh.* 1980;52:89-93. (English)

The degree of glycogenolysis in lymphocytes after incubation with adrenaline (epinephrine) was determined in 108 patients with preasthma and bronchial asthma of varying severity and in 32 healthy individuals. The basal and adrenaline stimulated level of cAMP was determined in leukocytes of 27 patients with bronchial asthma and 9 healthy individuals. The same methods were used to examine 5 patients with acute pneumonia. The cAMP/cGMP ratio of both and adrenaline and acetylcholine-stimulated levels was studied in 5 patients with bronchial asthma and 5 healthy individuals. The informativeness of the new indirect method of evaluation of adrenoreactivity of target cells--the degree of glycogenolysis--was emphasized. A statistically significant decrease in adrenaline response by the degree of glycogenolysis and by the growth of cAMP with aggravation of the disease was obtained. A decrease in the cAMP/cGMP coefficient was noted in the patients with bronchial asthma. The informativeness of the correlation of the basal and stimulated levels coefficients is emphasized. Possible causes of these changes are discussed.

Psychosocial Factors
and Immunity

Psychosocial factors and disease susceptibility

505
Anonymous. **New model sees immune system as cognitive process.** *Brain/Mind Bull.* 1978;3:1-2. (English) (no abstract)

506
Biggar RJ, Melbye M, Ebbesen P, Andersen HK, Vestergaard BF. **The immune suppression syndrome in homosexual men: an epidemiological study from the Cancer Research Institute in Arhus.** *Ugeskr Laeger.* 1982;144:777-80. (Danish) (unavailable at publication)

507
Bock OA. **Why some people become ill.** *S Afr Med J.* 1980;58:775-9. (English)

Tension is often responsible for the symptoms with which the patient presents to the doctor. By taking into account the age, sex, social standing and marital status of the patient, the doctor should have some idea of what the underlying causes might be.

508
Cobb S, Kasl SV. **Termination: the consequences of job loss.** *DHEW (NIOSH).* 1977;77:224. (English) (no abstract)

509
Cohen-Cole S, Cogen R, Stevens A, Kirk K, Gaitan E, Hain J, Freeman A. **Psychosocial, endocrine and immune factors in acute necrotizing ulcerative gingivitis.** *Psychosom Med.* 1981;43:91. (English)

To clarify a postulated role of "stress" and immunodepression in "trenchmouth" (ANUG), the authors studied psychosocial, endocrine and immune variables. ANUG is an acute infection associated with indigenous oral bacteria which are normally non-pathogenic. On presentation (T1), 35 patients and controls (matched for age, sex, and dental hygiene) filled out rating instruments, gave blood, and collected overnight and spot urines. Rating instruments and urine collections were repeated in two weeks (T2), after resolution of the infection. Results revealed that ANUG patients compared to controls: (1) experienced more negative life events in the previous 12 months (p<0.0002); (2) reported more state anxiety at T1 (p<0.0001) and T2 (p<0.0001); (3) were more likely to have significant emotional distress as measured by the General Health Questionnaire at T1 p<0.0003) and T2 (p<0.02); (4)

reported more symptoms of depression at T1 (p<0.004) but not at T2; (5) had higher scores on the D, PD, SC, and MA MMPI scales (p<0.009 - p<0.01) at T2 (the only time the MMPI was given); (6) had higher levels of overnight urine cortisol at T1 (p<0.1) and T2 (p<0.05); (7) had depressed lymphocyte function as measured after concanavalin A stimulation (p<0.0002); and (8) had depressed PMN leukotaxis (p<0.006) and phagocytosis (p<0.006). There were no statistically significant differences between patients and controls in serum cortisol, prolactin, growth hormone, or thyroid levels, nor in urine catecholamines. Other findings included associations between: (1) prolactin and symptoms of depression (p<0.02); (2) growth hormone and negative life events (p<0.01); overnight cortisol and HS (p<0.01) and HY (p<0.02) MMPI scales; and (4) overnight cortisol (p<0.0001) and low social support (p<0.02). These results demonstrate that several psychosocial, endocrine, and immune variables were significantly associated with ANUG, and may all contribute to its pathogenesis.

510
Cramer I, Blohmke M, Bahnson CB, Bahnson MB, Scherg H, Weinhold M. **Psychosocial factors and cancer: a study of 80 women by means of a psychosocial questionnaire** (author's transl). *Munch Med Wochenschr.* 1977;119:1387-92. (German)

The psychosocial questionnaire compiled by C.B. Bahnson and M.B. Bahnson and adapted for the German-speaking area was used to question 40 female cancer patients (30 mammary, 6 gastric and 4 pulmonary carcinomata) aged between 36 and 64 years and 40 control subjects selected by the matched pairs method. The cross section examination showed significant differences (p≤0.05) between cancer patients and control subjects on single variate examination in 10 individual variables. Discriminant analysis (multivariate examination) revealed a discriminant function of 12 variables which enabled the classification of the entire collective of subjects with 95 percent accuracy in the carcinoma and control groups. Our results confirm largely the hypotheses developed in the USA.

511
Czubalski K, Zawisza E. **The role of psychic factors in patients with allergic rhinitis.** *Acta Otolaryngol.* 1976;81:484-8. (English)

Psychosomatic studies were made in 128 patients with allergic rhinitis. After the allergic and clinical anamnesis, the patients were divided into two groups: those ill with hay fever (91 patients) and those suffering from perennial allergic rhinitis (37 patients). The assessment of the role of psychogenous factors in both varieties of allergic rhinitis was the main purpose of the investigation. The investigation showed that psychogenous factors are practically of no importance in hay fevers. Their role is great, however, when perennial allergic rhinitis is involved.

512

Drew WL, Conant MA, Miner RC, Huang ES, Ziegler JL, Groundwater JR, Gullett JG, Volberding P, Abrams DI, Mintz L. **Cytomegalovirus and Kaposi's sarcoma in young homosexual men.** *Lancet.* 1982;2:125-7. (English)

10 homosexual men with Kaposi's sarcoma (KS) were studied for evidence of cytomegalovirus (CMV) infection. IgG and IgM antibodies to CMV were detected in 9 out of 9 and in 7 out of 9 of these patients, respectively. CMV was recovered from body secretions or peripheral blood of 7 patients. Viral cultures of KS tumour biopsy specimens were negative in 8 out of 8 patients, but CMV RNA was detected by in-situ hybridisation in 2 out of 3 and CMV antigen(s) by immuno-fluorescence in 6 out of 9. Normal tissue specimens from 3 KS patients were negative for CMV antigen. These observations suggest an association of CMV with KS.

513

Durack DT. **Opportunistic infections and Kaposi's sarcoma in homosexual men** (editorial). *N Engl J Med.* 1981;305:1465-7. (English)

514

Eisenberg L. **Is health a state of mind?** (editorial). *N Engl J Med.* 1979;301:1282-3. (English)

515

Engle GL. **The predictive value of psychological variables for disease and death** (editorial). *Ann Intern Med.* 1976;85:673-74. (English)

516

Follansbee SE, Busch DF, Wofsy CB, Coleman DL, Gullet J, Aurigemma GP, Ross T, Hadley WK, Drew WL. **An outbreak of *Pneumocystic carinii* pneumonia in homosexual men.** *Ann Intern Med.* 1982;96:705-13. (English)

Pneumocystic carinii pneumonia has rarely been reported in previously healthy persons over the age of 6 months. Five cases of *P. carinii* pneumonia in adult homosexual men, confirmed by biopsy results, are reported. All five patients were seropositive when tested for antibodies to cytomegalovirus and four had evidence of active concurrent cytomegalovirus infections. Kaposi's sarcoma was shown in two of the patients and one had possible *Pneumocystis* infection of the central nervous system as well as *P. carinii* pneumonia. Four of the five patients have died. Past or concurrent cytomegalovirus infection and homosexuality were the only common epidemiologic features in all five patients.

517

Friedman AH, Freeman WR, Orellana J, Krausher MF, Starr MB, Luntz MH. **Cytomegalovirus retinitis and immunodeficiency in homosexual males** (letter). *Lancet.* 1982;1:958. (English)

518

Friedman E, Katcher AH, Brightman VJ. **Incidence of recurrent herpes labialis and upper respiratory infection: a prospective study of the influence of biologic, social and psychologic predictors.** *Oral Surg.* 1977; 43:873-8. (English)

In a 3-year prospective study of recurrent herpes labialis (RHL) in a population of 149 student nurses, 40 to 50 per cent of the variance in incidence could be explained by a small group of variables. Measures of previous experience with RHL accounted for the largest fraction of the explained variance, followed by upper respiratory infection (URI) rate, socioeconomic status, and mood trait, in order of declining influence. Timing of RHL episodes was not related to phase of the menstrual cycle.

519

Friedman-Kien AE, Laubenstein LJ, Rubinstein P, Buimovici-Klein E, Marmor M, Stahl R, Spigland I, Kim KS, Zolla-Pazner S. **Disseminated Kaposi's sarcoma in homosexual men.** *Ann Intern Med.* 1982;96:693-700. (English)

Nineteen cases from an epidemic of disseminated Kaposi's sarcoma in homosexual men were studied by clinical, virologic, immunologic, and genetic methods. The patients were all male homosexuals ranging in age from 29 to 52 years, with histories of multiple sexually transmitted diseases and exposure to both prescription and recreational drugs. Sites of disease included skin (16 of 19 patients), lymph nodes (13 patients), gastrointestinal tract (12 patients), spleen (three patients), and lung (one patient). Most patients had elevated levels of serum immunoglobins, positive antibody titers to hepatitis A and B virus, cytomegalovirus and Epstein-Barr virus, and impairment of cell-mediated immunologic reactions. The frequency of HLA-Dr5 in these patients is significantly elevated. Two of the 19 patients died. Although the precise cause of this epidemic is unknown, it is likely that a genetic predisposition, an acquired immunoregulatory defect, and one or more infectious agents and drugs may be involved.

520

Greene WA, Betts RF, Ochitill HN, Iker HP, Douglas RG. **Psychosocial factors and immunity: preliminary report** (abstract). *Psychosom Med.* 1978;40:87. (English)

Effects of social stress and mood on immune status were observed in a study of drug (isoprinosine) effects on influenza in 33 Ss, age 18-35, 18 male, 15 female, confined in a motel for 7 days. Symptoms and signs were rated on day 1 and twice daily thereafter. On day 1 the College Schedule of Recent Experience (CSRE) with derived Life Change Units (LCU) and the Profile of Mood States (POMS) were administered. On day 2, Ss were inoculated intranasally with influenza A/Victor/75H3N2 virus. Immune measures on all 33 Ss included nasal virus shed; nasal wash interferon (INF), and Hemagglutination Inhibition antibody titer (HAI). On 25 Ss Lymphocyte Transformation (LTN) and Lymphocyte Cytotoxicity (LCT) response rates were obtained. The LCU score as well as the POMS, Tension-, Depression-, Anger-, Vigor-, Fatigue- and Confusion- factor scores were standardized. Correlations of clinical and immune measures with age, sex, or drug were nonsignificant. So, all Ss were considered for psychosocial-immune variable analyses. Vigor was negatively correlated with Tension, $p<0.005$, Fatigue, $p<0.05$, Confusion $p<0.02$. There was a negative correlation between LCUs and LCT, $r= -.42$, $p<0.035$. LTN was the only other immune measure suggesting a relation with LCU, $r= -.28$, $p<0.18$. The only mood indicating a positive correlation with immunity was Tension with INF, another index of cellular immunity $r=.31$, $p<0.08$. Vigor showed a suggested negative correlation with LCT, $r= -.32$, $p<0.12$. Our hypothesis assumed a correlation of high LCU and/or negative moods with reduced immune response. Rather there was a significant correlation between a combined LCU and Vigor score with LCT, $r= -.54$, $p<0.006$ and with HAI $r= -.35$, $p<0.045$. Studies of psychosocial and immune measures should include 1) determination of expressed positive as well as negative moods, 2) measures of cellular immunity as well as humoral antibodies. The negative correlation between cellular immunity and the LCU-Vigor score suggests a psychophysiologic stance involving attenuated affect response to high social change and an attenuated immune response to influenza virus.

521

Grossarth-Maticek R. **Synergetic effects of cigarette smoking, systolic blood pressure, and psychosocial risk factors for lung cancer, cardiac infarct and apoplexy cerebri.** *Psychother Psychosom.* 1980;34:267-72. (English)

Determined the physical and psychosocial risk factors for cancer and other internal diseases for 1,353 Yugoslavians and the incidence of these diseases over a 10-year period. The strongest physical and psychosocial risk factors for lung cancer, cardiac infarct, and apoplexia cerebri were investigated with respect to synergetic effects (interaction nonlinearities)--a dependence of the effect of one variable upon the value of another. The efficacy of physical risk factors was wholly dependent upon the presence of psychosocial risk factors, while the latter were sometimes effective even in the absence of physical ones.

522

Henoch MJ, Batson JW, Baum J. **Psychosocial factors in juvenile rheumatoid arthritis.** *Arthr Rheum.* 1978;21:299-33. (English)

A detailed survey of 88 children with juvenile rheumatoid arthritis (JRA) was made in an attempt to elucidate characteristics that may participate in the etiologic mechanism. Data from a random pediatric population from the same geographic area were also included for comparisons. The most striking findings were psychosocial factors. Children whose parents were unmarried as a result of divorce, separation or death comprised 28.4% of the JRA population, compared to 10.6% of the comparison group. In addition, adoption occurred three times more often in the JRA population. Fifty-one percent of these events (divorce, separation, death, or adoption) occurred near the date of onset of the disease.

523

Horne RL, Picard RS. **Psychosocial risk factors for lung cancer.** *Psychosom Med.* 1979;41:503-14. (English)

The existence of psychosocial risk factors for the development of malignancy has been postulated by many investigators. This study investigated selected psychosocial factors as predictors of malignancy. 110 male patients with undiagnosed subacute or chronic pulmonary x-ray lesions participated in a semistructured interview. Ratings were made of 5 subscales: 1) childhood instability, 2) job stability, 3) marriage stability, 4) lack of plans for the future, and 5) recent significant loss. The composite scale correctly predicted the diagnosis of 53 (80%) of the 66 patients with benign disease and 27 (61%) of the 44 with lung cancer. The scale was at least as important as smoking history in predicting diagnoses. Thus, significant psychosocial risk factors for the development of malignant disease might well be incorporated in selecting high-risk individuals for cytological or other screening for lung cancer.

524

Johnson SB. **Psychosocial factors in juvenile diabetes: a review.** *J Behav Med.* 1980;3:95-116. (English)

Studies assessing (1) the influence of psychosocial factors on the onset of juvenile diabetes (2) the influence of psychosocial factors on the course of this disease, and (3) the influence of diabetes on the psychosocial development of the child are reviewed. Directions for future research are suggested.

525

Kasl SV, Evans AS, Niederman JC. **Psychosocial risk factors in the development of infectious mononucleosis.** *Psychosom Med.* 1979;41:445-66. (English)

In a 4-year prospective seroepidemiological study of infectious mononucleosis (IM) of one class of some 1400 cadets at the West Point Military Academy, susceptibles and immunes were identified by the absence or presence of antibody to Epstein-Barr virus (EBV), the causative agent, and new infections by the appearance of antibody (seroconversion). On entry, about one-third lacked EBV antibody, of whom some 20% became infected (seroconverted); about one-quarter of seroconverters developed definite, clinical and recognized IM. Psychosocial factors that significantly increased the risk of clinical IM among seroconverters included: 1) having fathers who were "overachievers"; 2) having a high level of motivation; 3) doing relatively poorly academically. The combination of high motivation and poor academic performance interacted in predicting clinical IM. Additional data on presence of elevated titres among seroconverters with inapparent disease and on length of hospitalization among cases of clinical IM revealed that these two additional indices of infection or illness could also be predicted from the same set of psychosocial risk factors.

526

Marmor M, Friedman-Kien AE, Laubenstein LJ, Byrum RD, William DC, Donofrio S, Dubin N. **Risk factors for Kaposi's sarcoma in homosexual men.** *Lancet.* 1982; 1:1083-7. (English)

An investigation of 20 homosexual men with histologically confirmed Kaposi's sarcoma and 40 controls revealed significant associations between Kaposi's sarcoma and use of a number of drugs (amyl nitrite, ethyl chloride, cocaine, phencyclidine, methaqualone, and amphetamine), history of mononucleosis, and sexual activity in the year before onset of the disease. Patients with Kaposi's sarcoma also reported substantially higher rates of sexually transmitted infections than did controls. Multivariate analysis indicated independent significant associations for amyl nitrite and sexual activity and showed use of phencyclidine, methaqualone, and ethyl chloride to be non-significant. Evaluated at the median exposure for patients, the analysis yielded risk-ratio estimates of 12.3 for amyl nitrite (95% confidence limits 4.2, 35.8) and 2.0 for sexual activity (95% confidence limits 1.3, 3.1).

527

McFarlane AH, Norman GR, Streiner DL, Roy R, Scott DJ. **A longitudinal study of the influence of the psychosocial environment on health status: a preliminary report.** *J Health Soc Behav.* 1980;21:124-33. (English)

This paper describes a prospective study to be completed in May of 1980, that is examining various aspects of the psychosocial environment and their relationship to health status. Over a two-year period, measures are being taken on a sample of 500 subjects of (1) social relationship networks; (2) extent to which subjects perceive themselves as having some control over their environment; (3) accumulating life changes; (4) subjective strain; and (5) health status. The research hypothesis states that the extent to which individuals are successful in coping with changes in their lives will be reflected in the degree to which they report distress or strain. It is this cost in the coping struggle that results in an increase in the likelihood of health problems. Although the study does not as yet have an adequate data base on the health status measures, the preliminary results reported in this paper indicate that positive (desirable) life events do not have significant statistical correlation with the measure of strain, whereas negative (undesirable) life events do. Furthermore, two dimensions of life events, anticipation and control, add substantial and interactional information about these relationships.

528

McMahon CE, Hastrup JL. **The role of imagination in the disease process: post-Cartesian history.** *J Behav Med.* 1980;3:205-17. (English)

A previous paper traced the pre-Cartesian history of the concept of imagination as a causal variable in physiopathology. The present continues that history, showing the prohibitive impact of mind-body dualism and sampling the views of some eighteenth-and nineteenth- century supporters of the theory. Contemporary research has produced abundant evidence supporting the historic belief that imagination has an arousal function and a direct link to physiopathology. This literatuare is surveyed and possible therapeutic applications are discussed.

529

Mildvan D, Mathur U, Enlow RW, Romain PL, Winchester RJ, Colp C, Singman H, Adelsberg BR, Spigland I. **Opportunistic infections and immune deficiency in homosexual men.** *Ann Intern Med.* 1982;96:700-4. (English)

A syndrome of opportunistic infections and acquired immune deficiency occurred among four previously healthy homosexual men. Fever, leukopenia, and diminished delayed hypersensitivity were accompanied by various degrees of proctitis, perianal ulcerations, and lymphadenopathy. The infectious agents included Pneumocystis carinii, Cryptococcus neoformans, Candida albicans, herpes simplex virus, and cytomegalovirus. The immune deficiency was characterized as a persistent and profound selective decrease in the function as well as number of T lymphocytes of the helper/inducer subset and a possible activation of the suppressor/cytotoxic subset. Three patients died despite aggressive anti-infective therapy.

530

Morris L, Distenfeld A, Amorosi E, Karpatkin S. **Autoimmune thrombocytopenic purpura in homosexual men.** *Ann Intern Med.* 1982;96:714-7. (English)

Since November 1980 we have diagnosed 11 cases of severe autoimmune thrombocytopenic purpura in homosexual men; their mean platelet count ($\pm$ SE) was 16,000 $\pm$ 3000/mm^3. All patients have been sexually active with multiple partners and exposed to numerous viruses and drugs. During this period we also have diagnosed 20 cases of classic autoimmune thrombocytopenic purpura in heterosexual persons, with a normal women to men ratio of 3:1. Eight of nine homosexual patients had elevated platelet IgG compared with normal values in eight of 10 homosexual control subjects having normal hemograms (p<0.01). All responded moderately or completely to steroids. The three patients who had splenectomy had excellent responses. Four of five patients had a decreased helper/suppressor T cell ratio compared to healthy controls (p<0.001). Circulating immune complexes and total gamma globulin levels were elevated and lymphocytes relatively decreased in homosexual patients compared with homosexual controls (p<0.05). Thus, some sexually-active homosexual men seem to have an increased incidence of an immune regulation disorder directed against platelets.

531

Pierloot RA. **Psychogenesis of somatic disorders.** *Psychother Psychosom.* 1979;32:27-40. (English)

Psychogenesis, considered as a linear sequential process by which psychological influences lead to somatic disturbances, is only a link in a larger bio-psycho-social interactional field. Therefore, in practice, a multilateral approach of the whole person, in his psychological, social and somatic aspects, in health and disease, in his habitual and his therapeutical contacts, should be stressed. It seems unlikely that the somatic symptoms we are confronted with can be considered as pure psychogenetically determined phenomena. This does not exclude that in the psychosomatic interaction, there exists at one or more stages a transition from the sphere of psychological functioning to the somatic area, ending up in somatic symptoms. This process, which we call psychogenesis, is not a single event but should be considered as an abstraction, grouping a number of component processes possibly occurring at different moments in the total system. We have distinguished four components: a psychopathological component, a psychophysiological component, a physiopathological component and a "somatic illness experience" component. For each of these components, a number of conceptions are proposed according to the different theoretical models of psychosomatic connections. Most of these formulations are largely hypothetical or based on fragmentary observations. Still, they offer guidelines for further research.

532
Rasmussen EO, Cooper KD, Kang K, White CR Jr, Regan DH, Hanifin JM. **Immunosuppression in a homosexual man with Kaposi's sarcoma.** *J Am Acad Dermatol.* 1982;6:870-9. (English)

The occurrence of Kaposi's sarcoma in young homosexual men is a recently reported condition. The same individuals are at risk for the development of Pneumocystis carinii pneumonia and other unusual infections. These associations suggest these persons are somehow immunocompromised. Evidence of current or prior cytomegalovirus (CMV) infection is seen in a high percentage of these and other homosexual men. CMV infections are known to induce alterations in the immunoregulatory suppressor and helper T lymphocyte populations. The CMV infection is suspect as the cause of immunosuppression in these individuals. We present a case of Kaposi's sarcoma in a homosexual man with CMV cultured from his urine and semen. He showed a marked increase in his suppressor/cytotoxic cell (OKT8-positive) population, as well as a marked decrease in his helper cell (OKT4-positive) population. Mitogen and antigen studies demonstrated absent or markedly diminished response both *in vitro* and *in vivo*. Pokeweed mitogen (PWM)-induced IgG synthesis appeared normal. This patient, as well as the majority of other reported patients with this disease, manifested the HLA-Dr5 phenotype. The immunosuppression in this patient and possibly other similar men appears to be mediated by abnormalities in the immunoregulatory T lymphocytes.

533
Rimon R, Belmaker RH, Ebstein R. **Psychosomatic aspects of juvenile rheumatoid arthritis.** *Scand J Rheumatol.* 1977;6:1-10. (English)

Juvenile rheumatoid arthritis (JRA) is presently thought to represent a different expression of rheumatoid arthritis (RA) that is characteristic of the age group under sixteen. According to Halvard *et al.* the proportion of JRA amounts to 4 to 7% of all patients with RA. Thus JRA is a relatively rare rheumatoid disorder whose importance, however, lies in the fact that it cripples more children than any other musculoskeletal disease. Even though rarely fatal, it may lead to a slow accumulation of incapacitated adults. JRA is also a major cause of childhood blindness. The prevalence of JRA is estimated to be approximately one out of every 1700 children. Though a considerable body of reserach is available exploring the psychological, social and personality characteristics of adult arthritis, a search of the literature reveals few studies focusing on the psychological and psychiatric aspects of JRA. Even scantier references exist on the dynamic interrelationships between the affected children and their parents or siblings. The studies conducted so far indicate that the onset, recurrence and degree of eventual rehabilitation depend to an undefined extent on psychosomatic factors. These facts motivated us to conduct a psychosomatic study of JRA with the goal of reaching a more comprehensive understanding of the characteristics and development of the illness.

534
Selby JW, Calhoun LG. **Psychosomatic phenomena: an extension of Wright.** *So Am Psychol.* 1978;33:396-8. (English) (no abstract)

535
Sheldrake P. **Predispositions to illness: patterns in the reporting of psychosomatic illness.** *J Psychosom Res.* 1977;21:225-30. (English)

In a survey on the distribution of psychosomatic illnesses in 8,078 university students, variations in illness reporting were examined in relation to college major and birth order. Based on the theory that people may be either inner- or outer-directed, it was hypothesized that students in the arts or social sciences or who were later-borns would be more likely to report illnesses where the role of stress is generally accepted as significant in causation than those in the sciences or professions or first borns. Results provide qualified support to these hypotheses: Ss reporting more than one illness tended to report illnesses from either the stress-related group or from the set of "non-stress-related" which had the further characteristic that they were associated with manifest physical symptoms.

536
Shuval JT. **The contribution of psychological and social phenomena to an understanding of the aetiology of disease and illness.** *Soc Sci Med A.* 1981;15:337-42. (English)

The influence of psychosocial factors in the general aetiology of disease is examined with particular reference to the notions of vulnerability and susceptibility. Cultural definitions are considered as well as cultural variations in help-seeking behaviour. Analysis concludes by looking at eight patterns of help-seeking behavior.

537
Spiers AS, Robbins CL. **Cytomegalovirus infection simulating lymphoma in a homosexual man** (letter). *Lancet.* 1982;1:1248-9. (English)

538
Stahle J. **Meniere's disease: allergy, immunology, psychosomatic, hypo- and hypertonus.** *Arch Otorhinolaryngol (NY).* 1976;212:287-92. (English) (no English abstract)

539
Swenson WM. **Psychological correlates of medical illness.** *Psychosomatics.* 1981;22:384-91. (English) (no abstract)

540

Thomas CB, Duszynski KR, Shaffer JW. **Family attitudes reported in youth as potential pedictors of cancer.** *Psychosom Med.* 1979;41:287-302. (English)

In a long-term prospective study of a cohort of former medical students, men who later developed cancer reported different family attitudes in youth from those of their healthy classmates. The items checked on a Family Attitude Questionnaire by the future cancer group indicated a lack of closeness to parents compared with the items checked by the healthy group. These prospective findings appear to fit with those of retrospective studies concerning early family relationships in cancer patients.

541

Thomas CB. **Precursors of premature disease and death: the predictive potential of habits and family attitudes.** *Ann Intern Med.* 1976;85:653-8. (English)

The youthful habits and family attitudes of medical students who later developed and died from one of five disease states were different from those of healthy classmate controls to begin with. In medical school, the total disorder group had significantly more nervous tension, anxiety, and anger under stress, had more insomnia, smoked more cigarettes, and took alcoholic drinks more frequently. Individual disorder group means were significantly different from each other. The mental illness group showed the most nervous tension, depression, and anger under stress and the malignant tumor the least. The malignant tumor group resembled the healthy control group in these respects. The suicide, mental illness, and malignant tumor groups had low mean scores for closeness to parents, while the hypertension and coronary occlusion group means were slightly higher than the control group mean. Thus psychologic differences in youth have predictive potential in regard to premature disease and death.

542

Turns D, Newby LG. **Cancer of the breast: psychosocial factors.** *Major Probl Clin Surg.* 1979;5:568-86. (English) (unavailable at publication)

543

Vaillant GE. **Natural history of male psychological health: effects of mental health on physical health.** *N Engl J Med.* 1979;301:1249-54. (English)

Four decades ago 204 men were selected as adolescents for an interdisciplinary study of health; since then they have been followed biennially. Of the 185 men who remained in the study and in good health until 1964 (age, 42 ± 1 years), 100 men remained in excellent physical health over the next 11 years, 54 acquired minor problems, and 31 acquired serious chronic illness or died. Of 59 men with the best mental health, assessed from the age of 21 to 46 years, only two became chronically ill or died by the age of 53. Of the 48 men with the worst mental health from the age of 21 to 46, 18 became chronically ill or died. The relation between previous mental health and subsequent physical health remained statistically significant when the effects on health of alcohol, tobacco use, obesity, and longevity of ancestors were excluded by multiple regression analysis. The data suggest that good mental health retards midlife deterioration in physical health.

544

Vanley GT, Huberman R, Lufkin RB. **Atypical pneumocystis carinii pneumonia in homosexual men with unusual immunodeficiency.** *AJR.* 1982;138:1037-41. (English)

Pneumocystis carinii pneumonia is a well known opportunistic infection whose radiographic presentation and association with cytomegalovirus (CMV) have been well described. Recently nine young homosexual men with chronic flulike illnesses were seen. Bronchoscopy in six cases demonstrated evidence of CMV infection with pneumocystis pneumonia. The radiographic presentation was atypical. Immunologic evaluation revealed T-cell abnormalities. CMV infections altering immunologic mechanisms has been postulated as the underlying cause of this and other uncommon infections in homosexual men.

545

Williams RC Jr. **Host factors in rheumatic fever and heart disease.** *Hosp Pract.* 1982;17:125-9, 135-8. (English) (no abstract)

Stress and immunity
Clinical studies
Stress and illness

546

Boyd GW. **Stress and disease, the missing link: a vasospastic theory; III--Stress, vasospasm and general disease.** *Med Hypotheses.* 1978;4:432-44. (English)

The potential importance of vasospasm, with or without consequent thrombosis, as a mechanism in general disease is discussed and the evidence examined in one organ, namely the brain, It is concluded that vasospasm might be important in a number of neurologial disorders, including migraine, epilepsy, and even some of the schizophrenia-like illnesses. Repeated ischaemic cell damage from vasospasm is also discussed as a possible factor initiating qutoimmune disease and cancer. The similarities between viral transformation and neoplasia have led to the proposition that much cancer might be explained if as a species we have evolved by the gradual build-up of viruses.

547

Dutz W, Kohout E, Rossipal E, Vessel K. **Infantile stress, immune modulations, and disease patterns.** *Pathol Ann.* 1976;11:415-54. (English) (no abstract)

548

Fairbank DT Hough RL. **Life event classifications and the event-illness relationship.** *J Hum Stress.* 1979;5:41-7. (English) (unavailable at publication)

549

Frederick JF. **Grief as a disease process.** *Omega:Journal of Death and Dying.* 1976-7;7:297-305. (English)

Many years ago, Engel pointed out that grief fulfills all the requirements of a disease process. Despite the current interest in grief, most studies have concentrated on the psychological results of grief and the dysfunction associated with it; the physiological consequences have been largely ignored. The persistent reports of infection and neoplasia following shortly after a grief experience makes it mandatory that the relationship between grief as a stress mechanism and its consequences via the pituitary-adrenal axis on the depression of the immune response be explored on a physiological level.

550

Garrity TF, Marx MB, Somes GW. **The relationship of recent life change to seriousness of later illness.** *J Psychosom Res.* 1978;22:7-12. (English)

A sample of 313 college freshmen was prospectively studied to determine whether recent life change predicted the seriousness of subsequent illness. Using the Seriousness of Illness Rating Scale as the measure of seriousness, it was found that recent life change correlated at 0.33 with seriousness. This measure of seriousness also correlated with several other measures of severity and seriousness. However, the fact that seriousness was highly correlated (0.80) with the number of new health problems experienced, raises questions about the value of using both as outcome measures in life change research.

551

Goldberg EL, Comstock GW. **Life events and subsequent illness.** *Am J Epidemiology.* 1976;104:146-58. (English)

The objective was to examine for relationships between stress, as measured by life events, and hospitalization or death during the following 6 to 12 months, using a case-control design. As part of the Community Mental Epidemiology Program, life events data for the preceding year were gathered on a random sample of the population at two sites, and health data for the interval between interviews were collected at follow-up. A case is defined as anyone becoming ill and being hospitalized or dying during the interval between interviews. Each case was individually matched by several variables to a control who had neither been sick nor hospitalized. There were no significant demographic differences between cases and controls in either site or between sites. When life events were examined by various scoring methods, there were no differences between cases and controls. This finding is important since most longitudinal studies that have shown a positive relationship between life events and subsequent illness have had methodologic limitations or have been based on healthy, young, male populations who generally did not become seriously ill during the study period. The results of this study plus the lack of generalizability of previous findings and their somewhat conflicting results raise serious questions about the etiologic relationship of life events to subsequent illness.

552

Haynes SG, McMichael AJ, Tyroler HA. **The relationship of normal, involuntary retirement to early mortality among U.S. rubber workers.** *Soc Sci Med.* 1977;11:105-14. (English)

This paper describes an epidemiologic study of the patterns and correlates of mortality around compulsory retirement (age 65) among U.S. rubber tire workers. Death rates were significantly decreased before retirement, and were elevated 3-4 years after retirement. Lower status workers were more likely to die within 3 years of retirement than higher status workers. Higher status workers were more predominant among deaths 4-5 years after retirement. Risks of dying were greater among men with a pre-retirement history of repeated non-medical absences. The findings are discussed with respect to stress, retirement adaptation, and longevity theories.

553

Hull D. **Life circumstances and physical illness: a cross disciplinary survey of research content and method for the decade 1965-75.** *J Psychosom Res.* 1977;21:115-39. (English)

This study contributes a 10 factor 95 category schema for analyzing the content and method of 329 research articles dealing with the social, psychological and life event antecedents of physical illness. The form of this research was an inclusive archival survey of the primary literature. Selection was based on content, and articles and their distribution, based on a pilot study, were found to be accurate. Nineteen journals were surveyed for the period 1965-74, and the differing interests of 8 separate disciplines in various illnesses, preconditions, and methods is demonstrated. The results also indicated what antecedents were studied with reference to specific illnesses and illness groups. The findings suggest that the historic origins of the various disciplines remain influential in the selection of content, and that tradition also guides journals in their selection of articles for publication. The sources of data for the project on the social preconditions and precipitators of physical illness were 19 journals thought to represent the primary literature in this area. Each eligible study was regarded as a unit from which information in 10 categories, including content, method, discipline of authorship, journal, and year of publication were retrieved in accordance with a pre-established plan. The data sets were then subjected to cross-tabulation and trend analysis.

554

Hurst MW, Jenkins CD, Rose RM. **The relation of psychological stress to onset of medical illness.** *Annu Rev Med.* 1976;27:301-12. (English) (no abstract)

555

Jacobs S, Ostfeld A. **An epidemiological review of the mortality of bereavement.** *Psychosom Med.* 1977;39:344-57. (English)

Epidemiological literature revealing excess mortality in the newly widowed is reviewed. The risk varies by age and sex. Younger persons and men are at higher risk. There are manifold specific causes of death characterized by conditions manifest in middle and late life. Cause specificity also varies by sex. Methodological problems in this literature are mitigated by application of varied methodology and replication of basic findings. Socioeconomic status and "social" stress are not well controlled as independent variables. Nevertheless, they probably do not explain the large relative risk of mortal-

ity among the bereaved. Pathogenetic mechanisms resulting from a loss are probably twofold: physiologic changes associated with the loss response and behavioral changes that comprise health maintenance or chronic disease management. Because of its importance as a health problem, as a fundamental human reaction, and as a research strategy for the basic psychosomatic hypothesis, bereavement is a prime target of investigation.

556

Kobasa SC. **Stressful life events, personality and health: an inquiry into hardiness.** *J Pers Soc Psych.* 1979;37:1-11. (English)

Personality was studied as a conditioner of the effects of stressful life events on illness onset. Two groups of middle and upper level executives had comparably high degrees of stressful life events in the previous 3 years, as measured by the Holmes and Rahe Schedule of Recent Life Events. One group (n=86) suffered high stress without falling ill, whereas the other (n=75) reported becoming sick after their encounter with stressful life events. Illness was measured by Wyler, Masuda, and Holmes Seriousness of Illness Survey. Discriminant function analysis, run on half of the subjects in each group and cross-validated on the remaining cases, supported the prediction that high stress/low illness executives show, by comparison with high stress/high illness executives, more hardiness, that is have a stronger commitment to self, an attitude of vigorousness toward the environment, a sense of meaningfulness, and an internal locus of control.

557

Manhold JH. **Stress, oral disease and general illness** (presidential address). *Psychosomatics.* 1979;20:77-83. (English)

558

McClelland DC, Alexander C, Marks E. **The need for power, stress, immune function, and illness among male prisoners.** *J Abnormal Psychol.* 1982;91:61-70. (English)

Previous studies have demonstrated that a strong power motive in college students as assessed by the TAT (n Power), if inhibited and/or stressed, is associated with impaired immune-function reports of more serious illnesses. Subjects in this study were 133 male prisoners varying widely in age, ethnicity, and educational background. Motives were assessed from the TAT, stress and illness from self-report inventories, and immune function from concentrations of immunoglobulin A in saliva (S-IgA). Those high in n Power and in reported stress showed the highest levels of reported illness and the lowest concentrations of S-IgA, significantly different from those high in n Power and low in stress, or from all other subjects, but not from those simply high in stress. Although the stress-illness association may be due to a response bias to complain about everything, the motive/stress and lowered immune function connection cannot be attributed to this response bias. Among prisoners the effect of motive type is less and the effect of stress is greater than among college students perhaps because stress in prison is stronger. As expected, high concentrations of S-IgA were associated with reports of fewer upper respiratory infections supporting the hypothesis that some motive/stress and illness connections may be mediated by impaired immune-functions.

559
McClelland DC, Jemmott JB. **Power motivation, stress and physical illness.** *J Hum Stress.* 1980;6:6-15. (English)

College students reporting a larger number of life change events in the past six months also reported significantly more frequent and more severe instances of physical illness and more affective symptoms in the same time period. These relationships, however, were modified in an interesting way by type of life change and by individual differences. Life change events were classified as involving power, affiliative or other stresses. Individuals scoring high in the need for Power (n Power), in inhibition, and in the number of power stresses (HHH subjects), reported more severe physical ilness and affective synptoms than all subjects or, in particular, subjects low in n Power, power stress and inhibition (LLL subjects). Individuals scoring high in n Power and high in either inhibition or power stress also reported significantly more severe physical illness than other subjects. Among subjects high in inhibition, affiliative stress in combination with high n Power was associated with more severe physical illness, but, among subjects low in inhibition, affiliative stress in combination with high n Affiliation was associated with more physical illness. Affiliative stress was unrelated to affective symptoms. The findings are interpreted as consistent with the hypothesis that subjects in the HHH category compared with other subjects are characterized by chronically high sympathetic activity which has immunosuppressive effects, making them more illness prone.

560
Mehrabian A, Ross M. **Quality of life change and individual differences in stimulus screening in relation to incidence of illness.** *Psychol Rep.* 1977;41:367-78. (English)

A considerable amount of evidence indicates that a high rate of life changes--a source of continued and unavoidable arousal--is detrimental to health and psychological well-being. The present study hypothesized that sustained high-arousal states are unpreferred and that the persistence of unpreferred emotional states is harmful. Using a conceptual framework for a comprehensive description of emotional states and the differential preferences for these, it is possible to make more precise predictions on the illness consequences of emotionally unpreferred life changes. Particular hypotheses which received support were that more arousing life changes are more conducive to illness; that among the more arousing life changes, unpleasant changes are associated with more illness than pleasant ones; that unpleasant life changes are more detrimental to health when combined with dominance-inducing life changes; and that arousing life changes are particularly harmful to more arousable (non-screening) individuals.

561
Miller NE. **Learning, stress and psychosomatic symptoms.** *Acta Neurobiol Exp.* 1976;36:141-56. (English) (unavailable at publication)

562
Minter RE, Kimball CP. **Life events and illness onset: a review.** *Psychosomatics.* 1978;19:334-9. (English)

Investigations attempting to show a correlation between life events and onset of any illness are reviewed. A brief discussion of the main methodologic problems in this area of research is also presented. Investigations of the sick role and the effect of stress upon illness behavior indicate that greater control of these variables is desirable. To gain this, it is suggested that in future studies, illnesses be more adequately documented than it has been to date. In the studies reviewed here, the data are not sufficiently sound to warrant any firm conclusions concerning the relationship between life events and illness onset.

563
Murphy E, Brown GW. **Life events, psychiatric disturbance and physical illness.** *Brit J Psychiatr.* 1980;136:326-38. (English)

The relationship between life events and the onset of organic physical illness has been studied in a group of women in the general population. The link between severe events and the onset of organic illness, which held only for women of 50 years or younger, was not a direct causal association but mediated by an in evening psychiatric disturbance of an affective kind, all occurring within a six month period. The findings are discussed in the light of the high psychiatric morbidity found in physically ill patients.

564
Petrich J, Holmes TH. **Life change and onset of illness.** *Med Clinics N Am.* 1977;61:825-38. (English)

Stress, a popular term in lay and professional literature, is a concept shrouded in confusion and disagreement. The measurement of life change addresses the relationship of environmental events and health changes. This approach first crystallized in the "Life Chart" of Adolf Meyer. The Life Chart provided a unique method of organizing medical data into a dynamic biography. Concepts of Freud, Pavlov, Cannon and others were incorporated into the Meyerian schema by Harold Wolff and his associates. The research adduced powerful evidence that life events, by evoking psychophysiological reactions, played an important role in the natural history of many diseases. The purpose of this paper is to describe the measurement of life change and review its relationship to the study of onset of illness. Illness refers to any change in health status and includes the spectrum of medical, surgical and psychiatric disorders.

565
Rabkin JG, Struening EL. **Life events, stress and illness.** *Science.* 1976;194:1013-20. (English)

Although conceptual and theoretical orientations should play an important preparatory role in the design and execution of empirical studies, this does not often appear to be the case in the literature reviewed on the relation of life events, stress and illness. It is clearly recognized that illness onset is the outcome of multiple characteristics of the individual interacting with a number of interdependent factors in the individual's social context in the presence of a disease agent. The conceptual model is comprehensive, multicausal and interactive; empirical designs should consider this complexity. In spite of the repeatedly observed trivial relationships between measures of change in life events and illness onset (or care-seeking behavior), many investigators continue to focus on linear relationships between independent and dependent variables without consideration or control of intervening and mediating variables, some of which easily lend themselves to standard measurement procedures. To advance the accurate prediction and understanding of illness onset, the design and execution of empirical studies must be taken into account as Mechanic and others have stressed, the complexity of the phenomena being studied. Crucial in the measurement process are the psychometric properties of the measures used and the methods of collecting data that are employed. Investigators in the area of life events research are vulnerable in their operational definitions of both independent and dependent variables. More emphasis should be placed on a thorough conceptualization and sampling of the universe of life events, followed by multidimensional scaling of item samples in a variety of respondent samples drawn from theoretically meaningful populations to identify common dimensions of life events. The internal consistency and test-retest reliability of summary scales derived from those analyses should be studied across samples to determine true variance and stability of these measures over a variety of populations. The use of unidimensional scales with questionable content validity continues to be a problem in the operational definition of such complex domains as reported symptoms of illness or mental illness. The continued use of one measure to represent an obviously complex domain of symptoms will frequently lead to limited and erroneous conclusions. An extensive literature also indicates that symptoms of mental and physical illness are not unidimensional. In retrospective studies important sources of error in the measurement of life events include selective memory, denial of certain events, and overreporting to justify a current illness. In prospective studies, the subjective evaluation of the significance of a life event to the respondent has been neglected. The data analytic procedures used in life events research do not adequately inform the reader of the nature of obtained results. Certain procedures crucial to the understanding of results seldom have been undertaken. For example, not one instance of an estimate of the internal consistency reliability of a life events scale was discovered in this review, though such values are important in the evaluation of measures and in the interpretation of the magnitude of relationships. Further, the application of similar data analytic procedures to the data of a number of studies would enhance the comparability and communication of results and the possibility of making generalizations. It is concluded that improvement in data analytic procedures remains a major challenge for life events investigators. Refinements of method and content in this field are to be encouraged, in the expectation that they will contribute to a better understanding of the disease process and also to the development of techniques of primary prevention of illness and rehabilitation of the chronically ill.

566
Racy J. **Stress and human disease: an overview and background.** *Ariz Med.* 1980;37:352-4. (English) (no abstract)

567
Rahe RH, Arthur RJ. **Life change and illness studies: past history and future directions.** *J Hum Stress.* 1978;4:3-15. (English)

A selected review of life changes and illness studies is presented which illustrates both the diversity of samples that have been tested in these studies and the generally positive results which have been obtained. Although early (retrospective) work in this field led to simplistic explanations, later (prospective) studies have begun to document the several intervening variables which occur between subjects' recent life change exeriences and their subsequent symptomatology and disease. A life change and illness model is presented to illustrate key intervening variables. The authors believe that future research in the field of life change and illness should concentrate on further delineations of these intervening variables — an effort necessitating active collaboration between social and medical scientists.

568
Rahe RH, Holmes TH. **Life crisis and disease onset; II--Qualitative and quantitative definition of the life crisis and its association with health change.** (unpublished manuscript) (English) (no abstract)

569
Rahe RH, Holmes TH. **Life crisis and disease onset; III--A prospective study of life crises and health changes.** (unpublished manuscript) (English) (no abstract)

570
Rees WL. **Stress, distress and disease: the Presidential Address at the annual meeting of the Royal College of Psychiatrists, held in London, 9 July 1975.** *Brit J Psychiatr.* 1976;128:3-18. (English) (no abstract)

571
Rosch PJ. **Stress and illness** (editorial). *JAMA.* 1979;242:427-8 (English)

572
Rose RM, Jenkins CD, Hurst MW. **Health change in air traffic controllers: a prospective study; I--Background and description.** *Psychosom Med.* 1978;40:142-65. (English)

The background, rationale, and design of a 3-year prospective study of health change in 416 air traffic controllers is described. This study was designed to assess the relevant variables that might predict future physical and psychological health change. This report describes the major variables that were assessed in all participants, which included endocrine, cardiovascular, and behavioral differences in response to work, the occurrence of significant life events, work attitude and morale, availability and usefulness of psychosocial supports, and job commitment and performance. Future reports will describe the contribution, both individually and interactively, of these various factors to the risk for future illness. A major hypothesis to be tested by this study is that health change among air traffic controllers can be predicted by differential responsivity to work.

573
Schuman SH, Jebaily GC, Samuelson DC. **Life events in a family with life-threatening illness.** *Psychosomatics.* 1977;18:34-9. (English) (no abstract)

574
Siegrist J. **The significance of life changes for the outbreak of a disease.** *Med Klin.* 1980;75:770-7. (German) (no abstract)

575
Suls J, Mullen B. **Life events, perceived control and illness: the role of uncertainty.** *J Hum Stress.* 1981;7:30-4. (English)

The health implications of recognizing the difference between situations that are controllable and those that are not has been noted by a variety of sources. With this notion in mind, the present study examined the relationship between perceptions of control and desirability of life events and subsequent health in a college student sample. Subjects indicated which of a list of life events had occurred to them over a three-month span and also specified how desirable each was and to what extent they were in control of its occurrence. Illness was reported for the following month. The results indicated that both undesirable uncontrollable events and undesirable events of uncertain controllability were significantly related to the occurence of illness. Of greater interest was the finding that the occurrence of events of uncertain controllability was more strongly related to illness than events perceived as totally uncontrollable. The results are discussed in terms of research and theory stressing the adaptive significance of the ability to discriminate controllable situations from uncontrollable ones.

Stress and cancer

576
Achterberg J, Lawlis GF, Simonton OC, Matthews-Simonton S. **Psychological factors, blood factors and blood chemistries as disease outcome predictors for cancer patients.** *Multivar Exp Clin Res.* 1977;3:107-22. (English)

Studied the relationship between blood chemistries and psychological variables in 126 15-71 yr old incurable cancer patients. An intensive battery of psychodiagnostics was administered (including MMPI, Bem Sex-Role Inventory, FIRO-B, and Profile of Mood States), and blood analyses were conducted. Criterion vairables (i.e., median life expectancy and disease and rehabilitation status) were included in the analyses. Initially, blood chemistries were clustered according to common variance via factor analysis, and the factors were used to predict present and follow-up disease status. Psychological variables were utilized to predict respective variances within the blood chemistries. Psychological variables were then factor analyzed and utilized to determine whether disease processer were related. Results yield at least 3 basic conclusions: (a) Blood chemistries tended to reflect ongoing or concurrent disease state. (b) There was a statistical relationship between psychological variables and blood chemistries. (c) Psychological factors were predictive of subsequent disease status. However, these relationships were multidimen-

sional and too complex to be considered either causative or reactive at this time. Findings are impressive in that blood chemistries offered information only about the current state of the disease, whereas the psychological variables offered future insights.

577
Achterberg J, Lawlis GF. **A canonical analysis of blood chemistry variables related to psychological measures of cancer patients.** *Multivar Exp Clin Res.* 1979;4:1-10. (English)

Performed a canonical analysis of data for 126 cancer patients who completed the MMPI, IMAGE-CA, H. Levenson's (1973) revision of Rotter's Internal-External Locus of Control Scale, the Profile of Mood States, and the FIRO-B. Disease status, rehabilitation status, and blood chemistries were also determined. Canonical coefficients ranged from .98 to .82. The 3 most stable factors were interpreted as Resignation, Nondirected struggle, and Purposeful action. No single factor contained a predominance of a type of medical treatment, but the factors were related to the severity of the disease.

578
Bahnson CB. **Stress and cancer: the state of the art, part 1.** *Psychosomatics.* 1980;21:975-81. (English)

Although it has been repeatedly recognized from antiquity that melancholy and grief may precede the development of cancer, a body of evidence has now accumulated of a common personal background and personality makeup in many cancer patients. A recurrent theme is a feeling of loneliness and hopelessness stemming from the lack of a protected and loving childhood. Such persons harbor chronic underlying feelings of depletion, emptiness, and resentment because they are unloved. Development of a personality marked by self-containment, inhibition, rigidity, repression, and regression precedes cancer, which may involve somatic (cellular) "regression." The author surveys the literature and provides an illustrative case report to support his hypothesis.

579
Bahnson CB. **Stress and cancer: the state of the art, part 2.** *Psychosomatics.* 1981;22:207-20. (English).

This paper reviews the evidence for specific personality and ego-defensive characteristics of cancer patients. The stress of loss and depression when combined with these personality factors seems to increase vulnerability to clinical cancer. A blind statistical sorting of cancer patients versus matched control patients on psychological items alone yielded results that bear promise for future psychological screening procedures. Three possible psychosomatic intervening processes are reviewed in order to provide suggestions for more specific research into the effects of personality and the stress of depression on vulnerability to cancer: relevant neurologic, endocrine, and immunologic data are reviewed in this perspective.

580
Carroll RM. **Stress and cancer: etiological significance**

and implications. *Cancer Nurs.* 1981;4:467-73. (English) (unavailable at publication)

581
Conti C, Biondi M, Pancheri P. **A statistical evaluation of stressful events in 144 neoplastic and psychiatric patients.** *Riv Psichiat.* 1981;16:357-77. (Italian)

Administered the Schedule of Recent Experience and the Life Experiences Survey to 144 women with breast or uterine cancer, fibrocystic mastopathy or uterine fibroma, or neurotic pathology. The analysis of life stress events for the 10 years preceding the diagnosis yielded a statistically significant difference between the psychiatric group and the groups with cancer and benign pathology. Neurotic Ss had higher scores for all 4 measures of stress: positive change, negative change, total change, and life change units. The discrepancy in the total number of events reported by the cancer and benign groups on the one hand, and by the neurotic group on the other hand, may be due to the greater tendency of the neurotic group to report events since they are more closely in touch with their emotional lives.

582
Duszynski DR, Shaffer JW, Thomas CB. **Neoplasm and traumatic events in childhood: are they related?** *Arch Gen Psychiat.* 1981;38:327-31. (English) (unavailable at publication)

Previous research has suggested that certain objectively defined traumatic events occuring in childhood and/or adolescence may be linked to the appearance of neoplasm later in life. The present report examines four such events—parental death, parental divorce, sibling death, and having been the youngest child for less than two years—for their frequency of occurrence within four groups of physician subjects classified according to current health status as follows: major cancer, skin cancer, benign tumor, and healthy controls. All data had been collected while the subjects were in medical school within the context of a long-term, prospectively oriented study. Major cancer subjects were also compared with their cancer-free siblings with respect to length of time spent as youngest child. Although there was a slight tendency for the trend of the findings to be in accord with the hypotheses tested, no statistically significant differences among groups could be demonstrated.

583
Fox BH. **Premorbid psychological factors as related to cancer incidence.** *J Behav Med.* 1978;1:45-134. (English)

In planning for studies relating psychological factors and/or stress (PF&/OS) to cancer, one should be aware of epidemiological findings that might contribute to or even account wholly for any found relationships. Most studies have not examined the known biological causes of cancer, nor have they described a rationale for relationships sought. The two broad mechanisms leading to cancer, carcinogens and lowered resistance to it, include physical and chemical causes, viruses and chronic infection, medication, genetic predisposition, hormonal stimuli, and aging. Interfering variables may bias or dilute a real relationship. Validity and reliability of instruments measuring PF&/OS are so variable as to warrant

considerable care in their use. The latent periods of different cancers are measured in years, not months, with consequent potent impact on possible inferences drawn from prebiopsy and short prospective studies. In these and in retrospective studies, cancer can have strong and biasing effects on apparently straightforward PF&/OS measurements, as can iatrogenic effects. Some theoretical issues are discussed. The known prospective studies are discussed and reasons are given for the view that they are less convincing than many seem to think. A sketch of a model relating PF&/OS to cancer appearance is outlined, with some theoretical implications, and issues in research design are addressed.

584
Girstenbrey W. **Stress resulting in cancer?** *Med Welt.* 1980;31:III. (German) (no English abstract)

585
Jacobs TJ, Charles E. **Life events and the occurrence of cancer in children.** *Psychosom Med.* 1980;42:11-24. (English)

Over a two-year period the families of twenty-five children with cancer and of a comparison group of children brought to a general pediatric clinic were studied by means of the Holmes-Rahe Life Schedule of Recent Events and by personal interviews. Results obtained by use of the Holmes-Rahe questionnaire revealed significant differences between the patient and control groups. Histories obtained from families in both groups also revealed that in the cancer group certain important life events were found to have occurred with greater frequency in the year prior to the onset of the disease. The relevance of these findings to previous work done in the field and to some current theories concerning the relationship of genetic, viral, endocrine, and psychological factors in the development of cancer are discussed.

586
Lecompte D. **Critical review of the literature on psychogenetic factors in cancer diseases** (author's transl). *Acta Paediatr Belg.* 1979;79:144-55. (French)

The author reviews the literature on various psychic etiopathogenic approaches of cancer and reminds the main methodological critics. He comes to the conclusion that these criticisms are similar to those in psychosomatic medicine. He believes the monistic psychobiological theory to be the most pertinent at present. The technique of associative investigations, of a dialectic nature, is proposed as a methodological instrument in the frame of psychosomatic research in cancer.

587
Lehrer S. **Life change and gastric cancer.** *Psychosom Med.* 1980;42:499-502. (English)

Forty colorectal cancer patients, 14 gastric patients, and 10 normal controls were tested with the Social Readjustment Rating Scale. The gastric cancer patients had a significantly higher amount of life change (p<0.05) in the two-year period preceding the onset of the first symptoms of their illness. Moreover, there was a significant (p<0.01) negative correlation between amount of life change and age at onset of symptoms in gastric cancer, but not in colorectal cancer. There was also no correlation between age and life changes in the normal controls. These findings suggest that emotional stress may be a predisposing factor in gastric cancer.

588
Lehrer S. **Life change and lung cancer.** *J Hum Stress.* 1981;7:7-11. (English)

Seventy-four lung cancer patients were studied with the Social Readjustment Rating Scale. There was a significantly higher association of recent life change with younger cancer patients than with older ones. There was no such difference in a control group of colorectal cancer patients. These results imply that lung cancer patients fall into two groups: a younger group, in which life change is a promoting factor, and an older group, in which life change has little or no effect in precipitating the onset of the disease.

589
Levy SM. **Health psychology and cancer research.** *The Health Psychologist.* 1981;3:3-4. (English) (no abstract)

590
Locke SE. **Brain, behavior and human immunity** (abstract). *Proceedings, 13th International Cancer Congress.* 1982;p.478. (English)

Evidence for direct influences of brain and behavior on immune function is accumulating. Studies in humans of the effects of experimental and naturally-occurring stress on parameters of humoral and cell-mediated immunity suggest that stress can be either immunosuppressive or immunoenhancing, depending upon certain critical factors. These factors include: 1) the specific parameter of immunity measured, 2) the duration and timing of the stressor, 3) coping ability and 4) personality traits. Finally, certain behavioral factors, especially depressive personality traits, have been reported to be associated both with increased risk of developing cancer and a poorer reponse of cancer patients to treatment in prospective, longitudinal studies. Demonstrated anatomical and functional links between the nervous and immune systems provide a basis for speculative formulations about the role of brain and behavior in the modification of host resistance to cancer. Recently, there have been widely publicized claims of efficacy for behavioral treatments designed to modify the clinical course of human cancer through behavioral modification of immune function. However, at present there is no experimental evidence to support these claims. Whether behavioral treatments have a role in the control of malignancy remains to be proven. Such treatments are not without side effects and may have adverse effects by leading to increased guilt and depression.

591
Mackintosh SL. **Incidence of breast and cervical cancer among women and selected social and psychological variables.** *Diss Abstr Int.* 1980;40:3091. (English) (unavailable at publication)

592
Miller TR. **Psychophysiologic aspects of cancer.** *Cancer.* 1977;39:413-8. (English)

Clinicians have long been aware of the neuro-endocrine axis and the action of the hypothalmus on the humoral immune response in the origin and course of cancer. Little attention has been paid, however, to the psychophysiologic aspects of cancer. These psycho-social effects may be related to hypothalmic activity, the autonomic nervous system, and neuro-endocrine activity. More attention should be paid to the manipulation of the psyche in the prevention and management of cancer.

593
Riley V, Spackman DH, McClanahan H, Santisteban GA. **The role of stress in malignancy.** *Cancer Detect Prev.* 1979;2:235-55. (English)

Either emotional or psychosocial stress in mice produces both biochemical and cellular changes in the host, which can be quantitatively measured providing that truly quiescent, nonstressful conditions can be maintained by the use of protective housing and special handling. Typical environmentally related stress symptoms can be imitated by the direct administration of either natural or synthetic hormones. The resulting physiological alterations induced in the experimental animal by either procedure modify important elements of the immunological and surveillance apparatus. Such effects of stress may change either the incidence or the course of neoplastic and other pathological processes.

594
Seifter E, Cohen MH, Riley V. **Of stress, vitamin A, and tumors** (letter). *Science.* 1976;193:74-5. (English)

595
Selye H. **Correlating stress and cancer.** *Am J Proctol Gastroenterol Colon Rectal Surg.* 1979;30:18-20, 25-8. (English) (no abstract)

596
Solomon GF, Amkraut AA. **Neuroendocrine aspects of the immune response and their implications for stress effects on tumor immunity.** *Cancer Detect Prev.* 1979; 2:197-224. (English)

Personality, emotions and stress appear to affect the immunologic system, which likely is regulated by the central nervous system via neuroendocrine mediation, with implications for the etiology and course of cancer, as well as infectious, autoimmune and possibly some mental diseases. Stress appears to affect chiefly the efferent and, to some extent, the afferent limbs of the immune system; macrophage activities are probably a major, if not the most important, target. We restate our belief, stemming from experimental observation, that stress-induced changes in the immune systems are generally small and determine the course of disease chiefly by shifting the balance between toxic factors and defense mechanisms in disease processes. The methods chosen for detecting such changes must, therefore, be the most sensitive and reproducible available. Experimental measurements must include levels of at least one hormone, but should cover as many hormonal systems as is reasonably practicable.

597
Zee HJ. **Stress and cancer.** *J Med Assoc Ga.* 1979;68:845-7. (English) (no abstract)

Stress and infectious disease

598
Boyce WT, Cassel JC, Collier AM, Jensen EW, Ramey CT, Smith AH. **Influence of life events and family routines on childhood respiratory tract illness.** *Pediatrics.* 1977; 60:609-15. (English) (unavailable at publication)

599
Totman R, Kiff J, Reed SE, Craig JW. **Predicting experimental colds in volunteers from different measures of recent life stress.** *J Psychosom Res.* 1980;24:155-63. (English)

Induced experimental colds by nasal inoculation with rhinoviruses during the course of a 10-day residental stay in 52 18-49 yr olds. Prior to inoculation, Ss were assessed on 5 different measures (e.g., the Schedule of Recent Experience and a loss index) of recent life stress and the Eysenck Personality Inventory (EPI). Clear evidence of a psychosomatic component in colds was obtained. Introverts developed significantly worse symptoms and infections than extraverts. Life Events, when they involved change in the S's general level of activity, were significantly related to magnitude of infection. Findings indicate that net changes in the level of social activity and scores on the Extraversion scale of the EPI are independently predictive of the extent of infection with rhinovirus. It is concluded that continuing life difficulties do not appear to contribute to the risk of infection.

600
Totman R, Reed SE, Craig JW. **Cognitive dissonance, stress and virus-induced common colds.** *J Psychosom Res.* 1977;21:55-63. (English)

A study of the effect of cognitive dissonance on symptoms of rhinovirus-induced common colds and their infectivity in 48 volunteers is presented. Subjects, about to be experimentally infected with two common cold viruses (rhinoviruses), were given a choice as to whether or not to receive a "trial anti-viral drug" (in fact a placebo) during the course of their infection. To make this choice difficult, they were also told that if they received the "drug", their gastric juices would have to be sampled by means of a stomach tube at the end of this experiment. It was predicted from Cognitive Dissonance Theory that all those making this choice, irrespective of the alternative chosen, would justify their decisions by "attenuating" the experienced severity of their colds, and that this effect would be evidenced in their symptoms and possibly in the amount of virus shed as compared to controls who were neither given the placebo nor the choice concerning it. An effect exactly opposite to that predicted was obtained. Symptoms, but not virus shedding, were significantly influenced by the psychological manipulations involved, the symptoms of subjects given a choice being more severe than those of subjects not choosing. Interpretations of this are explored.

Stress and autoimmune disorders

601
Linn MW, Linn BS, Skyler J, Jensen J. **Stress and immune functioning in diabetes** (abstract). *Psychosom Med.* 1982;44:128. (English)

Stressful life events are being recorded in insulin dependent (IDDM) and non-insulin dependent (NIDDM) diabetics at 6-month intervals in a prospective longitudinal study. All are males matched for age and sex. Stress data include number of stressful events, and ratings on 0-9 scales of the degree of perceived stress, anticipation of events, responsibility in precipitating events, and amount of support received in coping with events. Psychological and physiological data are also collected. The question here was whether stress variables differed between ADDM and NIDDM groups, whether perceived stress was related to immunological status, and if immune functioning differed between the 2 groups. Twenty IDDM patients were compared with 20 NIDDM by analysis of variance. IDDM patients reported significantly more stressful events (p<0.01), and more perceived stress, anticipation of stress, and responsibility for events (p<0.05). Amount of support received in coping with events did not differ between groups. Correlations between perceived stress and immune responsiveness were inverse and higher for IDDM than for NIDDM. The IDDM patients differed significantly on several immunological parameters. IDDM patients had less chemotactic responsiveness and fewer positive reactions to delayed hypersensitivity skin tests (p<0.05). Although lymphocyte responses to mitogens were less vigorous in IDDM than in NIDDM, these did not reach statistical significance. Others have noted that juvenile-onset diabetes has immunological features. Some have reported associations between stress and immune functioning in general. The relationship between perceived stress and immune function being greater in IDDM than NIDDM patients has not, to our knowledge, been reported. Helping these patients cope better with stress might influence their immunological responses favorably and thus lead to fewer problems in control and complications of the disease.

602
Morillo E, Gardner LI. **Activation of latent Graves' disease in children: review of possible psychosomatic mechanisms.** *Clin Pediatr.* 1980;19:160-3. (English)

In some children, psychological events have appeared to be important in the triggering of Graves' disease. This report examines the case histories of three children in whom the appearance of symptomatology of Graves' disease was associated with depression following the death of a loved one. An analysis of neuroendocrine and immunologic pathways suggests that depression, set off by bereavement, causes low levels of norepinephrine in the brain. The latter in turn may mediate an increase in ACTH and cortisol, leading to reductions in immune surveillance and resultant production of thyroid-stimulating immunoglobulins, hence the development of Graves' disease.

603
Morillo E, Gardner LI. **Bereavement as an antecedent factor in thyrotoxicosis of childhood: four case studies**

with survey of possible metabolic pathways. *Psychosom Med.* 1979;41:545-55. (English)

Various organic and psychosomatic factors have been postulated over the years as etiologic events antedating the onset of Graves' disease. In some patients psychological events have appeared to be important in the evocation of symptoms. Although examples of the latter have been described in adults for many years, there is little published on this phenomenon in children. The present study delineates findings in two boys and two girls with an age range of 8 to 14 years. Separating experiences appeared to be related to the onset or relapse of Graves' disease in these particular cases. In three of the patients the trigger event was represented by bereavement after loss of a close relative; in the fourth case the boy's loss was enforced and traumatic separation from his mother figure. In all these children depression was the common response to loss. The observed relationship between the affective disturbance and Graves' disease is compatible with one or more hypothetical models. One such pathway, via depletion of brain monoamines associated with the state of depression, could cause an activation of the hypothalamic-pituitary-adrenal axis with resultant suppression of immune surveillance. This could permit the formation of thyroid-stimulating immunoglobulins (TSI) and hence Graves' disease in genetically susceptible (HLA B8) persons.

604
Olhagen B. **Etiology and pathogenesis of chronic arthritis.** *Lakartidningen.* 1977;74:4484-90. (Swedish)

The discovery that 90 per cent of patients with certain forms of sero-negative arthritis, such as uro-arthritis and pelvospondylitis, have a genetically caused condition marked by tissue type HLA-B27 opened new ways to understanding of the mechanism of origin of these diseases. The etiology of rheumatoid arthritis (RA) is still unknown. The author discusses various pathogenetic factors: genetic disposition, microbial agents, immunological mechanisms, gastrointestinal genesis, and stress. RA is regarded as a syndrome with probably multiple etiology, in which a combination of pathogenetic factors is needed for the disease to appear.

605
Perini GI, Fornasa CV, Cipriani R, Pesserico R. **Stressful life events in alopecia areata** (abstract). *Psychosom Med.* 1982;44:125-6. (English)

The role of stressful life events in alopecia areata (A.A.), although stated by many authors, is still controversial. This study investigated life events in alopecic patients according to Paykel methodology. Forty-eight patients with A.A. (common type), 30 with common baldness, 30 with fungal infections underwent the Paykel's revised interview for Recent Life Events. In the 6 months preceding onset, alopecic patients reported a total of 123 events (2.56 per patient), patients with common baldness 22 (0.73) and those with fungal infection 15 (0.50) (p<0.001). Events with negative impact (p<0.001), exits from social field (p<0.05), uncontrolled events (p<0.01), and socially undesirable events (p<0.001) were significantly more frequent in A.A. than in controls. Work, finance, family and social relationships were the most involved areas. The results

of this study are consistent with the most recent view of A.A. as an autoimmune disorder related to reduced T-cell functions. In fact, there exists evidence that stressful events, such as bereavement, in men can influence the cellular immune system by means of hypothalamus, endocrine and autonomic systems whose diseases are often associated with A.A.

606
Rimon R, Viukari M, Halonen P. **Relationship between life stress factors and viral antibody levels in patients with juvenile rheumatoid arthritis.** *Scand J Rheumatol.* 1979;8:62-4. (English)

Serum specimens from 46 patients with JRA were tested for measles CF, HI, HLI, and RNP-GP antibodies, for rubella HI antibodies, and for adenovirus and herpes simplex virus CF antibodies. The mean antibody titres of the 16 JRA patients of the major conflict group (14) were generally higher than those of the 30 patients of the non-conflict group, although the differences do not reach the level of statistical significance. The interrelationships between life stress, emotions and immunological changes in JRA are discussed.

607
Volpe R. **The pathogenesis of Graves' disease: an overview.** *Clin Endocrinol Metab.* 1978;7:3-29. (English)

It is the author's view that Graves' hyperthyroidism, exophthalmos, and Hashimoto's thyroiditis (as well as other closely related organ-specific autoimmune diseases) may each be due to separate, albeit very closely related, inherited isolated defects in immune surveillance (presumably isolated defects in suppressor T lymphocytes). Each of these defects would permit the specific randomly mutating self-reactive 'forbidden' clone of helper T lymphocytes to survive, if it chanced to appear, interact with its complementary antigen, and induce a cell-mediated immune response. This clone of self-reactive T lymphocytes would presumably expand following interaction with its antigen, and consequently direct and co-operate with appropriate groups of (already present) B lymphocytes which in turn would produce specific immunoglobulins that appear to be necessary for the full expression of these disorders. The role of stress in the induction of hyperthyroidism may be by means of its effect in further reducing immune surveillance in those persons with only a partial isolated defect; remissions may be brought about by restoring the capacity for surveillance to its previous state. Those persons having an isolated complete defect in immune surveillance would not be expected to achieve remissions, except by destruction of thyroid parenchyma.

608
Zeitlin DJ. **Psychological issues in the management of rheumatoid arthritis.** *Psychosomatics.* 1977;18:7-14. (English)

The weight of research suggests a multicausal hypothesis in which genetic, autoimmune, infectious, and psychosocial factors interact to varying degrees to create a "predisposition matrix." A triggering factor (for some, a psychological event) then leads to clinical rheumatoid arthritis. The clinical course both affects and is affected by the patient's psychological state. An approach to the patient is outlined in which he is viewed not as a "rheumatoid personality" but as a unique human being facing acute and chronic stress, which sets up reverberations within and among all the systems of which he is a part: family, interpersonal, intrapsychic, occupational, and the comprehensive health care team. Specific psychological issues in these systems are discussed, with particular emphasis on the work of mourning in both patient and staff. Successful completion of mourning entails compromise and "rebirth." Incomplete mourning often leads to depression. Differential diagnosis and kinds of psychotherapeutic intervention are discussed for the acute and chronic situation, and some studies of psychological management are presented.

Stress and allergic disorders

609
Levenson RW. **Effects of thematically relevant and general stressors on specificity of responding in asthmatic and nonasthmatic subjects.** *Psychosom Med.* 1979;41:28-39. (English)

Twenty-nine mild asthmatics and 12 nonasthmatics were exposed to three films of varying emotional content to assess differential patterns of physiological response in the cardiac, ventilatory, and bronchial systems. Results indicated that only cardiac interbeat interval (IBI) and total respiratory resistance (RT) were reliable indices of reactivity. In a film of thematic relevance to asthmatics which depicted asthmatic children in a hospital setting, asthmatics evidenced sustained elevation of RT throughout the entire film with no reactivity in IBI. Nonasthmatics did not evidence any significant reactivity to the film. In a film of a generally stressful nature which depicted industrial accidents, asthmatics evidenced elevated RT in response to the accident scenes. Both asthmatic and nonasthmatic subjects responded to the post-accident periods with increases in IBI. In a film depicting a mother giving up her child for adoption, asthmatics responded to the relinquishing of the child with elevated RT. These results are discussed in terms of the necessity of evolving a comprehensive theory of specificity patterns in psychosomatic disorders which goes beyond models of symptom specificity and stimulus-response specificity, neither of which can adequately account for these results. The results are further seen as supporting the utility of selecting stressors of thematic relevance to asthmatics and measuring symptom-relevant indices of physiological reactivity to isolate these specificity patterns in response to stress.

610
McAndrew I. **Facts and fallacies in a sociological study of asthma.** *Aust Paediatr.* 1976;12:88-91. (English)

A number of the more popular beliefs about the characteristics of the asthmatic child, fostered by previous studies of select populations, were not born out in a study of a randomly selected population covering the whole range of wheezing children. It appears that there are no characteristics or trends which pertain to the whole asthmatic group. Some factors of stress, and some behavioural disturbances and developmental delays, are common in the small group of severely affected children, as is the child's close bond with the mother and a basic fear of separation.

611
Seville RH. **Psoriasis and stress.** *Brit J Dermatol.* 1978; 98:151-3. (English) (unavailable at publication)

612
Weiss JH, Lyness J, Molk L, Riley J. **Induced respiratory change in asthmatic children.** *J Psychosom Res.* 1976; 20:115-23. (English)

Tested a laboratory analog approach to studying emotionally precipitated asthma, using 28 12-15 yr old chronic asthmatics. The stimulus was a motion picture of children in severe asthmatic distress and was derived from patient reports that thinking about their breathing could trigger or aggravate their symptoms. Effects of viewing the film were compared with those of an avoidance learning condition, being exposed to the sounds of nonasthmatic breathing, and of listneing to music. There were 3 experimental sessions: Adapatation, in which Ss listened to music; Control, in which Ss were required to learn to avoid a moderately painful stimulus or to listen to simulated breathing sounds; and Film. On the measure of expiration flow rate, significantly more Ss showed a decrease in response to the Film than was the case for the Adaptation or Control conditions. Significantly fewer Ss showed no expiratory rate change in response to the Film than was true for the Adaptation or Control conditions. Ss whose expiratory flow rate decreased in response to the Film (D subgroup) also had significantly greater increases in expiratory duration during the film than did the remaining Ss (ND subgroup). Expiration duration increases for the D subgroup were significantly greater in response to the Film than to the Adaptation or Control conditions. Measures of subjective response show that the total group reported significantly increased asthma during the film. Results are discussed in terms of the uses and limitations of analog approaches and the properties of the induction stimulus.

613
Weston WL, Huff JC. **Atopic dermatitis: etiology and pathogenesis.** *Pediatr Ann.* 1976;5:759-62. (English)

Atopic dermatitis is a recognizable phenotype that most likely results from several mechanisms. An increasing number of children with atopic dermatitis are recognized as having immune defects, although the exact incidence of such immunodeficiency states among patients with atopic dermatitis is unknown. Children with atopic dermatitis who suffer recurrent or persistent infections should undergo immunologic evaluation. Ideally, this should include evaluation of cell-mediated immunity as well as neutrophil and monocyte chemotaxis. Further investigation into the beta-blockade theory may enhance our understanding of atopic dermatitis. Careful attention to factors exacerbating atopic dermatitis is essential in understanding this problem. Abnormal sweating, dry skin, sensitivity to contactants, and emotional stress should always be considered in evaluation of children with atopic dermatitis.

Stress, neuroendocrine changes and immunity

614

Abplanalp JM, Livingston L, Rose RM, Sandwisch D. **Cortisol and growth hormone responses to psychological stress during the menstrual cycle.** *Psychosom Med.* 1977;39:158-77. (English)

Twenty-one healthy women were studied during one menstrual cycle in order to determine whether cortisol and growth hormone responsivity to psychological stress was related to estrogen levels. Blood was drawn approximatelly three times per week for analysis of estradiol, progesterone, cortisol, and human growth hormone. During either the menstrual or intermenstrual phase, each subject participated in an interview that was designed to be mildly stressful. State and trait anxiet were assessed using the Speilberger State-Trait Anxiety Inventory. Anxiety state was measured prior to and immediately following exposure to the psychological stress; trait anxiety was assessed at the end of the study. Cortisol and growth hormone responses to the psychological stress were not related to menstrual cycle phase. Anxiety levels were also independent of menstrual cycle phase. Subjects who displayed significant cortisol and/or growth hormone responsisivity to the interview had significantly higher anxiety levels post stress than did nonresponders, although anxiety level prior to the interview was not different for the two groups.

615

Brown WA, Heninger G. **Stress-induced growth hormone release: psychologic and physiologic correlates.** *Psychosom Med.* 1976;38:145-7. (English) (unavailable at publication)

616

Corenblum B, Whitaker M. **Inhibition of stress-induced hyperprolactinemia.** *Br Med J.* 1977;2:1328. (English)

Evidence suggests that there is dual control of inhibition and stimulation of prolactin secretion. Inhibition appears to predominate under basal conditions and is probably mediated through dopamine. There is less certainty about the stimulatory pathway, but surges of prolactin secretion occur in some physiological and stressful states, such as sleep, nipple stimulation, general anaesthesia, and hypoglycaemia. This stimulatory pathway may include serotonin neurotransmission, since administration of L-tryptophan or 5-hydroxytryptamine--precursors in central serotonin synthesis-noticeably increased the serum prolactin concentration, which is blunted by serotonin antagonists. Furthermore, the stress release of adrenocorticotrophic hormone by hypoglycaemia may be serotonin mediated. We therefore investigated whether serotonin neurotransmission mediated the release of prolactin in a young woman with stress-induced galactorrhoea.

617

Dimsdale JE, Moss J. **Plasma catecholamine in stress and exercise.** *JAMA.* 1980;243:340-2. (English)

A technique was devised to monitor plasma catecholamines in a minimally obtrusive fashion in subjects going about their working activities. There was a disparity between plasma norepinephrine and epinephrine levels in different situations. During public speaking, epinephrine levels increase twofold, whereas during physical exercise, norepinephrine levels increase threefold. It seemed that while exercise induces a response of the sympathetic nervous system, psychological stress induces primarily an adrenal response.

618

Dimsdale JE, Moss J. **Short-term catecholamine response to psychological stress.** *Psychosom Med.* 1980;42:493-7. (English)

The recent development of radioenzymatic assays for plasma catecholamines and of highly portable nonobtrusive blood withdrawal pumps makes possible the investigation of the physiological response to actual stress. However, because the half-life of plasma catecholamines is so brief, meticulous care must be taken to obtain blood samples consistently vis-a-vis the stress immersion experience. These points are demonstrated in a study of ten young physicians under the stress of public speaking. Plasma epinephrine levels differ significantly between the initial moments of public speaking and the middle moments of speaking. These differences are large enough to affect the conclusions reached in comparing public speaking values with baseline values.

619

Felsl I, Gottsmann M, Eversmann T, Jehle W, Uhlich E. **Influence of various stress situations on vasopressin secretion in man.** *Acta Endocrinol Suppl.* 1978;215:122-3. (English)

An increase of arginine vasopressin (AVP) plasma levels under the influence of various stress situations is well documented. However, nothing is known about a possible quantitative correlation between the amount of AVP released and stress intensity. Therefore a stress grading was performed in human volunteers according to the scheme of Miller and Graybiel. In a second series AVP levels were determined before, during and after major surgery. Five male subjects were exposed to stepwise increased angular velocity in a vertical axis on a stille rotatory chair. Head tilt movements had to be carried out in the four cardinal directions. The stress grading scheme consists of one control and three test periods, each of them similar in principle but different in terms of the stress intensity produced during the experiments (M/O=control test without symptoms; M/IV=frank motion sickness with vomiting). AVP (measured radioimmunologically), sodium, potassium and osmolality in the serum were determined before, during and after each test. In nine patients the same parameters were measured before and during a surgical procedure. The test persons showed a stepwise increase of AVP plasma levels in relation to stress intensity. Basal levels of AVP were 1.2 pg/ml, maximal levels reached 31 pg/ml (condition M/IV). After cessation of angular velocity in the series M/II and M/III the test persons developed all clinical signs of M/IV and correspondingly a further increase in AVP release could be demonstrated. Sodium, potassium and osmolality remained unchanged. In surgical patients undergoing thyroidectomy AVP levels were slightly elevated after initiating anaesthesia (2.4 ± 1.0 pg/ml compared to basal controls with 1.1 ± 0.3 pg/ml), but increased dramatically during preparation and removal of the organ (15.6 ± 6.9 pg/ml), while sodium, potassium and osmolality again remained constant. Extremely high plasma AVP levels were found under a variety of experimental and clinical stress situations.

620
Frankenhaeuser M, Rauste von Wright M, Collins A, Von Wright J, Sedvall G, Swahn CG. **Sex differences in psychoneuroendocrine reactions to examination stress.** *Psychosom Med.* 1978;40:334-43. (English)

Sex differences in adaptation and coping were studied by comparing neuroendocrine and psychological functions in male and female high-school students during 2-3 hr of routine school work (control condition) and a 6-hr matriculation examination (stress condition). In the control condition sex differences were slight and nonsignificant. During examination stress, the urinary excretion of cortisol, adrenaline, noradrenaline, and 3-methoxy-4-hydroxyphenylethylene glycol (MOPEG or MHPG) increased in both sexes, but to a consistently greater extent in the male group, significantly so for adrenaline and MOPEG. Both sexes performed equally well in the examination, but self-reports showed that feelings of success and confidence were common among males, whereas feelings of discomfort and failure dominated in the female group. High discomfort correlated with poor performance in the males but with good performance in the females.

621
Kopin IJ. **Catecholamines, adrenal hormones and stress.** *Hosp Prac.* 1976;11:49-55. (English)

From its beginnings about a century ago, research into the mechanisms underlying the stress response has led by many avenues to the adrenal medulla and its chromaffin cells. The latter possess cholinergic synapses that, when activated by a wide variety of stimuli, trigger discharge of catecholamines directly into the blood. Control of the response is mediated by a final common pathway arising in the hypothalamus and/or midbrain.

622
Kurokawa N. et al. **Effect of emotional stress on human growth hormone secretion.** *J Psychosom Res.* 1977; 21:231-5. (English) (unavailable at publication)

623
Mikhail A. **Stress: a psychophysiological conception.** *J Hum Stress.* 1981;7:9-16. (English)

Physiological and psychological conceptions of stress have evolved independently within their respective fields. An attempt has been made to integrate the salient theoretical features of stress in a definition which accomodates them. The merits of this integration have been outlined. It is believed that the integrated approach will lead to interdisciplinary understanding among theoreticians, writers, and researchers and will allow a unified theoretical structure to grow.

624
Miyabo S, Asato T, Mizushima N. **Prolactin and growth hormone responses to psychological stress in normal and neurotic subjects.** *J Clin Endocrinol Metab.* 1977; 44:947-51. (English)

In order to study the response of plasma prolactin (PRL) to acute psychological stress and to compare it with that of growth hormone (GH), the mirror drawing test (MDT) was performed in 20 normal controls (11 male, 9 female) and 22 neurotic patients (12 male, 10 female). Plasma PRL and GH were measured serially before, during, and after the test. In controls, the test caused no significant change in plasma levels of either hormone. In neurotic males, the response of PRL to the test was not consistent, whereas, in neurotic females plasma PRL level rose significantly following the test. Increase of GH, on the other hand, was apparent in the neurotics of both sexes. The correlation between the responses of two hormones in the neurotics was low and nonsignificant. The results indicate that although the psychoendocrine coping mechanism in the neurotics works less effectively for both PRL and GH, the two hormones may have different psychological correlates.

625
Miyabo S, Hisada T, Asato T, Mizushima N, Ueno K. **Growth hormone and cortisol responses to psychological stress: comparison of normal and neurotic subjects.** *J Clin Endocrinol Metab.* 1976;42:1158-62. (English)

The mirror drawing test (MDT) was performed to induce acute psychological stress in 9 normal controls and 10 neurotic subjects. Plasma growth hormone (GH) and cortisol were determined serially before, during, and after the test. In controls the MDT caused no significant change in plasma GH level, while in neurotics plasma GH increased progressively following the test. The increase of cortisol also tended to be greater in neurotics as a group, but there was a considerable overlap in individual responses. The maximum increments of GH in neurotics correlated inversely with those of cortisol. The results indicate: 1) effective psychological coping mechanisms operate in normal man to keep the hormonal response minimum. 2) GH response is a more adequate indicator than cortisol response to psychological stress in neurotics. 3) GH and cortisol may have different psychological correlates in neurotics.

626
Noel GL. et al. **Prolactin, thyrotropin and growth hormone release during stress associated with parachute jumping.** *Aviat Space Environ Med.* 1976;47:543-7. (English) (unavailable at publication)

627
Palmblad J, Cantell K, Strander H, Froberg J, Karlsson CG, Levi L, Granstrom M, Unger P. **Stressor exposure and immunological response in man: interferon-producing capacity and phagocytosis.** *J Psychosom Res.* 1976; 20:193-9. (English)

Exposure of 8 healthy human females to a moderately stressful 77-hour vigil under strictly controlled conditions was accompanied by changes in adrenal cortical and medullary hormones compatible with stress reaction. The ability of the lymphocytes to produce interferon in response to the addition of Sendai virus to blood samples rose during the stressor exposure and was highest after this. Phagocytosis by peripheral blood phagocytes showed a decrease during the vigil and was followed in post-exposure samples by a rise to levels above pre-exposure values.

628
Rose RM. **Endocrine responses to stressful psychological events.** *Psychiat Clin N Amer.* 1980;3:251-76. (English)

Early work in the field emphasized the ubiquity of endocrine responses to a wide variety of stressful stimuli, as if stress response represented one final common pathway. This conclusion fails to take into account the very large role that novelty played even when exposing individuals to presumably physical stimuli, such as heat or cold. Since different physical demands would require different metabolic responses for adaptation, it is unlikely that just one pattern of endocrine responses for all stressful stimuli. Rather, much of the early work can be characterized by observing the psychoendocrine response to novelty. The other "lesson" learned from observations of how individuals differ in response to the same stressful stimuli emphasizes the relevance of whether or not the individual perceives the event as potentially threatening or challenging. If this is not so, he fails to become aroused and there is no endocrine response. The now well established critical role of the brain in controlling endocrine secretion not only makes the interpretation of the importance of psychological events influencing endocrine activity not only feasible, but establishes hormonal response as one of the three major affector systems of the central nervous system (motor, autonomic, endocrine).

629
Syvalahti E, Lammintausta R, Pekkarinen A. **Effect of psychic stress of examination on serum growth hormone, serum insulin and plasma renin activity.** *Acta Pharmac Tox.* 1976;38:344-52. (English)

The levels of serum human growth hormone (HGH), immunoreactive insulin (IRI), blood glucose (BG), and plasma renin activity (PRA) in a total of 131 healthy medical student volunteers and 83 controls were studied to find out whether the psychic stress of examination in pharmacology can affect the release of these hormones. The mean HGH level rose by 33% after a written interim examination and by 49% after a final oral examination. The mean IRI level rose by 45% after a written examination and by 43% after an oral examination. These results were statistically significant. The mean BG level did not vary significantly. The rise in HGH and IRI was higher after short than after long examinations. The mean PRA rose significantly by 44% after a written and by 27% after an oral examination, but the mean values of PRA after an examination were within the normal range.

Stress and measures of immunity

630
Bartrop RW, Luckhurst E, Lazarus L, Kiloh LG, Penny R. **Depressed lymphocyte function after bereavement.** *Lancet.* 1977;1:834-6. (English)

During 1975 twenty-six bereaved spouses took part in a detailed prospective investigation of the effects of severe stress on the immune system. T and B cell numbers and function, and hormone concentrations were studied approximately 2 weeks after bereavement and 6 weeks thereafter. The response to phytohaemagglutinin was significantly depressed in the bereaved group on the second occasion, as was the response to concanavalin A at 6 weeks. There was no difference in T and B cell numbers, protein concentrations, the presence of autoantibodies and delayed hypersensitivity, and in cortisol, prolactin, growth hormone, and thyroid hormone assays between the bereaved group and the controls. This was the first time severe psychological stress has been shown to produce a measurable abnormality in immune function which is not obviously caused by hormonal changes.

631
Biondi M, Conti C, Pancheri P, Sega FM, Sega E. **Emotional reactivity and immune reactivity: a preliminary study of patients in a situation of pre-operatory stress.** *Rivista di Psichiatria.* 1981;16:378-94. (Italian)

The purpose of this study has been to evaluate the relationship between emotional reactivity and immune reactivity in a group of patients waiting for a surgical operation for a possible life threatening disease. In this context, the pre-operative situation was utilized in the experimental design as a real life stressor capable of generating differential emotional reactions according to individual personalities and coping styles.

632
Dorian BJ, Keystone E, Garfinkel PE, Brown GM. **Immune mechanisms in acute psychological stress** (abstract). *Psychosom Med.* 1981;43:84. (English)

There is evidence that illness may be precipitated by stressful life events. Experiential and psychological conditions may influence the function of the immune system via central nervous system and endocrine pathways and thereby increase susceptibility to disease. The aim of this study was to measure changes in immune and endocrine function in a group of stressed individuals and then to relate these to measures of psychological distress, personality style and coping strategies. The acute stressor was an Oral Fellowship Examination for residents in Psychiatry. Nine experimental subjects and 17 age- and sex-matched physician controls were studied on a variety of measures of cellular immunity and a neuroendocrine function on two occasions approximately 1 week before the Exam and again on two occasions 2 weeks after. Psychological tests included the General Health Questionnaire (GHQ), measures of coping style, recent life changes and personality. Data were analyzed between experimental and control groups overall and between high stress experimental group (GHQ $\geq$ 12) and low stress controls (GHQ $\leq$ 5). Results were analyzed by analysis of variance, with significant cell differences subject to Duncan's Multiple Range Test. The experimental group displayed significantly reduced mitogens (PHA, PWM and total mitogens) before the exam, in comparison to controls; these were significantly elevated after the stressor. Cortisol levels were significantly lower in the experimental group before and after the Exam. Five of the nine experimental subjects were defined as subjectively highly stressed (GHQ $\geq$ 12) and 9 of the 17 control subjects were extremely low on subjective distress score (GHQ $\leq$ 5). When these groups were compared, the mitogen changes displayed by a sample as a whole was again seen. In addition the high stress subjects had significantly increased % late rosettes which fell to normal after the Exam. These results document significant changes in measures of cellular immunity (mitogens and late rosettes) in people under psychological stress.

633

Dostoevskaia LP, Shkhinek EK. **Episodic stress and immune reactions.** *(Russian) (in press)*

634

Eskola J, Ruuskanen O, Soppi E. et al.: **Effect of sport stress on lymphocyte transformation and antibody formation.** *Clin Exp Immunol.* 1978;32:339-45. (English) (unavailable at publication)

635

Goodwin JS, Bromberg S, Staszak C, Kaszubowski PA, Messner RP, Neal JF. **Effect of physical stress on sensitivity of lymphocytes to inhibition by prostagladin E$_2$** *J Immunol.* 1981;127:518-22. (English)

Physical stress is associated with depressed cellular immune function. We have found that lymphocytes from subjects undergoing either of 2 stressful events, cardiac surgery or childbirth, are more sensitive to inhibition by PGE$_2$. For example, the concentration of PGE$_2$ required for 50% inhibition of ^{3}H-thymidine incorporation (ID$_{50}$) into phytohemagglutinin-stimulated lymphocytes from patients undergoing cardiac surgery went from 1.5 X 10^{-8} M on the day before surgery to 3 X 10^{-9} M on the day after surgery. This increase in sensitivity to PGE$_2$ was accompanied by a significantly decreased lymphocyte proliferative response (27 to 68% of control, depending on mitogen dose) and a 50% increase in the percentage of E rosette-positive cells with receptors for the Fc portion of IgG. The increased sensitivity to PGE and the depressed mitogen responses returned to preoperative values by day 10. The depressed mitogen responses of the postoperative patients were completely restored to normal by removal of glass-adherent cells before culture. In addition, the responses of the postoperative patients and the women in labor were partially restored by the addition of indomethacin, a prostaglandin synthetase inhibitor, to the cultures. Thus it would appear that physical stress causes lymphocytes to become more sensitive to prostaglandin E$_2$, and the increased sensitivity to inhibition by this immunomodulator is responsible in part for the depressed cellular immune function after physical stress.

636

Handel AD, Balish E. **Effect of space flight on cell-mediated immunity.** *Aviat Space Environ Med.* 1977; 48:1051-7. (English)

The cell-mediated immune response to *Listeria monocytogenes* was studied in rats subjected to 20 d of flight aboard the Soviet biosatellite Kosmos 47820. Groups of rats were immunized with 1 x 10^6 formalin-killed *Listeria* suspended in Freunds Complete Adjuvant, 5 d prior to flight. Immunized rats subjected to the same environmental factors as the flight rats, except flight itself, and immunized and nonimmunized rats held in a normal animal colony served as controls. Following recovery, lymphocyte cultures were harvested from spleens of all rats, cultured *in vitro* in the presence of *L. monocytogenes* antigens, phytohemagglutinin (PHA), concanavalin A (Con A), or purified protein derivative (PPD), and measured for their uptake of ^{3}H-thymidine. The lymphocytes of all rats gave a blastogenic response to PHA and Con A. Although individual rats varied considerably, all flight and immunized control rats gave a blastogenic response to the *Listeria* antigens and PPD. With several mitogens, the lymphocytes of flight rats showed a significantly increased blastogenic response over the controls. The results of this study do not support a hypothesis of a detrimental effect of space flight on cell-mediated immunity; the data do suggest a possible suppressive effect of stress and gravity on an *in vitro* correlate of cell-mediated immunity.

637

Holdeman LV, Good IJ, Moore WEC. **Human fecal flora: Variation in bacterial composition within individuals and a possible effect of emotional stress.** *Appl Envir Microbiol.* 1976;31:359-75. (English)

Data presented on the distribution of 101 bacterial species and subspecies among 1,442 isolates from 25 fecal specimens from three men on: (i) their normal diet and normal living conditions, (ii) normal living conditions but eating the controlled metabolic diet designed for use in the Skylab simulation and missions, and (iii) the Skylab diet simulated in Skylab (isolation) conditions. These kinds of bacteria from each astronaut during the 5-month period showed more variation in the composition of the flora among the individual astronauts than among the eight or nine samples from each person. This observation indicates the variations in fecal flora reported previously, but based on the study of only one specimen from each person, more certainly reflect real differences (and not daily variation) in the types of bacteria maintained by individual people. The proportions of the predominant fecal species in the astronauts were similar to those reported earlier from a Japanese-Hawaiian population and were generally insensitive to changes from the normal North American diet to the Skylab diet; only two of the most common species were affected by changes in diet. However, one of the predominant species (Bacteroides fragilis subsp. thetaiotamicron) appeared to be affected during confinement of the men in the Skylab test chamber. Evidence is presented suggesting that an anger stress situation may have been responsible for the increase of this species simultaneously in all of the subjects studied. Phenotypic characteristics of some of the less common isolates are given. The statistical analyses used in interpretation of the results are discussed.

638

Kimzey SL, Johnson PC, Ritzmann SE, Mengel CE. **Hematology and immunology studies: the second manned Skylab mission.** *Aviat Space Environ Med.* 1976;47:383-90. (English)

The hematologic and immunologic functions of the Skylab 3 (second manned mission) astronauts were examined during the preflight, inflight, and postflight phases of the 59 d mission in order to evaluate the response to and/or the influence of the space flight environment. Most changes observed were subtle and did not represent a threat to the health and safety of the crewmen during orbital flight. Even the most significant change observed, a reduction in the circulating red cell mass, did not have a detrimental influence on the astronaut cardiovascular or exercise responses as evaluated by other experiment protocols. Considering the facts that the data were not collected under ideally controlled conditions and that the astronauts were in excellent physical condition, the results of these studies would seem to indicate that man can function quite well in the space flight environment of the Skylab orbiting workshop for extended periods of time.

639

Locke SE, Heisel JS. **The influence of stress and emotions on the human immune response** (abstract). *Biofeedback Self-Regul.* 1977;2:320. (English)

Many physicians believe that there is a relationship between stress, emotions, and susceptibility to illness. Experimental stress is capable of altering immune function in animals (Stein, 1976), but there are few prospective studies in humans on the relationship between psychological factors and immunity. We studied 124 subjects who received the A/NJ/76 ("swine") flu vaccine and completed the Schedule of Recent Experiences (Holmes & Rahe) and the Profile of Mood States (POMS). Hemagglutination inhibition antibody titers were determined before and 2 weeks after immunization. We found no relationship between postimmunization antibody levels and the following psychosocial variables: (1) life stress for either the antecedent month or year (Social Readjustment Rating Scale); (2) depression or anxiety scales (POMS); (3) repressed hostility, social withdrawal, or feelings of helplessness and hopelessness on scales derived from selected POMS items. Our data suggest that there is no apparent influence of these psychosocial factors on the antibody response to a viral immunogen. Possibly, either we chose to study the wrong time period and missed an effect, or, more likely, the major impact of stress and emotions is on the *cellular* as opposed to the *humoral* immune system. This latter possibility is currently under investigation.

640

Locke SE, Hurst MW, Leserman JM, Heisel JS, Kraus LJ, Williams RM. **Life change stress and human natural killer cell activity.** *Submitted for Publication.* (English)

Life change stress (LCS) has been reported to be linked with adverse health change, but the mechanisms mediating these changes remain poorly understood. To test the idea that stress is associated with alterations of cell-mediated immunity (CMI) in humans, we measured natural killer cell activity (NKCA), a type of lymphocyte-mediated cytotoxicity, in 108 healthy subjects who were also assessed using standard measures of LCS and psychiatric symptoms. From a single sample of whole blood, lymphocytes were isolated using a density-gradient separation method, cryopreserved, and later tested for NKCA using the K562 chronic myelogenous leukemia cell as the target. Subjects with high levels of LCS who reported high levels of psychiatric symptoms had the

lowest levels of NKCA. Those with high levels of LCS who reported relatively few symptoms had the highest levels of NKCA. These differences were significant ($p<0.005$). Additionally, subjects at the extremes of the NKCA distribution differed significantly in the amount of self-reported psychiatric symptoms under stress. These preliminary findings suggest a possible influence of stress and emotions on a measure of human CMI.

641

Locke SE. **Looking ahead: possible mechanisms of stress effects on immunity** (abstract). *The Gerontologist.* 1982;22:204. (English)

Evidence for direct influences of brain and behavior on immunity is accumulating. Studies in humans of the effects of stress on parameters of humoral and cell-mediated immunity suggest that stress can be either immunosuppressive or immunoenhancing, depending upon certain critical factors. These factors include: 1) the parameter of immunity measured, 2) the duration and timing of the stressor, 3) coping ability and 4) personality traits. Demonstrated anatomical and functional links between the nervous and the immune systems provide a basis for speculative formulations about the role of brain and behavior in determining host resistance. The recent demonstration that epinephrine and norepinephrine can alter parameters of human cellular immunity *in vivo* suggests a role for catecholamines in mediating stress effects on immune function. However, the popular notion that stress primarily causes elevated catecholamines and corticosteroids is oversimplified; the psychoendocrinology of stress is far more complex than previously understood.

642

Locke SE. **Stress, adaptation, and immunity: studies in humans.** *Gen Hosp Psychiatry.* 1982;4:49-58. (English)

The notion that some combination of excessive "stress" and inadequate coping may increase susceptibility to illness has long been part of our conventional wisdom. Yet until recently, there have been few data to support this contention. During the past decade, the relationship between stress, adaptation, and human immunity has come under closer scrutiny. There is now considerable evidence that certain types of experimental and naturally-occurring stress are associated with alterations of human cellular immune function. Furthermore, these observed changes are generally immunosuppressive. However, the mediating mechanisms underlying this relationship remain poorly understood. Critical factors in the stress-adaptation-immunity relationship are: the duration and proximity of the stressor, the adaptive capacity of the individual, and the differential effects of certain stressors on immunologic components.

643

Macek C. **Of mind and morbidity: can stress and grief depress immunity?** (medical news) *JAMA.* 1982;248:405-7. (English)

644

McClelland DC, Floor E, Davidson RJ, Saron C. **Stressed power motivation, sympathetic activation, immune function, and illness.** *J Hum Stress.* 1980;6:11-19. (English)

Previous research has reported that individuals high in the need for power, high in inhibition, and high in power stress (the HHH group) are more likely than other individuals to report more severe illnesses. The present study investigates the possibility that the mechanism underlying this relationship is greater sympathetic activation in the HHH group which has an immunosuppressive effect. College males with the HHH syndrome reported more frequent and more severe illnesses than other individuals, as in previous studies. More of the HHH than other subjects also showed above average epinephrine excretion rates in urine and below average concentrations of immunoglobulin A in saliva (s-IgA). Furthermore, higher rates of epinephrine excretion were significantly associated with lower s-IgA concentrations, and lower s-IgA concentrations were significantly associated with reports of more frequent illnesses. The findings are interpreted as consistent with the hypothesis that a strong need for power, if inhibited and stressed, leads to chronic sympathetic overactivity which has an immunosuppresive effect making indiviuals characterized by this syndrome more susceptible to illness.

645
Munster AM. **Post-traumatic immunosuppression is due to activation of suppressor T cells.** *Lancet.* 1976;1:1329-30. (English)

Severe immunosuppression occurs after major thermal burns, accidental injuries, and extensive surgical operations, and probably contributes substantially to patient morbidity and mortality. The mechanism of immunosuppression is unknown and attempts to explain it are contradictory. The contradictions can be resolved by assuming the activation by injury of the suppressor T-cell system, which is involved in normal immunoregulation. If this is true, then generalised, nonspecific attempts to bolster the immune response in these patients may be inappropriate.

646
Palmblad J, Blomback M, Egberg N, Froberg J, Karlsson CG, Levi L. **Experimentally induced stress in man: effects on blood coagulation and fibrinolysis.** *J Psychosom Res.* 1977;21:87-92. (English)

Sixteen healthy human females were exposed to a 77 hr vigil under strictly controlled conditions. Blood coagulation factors V, VIII and IX and fibrinogen decreased significantly during the vigil. Only the latter had returned to preexposure values within 5 days after the vigil. No increased fibrinolytic activity was detected. Concomitant adrenal reactions, interpreted as indices of stress, are reported and discussed in relation to these results. It is concluded that the decrease of coagulation factor activity might be interpreted as an expression of adaptation to prolonged stressor exposure.

647
Palmblad J, Petrini B, Wasserman J, Akerstedt T. **Lymphocyte and granulocyte reactions during sleep deprivation.** *Psychosom Med.* 1979;41:273-8. (English)

The possible influence of 48 hr of sleep deprivation on *in vitro* DNA synthesis of blood lymphocytes and on adhesiveness and intracellular, stainable activity of alkaline phosphatase in blood granulocytes was studied in twelve young male volunteers. Following the sleep deprivation, all 12 subjects showed marked reduction of DNA synthesis after stimulation with phytohemagglutinin. Pre-exposure levels were regained 5 days after terminating the vigil. No changes were noted in granulocyte adherence of alkaline phosphatase activity. The results suggest that sleep deprivation may decrease cell-mediated immune reactions and thereby impair some aspects of host defense.

648
Solomon GF, Amkraut AA, Rubin RT. **Stress and psycho-immunological response.** (in press) (English)

Animal models
Stress and disease

649
Gorizontov PD, Fedotova MI, Belousova OI, Khaitov RM, Chermeneva LI. **Role of T and B lymphocytes in the hematopoietic system response to stress.** *Biull Eksp Biol Med.* 1980;89:415-17. (Russian)

Cellular composition of the bone marrow, spleen, and peripheral blood was studied after 6-hour immobilization on the back in experiments on 4 groups of (CBAxC57Bl)F_1 mice with varying degree of T lymphocyte deficiency (thymectomy, sham thymectomy, administration of antilymphocytic serum, B mice). The evidence obtained shows that the "lymphoid peak" recorded in the bone marrow during stress is likely to be formed at the expense of T and B lymphocyte migration from the peripheral lymphoid organs. The data have been also obtained indicating that T lymphocytes migrating to the bone marrow during the first 6-9 hours after the exposure to stress may participate in granulocytopoiesis activation.

650
Hara C, Manabe K, Ogawa N. **Influence of activity stress on thymus, spleen and adrenal weight of rats: possibility for an immunodeficiency model.** *Physiol Behav.* 1981;27:243-8. (English)

64 Wistar rats were housed in laboratory or activity-wheel cages and fed either 1 or 24 hours/day. The incidence of ulcers was higher in Ss fed 1 hour at night than those fed 1 hour in the daytime though their mortality rate was similar. Thymus and spleen weights of Ss exposed to activity-stress (AS) decreased, while adrenal weights increased. Victims always revealed pulmonary infection and lack of immunologically competent cells. Results suggest that rats exposed to AS reveal, not only ulceration, but also immunosuppression. Stress factors and utilization of the AS rat for an immunodeficiency model are discussed.

651
Lattime EC, Strausser HR. **Arteriosclerosis: is stress-induced immune suppression a risk factor?** *Science.* 1977;198:302-3. (English)

Female Sprague-Dawley rats, purchased as retired breeders, developed arteriosclerosis that was accompanied by immune complex deposition in the arterial lesion and depressed immune responsiveness to T cell mitogens.

652

Monjan AA, Collector MI. **Stress-induced modulation of the immune response.** *Science.* 1977;197:307-8. (English)

After mice were exposed to a daily auditory stressor for varying lengths of time, the responses of their splenic lymphoid cells *in vitro* were assessed. Both the blastogenic activity of concanavalin A or lipopolysaccharide and the ability of immune lymphocytes to lyse P815 target cells showed the same patterns of immunosuppression and enhancement.

653

Petz R, Jezkova Z. **Stress and experimental atherosclerosis.** *Physiologia Bohemoslovaca.* 1976;25:375-9. (English) (no abstract)

654

Plaut SM, Huang SW, Taylor G, Wareheim LE, Sevdalian DA. **Effect of light-shock stimulation on resistance to diabetes in mice** (abstract). *Psychosom Med.* 1981;43:90-1. (English)

As part of an investigation of the role of psychosocial factors in resistance to insulin-dependent diabetes (DD), groups of 8-18, 45-day-old male CD-1 mice were injected with single 60 mg/kg doses of streptozotocin (STZ). Some groups were exposed to random 10 sec periods of light each followed by a 0.6 mA 2 sec scrambled footshock. Stimulation sessions occurred 24 hr/day during 6 equally-spaced 1 hour periods and involved an average of 12 stimulus presentations per hour. Three experiments were done in which stimulus presentations began and ended at various times after STZ injection, and blood samples were taken bi-weekly from the retroorbital sinus of all mice. Blood glucose increases were significantly attenuated over a 22 wk period in mice which were stimulated during the first 72 hr after STZ injection ($F = 4.68$; $df = 14/231$; $p<0.01$). The proportions of mice with IDD (blood glucose levels over 150 4mg %) after this period were 25% and 84% in the stimulated and non-stimulated mice, respectively ($X_2 = 8.24$; $df = 1$; $p<0.01$). Progressively increasing correlations between sampling order and blood glucose levels, which were significant over the last 12 wk of one experiment indicated that blood glucose levels of caged diabetic animals responded markedly to laboratory procedures. In a fourth experiment, plasma corticosterone responses to a single light-shock pairing were observed in STZ and buffer-injected mice which either had or had not experienced 48 hr of light-shock stimulation after injection. Corticosterone increases in response to the single stimulus were sharply attenuated in previously stimulated mice ($F = 17.3$; $df = 1/31$; $p<0.01$), and were not affected by STZ. Thus, the ability of light-shock stimulation during the first 72 hr after STZ injection to decrease the incidence of IDD may be related to high corticosterone levels induced by initial stimulation sessions.

655

Rogers MP, Trentham DE, Dynesius RA, Reich P, David JR.

Exacerbation of type II collagen-induced arthritis by auditory stress (abstract). *Clin Res.* 1980;28:508A. (English)

Predator stress can abrogate the development of arthritis in rats immunized with type II collagen. To evaluate further the effects of stress on this model, we performed the following experiment three times and combined the data: A total of 69 female Wistar rats were subjected to a 100 decibel noise for 5 seconds every minute for a 1-hour period beginning at 2 AM for 7 days commencing 3 days prior to injection of collagen (Group A). Sixty-nine rats received simultaneous immunizations but were otherwise left undisturbed (Group B). Auditory stress exacerbated the early course of arthritis. Maximal differences in the incidence of arthritis [33 of 69 (48%) arthritic in Group A vs. 20 of 69 (29%) in Group B, p<0.02] and severity of arthritis in involved rats (mean ± SEM arthritic index for arthritic rats 5.9 ± 0.5 in Group A vs. 3.8 ± 0.5 in group B, p<0.005), as well as summated arthritic indices (195 for Group A vs. 76 for Group B, p<0.001), occurred 15 days after immunization. Although the incidence of arthritis remained higher in Group A when the study was terminated on Day 32 [39 of 69 (56%) for Group A vs 26 out of 69 (38%) for Group B, p<0.02], there was no difference in the severity of arthritis in involved rats at this time (mean arthritic index 4.2 ± 0.4 for Group A vs. 4.0 ± 0.4 for Group B.) Auditory stress produced agitation but, unlike predator exposure, did not stimulate defecation. While the reason(s) for the dichotomous effects of different stress protocols is unclear, these data provide further evidence that stress can modulate profoundly the expression of this autoimmune disease.

656

Rogers MP, Trentham DE, McCune WJ, Ginsberg BI, Reich P, David JR. **Abrogation of type II collagen-induced arthritis in rats by psychological stress.** *Trans Assoc Am Physicians.* 1979;92:218-28. (English)

This study shows that psychological stress, produced either by exposure to a predator or by movement and handling, can profoundly suppress the clinical and histologic manifestations of collagen-induced arthritis. In addition, stress can disassociate the development of humoral and cellular sensitivity to collagen from the occurrence of arthritis. Thus stress modalities provide a means of acquiring additional insights into the pathogenesis of collagen-induced arthritis in rats. Such studies may lead to a further understanding of the relationship between emotional states and the functioning of the immunologic system. This study further illustrates the need to identify and control for the effects of stress in animal studies of immunopathology. Finally, the therapeutic implications of this study for autoimmune diseases would appear self-evident.

657

Rogers MP, Trentham DE, McCune WJ, Ginsberg BI, Rennke HG, Reich P, David JR. **Effect of psychological stress on the induction of arthritis in rats.** *Arthr Rheum.* 1980;23:1337-42. (English)

To determine whether emotional states could influence susceptibility to type II collagen-induced arthritis in rats, we studied the effects of experimentally produced psychological stress on the clinical, histologic, and immunologic manifestations of this autoimmune disease. Stress, induced by exposure to a cat, abrogated the development of arthritis in rats immunized with type II collagen. The incidence of arthritis was also decreased in rats subjected to transportation and handling. These environmental factors dissociated the development of humoral and cellular sensitivity to collagen from the occurrence of arthritis. This study provides a unique demonstration that psychosomatic processes can influence an animal model of autoimmunity.

658
Rogers MP, Trentham DE, Reich P. **Modulation of collagen-induced arthritis by different stress protocols** (abstract). *Psychosom Med.* 1980;42:72. (English)

We investigated the effects of different stress protocols on the clinical and immunologic manifestation of a new animal model of autoimmune arthritis. Approximately 10% of inbred and outbred rats develop arthritis 11-21 days after the intradermal injection of native type II collagen. Previously we have shown that exposure to a cat abrogates the development of arthritis without suppressing either the humoral or cellular response to collagen. To evaluate further the effects of stress on this model, we performed the following experiment: 23 female Wistar rats were subjected to a 100 decibel noise for 5 seconds every minute for a 1 hour period beginning at 2 ASM for 7 days commencing 3 days prior to the injection of collagen (Group A). Twenty-three were otherwise left undisturbed (Group B). We repeated this experiment 3 times and combined the data. Auditory stress exacerbated the early course of arthritis, as seen by the increased incidence of arthritis [33 of 69 (49%) arthritis in Group A vs. 20 of 69 (29%) in Group B, p<0.02], greater severity of arthritis in involved rats (mean $\pm$ SEM arthritic index for arthritic rats 5.9 $\pm$ 0.5 in Group A vs. 3.8 + 0.5 in Group B, p<0.005), and higher summated arthritic indices (195 for Group A vs. 76 for Group B, p<0.001) in the stressed animals. These maximal differences occurred 15 days after immunization. Although the incidence of arthritis remained higher in Group A when the study was terminated on Day 32 [39 of 69 (56% for Group A vs. 26 of 69 (38%) for Group B, p<0.02], there was no difference in the severity of arthritis in involved rats at this time (mean arthritic index 4.2 $\pm$ 0.4 for Group A vs. 4.0 $\pm$ 0.1 for Group B). Auditory stress produced agitation but, unlike predator exposure, did not stimulate defecation. Thus, unlike predator stress which abrogated arthritis, auditory stress exacerbated it. Although the reason(s) for these dichotomous effects is unclear, these data provide further evidence that stress can modulate profoundly the expression of this autoimmune disease.

659
Tsuda A, et al. **Effects of divided feeding on activity-stress ulcer and the thymus weight in the rat.** *Physiol Behav.* 1981;27:349-53. (English)

80 male Wistar rats housed in running-wheel activity cages and fed 1 or 2 hours daily exhibited excessive running and subsequently died revealing large stomach ulcers, reduced absolute thymus weight, and an increase in relative weight of adrenal glands. However, 2 0.5-hr or 2 1-hr daily feedings did

significantly reduce ulcer incidence. Controls for the 4 feeding schedules did not die, were ulcer free, and did not exhibit the changes in thymus and adrenal weight observed in experimental Ss. Results suggest that the divided daily feeding ameliorates the ulcerogenic and immune processes in activity-stress rats.

660
Zaks AS, Bykova AA. **Participation of the autoimmune mechanism of chemical homeostasis regulation in reactions to stress factors.** *Patol Fiziol Eksp Ter.* 1979;4:23-28. (Russian)

Antibodies against histamine, serotonin, adrenalin, insulin, and acetylcholine disappeared from serum 45 minutes after electrostimulation. In actively immunized animals subjected to electrostress, antibodies were not detected for 30 days. Lymphoid cells of organs of immune animals exposed to the effect of the current lost their capacity for antibody synthesis in culture *in vitro*. In immunization with haptene-protein conjugates against the background of periodical exposure to the current, immunity to the haptenes did not develop. After centrifugation and flotation, antibodies disappeared in the immune animals and none were demonstrated for 14 days. Formalin and immobilization stress were attended by a decrease in the titer of antibodies or their disappearance during acute exudative manifestations. By the 7th-14th day immunogenesis was activated. Recurrent inflammation was marked by earlier intensification of antibody synthesis. The data indicate an active participation of the immune mechanism of regulation of the homeostasis of neurohumoral factors in the organism's reaction to pathological effects.

Stress and cancer

661
Bammer K. **Psychosocial stress and the occurrence of cancer--animal experiment results and problems.** *Z Psychosom Med Psychoanal.* 1981;27:253-62. (German)

A review of the problems and results of experiments on animals with regard to psycho-social stress and the occurrence of cancer is presented. To a large extent the conflicting results of many studies derive from the problems involved in setting up and establishing reliable experimental conditions for experiments on animals. It is the prerogative of future research to refine experimental design so that an insight can be gained into hitherto unknown relationships. Nevertheless, in spite of varied and conflicting results the available facts provide proof that psycho-social stress factors are capable of influencing the occurrence and progress of carcinogenic illness. Our present state of knowledge about these processes, is, however, still very slight. The significance of this problem is worthy of more intensive and systematic investigatory experiments on animals within the area of psychosomatic cancer research than has been the case up until now.

662
Burchfield SR, Woods SC, Elich MS. **Effects of cold stress on tumor growth.** *Physiol Behav.* 1978;21:537-40. (English)

Assessed the relationship between stress and tumor growth in experiments in which the paradigm was held constant while type of tumor and sex of rats were varied. 764 singly housed male and female W/Fu rats were given cold stress before and/or after injection of tumor cells, or received no stress at all. Ss stressed only before receiving the tumor cells developed significantly smaller tumors than the nonstressed control group. Tumors of the other 2 groups were only slightly smaller than those of the nonstressed control group. The results indicate that being stressed before disease may provide an inoculation effect, whereas stress occurring after disease onset (or no stress at all) leads to increased severity of the illness.

663
Cooley B, Henry JP, Stephens PM. **Enhancing effects of psychosocial stimulation on experimental mammary tumors.** *Abstr, Int Symp Detect Prev Cancer, 3rd.* 1976. (English) (unavailable at publication)

664
Crispens CC Jr. **Apparent inhibitory influence of stress on SJL/JDg neoplasia.** *Psychol & Psychiatry.* 1976;4:169. (English) (unavailable at publication)

665
Kalisnik M, Vraspir-Porenta O, Logonder-Mlinsek M, Zorc M, Pajntar M. **Stress and Ehrlich ascites tumor in mouse.** *Neoplasma.* 1979;26:483-91. (English)

The aim of the study was to investigate the interaction of the psychosomatic stress and the Ehrlich ascites tumor (EAT) growth in mice. The stressor consisted of combination of a light signal followed by a mild electric shock. The first experiment was performed on CBA mice irritated for 0, 2 and 4 weeks respectively, prior to intraperitoneal transplantation of the EAT. In the second study, mice of BALB/c strain were used. Stress was applied 4 weeks before the tumor transplantation and continued through the experiment. Both the irritated and nonirritated animals were subjected to either intraperitoneal or subcutaneous inoculation of the EAT. In both experiments, mice were left to live until their spontaneous death. In the first experiment, after a 2-week irritation the experimental animals showed a significantly longer survival time as compared to the controls. Longer or shorter duration of the irritation had no significant effect on the results obtained. Results yielded by the second experiment showed no sigificant difference in the survival of the irritated and nonirritated animals after the i.p. transplantation, whereas after the s.c. inoculation of the EAT, the irritation significantly increased the survival period. The EAT in irritated mice was observed to have invaded the vitals later and less frequently than in the nonirritated animals. Quantitative histological analysis of some endocrine and lymphatic organs revealed signs of stress in the experimental animals. The EAT transplant, *per se*, had a stressogenic effect too.

666
Newberry BH, Gildow J, Wogan J, Reese RL. **Inhibition of Huggins tumors by forced restraint.** *Psychosom Med.* 1976;38:155-62. (English)

Three experiments that demonstrated that chronically administered restraint inhibits the development of DBMA-induced tumors. The effect is exhibited in a lower proportion of positive responses, increased latency of tumor development, and lower number of tumors in positive animals when restrained animals are compared with controls. Organ weights failed to show a stress response to restraint. Molar activity data from Experiment III indicated that early in the experiment activity increased among the restrained animals on release from restraint. A fourth experiment, which employed a crystal accelerometer to assess activity, produced a similar activity pattern and also provided evidence of adrenal ascorbic acid depletion as a function of restraint.

667
Newberry BH, Sengbusch L. **Inhibitory effects of stress on experimental mammary tumors.** *Cancer Detect Prev.* 1979;2:225-33. (English)

Earlier studies in our laboratory demonstrated that both electric shock and forced restraint have the capacity to reduce the number of mammary tumors which develop in rats given 7,12-dimethylbenz(a)anthracene. There is little indication that the restraint manipulation which we have used produces a prolonged systemic stress response or prolonged changes in activity level--suggesting that the animals adapt to it well. Later studies indicated that restraint applied before the administration of the carcinogen or during the period in which initiation of neoplastic cells occurs does not inhibit tumor development, while post-induction restraint is effective. The present experiment demonstrated that the termination of the restraint treatment produces a brief increase in the rate of appearance of new tumors. Subsequently the rate of appearance drops, however, indicating that more than one process may be involved in the inhibitory effect. The experiment failed to provide evidence that restraint alters the proportion of hormone-dependent tumors.

668
Newberry BH. **Inhibitory effects of stress on experimental mammary tumors.** *Abstr, Int Symp Detect Prev Cancer, 3rd.* 1976:35. (English) (unavailable at publication)

669
Newberry BH. **Restraint-induced inhibition of 7,12-dimethylbenz-(a)anthracene-induced mammary tumors: relation to stages of tumor development.** *J Natl Cancer Inst.* 1978;61:725-9. (English)

Experiments on the use of chronically applied restraint to reduce the number of mammary tumors developing in response to treatment of rats with 7,12-dimethylbenz-[a]anthracene indicated that this inhibitory effect was largely due to restraint applied after the induction period; preinduction restraint and induction period restraint had no significant effect on tumor development. After termination of the restraint treatment, the rate at which new tumors appeared first increased and then decreased. Restraint did not affect the proportion of tumors regressing after ovariectomy.

670
Nieburgs HE, Weiss J, Navarrete M, Grillione G, Siedlecki B.

Inhibitory and enhancing effects of various stresses on experimental mammary tumorigenesis. *Abstr, Int Symp Detect Prev Cancer, 3rd.* 1976;50. (English) (unavailable at publication)

671

Nieburgs HE, Weiss J, Navarrete M, Strax P, Teirstein A, Grillione G, Siedlecki B. **The role of stress in human and experimental oncogenesis.** *Cancer Detect Prev.* 1979; 2:307-36. (English)

A series of experiments were carried out to determine the effects of stress at the cellular level. This report is based upon the action of electric shock, forced cold swim, and handling on cellular changes in the gastric mucosa, liver, thymus, adrenals and blood lymphocytes. Two hour electric shock was associated with increased secretory granules in gastric chief cells, liver mitoses and marked lymphopenia. Use of 24-hour shock revealed less secretory granules, absence of liver mitoses, and only slight lymphopenia with delayed but longer lasting effects. Stress consistently produced a marked decrease in the number of small lymphocytes, with an increase in medium-sized lymphocytes and usually also in large lymphocytes, the latter depending upon the kind of stressor and the length of period following cessation of stress. Changes in the proportion of lymphocytes, particularly the decreased percentage of small lymphocytes, was closely related to the increase in liver mitoses. Control animals also revealed blood lymphocyte changes following repeated removal of rats from the same environment. Stress-induced effects from transportation of rats were evident by changes in gastric chief cells and liver mitoses for 12 to 16 days after shipment. Stress by electric shock immediately after transportation produced less effects than shock applied at least 21 days following animal transportation. Comparison of effects from various stressors revealed that lymphocyte changes persisted for 72 hours following handling and cold swim. Whereas liver mitoses were present in all rats at 96 hours, thymus involution was noted at 72 hours following handling, 48 hours after cold swim and 96 hours after electric shock. Slight adrenal hypertrophy persisted for 96 hours following handling and shock and for 24 hours after cold swim. The effect of stress on DMBA mammary tumorigenesis differed in relation to the kind of stressor and the length of the stress period following DMBA administration. At 90 days, cold swim and handling enhanced tumor induction, whereas, electric shock inhibited tumor induction but enhanced the rate of tumor growth. At 150 days, the number of rats with tumors was slightly greater and the tumor size considerably smaller in stressed rats than in those without stress following DMBA administration. The inhibited tumor growth of DMBA treated rats that were stressed for 150 days by handling and cold swim was associated with an increase in large- and medium-sized lymphocytes, and a marked decrease in small lymphocytes. The same increase in large- and medium-sized lymphocytes, and the marked decrease in small lymphocytes, also occurred in women with repressed hostility and in patients with a family history of cancer, as well as in patients with breast cancer and with poorly differentiated and metastatic lung cancer. The close relationship between a decrease in small lymphocytes and increase in identifiable liver mitoses points to a regulatory function of small lymphocytes (T lymphocytes) on cell kinetics. Possibly the entire imbalance of decreased small lymphocytes with markedly increased medium-sized and large lymphocytes may be responsible for the prolonged mitotic phases as evidenced from presence of mitoses. The imbalance in the proportion of lymphocytes as a result of stress, and the consistently found decrease of small lymphocytes with an increase in medium sized and large lymphocytes in cancer patients suggests a possible role of stress in the multifactorial etiology of neoplastic disease.

672

Peters LJ, Kelly H. **The influence of stress and stress hormones on the transplantability of a non-immunogenic syngeneic murine tumor.** *Cancer.* 1977;39:1482-8. (English)

Quantitative transplantation assays of a syngeneic murine adenocarcinoma have been used to investigate the effects of stress hormones on tumor take probability. Cortisol, injected intraperitoneally one hour before and 3 hours after tumor cells, caused a dose-dependent reduction of TD_{50} (number of tumor cells required for 50% takes) by factors of from 4 at a total dose 4 microg/g to 68 at 400 microg/g. ACTH, given at 0.2 I.U. daily for 49 days spanning the time of tumor cell injection, reduced the TD_{50} 2.5-fold, indicating that the peak gluco-corticoid level achieved, rather than its duration, was of greater significance. Adrenaline, while much less effective than cortisol, produced an 8-fold reduction in TD_{50} at its maximum tolerable dose. The effect of cortisol simulated that of whole body irradiation (WBI), and while both these agents depress immune reactivity, evidence is presented to suggest that immunological mechanisms are not responsible for their effect. WBI constitutes a systemic stress, and the demonstration that surgical trauma (laparotomy) could also reduce the TD_{50} for this tumor suggested that both might act via endogenous glucocorticoids. However, the failure of prior total adrenalectomy of mice to abrogate the effect of either WBI or laparotomy indicated that stress hormones were not essential intermediaries. It is concluded that both stress hormones, especially glucocorticoids, and stressful procedures acting independently of stress hormones, can facilitate tumor transplantation.

673

Plaut SM, Esterhay RJ, Sutherland JC, Wareheim LE, Friedman SB, Schnaper N, Wiernik PH. **Psychological effects on resistance to spontaneous AKR leukemia in mice** (abstract). *Psychosom Med.* 1980;42:72. (English)

Behavioral factors have been shown to alter the course of experimentally-induced disease. This study investigated the extent to which the anticipation of a noxious stimulus (shock preceded by a warning signal) can alter the natural course of AKR leukemia. Female AKR mice were subjected to one of four stimulation conditions beginning at age 7 mo. Mice (n = 5) receiving signaled shock were given random 10 sec periods of light followed by a mild, 2 sec scrambled footshock. Stimulation sessions occurred 24 hr/day during six equally-spaced 1 hr periods, and involved an average of 12 stimulus presentations per hour. Other groups of mice housed in similar cages received only shock (n = 4), only light (n = 5), or no stimulation (Mock, n = 5). Water and food consumption and body weight were recorded weekly. The mean number of weeks' survival after commencement of the study were: Light-Shock, 34.8 ± 3.4; Shock 24.8 ± 5.5; Light, 11.4 ± 2.9; Mock, 15.0 ± 3.7. (Analysis of Variance: F = 8.0; df = 3/15; p<0.01). Light-Shock animals differed from Light and Mock mice (p<0.01), whereas Shock animals did not differ from any of the other three groups. The incidence of leukemia in all animals was confirmed by post-mortem histological examination. The four groups did not differ in body weight or in consumption of food and water as a function of time prior to death. Of these three variables, water consumption was the most reliable predictor of mortality. As of the 11th week of a second replication, the number of deaths in each group of five mice was: Light-Shock, 1; Shock, 1; Light, 4; Mock, 3. Resistance to spontaneously occurring leukemia in AKR mice can thus be increased by unavoidable noxious stimulation, especially when preceded by a warning signal.

674

Riley V, Spackman DH, Hellstrom KE, Hellstrom I. **Growth enhancement of murine sarcoma by LDH-virus, adrenocorticoids, and anxiety stress** (abstract). *Proc Am Assoc Cancer Research.* 1978;19:57. (English)

Tumors induced by the Moloney murine sarcoma virus provide a sensitive model for immunological studies. Usually 80 to 90% of mice develop tumors at the virus injection site in about one week following subcutaneous inoculation of a standard dose of Moloney sarcoma virus into BALB/c mice. However, after progressive tumor development for an additional 4 to 5 days, all tumors proceed to regress. This immunological circumstance provides an experimental means for testing various potential modulating influences on the host immunological apparatus and upon the altered growth and/or regression of the tumors. Three immunological modulating factors were tested: The LDH-virus, adrenocorticoids, and anxiety stress. The latter was produced by a slow rotation of the mouse cage on an automatic rotating platform. Both anxiety stress and the LDH-virus increased plasma corticosterone, impaired immunocompetence, and produced enhanced tumour growth. Corticosterone, the natural murine corticoid, and dexamethasone produced similar immunosuppressions and tumor grwoth enhancements, and also delayed tumor regressions. Both the LDH-virus and the induced mild anxiety stress enhanced tumor growth rates 2 to 4-fold, while the exogenous, administered corticoids increased tumor growth 8 to 10-fold. Both stress and LDH-virus contamination are common, unappreciated elements in conventional environments, and thus may constitute both experimentally hazardous modulating factors as well as useful experimental instruments in immunological or neoplastic studies.

675

Riley V, Spackman DH. **Cage crowding stress: absence of effect on melanoma within protective facilities** (abstract). *Proc Am Assoc Cancer Res.* 1977;18:173. (English)

A number of reports have described the stressful effects of cage crowding, and the consequential influence on various neoplastic processes. We employed cage crowding as a simple means for the intentional induction of chronic stress, and compared the stress and tumor behavior in mice housed singly or 2, 3, 5, 10, 15, or 20 animals per cage. Unexpectedly, no tangible differences were observed. The critical difference between our experiments and those previously reported, was the protective environmental housing facilities observed in conventional animal facilities. In our experiments, all the mice exhibited normal low levels of plasma corticosterone (CSR) irrespective of the number of mice per cage. CSR is a good stress index and is rapidly elevated during or following anxiety-stress. To test for the influence of cage crowding on tumor behavior, we repeated the classical Dechambre and Gosse experiment by implanting all mice with a suspension of B-16 melanoma. In contrast to their experiment, the incidence, tumor growth rate, and mouse survival times were the same for all cage populations. These data clearly demonstrate that cage crowding per se is not stressful providing that the overall housing environment is not stressful, that no males are present, fighting does not occur, and pregnancy is not a factor.

676

Riley V. **Cancer and stress: overview and critique.** *Cancer Detect Prev.* 1979;2:163-95. (English)

This overview of research on stress and cancer includes an examination of representative papers. These published studies demonstrate the widespread contradictions in the experimental results obtained by various investigators. Such discordant findings testify to the complexity of the relationships between stress and disease processes. In an effort to better understand the reasons for these puzzling experimental differences, a number of experimental factors that may relate to these problems are discussed. Notwithstanding the experimental difficulties and conflicting results, the accumulative data demonstrate that stress is capable of influencing various disease processes, including some neoplastic diseases. The importance of the problem deserves a more intensive research effort, with a magnitude of support that will permit experimental activities to proceed on an appropriately broad front, and in sufficient depth, that the multiple factors responsible for the apparent contradictions can be resolved. It is conceivable that out of such studies a biochemical means for controlling the adverse consequences of physiological stress may result.

677

Riley V. **Introduction: stress-cancer contradictions--a continuing puzzlement.** *Cancer Detect Prev.* 1979;2:159-62. (English)

An intriguing aspect of stress-cancer research is the contradictory reports of various investigators. Such seemingly inconsistent findings are represented in several of the papers included in this cancer-stress consortium. Three laboratories reported an enhancement of tumor incidence, or of tumor growth, as an apparent consequence of the induction of experimental stress. In contrast, either the same or other investigators observed tumor inhibition following an exposure of experimental animals to certain varieties of stress. These conflicting observations are provocative and emphasize the importance of increasing our knowledge and understanding of basic stress processes as a prerequisite to the control, and possible therapeutic treatment of patients, or some form of prophylaxis for the general population.

678

Riley V. **Psychoneuroendocrine influences on immunocompetence and neoplasia.** *Science.* 1981;212:1100-9. (English)

Emotional, psychological, or anxiety-stimulated stress produces increased plasma concentrations of adrenal corticoids and other hormones through well-known neuroendocrine pathways. A direct consequence of these increased corticoid concentrations is injury to elements of the immunological apparatus, which may leave the subject vulnerable to the action of latent oncogenic viruses, newly transformed cancer cells, or other incipient pathological processes that are normally held in check by an intact immunological apparatus. This article describes studies that examine the adverse effects of increased plasma concentrations of adrenal corticoids on the thymus and thymus-dependent T cells, inasmuch as these elements constitute a major defense system against various neoplastic processes and other pathologies. The studies demonstrate that anxiety-stress can be quantitatively induced and the consequences measured through specific biochemical and cellular parameters, providing that authentic quiescent baselines of these conditions are obtained in the experimental animals by the use of low-stress protective housing and handling techniques.

679

Santisteban GA, Riley V, Spackman DH. **Stress-related factors in the neoplastic process** (abstract). *Proc Am Assoc Cancer Res.* 1977;18:172. (English)

The earliest detectable objective parameter associated with the stress syndrome in the rodent is plasma corticosterone (CSR) elevation. This corticoid elevation is followed by decreased numbers of circulating T and B cells, thymus involution, and weight loss in lymph nodes and spleen, and under some conditions, impairment of mouse immunological and surveillance capacities. Thus any sustained elevation of CSR may trigger physiological events that are capable of altering immunocompetence and neoplasia. Recent work in our laboratory has demonstrated that conventional animal facilities, and standard animal handling procedures, are inherently stressful and thus capable of altering experimental results, since plasma CSR values of such animals are 100 to 500 ng/ml compared with 30 to 60 ng/ml for quiescent animals maintained in protective facilities. Exposure of mice to the established stress of a population cage, where chronic psychosocial confrontations occur, produces animals with similar high levels, ranging from 200 to 600 ng/ml. This controlled chronic stress induces hypertension, cardiovascular lesions, and increased vulnerability to virus infections and latent neoplasia. Initiation of stress by the direct administration of corticoids enhances certain experimental neoplastic processes, and provides a practical model for examining the mechanisms of stress-associated malignancies.

680

Sklar LS, Anisman H. **Social stress influences tumor growth.** *Psychosom Med.* 1980;42:347-65. (English)

Growth of syngeneic P815 mastocytoma in DBA/2J male mice was evaluated following social and physical stress expo-

sure. Although social isolation following tumor cell transplantation enhanced tumor growth, it appeared that it was the abrupt change of social conditions, rather than the isolation *per se* which was responsible for the exacerbation of tumorigenicity. Moreover, it was found that the animals' behavior after social change could modify this effect. If mice engaged in persistent fighting, the tumorigenic consequences of social change were not apparent. In addition, it was observed that social conditions interacted with physical stress. Footshock enhanced tumor growth among group housed mice, but retarded tumor development among socially isolated mice.

681

Sklar LS, Anisman H. **Stress and cancer.** *Psychol Bull.* 1981;89:369-406. (English)

Data derived from infrahuman experimentation, consistent with the findings of human research suggesting that stress may influence the carcinogenic process, have revealed that aversive insults may potentiate or inhibit tumorigenicity. The nature of change, however, is dependent on a number of psychological, experiential, and organismic variables. Exacerbation of tumor growth is evidenced following acute exposure to uncontrollable, but not controllable, stress. Moreover, the effects of aversive stimuli vary as a function of the organism's prior stress history as well of social housing conditions. The fact that stress influences neurochemical, hormonal, and immunological functioning and that these changes are subject to many of the same manipulations that influenced the carcinogenic process suggests a relation between these three mechanisms and the stress-induced alterations of tumor growth. This contention is supported by the findings that pharmacologic manipulations that modify these endogenous substrates have predictable effects on tumorigenesis.

682

Sklar LS, Bruto V, Anisman H. **Adaptation to the tumor-enhancing effects of stress.** *Psychosom Med.* 1981;43:331-42. (English)

Growth of P815 mastocytoma in syngeneic DBA/2J male mice was evaluated following several stress regimens. Although escapable shock did not enhance tumor growth, an equivalent amount of inescapable shock applied in a yoked paradigm markedly augmented tumor development. If mice received repeated stress sessions on 5-10 consecutive days following tumor cell transplantation, the tumor-enhancing effects of an acute stress session were abrogated. This effect was not due to an antitumor effect exerted by a shock session applied several days after cell transplantation. It seems that the tumorigenic effects of stress are subject to adaptation since stress exposure prior to cell transplantation also inhibited the effects of an acute stress session. The data are discussed in relation to stress-induced neurochemical alterations.

683

Spackman DH, Riley V. **Modification of cancer by stress: effects of plasma corticosterone elevations on immunological system components in mice** (abstract). *Fed Proc, Fed Am Soc Exp Biol.* 1976;35:1693. (English)

Physiological and environmental stress modifies host susceptibility to infections and neoplasia. Although the complex mechanisms by which stress influences the host are incompletely understood, an early biochemical change is the elevation of adrenal corticoids. We are studying this response and its influence on tissues and cells of the immunological defense system in the mouse. Corticosterone levels are determined using a fluorimetric assay on duplicate 50 microl plasma samples from individual mice or pools. Mild stress induces an increase in plasma corticosterone from a normal, quiescent level of 30 to 50 ng/ml to approx. 600 ng/ml. When the stress is either sustained or repeated at appropriate intervals, such hormone elevations cause a lymphocytopenia and thymus involution. Rotation of quiescent mice on a turntable for 10 min at 45 rpm increases plasma corticosterone to 450 ng/ml. After peaking at 20 min, this level drops back to normal by 70 min, demonstrating a rapid re-equilibration. After rotation for 2 hours, or for 10 min intervals each hour for 4 hours, the WBC count dropped from 13,200 to 5,400/mm³. Similar intermittent rotation for 24 hours produces a thymus involution of 35 to 50%. Analogous stress, which causes a modestly sustained elevation of plasma corticosterone, modifies the Gardner lymphosarcoma toward an increased virulence. This tumor enhancement apparently results from a hormone-mediated suppression of cellular immune responses.

684

Udupa KN, Raq A, Prasad R, Khatri S, Patel V, Chansouria JPN. **Role of stress in cancer.** *Indian J Cancer.* 1980;17:7-10. (English)

Stress probably plays some definite role in the development and progress of carcinoma in various parts of the body. Psychic stress seems to produce its effect by releasing excess of catecholamines and cortisol into the blood. Excess cortisol causes immuno-suppression leading to proliferation of mutant cells which leads to tumor formation. Excess of catecholamine causes vasoconstriction of a weak organ leading to anaerobic conditions which may make the normal cells transform into abnormal cells. Such abnormal cells, with suppressed immunity, favors the development of cancer. This is in contrast to sarcoma, where it seems there is an excessive immunological reaction. It would be of interest to study the effect of various stress reducing measures such as the use of tranquilizers or combined practice of yoga which decrease the circulating levels of catecholamines and cortisol, in the prevention and control of cancer. These studies were performed on rats.

685

Van Den Brenk HA, Stone MG, Kelly H, Sharpington C. **Lowering of innate resistance of the lungs to the growth of blood-borne cancer cells in states of topical and systemic stress.** *Br J Cancer.* 1976;33:60-78. (English)

The survival and clonogenic growth (measured in terms of colony forming efficiency (CFE) of intravenously injected (i.v.) Walker (W256) tumour cells in the lungs of rats was greatly enhanced by states of topical and systemic stress induced by intrapperitoneal (i.p.) injection of rats with single dose of 10^{-5}- 10^{-3} mmol/g body weight of adrenaline and other beta-adrenergic agonists, inflammatory agents (including local x-irradiation), convulsive seizures, "tumbling" or physical restraint. Lowering of innate resistance of the host to growth of seeded tumour cells induced by states of topical and systemic stress, and by the addition of an excess of lethally irradiated (LI) tumour cells to i.v. injected intact tumour cells, were all potentiated by treatment of rats with aminophylline, an inhibitor of cyclic AMP phosphodiesterase. Enhancement of tumour growth by systemic stress was inhibited by bilateral total or medullary adrenalectomy and is attributed to the release and actions of endogenous adreno-medullary hormones. Alpha-adrenergic and most non-adrenergic agents administered in maximum tolerated doses did not significantly affect host resistance to tumour growth in the lungs. These findings, correlated with measurements of cyclic AMP in the lungs of normal and stressed rats, suggest that changes in the resistance of the host to tumour growth involve changes in cyclic nucleotide metabolism in the target tissues (tumour bed); possible mechanisms of action of cyclic nucleotides in this respect are discussed

686

Visintainer MA, Volpicelli JR, Seligman ME. **Tumor rejection in rats after inescapable or escapable shock.** *Science.* 1982;216:437-9. (English)

Rats experienced inescapable, escapable, or no electric shock 1 day after being implanted with a Walker 256 tumor preparation. Only 27 percent of the rats receiving inescapable shock rejected the tumor, whereas 63 percent of the rats receiving escapable shock and 54 percent of the rats receiving no shock rejected the tumor. These results imply that lack of control over stressors reduces tumor rejection and decreases survival.

Stress and infectious disease

687

Borysenko M, Turesky S, Borysenko J, Quimby F, Benson H. **Stress and dental caries in the rat.** *J Behav Med.* 1980;3:233-43. (English)

The stress of crowding and exposure to inescapable electric shock increased both the incidence and the severity of dental caries in rats housed in a conventional animal facility. Male Osborne-Mendel rats were inoculated intraorally with cariogenic bacteria, fed a high-sucrose diet, and housed in either a conventional or sheltered facility. Rats in both housing conditions were subdivided into control and stress groups. At the end of the 56-day trial period, stressed rats from conventional housing had a significant increase in both incidence and severity of dental caries in comparison to their controls. In contrast, stressed rats from sheltered housing had a trend toward increased cariogenesis which reached significance in only one of the five scores. These rats also failed to gain weight comparable to their controls, making it possible that stress-induced reduction in appetite partially offset stress-induced exacerbation in cariogenesis.

688

Mohamed MA, Hanson RP. **Effect of social stress on Newcastle disease virus (LaSota) infection.** *Avian Dis.* 1980;24:908-15. (English)

Individual immature chickens were socially stressed when

placed into an established group of chickens. The stress response was determined by periodic measurement of plasma cortisol and by determination of the relative regression of the bursa of Fabricius. Stressed chickens had elevated cortisol levels during the first 24 hours following the initiation of social stress. The bursa-to-body-weight ratios of stressed birds at 96 hours following stress were significantly lower than the ratios in control birds, and their tuberculin reaction was significantly depressed. Newcastle disease virus was more invasive and attained higher titers in stressed birds. The hemagglutination-inhibition (HI) response of the stressed birds was higher in one trial and lower in another.

689
Schlewinski E. **Changes in immunoreactivity dependent on psychic stresses: animal experiments.** *Z Psychosom Med Psychoanal.* 1980;26:336-46. (German)

White NMRI mice, separated according to sex, after different pretreatments (isolation, isolation combined with light deprivation, crowding) were exposed to an experimental infection with E. coli. The cumulative post-infectious mortality was significantly higher among the male test subjects in the isolation and the crowding experiments, whereas the female mice showed increased mortality after pre-treatment with isolation in combination with light deprivation. The results are discussed and compared to other findings in the literature.

690
Schlewinski E. **Studies on the influence of psychological factors on the immune system: changes in susceptibility to infection after infantile stimulation as a function of age.** *Z Psychosom Med Psychoanal.* 1976;22:370-7. (German)

NMRI mice of both sexes and in various stages of the suckling period were handled once a day for three minutes. They were intraperitoneally infected with E. coli O 111 on the eighteenth day of life. Handling was carried out daily from the first to the 18th day and led to a significantly higher mortality (p = 0.14) as compared to the control animals. Differences in mortality were not observed when the stimulation occurred on the 1st through 10th or 10th through 18th day of life. Weight determination carried out just prior to infection showed no remarkable differences between the experimental groups.

Stress and cell-mediated immunity

691
Bassett JR, Tait NN. **The effect of stress on the migration of leucocytes into the peritoneal cavity of rats following injection of an inflammatory agent.** *Aust J Exp Biol Med Sci.* 1981;59:651-66. (English)

Although previous studies have shown that the injection of exogenous corticosteroids suppresses the inflammatory response, no study has been made on the effect of inflammation of endogenous corticosteroids released in response to stress. In the present study a reduction was observed in the total number of leucocytes migrating into the peritoneal cavity of stressed rats in response to the injection of an inflammatory agent. The reduction of total counts was due to a stress-induced reduction of both polymorph and mononuclear cells. Permeability studies and blood leucocyte counts were conducted to determine the mode of action of the stress-induced reduction of leucocyte migration. In the case of the polymorphs, evidence is presented to implicate both a reduced release of these cells into the blood stream from storage sites and a blockade of the increased vascular permeability. The situation is not as clear for the mononuclear cells where no change in the circulating levels of these cells was observed in either stressed or control rats following induction of an inflammatory response.

692
Blecha F, Barry RA, Kelly KW. **Stress-induced alterations in cell-mediated immunity of mice *in vivo*** (abstract). *Fed Proc, Fed Am Soc Exp Biol.* 1980;39:479. (English)

Contact sensitivity to 2,4-dinitro, 1-fluorobenzene (DNFB) and delayed hypersensitivity (DH) to sheep erythrocytes (SRBC) were utilized to evaluate the effect of two stressors, cold and immobilization, on cell-mediated immunity (CMI). Swiss Webster mice were exposed to cold (5°C) or thermoneutral (25°C) air temperatures from sensitization through 72 hours post-challenge (PC). Cold stress increased (p<0.01) footpad swelling to SRBC at 48 and 72 hours PC in sensitized and non-sensitized mice. Sensitized mice were immobilized for 2.5 hours prior to challenge with DNFB or SRBC. Immobilization increased (p<0.01) the DNFB response and decreased (p<0.05) the SRBC response at 48 and 72 hours PC. These data indicate that immobilization stress influences expression of CMI or expression of DH reactions to SRBC. Further, these experiments suggest that two common indices of CMI yield differing results in stressed animals.

693
Boranic M, Pericic D, Poljak-Blazi M. **Immunological reactivity and concentration of neurotransmitters in the brain of mice stressed by overcrowding and treated with haloperidol.** *Period Biol.* 1980; 82:13-18. (English)

CBA mice were stressed by overcrowding. Their immune reactivity was determined 3, 7, 11 and 18 days after the beginning of the stress by counting the plaque-forming cells (PFC) in the spleens 4 days after the injection of sheep red blood cells (SRBC). On the same days, the concentrations of serotonin, 5-hydroxyindoleacetic acid [5-HIAA], noradrenaline [norepinephrine] and dopamine, were determined in their cerebra. There was a transient depression of the PFC response 3 and 7 days after the onset of the stress, a stimulation on day 11, and a decline on day 18. The level of 5-HIAA was significantly elevated throughout the period of stress, indicating an increased metabolism of serotonin. A neuroleptic drug, haloperidol (administered daily during the stress) blocked the stimulation of the PFC response observed on day 11. Neurotransmitter substances may be involved in the central regulation of the immune response during stress; this response can be blocked by neuroleptic drugs.

694
Borysenko M, Borysenko J. **Stress, behavior and immunity: animal models and mediating mechanisms.** *Gen Hosp Psychiat.* 1982;4:59-67. (English) (unavailable at publication)

695

Joasoo A, McKenzie JM. **Stress and the immune response in rats.** *Int Arch Allergy Appl Immunol.* 1976;50:659-63. (English)

The *in vitro* response of sensitized splenic lymphocytes to antigen (thyroglobulin) was increased by crowding and decreased by isolation in female rats. Both isolated and crowded male rats responded by a decrease in the *in vitro* reactivity of lymphocytes to antigen. The response of the lymphocytes to PHA was not altered in any consistent manner. Similar animals, both control and those immunized with thyroglobulin, were tested for an effect of *in vivo* injections of epinephrine on the *in vitro* reactivity of lymphocytes; epinephrine was given intraperitoneally 30 min before the rats were killed for removal of spleens. Incorporation of ^{3}H-thymidine by lymphocytes was greater in control cultures (neither PHA nor antigen present) but there was a decreased response to either PHA or antigen when epinephrine had been injected.

696

Keller SE, Weiss J, Schleifer SJ, Miller NE, Stein M. **Suppression of immunity by stress: effect of a graded series of stressors on lymphocyte stimulation in the rat.** *Science.* 1981;213:1397-1400. (English)

In rats a graded series of stressors produced progressively greater suppression of lymphocyte function, as measured by the number of circulating lymphocytes and by phytohemagglutinin stimulation of lymphocytes in whole blood and isolated cultures. This evidence suggests that stress suppresses immunity in proportion to the intensity of the stressor.

697

Keller SE, Weiss J, Schleifer SJ, Miller NE, Stein M. **Suppression of immunity by stress: effect of a graded series of stressors on lymphocyte stimulation in the rat** (abstract). *Psychosom Med.* 1981;43:91. (English)

A range of illnesses may be associated with stress-induced changes in immune function. The present study was undertaken to determine in the rat the relationship between a graded series of stressors and direct measures of *in vitro* cell-mediated immune function--number of lymphocytes, %T cells, phytohemagglutinin (PHA) lymphocyte stimulation in whole blood and with isolated peripheral blood lymphocytes. Four groups of 12 rats each were studied consisting in order of increasing levels of stress, home cage controls, apparatus controls, low-shock, and high-shock animals. There was a significantly graduated suppression of lymphocyte stimulation in the whole blood assay in response to graded increases in the intensity of the stressor. There was a mild suppression in the apparatus group as compared to the home cage rats. Low-shock further suppressed the response and the cells from the high-shock group approached levels of unstimulated cultures. There was no difference in the %T cells between the groups, however, a significant lymphocytopenia was induced by stressful conditions. The decreased PHA-induced lymphocyte stimulation in whole blood may, therefore, have been due to decreased numbers of available responding lymphocytes. Further studies were, therefore, conducted using a fixed number of lymphocytes in an isolated lymphocyte stimulation assay. The response of the lymphocytes from the apparatus control group was signficantly suppressed, and the responses of the lymphocytes from both the low-shock and high-shock groups were suppressed to the levels of unstimulated cultures. The present findings demonstrate that the cellular immune system responds differentially to stressful conditions. The effect of the stressful conditions on the lymphocyte response to PHA in the rat may be related to changes in hormone or neurotransmitter levels. It remains to be determined if the effects of stress results in a lymphocytopenia with concomitant functional impairment of the lymphocyte or is due to redistribution of subsets of lymphocytes producing selective decreases in PHA reactive cells.

698

Laudenslager M, Reite M, Harbeck R. **Suppressed immune response in infant monkeys associated with maternal separation.** *Behav Neural Biol.* 1982;36:40-8. (English)

The effect of maternal separation on an *in vitro* measure of the cellular immune response was studied in infant bonnet monkeys (*Macaca radiata*). Using a modified mixed-species separation paradigm, bonnet mother-infant pairs were each housed with a single adult female pigtailed monkey (*Macaca nemestrina*). Over a 14-day separation period, the infants showed a suppression of lymphocyte proliferation in response to mitogens relative to a 14-day baseline period which preceded separation. The lymphocyte response was restored following reunion. During separation, infants were initially agitated, and this was followed by observations of reduced activity and a slouched posture. Behaviors returned to baseline conditions following reunion. It was concluded that suppressed immunological functioning may be included among the pathophysiological consequences of maternal separation in infant monkeys.

699

Monjan AA, Collector MI. **Noise as a stressor in the laboratory rodent: modulation of lymphocyte reactivity.** *Cancer Res.* (in press) (English) (unavailable at publication)

700

Pavlidis N, Chirigos M. **Stress-induced impairment of macrophage tumoricidal function.** *Psychosom Med.* 1980;42:47-54. (English)

Several studies have shown the effect of stress on immune cells and their functions. The purpose of the present work was to investigate the influence of acute immobilization stress on macrophage nonspecific tumoricidal activity. Peritoneal macrophages were activated by specific immunopotentiators such as interferon or bacterial lipopolysaccharide (LPS) and the killing of MBL-2 leukemic target cells was measured. Macrophages from mice submitted to stress showed decreased responsiveness to interferon or LPS. In addition, the role of corticosteroids as mediators in the phenomenon was also studied. Indeed, we observed that corticosteroids were able to inhibit macrophage cytotoxicity and could at least play some role. This data could contribute to a better understanding of the effect of stress on the host immunosurveillance against tumor development.

702

Teshima H, Kubo C. Nagata S, Imada Y, Ago Y. **Influence of stress on phagocytic function of macrophages.** *Shinshin-Igaku.* 1981;21:99-103. (Japanese)

The evidence that the psychological factors influenced the prognosis of allergic diseases were observed by many clinicians and suggested the correlation between stress and the immune system. To clarify the correlation more in detail, the authors had carried out animal experiments whose results showed the effect of stress on plasminic activity, on Hageman's activity and cytotoxicity of killer T cells. In this paper, these studies were succeeded to the influence of stress on the function of macrophages, which had important roles in the immune system such as phagocytosis, recognition of antigen, etc. By using mice (AKR), the carbon clearance method was carried out to measure the activity of phagocytosis of macrophages. Stresses were given by immobilization and by the stress box where the stimuli of electricity, light and buzzer were given. Changes of the activity of phagocytosis were observed at the different durations of stress. The results showed that in the stress box group, the carbon clearance rates had been depressed during two to five days of stress, but at the sixth day, carbon clearance rates were rather recovered due to acclimatization of the mice to stress. In the immobilization group, the activity of phagocytosis was rather enhanced by stress until the eighth hour and then was suppressed strongly. Suppression of the function of macrophages was not recovered by infusion of serum of a control mouse. Corinebacterium can inhibit the suppression of phagocytosis by stress. Our experiments suggested that stress affected the phagocytic function of macrophage directly, not through the serum factors.

Stress and humoral immunity

703

Dadhich AP, Sharma VN, Godhwani JL. **Effect of restraint stress on immune response and its modification by chlorpromazine, diazepam and pentobarbitone.** *Indian J Exp Biol.* 1980;18:756-7. (English)

Antibody titre induced by Typhoid "H" antigen was determined by Widal agglutination technique in albino rats subjected to restraint stress by immobilization for 40 hr and compared with the groups of animals treated with chlorpromazine, diazepam and pentobarbitone. Restraint stress caused significant reduction of antibody titre. Chlorpromazine and diazepam induced significant inhibition of the antibody titre in stressed animals whereas pentobarbitone caused insignificant reduction of the antibody titre. Chlorpromazine and diazepam manifested significant depression of antibody titre in unstressed animals, and pentobarbitone caused an insignificant reduction of the antibody titre as compared to "controls." Inhibition of antibody titre in animals exposed to stress has been attributed to stimulation of pituitary-adrenal axis resulting in release of catecholamines and glucocorticoids. Reduction of antibodies with chlorpromazine, diazepam and pentobarbitone has been attributed to the denaturing effect of these drugs.

704

Edwards EA, Dean LM. **Effects of crowding of mice on humoral antibody formation and protection to lethal antigenic challenge.** *Psychosom Med.* 1977;39:19-24. (English)

The effects of grouping (crowding) on humoral antibody response to typhoid paratyphoid vaccine and subsequent protection from a minimal lethal challenge dose of salmonella typhimurium were studied in white Swiss-Webster mice. The data show a trend between the degree of crowding and antibody response. Geometric mean titers of high density grouped mice were significantly lower than the geometric mean titers of the less crowded mice. Also, there were significantly less antibody responders in the high density grouped mice than in the less crowded mice. However, challenged with a minimal LD_{50} dose of salmonella typhimurium, no deaths occurred in the immunized study group, regardless of measurable antibody level. In the nonimmunized controls, which were under the same stressor conditions, there was a significant difference between the level of crowding and death to challenge. The data show that nonimmunized mice in this study exhibited a marked increase in susceptibility to an infectious agent when under the stressor effect of crowding.

705

Edwards EA, Rahe RH, Stephens PM, Henry JP. **Antibody response to bovine serum albumin in mice: the effects of psychosocial environmental change.** *Proc Soc Exp Biol Med.* 1980;164:478-81. (English)

The effects of psychosocial environmental change upon circulating antibody response to antigenic challenge was investigated in CAB/USC mice. Mice were reared in isolation and selected groups were subsequently exposed to psychosocial stimulation. Antibody titers of mice that remained in isolation were significantly higher than the titers of mice exposed to psychosocial stimulation. One group of mice exposed to psychosocial stimulation and then returned to isolation showed titers significantly below those of mice exposed to psychosocial stimulation only. These data indicate that psychosocial environmental changes can be productive of significant suppression of antibody formation in mice.

706

Gross WB, Siegel PB. **Long-term exposure of chickens to three levels of social stress.** *Avian Dis.* 1981;25:312-25. (English)

Cockerels were kept in environments characterized by high (HSS), medium (MSS), or low (LSS) levels of social stress for 3 or 4 months. Chickens raised in an environment of low light intensity (LSS) gained more weight than did those raised under natural lighting. Ability of chickens to produce antibody in response to antigen was greatly reduced, 2(15.4) in the LSS group to 2(3.4) in the HSS group, 1 day after chickens were moved from the LSS environment into the HSS environment. Normal responsiveness returned within 1 week. No long-term environments affected antibody production. After 3 months, chickens in the LSS environment had reduced weight gain and resistance to Escherichia coli infection compared with birds in the HSS environment. Chickens in the MSS environment, compared with those on the HSS and LSS environments, had greater weight gains, superior feed efficiencies, medium plasma corticosterone levels, a better negative correlation between antibody responsiveness and RBC antigens, and better resistance to mycoplasma gallisepticum challenge. All parameters except antibody responsiveness were such that long-term exposure to HSS or LSS environments appears to be detrimental.

707

Hara C, Ogawa N, Imada Y. **The activity-stress ulcer and antibody production in rats.** *Physiol Behav.* 1981;27:609-13. (English)

Divided 40 male Wistar rats into 4 groups: a control group fed freely for 7 days and 3 stressed groups fed 1 hour each day for 3, 5 and 7 days. All Ss were housed in activity-wheel cages under a reversed light-dark cycle. They were immunized twice with sheep erythrocytes before beginning the stress schedule. After Ss were sacrificed, their stomach, lungs, thymus, spleen, and adrenals were removed and examined histologically. The incidence of Ss with ulcer reached 60% in the 3-day stress group, although antibody production was unaffected and no Ss died in this group. In the 5- and 7-day stress groups, the incidence of ulcer reached 90%, antibody production was significantly inhibited, and the degree of mortality increased to more than 50%. The severity of ulcer was in proportion to the length of stress periods. Data suggest that activity-stress Ss have 2 pathological phases: stomach ulcer and immunodeficiency. The present study emphasizes that immunological response can serve as an indicator of the biological response for stress.

708

Michaut R-J, et al. **Influence of early maternal deprivation on adult humoral immune response in mice.** *Physiol Behav.* 1981;26:189-91. (English)

10-wk-old mice were submitted to early maternal deprivation before weaning and were weaned earlier than the usual age. Upon reaching adulthood, Ss showed a decreased number of plaque-forming cells and a lowered level of seric immunoglobulins as compared to controls. Two etiogenic hypotheses are discussed: undernourishment and adrenal stress.

Stress, neuroendocrine changes and immunity

709

Bonnyns M, McKenzie JM. **Interactions of stress and endocrine status on rat peripheral lymphocyte responsiveness to phytomitogens.** *Psychoneuroendrocrinology.* 1979;4:67-73. (English)

(1) Rat peripheral blood lymphocyte responsiveness to phytohemagglutinin and to pokeweed mitogen was studied. The animals were intact or had undergone surgical removal of pituitary, thyroid, adrenals or gonads; half were subjected to non-traumatic stress for 7 consecutive days and the studies were performed with blood taken on days 1, 8 and 15. (2) In intact rats there was a significantly increased responsiveness to pokeweed mitogen 1 week after cessation of the stress. (3) In non-stressed animals, adrenalectomy was associated with lower responses to pokeweed mitogen. (4) There was no influence of stress on to pokeweed mitogen responsiveness in any of the surgically treated rats; however, in these rats, hypophysectomy and thyroidectomy were associated respectively with reduced and increased responsiveness to phytohemagglutinin. (5) Considering all stressed animals, i.e., intact and surgically treated, thyroidectomy, adrenalectomy and castration led to a greater responsiveness to phytohemagglutinin and hypophysectomy had the reverse effect. (6) The data support the concept that both stress and hormonal status may influence immune responses and may do so in an interrelated manner.

710

Monnet F, Lichtensteiger W. **Neuroendocrine regulation and central dopamine (DA) systems in physical and psychological stress.** *J Physiol* (Paris). 1980;76:273-5. (English)

Physical and psychological stress cause different patterns of changes in the fluorescence intensity of nigral and tuberoinfundibular DA neurons which point to changes in neuronal activity. In order to investigate possible interactions between alpha-MSH (alpha-melanotropin) and DA systems in stress, systemic and intraventricular injections of antiserum against alpha-MSH were made. The functional state of DA neurons was assessed by histochemical microfluorimetry and hormone levels were measured by radioimmunoassay. Antiserum against alpha-MSH was found to affect the functional state of DA neurons, but only through the intravenous route. Under physical stress i.v. injection of antiserum against alpha-MSH was accompanied by elevated levels of activity of the DA neurons of the substantia nigra. An intraventricular injection of the same antiserum was ineffective. In psychological stress, an effect was again seen only after intravenous injection of antiserum against alpha-MSH. In this situation, the activity in DA cell groups of the substantia nigra, ventral tegmental area and tubero-infundibular system was increased after antiserum injection. Possible influences from manipulations were checked; certain effects which depended upon experimental situation were noted. Our data suggest a modulatory influence of circulating alpha-MSH on the functional state of central DA systems.

Personality and immunity
Personality and disease susceptibility

711

Betz BJ, Thomas CB. **Individual temperament as a predictor of health or premature disease.** *Johns Hopkins Med J.* 1979;144:81-9. (English) (unavailable at publication)

712

Chauhan NS, Dhar U. **A psychodynamic study of children suffering from leprosy: a preliminary communication.** *Indian J Clin Psychol.* 1980;7:75-6. (English)

Data from 11 8-14 yr old leprosy patients indicate that Ss perceived their immediate environment as hostile and insecure and expressed a desire for love, security, courage, and freedom. Ss lacked ego integration, and the use of psychotherapeutic techniques is recommended.

713

Cohen JJ, Crnic LS, Dixon LK. **"Personality" and immune system function in mice: role of albinism** (abstract). *Psychosom Med.* 1982;44:121. (English)

We have previously shown that "emotionality" of seven inbred strains of mice, as measured by open field behavior, correlates highly with an immune system variable: the number of T cells in the bone marrow. Furthermore, mice selected over many generations for high or low activity in the open field show similar differences in bone marrow T cell levels. The selected low activity lines, and the low activity inbred strains, are albinos; so it was possible that the c coat-color locus controls both open field activity and T cell distribution. To test this hypothesis, we obtained normal black C57Bl/6J mice, and mutant C57Bl/6J$^{c/c}$ albinos, which are coisogenic with the black strain. Black and albino mice were tested in a standard open field, and the albinos were found to be somewhat less active than blacks (p<0.05) when tested in a lighted room; no difference between the two strains was seen when tested in the dark. Bone marrow T cell levels were essentially identical in the two strains, and much higher than those observed in low-activity albino mice. Thus the high activity and high T cell levels in the marrow of C57Bl/6J mice are not coat-color related, and T cell distribution and open field activity, while strongly correlated with each other, are not controlled by the c (albinism) locus. The true nature of the behavior/T cell distribution correlation in mice is not known, but may involve a single genetic locus, which we are investigating.

714

Garrity TF, Somes GW, Marx MB. **The relationship of personality, life change, psychophysiological strain and health status in a college population.** *Soc Sci Med.* 1977;11:257-63. (English)

A model which describes the process whereby recent life changes are translated to health changes through the agency of psychophysiological strain is put forward. The role of personality factors is appraised at three critical points in the process. Three personality measures are derived which seem to influence extent of reported life change, stress symptomatology and illness experience. The findings are examined in the light of both substantive and methodological interpretations.

715

Garrity TF. et al. **Personality factors in resistance to illness after recent life changes.** *J Psychosom Res.* 1977;21:23-32. (English)

Three personality dimensions, derived by factor analysis from the Omnibus Personality Inventory, are examined as possible intervening variables between recent life experience and subsequent health change in a college population. All three personality measures, social conformity, liberal intellectualism and emotional sensitivity are found to be independently and significantly predictive of health change: these relationships hold even when recent life experience is introduced as a significant predictor of health change. The addition of personality measures to information about recent life experience significantly improves the predictability of deleterious health change. The results are discussed in the context of factors which promote resistance to health breakdown after life changes.

716

Hong KM, Hopwood MA, Wirt RD, Yellin AM. **Psychological attributes, patterns of life change, and illness susceptibility.** *J Nerv Ment Dis.* 1979;167:275-81. (English)

Personality test data and patterns of life changes over a 3-year period were collected on 73 male medical students to determine the influence of these mediating variables on the occurrence of illness. The results showed that life change units tended to be stable over time within groups which had high and low scores and psychological attributes were significantly different in the two groups. It was found that the subjects who had sustained high life change in all 3 years (the Sustained Group) were associated with a significantly greater number of health changes of more serious kinds than the subjects who had high life change in year 1 but low life change in the subsequent 2 years (the Short Term Group) and that the Short Term Group had greater psychological strengths than the Sustained Group. These findings are congruent with the data from a slightly different analysis in which healthy subjects in the original High Life Change Group obtained lower scores in subsequent years while ill subjects maintained high scores and the healthy subjects showed greater psychological strengths than ill strengths. The data were interpreted to show evidence that psychological characteristics do influence the occurrence of illness and that health is more likely to be impaired by sustained stress than by a short term major crisis.

717

Pfitzner R. **The psychodynamics of psoriasis vulgaris as revealed in the Rorschach test.** *Z Psychosom Med Psychoanal.* 1976;22:190-7. (English)

Administered the Rorschach test to 9 adult psoriasis patients to test P. Vogel's model of the psychosomatic aspects of psoriasis vulgaris. Results show some similarities, particularly in sexualization of intentional and oral desires, and in the somatization of the conflicts between libidinous and aggressive impulses.

718

Vogel PG. **Psychodynamic aspects of psoriasis vulgaris.** *Z Psychosom Med Psychoanal.* 1976;22:177-89. (English)

A psychodynamic model for psoriasis vulgaris is developed, based on a case report of psychoanalytic treatment of a patient with a first manifestation of the disease. The probable significance of schizoid aggressive impulses is discussed.

719

Wenner FC. **Relationships between selected personality factors and types of physiological pathology exhibited.** *Diss Abstr Int.* 1980;40:5030-1. (English) (unavailable at publication)

Personality and cancer

720

Anonymous. **Breast cancer: fighters live longer.** *Med World News.* 1978;37. (English) (no abstract)

721

Anonymous. **Cancer and the mind: how are they connected?** (news and comment) *Science.* 1978;200:1363-5. (English)

722

Anonymous. **Cancer linked to personality traits.** *Med World News.* 1976;17-18. (English) (no abstract)

723

Anonymous. **Mind and cancer.** *Lancet.* 1979;1:706-7. (English) (no abstract)

724

Becker H. **Psychodynamic aspects of breast cancer-- differences in younger and older patients.** *Psychother Psychosom.* 1979;32:287-96. (English)

We looked into possible differences in the life history and reaction to illness to be observed in younger and older breast cancer patients. The patients, 49 in number, are between 29 and 69 years of age, average age 50. A semi-structured interview took place mostly in the final third of the post-irradiation phase. In the group of women, who developed cancer before the age of 48, some common aspects could be shown in their biography. These women lost an emotionally important person (e.g., a parent) more often in their early childhood. These patients describe an emotionally cold atmosphere in their families along with a missing pronounced basic trust. Also they were overstrained with responsibility too early for their age. The ideals of these patients are somewhat like those of the 'Amazons': they negate the typical female role and its consequences on the bodily, psychic and social level. They seem quite combative, achieving and to the point. As far as sexual responsiveness is concerned only 12% of the younger groups express a consistently positive attitude toward sexuality. Pregnancy, childbirth and breast-feeding are frequently accompanied by serious complications, but they have, in the majority of cases, children. When regarding the multi-causal genesis of cancer, it may be that psychic factors have less influence on the immune system in older patients than the overall ageing process with its weakening of the immunological defence system. The psychic component, if it exists, plays a greater role with the younger patients. The older patients in their life history and pre-morbid behaviour are nearer to what passes for the psychic norm. Other carcinogen factors play a more significant role in older patients: the cancer may have achieved greater autonomy from psychic factors.

725

Boranic M. **The psychophysiological theory of cancer (a review)** (author's transl). *Lijec Vjesn.* 1979;101:153-8. (Czechoslovakian)

The article presents a review of data and theories about the influence of psychogenic factors on the inception and growth of cancer. Patients with cancer are considered to have a personality structure characterized by diminished emotional outlet on the social level. For this reason, regressions of the libidinal energy due to frustrations that have reactivated latent conflicts (e.g., loss of an object), discharge on a more primitive somatic level. By weakening the immunological defense or by disturbing the endocrine function (presumably through the hypothalamus), this may permit the action of carcinogenic chemicals, viruses and other direct causes of malignant alteration (the "permissive" theory). According to more radical views, the psychic energy might manifest itself on the somatic level as a moving force of an aberrant, persistent cellular growth, the aim of which would be to replace the lost object in a primitive, biological form, so that even the localization of the tumor may serve a symbolic function (the "causative" theory). Cognizance of the psychogenic dimension in the etiology of cancer may find its place in medical measures aimed at prevention and therapy of this disease. For example, preventive actions might be directed toward high-risk individuals who are particularly liable to cancer because of professional, habitual, or personality factors, and the actions might be planned so as to meet their maximal response. On the therapeutic plane, an adequate psychological support to the patients which would promote their general psychophysiological state, might speed up recovery after an operation, irradiation or chemotherapy, and delay or retard the relapses and metastases.

726

Brainsky LS, et al. **Personality structure in patients with breast cancer; IV--Depression and cancer: a comparison.** *Rev Colomb Psiq.* 1977;6:255-73. (Spanish) (unavailable at publication)

727

Dattore PJ, Shontz FC, Coyne L. **Premorbid personality differentiation of cancer and noncancer groups: a test of the hypothesis of cancer proneness.** *J Consult Clin Psychol.* 1980;48:388-94. (English)

Although the question of a cancer-prone personality has been extensively researched, few if any studies have employed a premorbid data base. Thus, nearly all evidence has been confounded, most importantly by alterations of psychological functioning due to the disease itself. The present study provides a more equitable test of the cancer proneness hypothesis. Premorbid MMPI records were collected from 75 cancer and 125 noncancer patients of a VA hospital. It was reasoned that the hypothesis of the existence of psychologically related cancer proneness would gain some support if stepwise discriminant function analysis of the MMPI scores yielded a significant discrimination between the cancer and noncancer groups. Results support this contention. The group of men with cancer (irrespective of site) was significantly separated from the noncancer group primarily on the basis of lower scores on the Repression-Sensitization Scale (i.e., greater repression) and on the Depression scale of the MMPI (i.e., less self-report of depression). Results are discussed in terms of their theoretical, heuristic, and clinical relevance.

728

Dattore PJ. **Premorbid personality characteristics associated with neoplasms: an archival approach.** *Diss Abstr Int.* 1980;41:346. (English) (unavailable at publication)

729

Doll R, Peto R. **The causes of cancer: quantitative estimates of avoidable risks of cancer in the United States today.** *J Natl Cancer Inst.* 1981;66:1191-308. (English)

Evidence that the various common types of cancer are largely avoidable diseases is reviewed. Life-style and other environmental factors are divided into a dozen categories, and for each category the evidence relating those particular factors to cancer onset rates is summarized. Where possible, an estimate is made of the percentage of current U.S. cancer mortality that might have been caused or avoided by that category of factors. These estimates are based chiefly on evidence from epidemiology, as the available evidence from animal and

other laboratory studies cannot provide reliable human risk assessments. By far the largest reliably known percentage is the 30% of current U.S. cancer deaths that are due to tobacco, although it is possible that some nutritional factor(s) may eventually be found of comparable importance. The percentage of U.S. cancer deaths that are due to tobacco is still increasing, and must be expected to continue to increase for some years yet due to the delayed effects of the adoption of ciagarettes in earlier decades. Trends in mortality and in onset rates for many separate types of cancer are studied in detail in appendices to this paper. Biases in the available data on registration of new cases produce apparent trends in cancer incidence which are spurious. Biases also produce spurious trends in cancer death certification rates, especially among old people. In (and before) middle age, where the biases are smaller, there appear to be a few real increases and a few real decreases in mortality from some particular types of cancer, but there is no evidence of any generalized increase other than that due to tobacco. Moderate increases or decreases due to some new agent(s) or habit(s) might of course be overlooked in such large-scale analyses. But, such analyses do suggest that, apart from cancer of the respiratory tract, the types of cancer that are currently common are not peculiarly modern diseases and are likely to depend chiefly on some long-established factor(s). (A prospective study utilizing both questionnaires and stored blood and other biological materials might help elucidate these factors.) The proportion of current U.S. cancer deaths attributed to occupational factors is provisionally estimated as 4% (lung cancer being the major contributor to this). This is far smaller than has recently been suggested by various U.S. government agencies. The matter could be resolved directly by a "case-control" study of lung cancer two or three times larger than the recently completed U.S national bladder cancer study but similar to it in methodology and unit costs; there are also other reasons for such a study. A fuller summary of conclusions and recommendations comprises the final section of this report.

730

Dyregrov A. **Psychological factors in the development of cancer: a critical evaluation.** *Tidsskrift Norsk Psykologforening.* 1981;18:257-65. (Norwegian)

Discusses studies that propose a link between psychological factors and the development of cancer. Both a cancer-prone personality and adverse life-events had been considered as important in the etiological chain of cancer. The hypothesis of adverse life-events as a precursor of cancer does not find strong support in the literature. There seems to be more consensus that the cancer patient is emotionally stable, experiences little psychic and autonomous anxiety, and comes from a cold family of origin. However, the methodological designs used do not allow the conclusion that these personality characteristics are present premorbidly. Alternative theories are set forth, and the methods used are critically evaluated. It is concluded that there is currently no valid support for the theory that certain psychological factors preceded the development of cancer.

731

Frank SJ. **Personality correlates of breast cancer: an exploration of extraversion-introversion in women who**

have had breast cancer. *Diss Abstr Int.* 1978;38:5013-4. (English) (unavailable at publication)

732
Gorzynski JG, Holland JC. **Psychological aspects of testicular cancer.** *Sem Oncol.* 1979;6:125-9. (English) (unavailable at publication)

733
Gorzynski JG, Lebovits A, Holland J, Vurgrin D. **Psychosexual risk factors in testicular cancer.** *Psychosom Med.* 1981;43:89-90. (English)

We have compared 51 consecutive patients with germ cell neoplasms of the testis (T), with 51 males with acute leukemia (L). Mean age was 30.0 (T), and 30.2 years (L), all were within one year of diagnosis and were undergoing chemotherapy. Identical psychosexual development histories and semistructured interviews (Current and Past Psychopathology Scales of Spitzer and Endicott), were used to generate 18 scales of past psychologic adjustment (prior to illness) and 8 scales of present adjustment (within the past month). Mean onset of puberty was 14.3 years in T patients and 12.7 in L patients ($p<0.0005$). Overt psychiatric illness had occurred prior to onset of cancer in 25% of T patients and 8% of L ($p<0.03$). On scales rating adolescent behavior, T patients had less interest and emotional involvement in social and heterosexual relationships ($p<0.001$), were higher on measures of dependency ($p<0.002$) and prior levels of emotional distress (depression-anxiety) ($p<0.02$). They had been less successful and had achieved less in school/work role ($p<0.02$). Cryptorchidism had been present in 14% of the T patients and 2% of L patients ($p<0.05$). Despite both groups of patients facing equally stressful treatment and threat to life, present psychologic adjustment of T patients showed greater disturbance than L patients in impulse control ($p<0.01$), depression-anxiety ($p<0.04$), somatic concerns ($p<0.0001$), and reality testing ($p<0.001$). Psychiatric diagnoses were generated from scale scores resulting in diagnosis of a major psychiatric disorder in 14% of T patients and only 2% of L patients ($p<0.05$) (leukemic patient with steroid psychosis). These data indicate that delayed puberty, diminished sexual interests, and significant psychiatric disturbance in adolescence are psychosexual risk factors, which, along with cryptorchidism, suggest the presence of a developmental abnormality in the hypothalamic-pituitary-gonadal axis which is associated with testicular cancer.

734
Greenberg RP, Dattore PJ. **The relationship between dependency and the development of cancer.** *Psychosom Med.* 1981;43:35-43. (English)

Theoretical speculations have raised the possibility that oral-dependent traits may predispose certain individuals to cancer. Alternatively, some have suggested that such traits are more broadly predictive of an array of illnesses. This study sought to test whether dependency characteristics predispose men to illness in general or cancer in particular or whether such characteristics have no particular effect on the development of illness. Comparisons were made of the premorbid MMPI records of 58 VA male domiciliary residents who later developed cancer with the records of 104 residents who either remained disease free or developed 1 of 3 other conditions (benign tumors, hypertension, or gastrointestinal ulcers). Scores on 8 scales, demonstrated to measure dependency-related characteristics, were derived for all subjects. Results showed that 4 dependency measures predicted the later occurrence of illness. However, none of the measures specifically differentiated cancer from the other illness conditions or the no-disease group. Thus, while findings suggest that dependency may predispose males to illness, no support was found for a specific link between dependency and cancer.

735
Greer S. **Psychological enquiry: a contribution to cancer research.** *Psychol Med.* 1979;9:81-9. (English)

A review of psychological contributions to cancer research is presented and a theoretical framework of heuristic value for such investigations is suggested. The author's study of women with breast cancer is described and methodological limitations are considered. There is evidence that psychological and psychobiological studies can make a useful contribution to cancer reseach, providing they are based on rigorous scientific methods.

736
Grossarth-Maticek R. **Psychosocial predictors of cancer and internal diseases: an overview.** *Psychother Psychosom.* 1980;33:122-8. (English)

In 1965, questionnaire data were obtained for 1,353 inhabitants of a Yugoslavian town on the following variables: blocked expression of feelings and needs; psychosocial stress in the form of either lasting depression or hopelessness or lasting anger and irritation; harmonization and idealization, with negation of self; rational orientation with repression of emotions; psychopathological symptoms; "explosive behavior," including exposure to adverse environmental conditions, abuse of medicines, etc., ignoring signs of illness, hyperactivity. These variables were related to the incidence of cancer and internal diseases over the next 10 years. A discriminant analysis yielded 93% correct predictions. The results, beyond their theoretical significance, open up substantive possibilities of early recognition as well as preventive and curative sociopsychotherapy of cancer and internal diseases.

737
Haney CA. **Illness behavior and psychosocial correlates of cancer.** *Soc Sci Med.* 1977;11:223-8. (English)

A recurrent theme in the literature on cancer is that which reports various psychosocial precursors. These factors have ranged from those which focus upon the personality of the individual to those which are associated with various life events such as death of a loved one or divorce. Numerous explanations and interpretations have been offered to account for these findings. It has been asserted that these factors operate through their influence on such processes and mechanisms as the limbic system, endocrine system, hormone levels or the central nervous system. The explanation offered here however is that these events can determine the extent to which one attends to his body, and the nature of an individual's illness behavior, that is the ways in which the individual perceives, evaluates and acts upon the messages and sensations of his body.

738
Headley DB. **Premorbid psychological factors of cancer.** *Biol Psychol Bull.* 1977;5:1-16. (English)

Research on personality and cancer focuses on three issues-- the psychological reactions to knowledge of cancer, psychological changes caused by the underlying malignancy, and the effects of certain personality traits and life styles on the development of cancer. This article reviews the literature on the premorbid psychological factors of cancer; two major areas are reviewed: personality profile theory (e.g., poor emotional outlet), and significant life events (e.g., object loss, denial of events). Although deficiencies in methodology are noted, the results are suggestive enough to warrant the premorbid personality to be considered as a risk factor acting within a multiplicative framework. The postulated psychophysiological mechanism of action involves relationships between emotions, hormones, and immunological systems.

739
Helsing KJ, Comstock GW. **Psychosocial characteristics and cytologic screening for cervical cancer.** *Preventive Med.* 1978;7:550-60. (English) (unavailable at publication)

740
Hughson AVM, Cooper AF. **Psychological aspects of breast cancer and its treatment.** *The Practitioner.* 1982; 226:1429-. (English) (unavailable at publication)

741
Jenner C. **The psyche of the stomach cancer patient: cancer-releasing agent--a carcinogenic development.** *Z Psychosom Med Psychoanal.* 1981;27:73-83. (German)

24 patients with stomach cancer underwent a series of psychoanalytical interviews and tests (TAT). The method consisted of an analysis of early childhood conditions, personality structure, object relationships, and the psychic causes for the cancer. Results show that the loss of one parent or an equivalent early loss was significantly more frequent in cancer patients than in the average population and that their predominant sibling position was the so-called "sandwich position." In regard to personality structure, a persisting false assimilation of inner conflicts presented itself as the essential item of premorbid structure. Other features responsible for the formation of the cancer were a persisting problem of separation (Oedipus conflicts), a resignation in an apathetic reaction (excessive demands), and an inability to release aggression in a normal way and against the appropriate target.

742
Kellerman J. **A note on psychosomatic factors in the etiology of neoplasms.** *J Consult Clin Psychol.* 1978; 46:1522-3. (English)

Watson and Schuld attempted to study the relationship between psychopathology and subsequent development of neoplasms. Their results, which indicated no apparent connections between these variables, are limited due to methodological flaws, both relating to sample selection. The study sample, composed of psychiatric patients, was highly restricted along one of the variables studied--psychopathology-- and was further confounded by uneven distribution of a potentially carcinogenic factor--alcoholism. Though there is no empirical evidence of psychological causation of neoplasms, the Watson and Schuld study is not one to lay this issue to rest.

743
Lickiss JN. **Psychosocial aspects of cancer.** *Med J Austr.* 1980;1:297-. (English) (unavailable at publication)

744
Marcus MG. **The shady link between cancer and character.** *Psychology Today.* 1976;85:52-9. (English) (unavailable at publication)

745
Margarey CJ, Todd PB, Blizard PJ. **Psycho-social factors influencing delay and breast self-examination in women with symptoms of breast cancer.** *Soc Sci Med.* 1977; 11:229-32. (English)

90 women who were to undergo biopsy of their breast were interviewed concerning their fears about breast symptoms and impending surgery and asked questions concerning the time of reporting their first symptom (length of delay) and their practice of breast examination. Later Ss were also given the Spielberger Anxiety Inventory, Millimet's Manifest Anxiety-Defensiveness Scale, and the D scale of the MMPI. Results show that one-quarter of the Ss had delayed more than 4 months in reporting symptoms and half had never examined their own breasts. It is suggested that their delay was determined by unconscious psychological processes, including the use of the ego defenses of denial and suppression, the nonuse of the defense of intellectualization-isolation, the absence of anxiety reported verbally, the presence of anxiety shown nonverbally, and the presence of depression reported verbally. Together, these accounted for nearly half (43.4%) of all the variance in delay. Conscious factors, including age, education, knowledge about cancer, and fear (of death, disease, or breast loss) were not related to the length of delay, nor to the practice of breast self-examination. Furthermore, the evidence suggests that the presence of malignancy was related to a low level of conscious anxiety before biopsy.

746
McCoy JW. **Psychological variables and onset of cancer.** *Diss Abstr Int.* 1978;38:4471. (English) (unavailable at publication)

747
Meares A. **Cancer, psychosomatic illness, and hysteria.** *Lancet.* 1981;2:1037-8. (English)

The onset of cancer is sometimes preceded by psychological reactions similar to those seen in psychosomatic illness and conversion hysteria. Some cancers have regressed after treatment similar to, but more intense than, that used in psychosomatic illness and conversion hysteria. It is suggested that psychological mechanisms resembling those of psychosomatic illness and conversion hysteria may cause some cases of cancer when acting in conjunction with the known chemical, viral, and radiational causes of the disease.

748

Morrison FR. **Psychosocial factors in the etiology of cancer.** *Diss Abstr Int.* 1981;42:155B. (English)

This prospective, epidemiologic study utilized observations on former university students in an attempt to identify psychological or physiological characteristics in youth predictive of site-specific and total cancers later in life. The investigation was undertaken to substantiate a hypothesis suggested by the work of various behavioral scientists over the last 30 years, that basic (ingrained) personality traits or characteristics precede and in some way cause cancer. The study utilized files maintained on approximately 15,000 men and women former students of the University of Pennsylvania. Data on "potential cause" was collected at college entrance in 1931-1940, 36 to 45 years in advance of "observed effect"--the development of or death from cancer. During the follow-up period, the files were updated by information collected by mail questionnaire and by information obtained from official death records for those who died. The results of this investigation provide no evidence that psychological characteristics measured in youth are predictive of *all* cancers later in life. No differences in response to 71 psychophysiological items were found among former students who died of cancer, those who died of other causes and those alive. Relative risks based on death rates calculated separately for those who answered "yes" and those who answered "no" to 15 psychological items, demonstrated no increased risk for those who died of cancer or those who died of any other cause in either men or women. Further, response to these psychological items was not associated with a significantly increased risk for those who died of lung or pancreatic cancer in men, and breast cancer in women. No elevated risk, based on response to the psychological items, was noted in men with colorectal cancer or women with breast cancer who were alive in 1976. Elevated risks were found only for 34 men who died of colorectal cancer. In this group of men, 12 or 13 relative risks were greater than 1.0, and 7 of the 12 positive values were greater than 2.0. Of the elevated relative risks, 5 were statistically significant and 1 remained significant even after adjustment of the p-value for the 141 comparisons made in this study. The pattern of responses in these decedents suggested a group of men who were tense, anxious, and self-conscious with a tendency to translate psychological states into somatic symptoms. Questions about digestive tract function showed no increased risk of cancer for those who responded "yes" in either decedents or those alive with colorectal cancer. The disparity in results for colorectal cancer decedents and those alive with the disease is disquieting, but it is possible that those already dead may constitute a substantially different subgroup among those who develop cancer of the colon or rectum. Study data suggest that decedents were younger when the disease developed and that they differed in attendance at professional schools. They might well have differed in tumor histopathology, location within the involved organ, genetic predisposition, or host resistance. Alternatively, the results obtained

might be due to chance. It is not possible in the context of this explanatory study to choose either alternative as the more probable. The results of this study cannot be accepted without verification on other data sets. Of the 141 relative risks calculated, 8 would be expected to be statistically significant at the 95% level of confidence used in this study, and 8 significant results were obtained. The concentration of 5 of the 8 significant results in the group of men who died of colorectal cancer argues that view but only further research can provide the answer.

749

Niemi T, Jaaskelainen J. **Cancer morbidity in depressive persons.** *J Psychosom Res.* 1978;22:117-20. (English)

Cancer morbidity of people who earlier had had depressive illness was evaluated employing the division into unipolar and bipolar depressions. The material comprised 191 patients who had been hospitalized between 1954-1956 and 1964-1966, of whom 143 belonged to the unipolar and 48 to the bipolar group. The study failed to indicate that depression increased cancer morbidity.

750

Paffenbarger RS, Wing AI, Hyde RT. **Brief communication: characteristics in youth indicative of adult-onset Hodgkin's disease.** *J Natl Cancer Inst.* 1977;58:1489-91. (English)

From the college entrance health data of 50,000 male former students, the records of 45 who eventually died of Hodgkin's disease were compared with those of 180 surviving classmates with reference to certain indicator characteristics. Risk ratios of Hodgkin's disease tended to be lower for men who had experienced various common contagious diseases in childhood. This reduced incidence of clinical contagions may signify that: 1)Inadequate early challenge of immune mechanisms left subjects more susceptible to later Hodgkin's disease, whether or not it is of infectious origin; 2) heightened immune mechanisms that led to subclinical attacks of early contagious diseases promoted an autoimmune response that evolved as Hodgkin's disease; or 3) early childhood infections eliminated some subjects who otherwise would have attended college and ultimately developed adult-onset Hodgkin's disease. Also, Hodgkin's disease risk was higher for students who had reported early death of a parent, particularly from cancer. Moreover, the risk tended to be increased among collegians who were obese, heavy cigarette smokers, and coffee drinkers. None of these indicator characteristics was associated with 89 fatal lymphomas of other types that occurred in the same study population.

751

Pettingale KW, Philalithis A, Tee DE, Greer HS. **The biological correlates of psychological responses to breast cancer.** *J Psychosom Res.* 1981;25:453-8. (English)

A prospective, multidisciplinary, 5 year study of 69 consecutive women with early breast cancer was conducted. Patients' psychological responses to the diagnosis were assessed 3 months postoperatively and correlated with various histological, mammographic, hormonal and immunological investigations performed pre-operatively and at 3 months post-operatively. There was no statistically significant association between the type of psychological response and any of the biological measures studied pre-operatively. There is, therefore, no evidence that biological factors have biased the composition of the groups and accounted for observed differences in outcome. Serum levels of IgM, performed 3 months post-operatively, however, were significantly higher in patients who showed denial compared to those who responded with fighting spirit ($p<0.02$) or stoic acceptance ($p<0.02$). Also patients who showed fighting spirit had significantly lower serum levels of IgG than those who showed stoic acceptance ($p<0.025$). The mechanisms by which such immunoglobulin changes could influence survival in cancer remain hypothetical. A greater understanding of the neuroendocrine control of the immune system and much more sophisticated measurements will be needed to elucidate such mechanisms.

752
Pinderis GM. **Selected personality variables as contributing factors in cancer development.** *Diss Abstr Int.* 1982;42:3403. (English) (unavailable at publication)

753
Rassidakis NC, et al. **A contribution to the study of the personality of cancer patients: a preliminary report.** *Transnat Ment Health Res Newsletter.* 1978;20:10-12. (English) (no abstract)

754
Richter HE. **Psychological factors and cancer.** *Med Welt.* 1981;32:177-84. (German) (unavailable at publication)

755
Scurry MT, Levin EM. **Psychosocial factors related to the incidence of cancer.** *Int J Psychiatry Med.* 1978-79;9:159-77. (English)

The recent data concerning the relationship between psychosocial factors and the incidence of cancer have been reviewed covering life events, personality factors, psychiatric diagnoses, and loss-separation-hopelessness. The multiple methodological and design problems in this area of investigation are the factors that stand out and make interpretation difficult. Nevertheless, an association between oncogenesis and a number of factors such as extroversion, neuroticism, and lack of closeness to family is suggested. Many studies raise additional questions without providing definitive answers. A long-term prospective study which has been designed to look at cancer outcome and multiple psychosocial factors is needed to determine if such factors add to the risk of oncogenesis.

756
Seth M, Saksena NK. **Personality characteristics of lung cancer patients.** *Indian J Clin Psychol.* 1978;5:43-8. (English)

Compared the 16 PF results of 25 50-75 year old male lung cancer patients to those of 50 normal Ss who had not suffered from any ailment during the past year. Both groups were matched in terms of age, sex, and socioeconomic status. Factor B (Less intelligent versus more intelligent) was not taken into consideration. Results show that the cancer

patients differed significantly from controls in all but the following 4 factors: practical vs imaginative, forthright vs shrewd, group-dependent vs self-sufficiency, and undisciplined vs controlled. Cancer patients' sten norms were significantly lower than the general population on 5 factors, and controls were significantly lower on 3 factors.

757
Seth M, Saksena NK. **Personality differences between male and female cancer patients.** *Indian J Clin Psychol.* 1978;5:155-60. (English)

Administered the 16 PF to 50 male and 50 female cancer patients. The 2 groups differed significantly on 8 factors of the 16 PF. Female patients were emotionally less stable, more sober, more expedient, more tenderminded, more suspicious, more forthright, and more tense than their male counterparts.

758
Seth M, Saksena NK. **Personality of patients suffering from cancer, cardiovascular disorders, tuberculosis and minor ailments.** *Indian J Clin Psychol.* 1977;4:135-40. (English)

200 patients were matched with 400 normal Ss on age, sex, education, and socioeconomic status. All Ss were administered the Hindi version of the 16 PF. These 16 factors can also be scored for 4 broad 2nd-order personality factors: Factor I (Adjustment vs Anxiety), Factor II (Introversion vs Extraversion), Factor III (Tender-Minded Emotionality vs Alert Poise), and Factor IV (Subduedness vs Independence). Results reveal that cancer patients were significantly different from their controls on Factors I, II, and III, but not on Factor IV; from the tuberculosis patients on Factors I, II and IV but not on Factor III; and from the cardiovascular patients on Factors I, II, III, and IV. The clinical group of patients suffering from minor ailments did not differ significantly from their normal counterparts on any of the 2nd-order personality factors.

759
Shanfield SB. **On surviving cancer: psychological considerations.** *Compr Psychiatry.* 1980;21:128-34. (English) (unavailable at publication)

760
Sheehan TF. **Breast cancer and personality.** *Diss Abstr Int.* 1978;38:3908. (English) (unavailable at publication)

761
Spinetta JJ. **Behavioral and psychological research in childhood cancer: an overview.** *Cancer.* 1982;50:1939-43. (English) (unavailable at publication)

762
Stoll BA. **Psycho-physiologic aspects of breast cancer.** *Eur J Cancer.* 1980;1:221-2. (English)

A correlation has been suggested between the rate of growth of breast cancer on the one hand, and personality, emotional stress or affective disorders in the patient, on the other. Endocrine mechanisms could be involved in such a relationship and the hypothalamus may mediate it. Long continued stress could lead to high circulating levels of prolactin, growth hormone, thyrotropin, oestrogen and corticosteroids, some of which might affect the growth of breast cancer. There have been reports suggesting that the prognosis may be worse in breast cancer patients who are overanxious. It is possible that mental factors could activate the tumour or else that the toxic effects of a more active tumour could cause specific mental effects. There are also firm clinical impressions that giving up can shorten a patient's life expectancy, that optimism will improve the quality of life and that faith can cause placebo effects. None of these benefits need necessarily involve an effect on tumour growth, and the fact that a mechanism can be postulated for an effect by stress on tumour growth, does not prove that it occurs.

763
Veilleux F, Villard HP. **Cancer: A psychosomatic disease?** *Union Med Can.* 1981;110:159-69. (French)

Cancer is indeed a psychosomatic disorder if one considers the human being as a psychosomatic entity. There should not be any more attempts to reach a "scientific proof" of an etiological relationship since psychology and biology pertain to entirely different worlds. It is an everyday experience for every one that there are mutual influences. Many authors are still involved in the task of "comprehending" these influences on all kinds of diseases, cancer included.

764
Verns GP. **Psychological differences associated with primary location of cancer in women.** *Diss Abstr Int.* 1981;42:1224-5. (English) (unavailable at publication)

765
Voth HM. **Cancer and personality.** *Percept Mot Skills.* 1976;42:1131-7. (English)

Autokinesis (the apparent motion of a pinpoint of light in total darkness) been predictably related to a variety of personality variables and psychiatric syndromes. The present study reports a statistically significant relationship between cancer and autokinesis in 2 samples. The 1st sample of 17 females and 14 males was prospective, while the 2nd, with 26 females, was retrospective. In both samples, cancer Ss reported less autokinesis than controls, a finding which fits conceptually with prior work with autokinesis and also with the observation by many others that cancer is preceded by or associated with a sense of helplessness or hopelessness and some degree of resignation from life. A 2nd finding, but one which has not been replicated, showed that there was a statistically significant relationship between scores on the Embedded-Figures Test and cancer.

766
Watson CG, Schuld D. **Psychosomatic etiological factors in neoplasms: a response to Kellerman.** *J Consult Clin Psychol.* 1978;46:1524-5. (English)

Kellerman argues that our use of psychiatric patients in a study designed to search for psychosomatic etiological factors in neoplasms may have led to our negative results. However, we suggest that the use of psychiatric patients increased the heterogeneity of the sample and probably enhanced, not limited, the likelihood of positive findings. He also suggests that our inclusion of alcoholics in the study may have masked real differences between neoplasm and control subjects. However, new analyses run on subsets of our malignancy and malignancy-control samples from which alcoholics were first deleted failed to support his contention. New analyses run to test for differences between the frequencies of various high-scale Minnesota Multiphasic Personality Inventory types in neoplasm and control groups also failed to support the view that neoplasm patients are qualitatively different from controls on the inventory.

767
Watson CG, Schuld D. **Psychosomatic factors in the etiology of neoplasms.** *J Consult Clin Psychol.* 1977;45:455-561. (English)

Several psychogenic theories have been developed to explain the onset of cancer. Much of the research used to support them suffers from methodological weaknesses, particularly the absence of control groups and/or the use of criterion samples already suffering from malignancies. In the present study, the psychiatric diagnoses and Minnesota Multiphasic Personality Inventory (MMPI) performances of psychiatric patients who later developed malignant and benign neoplasms were compared to controls. No differences (beyond a chance level) appeared in the diagnostic composition, the MMPI clinical scale scores, or the individual MMPI-item performances of the groups. The results do not offer support for the major psychogenic-origin theories of the development of neoplasms.

768
Weinstock C. **Recent progress in cancer psychobiology and psychiatry.** *J Am Soc Psychosom Dent Med.* 1977; 24:4-14. (English)

Recent events in the fields of psychosomatic research and treatment (which are very much alive and progressing) are discussed. The chief areas of evidence are as follows: "spontaneous" regressions of cancer are frequent, and invariably when investigated show one of four favorable psychic processes having the common denominator of hope to have just preceded the shrinkage. (The most usual process is a basic favorable change in the psychosocial situation.) There are vertebrate oncology experiments demonstrating the linkage of an active, flexible cerebral cortex to adequate immune defenses against cancer. There is evidence pointing to the ubiquitousness of aborted or avoided grief and profound depression long before cancer, and of the partial somatization of the depression. There is striking regularity of organ specificity in terms of earlier loss, especially in carcinoma and sarcoma. ECT and insulin coma appear quite regularly to bring approximately simultaneous marked beneficial effects on the patients' depression and cancer. Preliminary formulations for a psychotherapeutic approach are outlined. The early findings of the Psychosomatic Cancer Study Group are described.

Personality and autoimmune diseases

769
Camerlain M, Myhal D. **Psychosomatic medicine and rheumatoid arthritis.** *Union Med Can.* 1979;108:289-92. (English)

The authors describe the various theories on the psychosomatic approach to rheumatoid arthritis. They reject the concept of a rheumatoid personality. A new holistic conception of the disease is proposed that should have a direct impact on the therapeutic approach of the patient.

770
Erwin WJ, Granacher RP Jr. **New behavioral data concerning the autoerythrocyte sensitization syndrome.** *South Med J.* 1977;70:876-8. (English)

A typical case of autoerythrocyte sensitization or the Gardner-Diamond syndrome as reviewed with respect to personality factors, hypnotic factors, hypnotic influence in general, the effect of controlled hypnosis under two variable conditions, and the measurement of certain psychophysiologic responses before and following hypnosis. In this case it was not possible to delineate a clear psychiatric syndrome and hypnotic suggestion induced the classical lesion only during the active phase of the disease. When the lesions were absent or quiescent, no changes in various psychophysiologic measurements taken were observed.

771
Gardiner BM. **Psychological aspects of rheumatoid arthritis.** *Psychol Med.* 1980;10:159-63. (English)

This study had 3 aims: to determine whether rheumatoid arthritics had certain personality traits; to examine the relationship between psychological factors and the presence of rheumatoid factor in blood serum; and to explore the prognostic significance of psychological factors in the management of rheumatoid arthritis. Within a few days of discharge, 129 in-patient rheumatoid arthritics were clinically and psychologically assessed and allocated at random to 1 of 3 forms of follow-up care. The psychological assessment included measures of personality, non-psychotic psychiatric disturbance, and attitudes and beliefs. A year later all patients were reassessed. It was found that rheumatoid arthritics were more neurotic in personality, more likely to give socially desirable responses, and more prone to psychiatric disturbance, than the general population. Seropositive patients were less susceptible to psychiatric disturbance than seronegative patients. None of the psychological variables predicted disease activity, but those patients who rated themselves as "slow, dependent, and weak" lost more time off work in the subsequent year.

772
Hanna WT, Fitzpatrick R, Krauss S, Machado E, Dunn CD. **Psychogenic purpura (autoerythrocyte sensitization).** *South Med J.* 1981;74:538-42. (English)

A 41-year-old woman has had a long history of repeated episodes of recurrent painful ecchymotic lesions. Results of coagulation tests were normal other than a slight decrease in antithrombin III. Skin tests were positive in response to the patient's own washed red cells. Light and electron microscopy of both the spontaneous and the induced lesions showed nonspecific changes but failed to reveal immunologic vasculitis. Psychologic evaluation showed hysterical and masochistic traits, depression, anxiety, and inability to deal appropriately with hostile impulses. Placebo was successful on several occasions in controlling or modifying the severity of the ecchymotic lesions.

773
Kammerer W, Reindell A. **Psychosomatic aspects of diabetes mellitus.** *Z Psychosom Med Psychoanal.* 1977;23:351-62. (German)

Based on the evidence of the available literature, we consider an exact differentiation between the elderly diabetic and the young diabetic--aside from the other classification possibilities--to be indispensable, not only for the diagnostics but also the therapy, especially the accompanying psychotherapy. In both types of diabetes, the emotionally vulnerable state of insecurity has a special pathoplastic meaning, whereas an unequivocal psychogenic cause does not seem to be apparent. Personality changes due to the disease vary not only in accordance to the severity of the illness and the difficulties involved in the application of the therapeutic measures, but also as a result of considerable differences in their cognitive, emotional, and physiological condition at the onset of the disease. Yet it appears improbable that a certain type of personality structures indicated a predetermined susceptibility to diabetes since personality traits can never be separated from the reaction to the illness. Rather, the necessity of a differentiated psychotherapy suited to the individual idiosyncrasies must be emphasized. Further studies, increasingly taking the social and familial context into consideration, will have to elucidate this approach. The abundant conditions leading to obesity apply as well to the adult diabetic. All told, there exists a preponderance for a depressed attitude in conjunction with a parasympathetic fundamental tension which enables the individual to accept the illness as fate. On the other hand, the juvenile diabetic very quickly loses for the most part his ability to produce body insulin and thereby falls into a chronic state of emergency. A sympathetic fundamental tension leads to an intense fight for independence manifested in rebellious resistance and paranoid projections.

774
Meister MM, Bodner AC. **Autoerythrocyte sensitization: a psychogenic purpura.** *Cutis.* 1977;19:221-4. (English)

There are two schools of thought regarding the pathogenesis of this syndrome. Gardner and Diamond and others demonstrated that these patients have a hypersensitivity to extravasated RBC's. They assumed that a fixed tissue antibody reacted with red blood cell stroma producing edema, increased capillary permeability, and further extravasation of blood into the tissues. Ratnoff, Agle, and others, however, believe the syndrome is a psychiatric disorder and that the ecchymotic lesions represent a form of conversion reaction--a mechanism that could explain the patient's myriad complaints. There is evidence that vascular beds are controlled by psychic processes. Neurogenically elaborated kinin-like agents might serve as humoral mediators between the central nervous system and the local tissue reaction. Regardless of the basic etiology, we think the syndrome is more common than has previously been considered and should be thought of in patients with recurrent purpuric eruptions of the extremities.

775
Radvila A, Eisenberg S, Nadel C, Schoenfeld M, Rechsman F. **Personality characteristics, affects and stressful life events in Graves' disease** (abstract). *Psychosom Med.* 1980;42:74. (English)

Personality and social features specific for Graves' disease were described by Alexander and others. Anecdotally stressful life events were reported to trigger its onset. In addition to testing these findings we hypothesized that these patients display affects, namely higher basal levels of anxiety (= trait anxiety) and of depression, which might increase their susceptibility to developing Graves' disease. We studied 37 patients, who had been treated successfully for Graves' disease and then were euthyroid for at least one year. Euthyroid patients with nodular goiter, matched for sex, age and duration of disease served as controls. Each patient was evaluated by means of a semi-structured interview, of the State-Trait-Anxiety Inventory (STAI), of the Multiple Affect Adjective Checklist (MAACL) and the Social Readjustment Rating Questionnaire (SRRQ). None of Alexander's characteristics showed a statistically significant difference between the two groups. In the STAI the post Graves' disease patients had a significantly higher ($p<0.05$) mean trait anxiety score (44.8 ± 7.1) than the controls (36.3 ± 6.9). In the MAACL and interview ratings the difference in the mean anxiety and depression scores only approached statistical significance ($p<0.075$). The patients with Graves' disease, for the period of 1 year preceding onset of illness, scored higher life change units on the SRRQ than the control group (189 ± 67 vs 107 ± 50, $p<0.05$). Our findings do not support Alexander's specificity theory for Graves' disease. They rather suggest that a chronic high anxiety proneness could be a psychophysiological predisposing factor in the pathogenesis of Graves' disease and that stressful life events indeed influence its onset.

776
Ratnoff OD. **The psychogenic purpuras: a review of autoerythrocyte sensitization, autosensitization to DNA, "hysterical" and factitial bleeding, and the religious stigmata.** *Semin Hematol.* 1980;17:192-213. (English) (no abstract)

777
Spalter L, On A, Ben-Assuly S. **Autoerythrocytotic sensitization in psychogenic purpura.** *Harefuah.* 1980;99:435-6. (Hebrew) (unavailable at publication)

Personality and allergic disorders

778
Agarwal K, Sethi JP. **A study of psychogenic factors in bronchial asthma.** *J Asthma Res.* 1978;15:191-8. (English)

A study of psychogenic factors in asthma was accomplished in 46 cases which included 10 normals, 20 asthmatics, 10 cases of allergy other than asthma, and 6 siblings of asthmatics. Apart from history, physical examination, general and special laboratory tests and special allergy tests, a battery of psychological tests was given which included IPAT's Neuroticism Scale, IPAT's Anxiety Scale, Sentence Completion Test, and IPAT's Sixteen Personality Factors Test. On the Sixteen Personality Factors Test, asthma subjects scored low on factor C (emotionally less stable) and factor F (sober, serious), and scored high on factor Q4 (tense, frustrated) as compared with normals. Allergic subjects were almost identical with asthmatic subjects except they in addition scored higher on factor I (tender-minded, dependent) than normals and siblings of asthma subjects. On the Neuroticism Scale a statistical difference was observed between normals and asthmatics and between normals and allergic subjects ($p<0.001$). Asthmatic subjects revealed high anxiety levels as compared with normals ($p<0.01$). No statistically significant difference was obtained between allergic subjects and normals. On the Sentence Completion Test, 70% of asthmatics and 60% of allergic subjects showed a disturbed attitude while only 20% of normals showed disturbance. Disturbance in attitude included disturbed attitude towards father, disturbed attitude towards heterosexual relationships, and disturbed attitude towards own abilities.

779
Ago Y, Teshima H, Nagata S, Inoue S, Ikemi Y. **Psychosomatic studies of allergic disorders.** *Psychother Psychosom.* 1979;31:197-204. (English)

It is generally conceded that allergic disorders occur in individuals who have a hereditary or congenital allergic constitution. Clinical symptoms of allergic disorders, however, often disappear due to changes of the individual's life situations and/or their adaptive patterns. In a comparative study of allergic predisposition in students with allergic disorder (asthmatics) and students who had become completely free from childhood asthma for more than 3 years, without specific treatment, there was no significant difference in allergic predisposition between the two groups. The same tendency was also found between adult patients with allergic disorder (asthmatics) and persons who had shown complete remission for more than 3 years, having had psychosomatic treatment. These findings suggest that allergic predisposition does not influence the prognosis of allergic disorders as much as do socio-psychological factors. It is thought that the effect of psychosomatic treatment reconditions these socio-psychological factors which disturb homeostatic balance and which facilitate the clinical manifestation based on the allergic predisposition.

780
Ahmar H, Kurban AK. **Psychological profile of patients with atopic dermatitis.** *Br J Dermatol.* 1976;95:373-7. (English)

Tests designed to measure psychopathological characteristics common to the neurotic population were administered to patients with atopic dermatitis, patients with other dermatological disorders and to a control group of normal individuals. The parameters tested were manifest anxiety, neurosis, extroversion, depression, hypochondriasis and hysteria. The scores were statistically analyzed. The results showed that the patients with atopic dermatitis responded significantly differently from patients with other dermatological diseases and from the control group in specific psychometric scales. Moreover, patients with skin conditions other than atopic dermatitis also responded significantly differently from the control group. The study clearly shows that patients with atopic dermatitis have a characteristic psychological profile not shared by the other two groups. The atopic dermatitis patients tend to be in a state of high manifest anxiety, depressed, neurotic and hypochondriac.

781
Benjamin S. **Is asthma a psychosomatic illness? I--A retrospective study of mental illness and social adjustment.** *J Psychosom Res.* 1977;21:463-9. (English)

A group of 53 asthmatics and 50 matched controls together with their first-degree relatives has been followed up retrospectively after an interval of 15 years. There was no evidence that the mental illness experienced by the asthma group differed significantly from that of controls during the follow up period either in period prevalence or diagnosis. The presence of mental illness amongst asthmatics was not related to the prognosis for asthma, nor to the age of onset, family history of asthma or other atopic conditions. The asthma group showed only slightly greater impairment in social adjustment than controls. These findings are discussed in the light of traditional views of asthma as a psychosomatic illness.

782
Benjamin S. **Is asthma a psychosomatic illness? II--A comparative study of respiratory impairment and mental health.** *J Psychosom Res.* 1977;21:471-81. (English)

The respiratory state and mental health of a group of 47 asthmatics and 43 matched non-asthmatic controls have been compared using standardised interview and respiratory function assessments. Despite physical impairment the asthma group failed to show any significant excess in point prevalence, or any difference in the diagnostic categories of mental illness suffered. There was a tendency for more positive ratings for psychopathology to be made for the asthma group but this was not related to greater physiological impairment. It is suggested that this trend arises mainly due to overreporting of symptoms of all kinds by some members of the asthma group. These results are considered in the light of similar findings in others with respiratory disorder. The importance of bias arising from selection of subjects in research into somatic and psychic relationships is emphasised and the implications for clinical management are discussed.

783
Berger D, Maack N, Nolte D. **Personality-structure in different kinds of bronchial asthma** (author's transl.). *Med Klin.* 1979;74:15-20. (German)

The "Giessen-test" is a psychological test in form of a questionnaire, basing on self-assessment. It was applied in 63 patients with bronchial asthma in order to get their "self-images" and their "ideal self-images". Except for higher values for depression the "self-images" of the asthmatics resembled

very closely those of normals. The ideals ("ideal-self-image") of the patients were uncharacteristic and reflected general trends. In contrast to these findings eleven physicians had a negative conception of asthmatic patients ("foreign image"). Physicians assessed the asthmatics to be disliked ("negative social resonant"), obstinate ("dominant") and depressive. Patients with high exogen-allergic asthma, intrinsic asthma and asthma of unknown origin differ from each other only within a few marks. These differences, however, are not sufficient, to allow to coordinate a specific personality-structure with one of the different kinds of asthma.

784
Byrne DG, Murrell TG. **Self descriptions of mothers of asthmatic children.** *Aust NZ J Psychiatry.* 1977;11:179-83. (English) (no abstract)

785
Chang BH. **Selected psychological and somatic variables in asthmatic children.** *Diss Abstr Int.* 1976;36:5783-4. (English) (unavailable at publication)

786
Chobotova Z. **Psychological factors in asthma.** *Psychol Patopsychol Dietata.* 1980;15:421-31. (Czech)

Discusses psychological factors related to bronchial asthma, especially in childhood. Recent findings from domestic and foreign literature are presented and the author discusses her experiences at a medical institution for asthmatic children.

787
Cornia G, Cornia C, Lorenzini R, Giammarruto R, Siani V, Mariotta S, Pasqua F. **Asthma as a psychosomatic disease and its treatment with tranquilizing agents.** *Minerva Med.* 1977;68:29-32. (Italian)

On the basis of personal research and experience, it is concluded that the majority of asthmatics also suffer from psychoneurosis and that psychological alterations are primary and not secondary to dyspnoea. Some hypotheses are put forward relating the onset of asthma and psychoneurosis.

788
Coyas A, Stavrou J, Antonakopoulos C. **Vasomotor rhinitis: Psychosomatic conditions and treatment.** *Rhinology.* 1976;14:177-80. (English)

The importance of the autonomic nervous system in vasomotor conditions of the nose was outlined. The symptoms, findings and differential diagnosis of the vasomotor rhinitis were reviewed. Reference is made to the applied treatment and results obtained with different antihistaminics in 2150 patients.

789
Czubalski K, Rudzki E. **Neuropsychic factors in physical urticaria.** *Dermatologica.* 1977;154:1-4. (English)

Psychosomatic investigations were made in 18 patients with dermographism, 17 with cold urticaria, and 13 with cholinergic urticaria. The Maudsley Personality Inventory was used and electroencephalograms were recorded from most patients. In the majority of cases of dermographism first symptoms coincided with frustrating situations and psychic stress-intensified manifestations. 81.8% of the patients with dermographism had abnormal electroencephalograms. In cold urticaria the role of psychic factors could not be demonstrated, whereas in cholinergic urticaria "brief" emotions provoked symptoms in three-quarters of the patients, although no other signs of the role of psychic factors were detected.

790

Dahlem NW, Kinsman RA, Horton DJ. **Panic-fear in asthma: Requests for as-needed medications in relation to pulmonary function measurements.** *J Allergy Clin Immunol.* 1977;60:295-300. (English)

Requests for as-needed medications and treatments (PRN's) by asthmatic patients scoring high, moderate, or low on the asthma symptom checklist panic-fear category were studied for days when patients were matched at normal, intermediate, and subnormal levels of pulmonary function. Low panic-fear patients were the least likely to request PRN's regardless of the pulmonary function level. In contrast, high panic-fear patients often requested PRN's at each level of pulmonary function. Only moderate panic-fear patients made progressively more PRN requests on days when pulmonary functions were lower. These observations and others concerning the adverse influence of extreme panic-fear coping styles upon the treatment of asthma were discussed.

791

Dahlem NW, Kinsman RA. **Panic-fear in asthma: a divergence between subjective report and behavioral patterns.** *Percept Mot Skills.* 1978;46:95-8. (English)

The reported frequency of occurrence of panic-fear symptoms during asthmatic attacks varies widely and is related to treatment response independently of the objective severity of asthma. In a previous study, symptom minimizers (low panic-fear) requested few as-needed (PRN) medications and treatments while hospitalized, even on days when significant airway obstruction was present. In contrast symptom emphasizers (high panic-fear) requested PRN's frequently, even on days when no airway obstruction was present. In the present study, these behavioral differences towards PRN's occurred despite the similar ability of patients in various panic-fear groups to perceive and report changes in airway obstruction. Together these results suggest that specific behavioral strategies, which do not derive from differences in symptom perception, influence the treatment response of asthmatic patients differing in panic-fear symptomatology.

792

Davis JB. **Neurotic illness in the families of children with asthma and wheezy bronchitis: a general practice population study.** *Psychol Med.* 1977;7:305-10. (English)

In a controlled population study 111 families of children with asthma and wheezy bronchitis were screened. The mothers of asthmatics suffered more depressive illness than controls. This correlates with the severity of the child's asthma. There was no difference in immunological status between depressive and non-depressive mothers of asthmatics.

793

Dirks JF, Fross KH, Evans NW. **Panic-fear in asthma: generalized personality trait vs specific situational state.** *J Asthma Res.* 1977;14:161-7. (English)

Previous studies have found that both ASC and MMPI panic-fear scale scores are related to the maintenance of the medical intractability of asthma. Despite the large overlap of these two scales, they measure somewhat different aspects of "panic-fear." The ASC measures a situational response (state variable) to breathing difficulties, while the MMPI measures a more stable, diffuse, and global personality characteristic (trait variable). The present study analyzes the relationship between these state and trait variables as they relate to the intensity of prescribed discharge medication. The results indicate that it is the trait variable which is more important in the maintenance of the medical intractability of asthma. The state variable is implicated in maintaining the illness only to the extent that it is a specific manifestation of the trait variable.

794

Dirks JF, Fross KH, Paley A. **Panic-fear in asthma: state-trait relationship and rehospitalization.** *J Chronic Dis.* 1978;31:605-9. (English)

Both the MMPI Panic-Fear scale (personality trait) and the ASC Panic-Fear symptom category (situational, state response to breathing difficulties) have shown important relationships to various medical outcome measures in chronic asthma. This paper furthers previous findings by investigating panic-fear state-trait relationships in terms of rehospitalization of asthmatics following intensive long-term treatment. Results indicate that the two measures of panic-fear interact in predicting important differences in rehospitalization rates.

795

Dirks JF, Jones NF, Fross KH. **Psychosexual aspects of the panic-fear personality types in asthma.** *Can J Psychiatry.* 1979;24:731-9. (English)

Numerous earlier studies have demonstrated the close relationship between MMPI panic-fear categories and various medical outcome measures in asthma. The present study relates MMPI panic-fear categories to psychosexual development. Specifically, high panic-fear patients demonstrate oral preoccupations, low panic-fear patients demonstrate anal preoccupations, while moderate panic-fear patients do not demonstrate pre-oedipal preoccupations. Thus, MMPI panic-fear categories, useful in predicting medical outcome measures, have now been related to developmental levels, with the explanatory power of developmental concepts as well as their implications for psychological treatment.

796

Dirks JF, Jones NF, Kinsman RA. **Panic-fear: a personality dimension related to intractability in asthma.** *Psychosom Med.* 1977;39:120-6. (English)

A 15-item MMPI scale has been developed that relates to the reported frequency of panic-fear symptoms on the Asthma Symptom Checklist (ASC). High scale scores describe fearful, emotionally labile individuals who profess to be more sensitive than others and unable or disinclined to persist in the face of difficulty. The relationship between the MMPI panic-fear scale and the ASC panic-fear symptoms is highly replicable and related to a crucial aspect of chronicity in asthma. High scoring asthmatic patients were prescribed more intensive discharge steroid regimens upon completion of residential treatment. This relationship was not mediated by available objective pulmonary function measurements used to index medical condition. Development of the MMPI panic-fear scale should enable further investigation of personality and behavioral aspects related to the perceived severity and intractability of other medical conditions and disabilities.

797

Dirks JF, Keliger JH, Evans NW. **ASC Panic-Fear and length of hospitalization in asthma.** *J Asthma Res.* 1978;15:95-7. (English)

A prior study has demonstrated the relationship between MMPI Panic-Fear scores and length of hospitalization in several respiratiory iullness groups, including asthma. *Mycobacterium tuberculosis, Mycobacterium intracellulare-avium,* and *Mycobacterium kansasii.* In general, MMPI Panic-Fear scores related linearly to length of hospitalization, with High MMPI Panic-Fear patients being hospitalized the longest and Low MMPI Panic-Fear patients being hospitalized the shortest length of time. These findings were found to be independent of pulmonary function measurements in asthma and of bacteriological type and drug resistance in tuberculosis. As the MMPI Panic-Fear scale was empirically derived from the Asthma Symptom Checklist (ASC) Panic-Fear cluster, it would appear reasonable to assume that ASC Panic-Fear scores would also relate to length of hospitalization in asthma. However, recent studies have found important differences between these two scales. Conceptually, MMPI Panic-Fear measures a personality trait associated with the reported frequency of subjective symptoms accompanying asthmatic attacks as feeling scared, panicky, worried, and frightened, while ASC Panic-Fear directly measures these subjective symptoms. A later formulation notes that ASC Panic-Fear defines a specific, situational Panic-Fear response to breathing difficulties experienced during an asthma attack, while MMPI Panic-Fear defines a personality trait which taps a general, diffuse anxiety. More recently, ASC Panic-Fear has been referred to as vigilance or signal anxiety about asthmatic attacks, while MMPI Panic-Fear assesses the patient's ego controls for dealing with that signal anxiety. Empirical findings suggest that ASC and MMPI Panic-Fear do not always relate in the same manner to either intensity of prescribed oral corticosteroids or to rehospitalization rates. Indeed, the best predictors of treatment outcome appear to be found in the interactions between ASC and MMPI Panic-Fear scores. Given the above, it was decided to investigate the relationship between ASC Panic-Fear scores and length of hospitalization for asthmatic patients in intensive long-term treatment.

798

Dirks JF, Kinsman RA, Horton DJ, Fross KH, Jones NF. **Panic-fear in asthma: rehospitalization following intensive long-term treatment.** *Psychosom Med.* 1978;40:5-13. (English)

The panic-fear personality scale related to rehospitalization rates of asthmatics during two successive 6-month periods following intensive long-term treatment. High and low panic-fear patients were nearly twice as likely as moderates to be rehospitalized. Neither longitudinal pulmonary function measurements, physicians' judgments about the medical severity of the asthma during treatment, nor the presence or absence of maintenance oral corticosteroids at discharge were related to rehospitalization. The available information suggests that high panic-fear patients react to asthma with symptom exaggeration and helplessness, while low panic-fear patients employ an equally maladaptive strategy best characterized as symptom minimization and denial. It is possible that both of these extreme response styles may affect adherence to prescribed medical regimens and are equally detrimental as indicated by rehospitalization following intensive long-term treatment.

799

Dirks JF, Kinsman RA, Jones NF, Fross KH. **New developments in panic-fear research in asthma: validity and stability of the MMPI Panic-Fear scale.** *Br J Med Psychol.* 1978;51:119-26. (English)

An earlier study (Dirks et al., 1977) described the development of a 15-item Minnesota Muliphasic Personality Inventory (MMPI) panic-fear scale relating to the reported frequency of panic-fear symptoms on the Asthma Symptom Checklist (ASC). High MMPI panic-fear scale scores describe fearful, highly emotional individuals who profess to have their feelings hurt more easily than others, to feel helpless and to give up easily in the face of difficulty. High scoring asthmatic patients were prescribed more intensive steroid regiments at discharge from a residential treatment facility months after psychological testing (Dirks et al., 1977) and required longer periods of hospitalization while in residential treatment (Dirks et al., 1976). These relationships were not attributable to differences in longitudinal pulmonary function measures during hospitalization. Consistent with earlier findings, the MMPI panic-fear scale was again shown to be significantly related to both ASC panic-fear scores and to recommended discharge steroid regiments for an enlarged sample of patients. Additionally, MMPI panic-fear scores were shown to be stable from admission to discharge despite two to four months of intervening medical treatment and to be independent both of age of asthma onset and longitudinal pulmonary function measures during treatment. These results suggest that the MMPI panic-fear scale measures a personality dimension which should be regarded as a stable character trait, unaffected by severity or duration of asthma or by intervening medical treatment for asthma. As such, MMPI panic-fear is not merely a product of the medical condition. Instead, it appears to be a consistent component of the patient's personality which influences medical intractability in asthma probably via associated behaviours, symptom reports, and attitudes during medical treatment. These considerations invite further inquiry.

800

Dirks JF, Kinsman RA, Staudenmayer H, Kleiger JH. **Panic-fear in asthma: symptomatology as an index of signal anxiety and personality as an index of ego**

resources. *J Nerv Ment Dis.* 1979;167:615-9. (English)

Clinical observations and studies of asthmatic patients have often concluded that there is a strong relationship between the degree of the patient's anxiety and the medical intractability of his illness. However, psychotherapeutic interventions designed to alleviate patient anxiety have been noticeably inconsistent in achieving meaningful alleviation of the patient's asthma. The present paper addresses this apparent paradox by positing the existence of two types of anxiety: a) asthma-specific anxiety, as indexed by panic-fear symptomatology scores of the Asthma Symptom Checklist; and b) characterological and pervasive anxiety, as indexed by panic-fear personality scores of the Minnesota Multiphasic Personality Inventory. In this study, long term medical outcome was found to be influenced by the combination of these types of anxiety. When high asthma-specific anxiety coexisted with high characterological anxiety, medical outcome following intensive long term medical treatment was exceptionally poor. In contrast, when high asthma-specific anxiety coexisted with average levels of characterological anxiety, medical outcome was exceptionally good. These results are discussed relative to the theoretical distinctions between signal anxiety and anxiety concomitant with a lack of basic ego resources.

801

Dirks JF, Kinsman RA. **Death in asthma: a psychosomatic autopsy.** *J Asthma.* 1982;19:177-87. (English)

In most, if not all, chronic illnesses, the patient is a participant in medical management. Attitudes and behaviors during treatment can influence medical outcome in important ways that are becoming increasingly understood. This case history illustrates how a personal style may have contributed to the worst possible outcome, death, in an illness that is usually not fatal. There is a need to unravel the complex interplay between the psychological and medical factors contributing to such extremes in medical treatment failure in order to permit timely and appropriate intervention.

802

Dirks JF, Paley A, Fross KH. **Panic-fear research in asthma and the nuclear conflict theory of asthma; similarities, differences and clinical implications.** *Br J Med Psychol.* 1979;52:71-6. (English)

Recent reseach with the MMPI panic-fear scale has identified personality traits implicated in the psychological maintenance of the medical intractability of asthma. Intensity of prescribed medication, length of hospitalization, and rates of rehospitalization have been found to relate to MMPI panic-fear scores independent of the objective medical severity of the illness as indexed by longitudinal pulmonary functions. In the present study, MMPI panic-fear scores are related to separation and protection conflicts arising in childhood. While the nuclear conflict theory of asthma maintains that such conflicts occur in nearly all asthmatics and form a genetic component of the asthma, the present study finds that childhood separation and protection conflicts occur in a minority of patients, but may be instrumental in maintaining the medical intractability of the illness.

803

Dirks JF, Schraa JC, Brown EL, Kinsman RA. **Psychomaintenance in asthma: hospitalization rates and financial impact.** *Br J Med Psychol.* 1980;53:349-54. (English)

Certain patient styles perpetuate chronic physical illness, defeat medical treatment, and increase the utilization of medical services. Two such extreme styles among asthmatic patients are indexed by the MMPI panic-fear scale, reflecting either (a) helpless dependency and anxiety, or (b) excessive inappropriate independence. The present findings indicate that both of these patient styles are related to excessively high hospitalization rates during the two 1-year periods after discharge from intensive treatment, even among patient groups having asthma of similar objective severity. The discussion centres upon the increased demand for medical services, and the need for early identification of patients whose personal styles contribute to the maintenance of illness.

804

Fava GA, Perini GI, Santonastaso P, Fornasa CV. **Life events and psychological distress in dermatologic disorders: psoriasis, chronic urticaria and fungal infections.** *Br J Med Psychol.* 1980;53:277-82. (English)

A consecutive unselected series of 60 in-patients suffering from dermatologic disorders (psoriasis, chronic urticaria and fungal infections of the skin) was examined. Twenty patients with each illness were included. Stressful life events immediately before illness onset, levels of psychological distress, and alexithymic traits were investigated. Patients with psoriasis and chronic urticaria were exposed to stressful life situations before disease onset and suffered from psychological distress (anxiety, depression, inadequacy) significantly more than those with fungal infections. Implications for psychosomatic research and treatment are discussed.

805

Fedosejew GB, Filippow WL. **Peculiarities of personality and neuro-psychical disturbances in bronchial asthma** (author's transl). *Z Erkr Atmungsorgane.* 1979;152:240-6. (German)

Premorbid peculiarities and types of reaction of personality in bronchial asthma are considered. Neuro-psychical disturbances in different stages of disease are demonstrated by the majority of explored patients (92 ± 47, $4 \pm 2.6\%$). The development of psychical disturbances is connected with the combined influence of psychogenic and somatogenic factors, that finds its expression in the clinical picture and in the current of these disturbances. The role [that] ethiopathogenic factors [take] is shown. It had been directed on the matter that the combined diagnosis and treatment of bronchial asthma by therapeutists and psychotherapeutists should be instilled in the practice of all large institutions.

806

Fickova E. **Personality profile of asthmatics in Cattell's 16 inventory.** *Studia Psychol.* 1980;22:306-10. (Russian)

In 2 groups of 53 asthmatic patients, 16 PF scores showed (a) depressed values for Factor E (submissiveness); (b) enhanced values for Factors G (strength of superego), N (sophistication), O (guilt proneness), and Q3 (strength of self-sentiment); and (c) concordant scores on Factors E-, G+, N+, and Q3+.

807

Fritz GK. **Psychological aspects of atopic dermatitis: a viewpoint.** *Clin Pediatr (Phila).* 1979;18:360-4. (English)

An overview of existing research on the psychological aspects of atopic dermatitis is presented. Conclusive evaluation of specificity hypotheses, relating to emotional conflict or personality types, is lacking, yet these theories continue to exert their influence. A reactive-interactive model is elaborated whereby a number of psychological processes exacerbate and maintain the disorder. Management strategies and psychiatric involvement are discussed.

808

Gauthier Y. **The "bad mother" and the vulnerability of the parent-child relationship.** *Can J Psychiatr.* 1979;24:633-43. (French)

A brief history of the development of the concept of the "bad mother," who has become the scapegoat not only in childhood asthma but in many illnesses encountered in child psychiatry is presented here. The question of vulnerability within parent-child relationships leading to the appearance of child psychopathology is examined and the development of methods that could help in its early detection discussed. Results from a longitudinal study on young asthmatic children and particularly on the mother-child relationship in this illness are given. Children were observed at 14-30 mo of age and again at 4-6 yrs. The majority of Ss appeared to be developing in an adequate manner in the areas of autonomy and opposition, and the mothers appeared adequate in the face of the child's illness. However, a certain vulnerability in the area of opposition was more marked in a few cases, more frequently between the ages of 4 and 6 yrs than between 14 and 30 mo of age.

809

Groen JJ. **The psychosomatic theory of bronchial asthma.** *Psychother Psychosom.* 1979;31:38-48. (English)

The author discusses the development of the psychosomatic asthma theory as a paradigm of theory formation in psychosomatic medicine. The first formulation of the theory was based on clinical and psychiatric observations. It was tested by psychological, physiological and experimental methods and as a result was reformulated and extended. In its present form it regards asthmatic breathing as a reaction of a predisposed personality structure (partly hereditary, partly acquired during a youth situation in which overprotection by a domineering parent played a large role), to an ambivalent conflict with a key figure. The resulting frustration is not acted out by aggressive, flight, or depressive behaviour, but inhibited; thereby the motoric and verbal discharges are displaced into (substituted by) a respiratory behaviour pattern, which is characterised by an abnormally forceful contraction of the abdominal muscles during the expiration. The resulting high intraabdominal pressure is transmitted into the thorax where it pushes the posterior membranaceous wall of the trachea

and large bronchi forward into the lumen and thus produces a long stretched obstruction of the large airways. The passage of the air through the compressed large air passages under high pressure and low velocity is the mechanism which causes the typical wheeze and other manifestations of the asthmatic airway obstruction. A hypothesis is suggested for ways in which the psychoneurogenic respiratory behavior contributes to the so-called bronchial hyper-reactivity and the secondary development of allergies.

810

Hansen O, Kuchler T, Lotz GR, Richter R, Wilckens A. **My fingers itch, but my hands are bound—an exploratory psychosomatic study of patients with dyshidrosis of the hands (cheiropompholyx).** *Z Psychosom Med Psychoanal.* 181;27:275-90. (German)

The purpose of a pilot study with 20 patients, suffering from dyshidrotic eczema of the hands, was to investigate the relevance of a psychosomatic approach for its etiology and therapy. A set of psychological and allergological tests revealed the following results. 10 patients suffered from a contact allergy (epicutaneous test), 6 of them were allergic to nickel--the patients were less aggressive and more permissive (Freiburger Personality Inventory; FPI) as compared to a standard population. They reported more somatic complaints (HHM) as healthy subjects. The results of a semistructured interview support the hypothesis that the dyshidrotic eczema often has an expressive function: the patients present their dependency conflict in a symbolic manner by means of their hands. They try to take their life into their own hands; autonomous actions however are hampered by their own dependency needs. The development of the dyshidrotic symptoms corresponds to the autonomy, which has been achieved with regard to the individual conflict of ambivalence. According to our findings the contact with nickel is not [a] predominant, neither causative nor triggering, factor. Following the psychosomatic concept of Engel Schmale, the authors discuss the pathogenesis of dyshidrosis with the meaning of a complication of (pregenital) conversion, with the hands as the part affected.

811

Hartung M-L, Lehrl S. **Psychological test results of female patients suffering from perioral dermatitis.** *Z Psychosom Med Psychoanal.* 1976;22:110-14. (German) (unavailable at publication)

812

Jackson M. **Psychopathology and psychotherapy in bronchial asthma.** *Br J Med Psychol.* 1976;49:249-55. (English)

The role of psychological factors in the genesis of bronchial asthma is much disputed, and hence the place of psychotherapy in its management is equally controversial. The opportunity to study a series of such patients and to attempt to provide psychotherapy for them has led the author to the view that significant psychopathology is more common in asthmatic subjects than is generally realized, and that psychotherapy has a vital part to play in management. Some case material is presented to support this contention, and the application of psychoanalytic concepts, evaluation and treatment are discussed.

813
Jones NF, Kinsman RA, Schum R, Resnikoff P. **Personality profiles in asthma.** *J Clin Psychol.* 1976;32:285-91. (English)

155 hospitalized asthma patients were administered the MMPI in order to evaluate the existence of common personality characteristics. When Ss were divided into subgroups according to age, sex, and duration of the illness, patterns emerged that appeared largely explicable by these variables rather than the asthma *per se*. The single most frequent pattern observed across these subgroups was a V-shaped configuration of a "neurotic triad" (Scales 1, 2, and 3). This pattern is not unique to asthma, but is also characteristic of other chronic illness populations and seems to represent a defensive stance in coping with the problems of chronic illness. Findings refute any stereotypic asthmatic personality. It appears more profitable to investigate individual personality patterns associated with coping styles and their relationship to the illness via behaviors that either maintain or delimit the effects of chronic asthma.

814
Karol C. **The role of primal scene and masochism in asthma.** *Int J Psychoanal Psychother.* 1980-81;8:577-92. (English)

Early investigators, such as French (1939), observed that asthma patients need to repress their sexual and aggresive impluses in an attempt to retain their mother's love. Early traumatic experiences (Brown and Goitein, 1946), illness, primal scene, death in the family, miscarriage or birth of a sibling have all been mentioned as precursors of asthmatic attacks. These factors are also of considerable relevance in the case material presented here. Emphasized in this presentation, in addition to the above-mentioned factors, are critical aspects of primal scene traumatic experiences and their role in the subsequent development of sadomasochistic character formation. This sadomasochism plays a considerable role in the later eruption of asthmatic symptomatology. The crucial factor in the asthmatic symptomatology arises from the effect of the traumatic experiences which are associatively linked to these sadomasochistic fantasies. Clinical material of an asthmatic girl with learning inhibitions and sleeping difficulties is presented. She demonstrates a clownish sadomasochistic type of behavior reflecting a disturbance in her object relationships. During the course of analysis, it was revealed that specific unconscious fantasies, associated with early traumatic experiences, played a predominant role in the development of her sadomasochistic attitudes. These, in turn, were linked to her asthmatic attacks.

815
Keegan DL. **Chronic urticaria: clinical psychophysiological and therapeutic aspects.** *Psychosomatics.* 1976; 17:160-3. (English)

A multifactorial and dynamic approach to the problem of chronic urticaria has been used to describe a prototype for other psychophysiologic disorders. Four clinical cases, of

nine studied, were examined in relationship to the present literature. Physicians must no longer deal with problems as though physical aspects of life occur in a psychological vacuum and must recognize the effect of the milieu on illness and the resultant effect of illness in their clinical practice. The family physician is key to this type of approach.

816
Kellum RE, Stone SP. **Psychodynamics of dyshidrotic hand eczema.** *Dialogues Dermatol.* 1978;4:Pside 2. (English) (unavailable at publication)

817
Kim SP, Ferrara A, Chess S. **Temperament of asthmatic children: a preliminary study.** *J Pediatr.* 1980;97:483-6. (English)

The temperamental profile of a group of 12 asthmatic chilren between 3 and 7 years of age was compared to those of two comparison groups, each consisting of 12 normal well children and 12 children of the same age range with chronic eczema, allergic rhinitis, or both, but without asthma. The children with asthma differed significantly from the comparison groups in their temperamental profile, which was characterized by lower rhythmicity (regularity), lower adaptability, lower intensity of reaction, lower mood value, and lower persistence. The results indicate the need for further longitudinal studies of large populations of children with asthma to explore the implications and behavioral consequences of "the asthma temperament," and its interaction with other development factors.

818
Kinsman RA, Dirks JF, Dahlem NW, Heller AS. **Anxiety in asthma: panic-fear symptomatology and personality in relation to manifest anxiety.** *Psychol Rep.* 1980;46:196-8. (English)

Anxiety in asthma has been measured in two ways. The MMPI Panic-Fear scale is a measure of general, nonillness specific anxiety and the Panic-Fear symptom scale of the Asthma Symptom Checklist is a measure of illness-specific anxiety focused on the asthma attack. Both measures relate to response styles in asthma which contribute to the maintenance of illness. In the present study of 140 asthmatic patients, MMPI Panic-Fear scores were highly related to trait-anxiety measured by the Taylor Manifest Anxiety Scale, even after partialling out checklist Panic-Fear symptom scores. In contrast, Panic-Fear symptomatology had a more moderate relationship to the Taylor Anxiety scores and was independent of the Taylor scores after partialling out MMPI Panic-Fear scores. The results support earlier findings suggesting that MMPI Panic-Fear measures trait anxiety. In contrast, checklist Panic-Fear reports measure an illness-specific state anxiety that is not *per se* a measure of trait anxiety.

819
Kinsman RA, Dirks JF, Jones NF, Dahlem NW. **Anxiety reduction in asthma: four catches to general application.** *Psychosom Med.* 1980;42:397-405. (English)

Anxiety reduction procedures as adjuncts to medical treatments have almost invariably been reported to benefit asthmatic patients in individual case studies. However, the results of more systematically controlled studies are clearly inconsistent. This discrepancy is understandable in view of what is now known about anxiety in asthma. Four catches, each based on what has been reported about the roles and forms of anxiety in asthma, are presented. Each catch argues against general, across-the-board application of anxiety reduction procedures in asthma. Careful evaluation leading to more problem-oriented treatment is needed in view of the different roles of anxiety in asthma.

820

Kinsman RA, Dirks JF, Jones NF. **Levels of psychological experience in asthma: general and illness-specific concomitants of panic-fear personality.** *J Clin Psychol.* 1980;36;552-61. (English)

Coping styles in asthma indexed by a panic-fear personality measure are known to influence physicians' medical decisions and long-term treatment outcome. Unusually high or low panic-fear personality styles are maladaptive, the former characterized by anxious, helpless dependency and the latter by extreme counterphobic independence. In this study (n=90), the psychological experiences among panic-fear personality groups (low, moderate, and high) of asthma patients are described at three levels of assessment: (1) general personality characteristics; (2) attitudes toward asthma and its treatment; and (3) the subjective symptoms reported during breathing difficulties. Comparisons among the groups delineated the linkages between panic-fear personality and more illness-specific attitudes, symptoms, and experiences in asthma. Discussion centered upon how general personality and illness-specific characteristics associated with extreme high and low panic-fear personality may contribute to the psychomaintenance of asthma.

821

Kleiger JH, Dirks JF. **Medication compliance in chronic asthmatic patients.** *J Asthma Res.* 1979;16:93-6. (English) (unavailable at publication)

822

Lindemayr H, Gathmann P, Cermak T, Grunberger J. **Is chronic recurrent urticaria a psychosomatic disease?** *Z Hautkr.* 1981;56:28-40. (German)

A random group of 37 patients with chronic recurrent urticaria, 26 female and 11 male, was subjected to multidimensional personality tests (Frieburg Personality Inventory, FPI; Freiburg Aggression Test, FAF) whereas, deviating from establishing standards, introversion, nervousness and psychosomatic disturbance were more pronounced in the urticaria group, the following traits in deviation from normal standards were not noted: depression, irritability, sociability, emotional instability, composure. Nevertheless, this group appeared to be less communicative, more inhibited, compliant, and less dominant and aggressive. Neither did they show signs of socially accepted expression of negative and annoyed emotions nor socially desirable signs of assertiveness. A high rate of coincidence with other psychosomatic disorders such as frequent headache (18/37), chronic gastritis (19 of 37) and

ulcus duodeni (5 of 37) and migrainous headache (6 of 37) was also found in this group. In all cases explorable latent conflictive situations (frequent ambivalence) and negative childhood experience are further indicative of psychosomatic diseases.

823

Margalit M. **Multivariate concept of psychosomatic illness: the self-concept of asthmatic children.** *Int J Soc Psychiatry.* 1982;28:145-8. (English)

The self-concept of asthmatic children was studied in order to demonstrate the complicated nature of the psychosomatic syndrome; that of 18 asthmatic children was compared to those of three other groups': 20 healthy children, 20 children with emotional difficulties and 11 children with cystic fibrosis. Measures reflecting the psychological self-acceptance differentiated the healthy children significantly from the two groups with emotional difficulties (asthmatics, and children with adjustment difficulties). Measures reflecting physical self acceptance differentiated the healthy group significantly from the two groups with somatic complaints (asthmatics and cystic fibrosis children).

824

Matus I. **Assessing the nature and clinical significance of psychological contributions to childhood asthma.** *Am J Orthopsychiatry.* 1981;51:327-41. (English)

Psychological factors can enter into and affect the course of childhood asthma in a variety of ways. An organizational schema is presented and guidelines suggested for the clinical assessment of the possible clinical significance of these factors.

825

Meijer A. **Psychosomatic research in childhood asthma.** *Acta Paedopsychiatr (Basel).* 1981;47:261-8. (English)

This paper provides a concise review of psychosomatic research in childhood asthma. Early findings were mainly reconstructions of childhood events of adult asthmatic patients. In the last four decades more data on direct observations of asthmatic children and their mothers became available. Comprehensive consideration of biological, psychological and social factors in the evaluation of asthma is extremely rare. The diagnostic value of skin-testing is highly controversial as is the assumption of a so-called asthmatic personality. Objective assessments of pulmonary function *in vivo* have not led to a better understanding of psychological precipitating factors in asthma. Attempts to differentiate between biological and psychological asthma have not been useful. Certain predictions could be made concerning the effect of separation from the family. Various trials of artificial induction of asthma have not shown unifocal results. The role of dependency and depression was discussed and their relation to inhibited aggressive impulses examined. The role of family relationships and particularly of the mother's childhood family seems important in the evaluation of childhood asthma. Given a constitutional allergic predisposition and a familial allergy history, statistically significant differences between asthmatic and non-asthmatic children and their families were found. These findings were discussed with regard to available data from other studies on childhood asthma. Longitudinal studies on high risk children for asthma are necessary in order to determine the predictive value of the presently available psychological data which were found to be closely associated with childhood asthma.

826
Meijer A. **Sources of dependence in asthmatic children.** *Psychosomatics.* 1978;19:351-5. (English)

The question of whether childhood asthma produces increased dependency is examined. Dependency scores of 60 asthmatic and non-asthmatic children with the same familial-constitutional allergic predisposition were divided into "low-dependent" and "high-dependent" groups. In each group, asthmatic and non-asthmatic children with the same familial-constitutional allergic predisposition were compared statistically for significant psychological differences. Dependency was not found to be associated with the severity of asthma, but was associated with family relationship patterns.

827
Mellett P. **The birth of asthma.** *J Psychosom Res.* 1978; 22:239-46. (English)

"Conditioning" procedures involving reciprocal inhibition, altered perception associated with hypnosis, etc., were successful in greatly reducing or eliminating asthma in many subjects. This was so whatever the trigger (including allergy) and in spite of the failure of previously-given orthodox treatments. A small fraction of patients treated as above showed no improvement--some even being unable to collaborate in relaxing procedures. Forty such unresponsive patients were referred to me and investigated by psychiatric interview; in most a few further psychotherapeutic interviews and/or treatment with anti-depressants followed. Most showed suppressed depression or aggression. The majority improved markedly when the depression was relieved and/or the expression of anger was facilitated. It was later suggested that the behavior pattern of asthmatic breathing had, in these subjects, in some way been locked on to the affective state. In an attempt to explain these concomitant physiological and psychological phenomena, theories of the initiation of an attack will be discussed with emphasis on the relationship between bronchial mucosal capillary dilation and bronchial smooth muscle contraction. The limitations and the surviving significance of the Dutch "heresy" regarding the initiation of the attack by the use of voluntary muscle, increasing intra-thoracic pressure and causing tracheal compression, will be critically examined. It will be argued that all the theories of initiation refer, in fact, to the immediate post-nasal breathing pattern of an infant, whose first gasps of air have been shown to be exhaled against upper respiratory tract resistance without effective contraction of the vocal cords--giving rise to the specific "unvoiced" birth cry. It will be noted that this innate reflex behavior is associated with pulmonary capillary dilatation and the affects of fear, anger and depression which may be associated with birth. It will be suggested that the "first cry" mechanism, switched briefly into play at birth, may subsequently not be totally extinguished but, in some individuals, revived as if "locked on" to physiological states of pulmonary capillary dilatation (e.g. associated with allergy) or psycholog-

ical states of anger or depression. The lack of extinction and "locking on" of the abnormal breathing pattern may be the result of immensely intense affect associated with the particular individual's intra-uterine, birth canal and birth experience.

828
Panides WC, Ziller RC. **The self-perceptions of children with asthma and asthma/enuresis.** *J Psychosom Res.* 1981;25:51-6. (English)

Three groups of children with asthma were studied to determine the differential effects of the disease upon their perception of the self and other psychosocial structures. The groups included a group of children with mild asthma, a group of children with severe asthma, and a group of children with mild or severe asthma and enuresis. Results suggest that children with asthma/enuresis appear to be a high risk for lower levels of self-esteem, quality of life in the past year, self-complexity, and parental preference vis-a-vis their siblings. Children with severe asthma appear to perceive themselves as significantly closer/dependent upon their mothers and have lower scores on the present quality of life indicator. Children with mild asthma appeared to be the healthiest of the three groups on the variables studied.

829
Pistiner M, Pitlik S, Rosenfeld J. **Psychogenic urticaria** (letter). *Lancet.* 1979;2:1383. (English)

830
Plutchik R, Williams MH Jr, Jerrett I, Karasu TB, Kane C. **Emotions, personality and life stresses in asthma.** *J Psychosom Res.* 1978;22:425-31. (English)
Forty asthma clinic patients completed a battery of tests designed to measure personality, emotional states and current life stresses as well as subjective reactions to asthma symptomatology. In addition, physician's severity ratings, based on the amount of steroid medication needed for symptom control, and Peak Expiratory Flow Rates (PEFR), assessing lung functioning, were obtained for each patient. Analysis of the data revealed significant correlations between measures of personality, self-esteem, life problems and severity of asthma when asthma severity was measured by patients' self-reports of symptoms, but not when measured by either physicians' ratings or PEFR scores. Although there were moderate correlations between objective and subjective measures of asthma severity, the subjective measures correlated to a greater degree with a larger number of psychological variables.

831
Purschel W. **Neurodermatitis and psyche.** *Z Psychosom Med Psychoanal.* 1976;22:62-70. (German) (unavailable at publication)

832
Rechenberger HG. **Psychosomatic aspects in the therapy of allergic disease of respiratory organs** (author's transl). *Psychother Med Psychol.* 1978;28:139-41. (German (unavailable at publication)

833
Rechenberger I. **Psychodynamic of a patient with atopic**

dermatitis. *Z Psychosom Med Psychoanal.* 1976;22:71-4. (German) (unavailable at publication)

834

Rechenberger I. **Psychosomatic aspects in the diagnosis of allergic diseases of the respiratory organs (author's transl).** *Psychother Med Psychol.* 1978;28:135-8. (German) (unavailable at publication)

835

Rees WL. **Etiological factors in asthma.** *Psychiatr J Univ Ottawa.* 1980;5:250-4. (English)

Reviews the variety of etiological factors involved in the development of asthma, including (a) the role of emotional distress in various age groups as a precipitant of asthma and (b) various personality factors. A unifying etiological concept of asthma, taking into account the homeostatic mechanisms that are invariably involved, is offered.

836

Sauer J, Schnetzer M. **Personality profile of asthmatics and its changes in the course of various treatment methods.** *Z Klin Psychol Psychother.* 1978;26:171-80. (German)

Our study of 30 asthmatics showed an increase in the neurotic triangle (MMPI-Saarbrucken) and good agreement with the personality profile of neurotics with psychosomatic tendencies. To measure the effect of a 4-week treatment-course on the personality structure of the patients, the FPI-scale was used, where only a slight change was found in the scale nervositat (FPI 1 measures psychosomatic conflicts). For those patients who were also treated with autogenic training, the change was somewhat larger but not statistically significant, as compared to a group of patients who did not receive autogenic training. The treatment-course itself, judging only by the medical evaluations, was proved to be highly effective with statistical significance. A possible explanation for the discrepancy between the two findings could be the difference between the methods of investigation and/or the attitude of the patients to their asthma because many of them emphasize the somatic aspect of their illnesses, wishing to ignore or deny a possible psychosomatic explanation.

837

Scheer P. **Endogenic eczema in childhood: etiopathogenesis from the view of psychosomatic medicine** (author's transl). *Munch Med Welt.* Welt 1981;123:1571-4. (German)

The etiopathogenesis of endogenous eczema in childhood is discussed on the basis of existent literature--mainly of European origin. In the treatment of two children with severe neurodermatitis the partial failure of existing immunological and allergological theories became evident. Therefore, the hypothesis offered by psychosomatic medicine is that a synergism of specific prenatal factors, a "susceptible" cutaneous system and a particular mother-child relationship is at least in part to be blamed for the occurrence and maintenance of the disease.

838

Sharma S, Nandkumar VK. **Personality structure and adjustment pattern in bronchial asthma.** *Acta Psychiatr Scand.* 1980;61:81-8. (English)

A controlled study was conducted on 25 bronchial asthma patients in order to understand their personality structure, interpersonal relationships, conflicts and adjustment patterns. Psychometric evaluation was done by administering Rorschach's test, Eysenck's rating scale for anxiety and neurasthenic tendency, and sentence completion test. The results revealed that the asthmatics were intelligent but inhibited. They had covert aggression, neurotic construction and marked affectional and dependency needs. They had considerable anxiety and were unable to use their energy for constructive work. Excessive dependency on the mother and sexual disturbance were prominently noticeable. They were possessed with irrational fears, guilt feelings and insecurity. Though high goals were set they were unable to achieve them. The present data suggest avenues for further research in the cross-cultural field.

839

Sharma S, Nandkumar VK. **Some psychological concomitants of bronchial asthma.** *J Assoc Physicians India.* 1981;29:373-8. (English) (unavailable at publication)

840

Singh SB, Nigam A, Srivastava JR. **An investigation into the personality structure of asthmatic children and their parents by use of High School Personality Questionnaire and the 16 PF.** *Indian J Clin Psychol.* 1977;4:9-14. (English) (unavailable at publication)

841

Staudenmayer H, Kinsman RA, Dirks JF, Spector SL, Wangaard C. **Medical outcome in asthmatic patients: effects of airways hyperreactivity and symptom-focused anxiety.** *Psychosom Med.* 1979;41:109-18. (English)

Hypotheses about medical outcome in asthma, indexed by rates of rehospitalization within 6 months after discharge from long-term intensive care, were evaluated. Predictions for rehospitalization were based on the levels of airways hyperreactivity, indexed by inhalation challenges with histamine or methacholine, and levels of anxiety focused upon and concurrent with periods of asthmatic distress, indexed by panic-fear symptomatology. Results indicated that, although some prediction could be made on the basis of levels of anxiety and airways hyperreactivity alone, the best predictions resulted from the combined effects of these factors. Almost half of the patients who had highly hyperreactive airways and a tendency to disregard symptoms of breathing difficulty were rehospitalized. By comparison, none of the patients who had less hyperreactive airways and a tendency to be vigilant about their symptoms were rehospitalized. The hypotheses and results were discussed with respect to symptom-focused and general, illness-dependent types of asthma. The results have implications for the application of anxiety-reducing forms of intervention in asthma.

842

Staudenmayer H, Kinsman R A, Jones N F. **Attitudes toward respiratory illness and hospitalization in asthma: relationships with personality, symptomatology, and treatment response.** *J Nerv Ment Dis.* 1978;166:624-34. (English)

In a previous study, the 2nd author *et al* described the development of the Respiratory Illness Opinion Survey (RIOS), which measures 6 categories describing attitudes toward respiratory illness and its treatment: Optimism, Negative Staff Regard, Specific Internal Awareness, External Control, Psychological Stigma, and Authoritarian Attitudes. In the present study, 159 14-72 yr old asthmatic inpatients hospitalized for long-term intensive therapy, were administered a battery of psychological tests within 3 wks after admission. Measures included the RIOS, Asthma Symptom Checklist, MMPI, and the Panic-fear Personality Scale, which is based on the MMPI. Results show that the 6 attitudes measured by the RIOS (a) relate more clearly to general personality characteristics than to illness-specific subjective symptomatology; (b) enable types of asthmatic patients to be described on the basis of the patterns of attitude category scores; and (c) provide information about treatment outcome in asthma as indexed by length of hospitalization during long term, intensive therapy, the need for prescribed oral corticosteroids, and rates of rehospitalization and judged severity following discharge from treatment.

843

Steiner H, Fritz G K, Hilliard J, Lewiston N J. **A psychosomatic approach to childhood asthma.** *J Asthma.* 1982;19:111-21. (English) (unavailable at publication)

844

Straker N, Bieber J. **Asthma and the vicissitudes of aggression: two case reports of childhood asthma.** *J Am Acad Child Psychiatry.* 1977;16:132-9. (English)

We report two children with childhood asthma who without prior evidence of psychosis manifested transient and completely reversible psychotic episodes in the course of psychotherapy. The dynamic conflicts which precipitated the transient psychosis would previously have precipitated an asthmatic episode had aggressive conflicts remained repressed. A brief review of the literature on the subjects of asthma and aggression and psychosis and asthma is presented. An attempt is made to explain the relationship between the observed psychotic episodes, the observed asthmatic episodes, and the vicissitudes of the aggression in these patients.

845

Studt H H. **Psycho- and somatoneuroses in comparison: anxiety neurosis/phobia--bronchial asthma; psychosomatic inquiry study.** *Fortschr Med.* 1976;94:1786-90. (German)

In order to answer the question of whether an interrater's stable facts make it possible to differentiate between neurosis, 50 psychosomatics (asthmatics) were compared with 50 psychoneurotics which included 25 cases of anxiety neurotics and 25 phobics. The age at the time the patient became ill, the age at the time of the scientific investigation, length of illness, psycho- and psychosomatic pre-illnesses, former hospitalizations, primordial and accompanying symptoms, social facts, types of conflict situation which triggered the illness and the results of intelligent tests were correlated with the main variabilities: neurosis, sex, character structure and tests for statistical significance were performed: psycho- and psychosomatic-neurosis as well as anxiety neurosis and phobia are different from one another in numerous variabilities.

846

Stuttgen G. **Physiology and pathophysiology of pruritis** (author's transl). *MMW.* 1981;123:987-91. (German)

The origins of pruritus, transmission of sensitivity and changes in the itch threshold are presented. Nociceptively, as protopathic quality of sensitivity and as a general concept for pain and itching, the elements of psychosomatic appraisal and comprehension of organic nervous complaints and neurohormonal disturbances are given.

847

Teiramaa E. **Asthma, psychic disturbances and family history of atopic disorders.** *J Psychosom Res.* 1979;23:209-17. (English)

One hundred asthmatic patients, divided into groups with/-without a family history of atopic disorders (n = 62 and 38 respectively), underwent a semi-structured psychiatric interview and questionnaire and psychological investigations (MMPI, Wartegg test, Self-image test, Beck Depression Inventory). The study revealed a sub-group of 24 patients who were more likely than the others to have been extroverted and/or dominant in childhood and who were in sharp contrast with the remainder of the series showing less or no introversion or depression. Twenty-three of these patients (96%) had a family history of atopic disorders, with an asthmatic parent more frequently among these than among the other cases. The patients with no atopic disorders in their relatives showed introversion in particular more frequently than the others, this being at least predominantly a precursor of asthma (long before the onset), but phobic symptoms were less frequent in this group. When asthma is viewed as a disease of multifactorial origin, the present results (and the differences in psychic and psychosocial factors between the present asthmatics and the non-asthmatic controls referred to in an earlier study) suggest that among the psychic factors introversion in particular is probably important within the combination of factors affecting the inception of asthma.

848

Teiramaa E. **Psychic disturbances and duration of asthma.** *J Psychosom Res.* 1978;22:127-32. (English)

One hundred adult asthmatic patients, divided into four groups by duration of the disease, underwent a psychiatric interview and psychological investigations. Contrary to certain previous results, no marked interdependences were observed between psychic disturbances and the duration of asthma. In a previous study with the same patients, psychic disturbances and introversion correlated positively with a failure to show any improvement in the asthma condition.

The results of the present study suggest that such psychic properties can scarcely be explained as consequences of asthma, as individual personality characteristics and psychic disturbances will probably have their origin, to a large extent at least, in the pre-asthmatic phase.

849

Teiramaa E. **Psychic disturbances and severity of asthma.** *J Psychosom Res.* 1978;22:401-8. (English)

One hundred adult asthmatic patients, divided into four groups by the nature and amount of medication for the disease, underwent a psychiatric interview and questionnaire and psychological investigations. The patients in the first group did not regularly need drugs for asthma, those in the third group used beta$_2$-receptor-stimulating inhalants, which were not used in the second group, and those in the fourth group continuously used corticoids. The patients in the first and second groups were healthier psychically than those in the third and fourth groups. Neurotic features and psychosomatic and neurotic symptoms were shown most frequently in the third group, and introversion and strong repression by the patients on corticoids, who were more likely to have been withdrawn in childhood. In a previous study the same patients had been divided into two groups, one with improving asthma and the other with a static or deteriorating condition. The patients in the first group were healthier psychically, showed better psychosocial adaptation and were more often extroverted than those in the latter, the differences being more distinct than in the present instance.

850

Teiramaa E. **Psychic factors and the inception of asthma.** *J Psychosom Res.* 1979;23:253-62. (English)

One hundred adult asthmatics and one hundred nonasthmatic subjects answered a questionnaire and underwent psychological investigations. Sixty-two percent of the asthmatics and 30% of the controls had near relatives with atopic disorders, but psychic factors, especially those referring to the dichotomy introversion/extroversion, also had a high explanatory power for the group code asthmatic/control. This was conspicuous for "the number of hobbies when of school age" in particular, in which asthmatics with a negative family history of atopic disorders obtained especially low values not connected with the onset of asthma in childhood. The controls with a positive family history of atopic disorders obtained the highest values, which might suggest that psychic properties connected with marked extroverted tendencies and behavioural activities may have a certain preventive effect against the inception of asthma, lessening the possibility of a manifestation of the disease in "potential asthmatics". Inhibition, disturbances in self-esteem, problems in handling anxiety, fears (particularly in the women) and depression were typical of the asthmatics, whereas the male controls showed emotionality, energeticness and dominance more frequently than did the asthmatic men. The patients with a negative family history of atopic disorders in particular showed schizothymia and had difficulties in the expression of depressive feelings, although the investigation uncovered a high degree of depression in them.

851

Teiramaa E. **Psychosocial and psychic factors and age at onset of asthma.** *J Psychosom Res.* 1979;23:27-37. (English)

100 adult asthmatic patients, divided into 4 groups by age at onset (0-16, 17-27, 28-35, and 36-48 yrs), underwent a semistructured, psychiatric interview and questionnaire and psychological investigations, including the MMPI and the Beck Depression Inventory. Ss in the first and third groups most often belonged to the highest or lowest social strata and most frequently showed psychic disturbances, while Ss in the second group had these least often. Ss in the first group had most often been either very lively or quiet and with neurotic symptoms as children. Ss in the second group most often showed an improvement in their asthma and least often suffered from depression or obsession, inhibition, or psychasthenia, whereas obsession or depression and schizothymia were characteristic of the third group. The third group had the fewest patients with near relatives with atopic disorders. Disappointments within a year before asthma had been experienced most often by Ss in the fourth goup. Results indicate that the onset of asthma may be the end-product of the synergic effects of various factors, the contribution of each group (somatic, psychic, and psychosocial) probably differing according to age at onset.

852

Teiramaa E. **Psychosocial and psychic factors in the course of asthma.** *J Psychosom Res.* 1978;22:121-5. (English)

100 asthmatic patients aged 16-52 yrs were divided into 2 groups, favorable vs unfavorable prognoses. The patients who were most extraverted and/or lacked psychic symptoms almost always fell into the favorable group, and amnestic data suggested that these patients already differed psychically from the other asthmatics in the preasthmatic phase by showing more extraverted tendencies and better psychosocial adaptation. In general, poor psychosocial adaptation, obsessive neurosis, immature personality, and alcohol problems were associated with static or deteriorating trends in asthma.

853

Teiramaa E. **Psychosocial factors in the onset and course of asthma: a clinical study on 100 patients.** *Acta Univ Ouluensis.* 1977;D-14:135. (English)

Compared the mental health of 58 female and 42 male 16-52 yr old asthmatics with that of 100 adults matched for age, sex and marital status. Ss were given a psychiatric interview, the MMPI, the Beck Depression Inventory, the Wartegg test, and tests of self-image and identity diffusion. Among the results, it was found that the asthmatics had childhood milieux less favorable for personality development than controls. The asthmatics were more psychicallly disturbed than the controls, and the male asthmatics differed more from the male controls than the female asthmatics did from the female controls. The females with an improving asthmatic condition were the least disturbed of those studied. The asthmatics were more introverted than the controls. Ss had had introversion tendencies and a tendency for respiratory symptoms even before the manifestation of asthma. Introversion and psychic disturbance were associated with a deteriorating or static asthmatic condition. 19% of the female asthmatics had contracted asthma during pregnancy or after delivery, and 19% of the male asthmatics had done so during their wife's pregnancy or after her delivery. Other situations in which asthma had begun included occupational stress and marital conflicts.

854
Teiramaa E. **Psychosocial factors, personality and acute-insidious asthma.** *J Psychosom Res.* 1981;25:43-50. (English)

One hundred adult asthmatics, divided into groups by duration of the prodromal phase, i.e., 'acute', 'subacute' or 'insidious' onset (0-1, 2-11, and ≥ 12 months), underwent a semistructured psychiatric interview and questionnaire and psychological investigation (MMPI, Wartegg test, Beck Depression Inventory). Disappointments prior to asthma were associated with a close personal relationship in the acute cases in particular, and to progress at work and/or economic matters in cases of subacute onset. The arrival of a new family member or a period of 0-3 years in marriage were connected with insidious asthma most frequently. The present findings suggest that the duration of asthmatic prodomi may be largely dependent on the nature of psychosocial stress factors (in connection with individual psychic properties: 'key and lock'), which may be of practical significance in the early evaluation of the patient.

855
Thurn A. **Psychogenic aspects of perioral dermatitis.** *Z Psychosom Med Psychoanal.* 1976;22:99-109. (German) (unavailable at publication)

856
Werth GR. **The hives dilemma.** *Am Fam Physician.* 1978;17:139-43. (English)

Recurrent or persistent hives may sometimes be due to an apparently insoluble emotional dilemma. Five case studies demonstrate this association. They show that resolution of the dilemma can be curative. When the dilemma is unalterable, explaining this insoluble conflict-hives phenomenon to the patient will ameliorate symptoms. Such an emotional history should be sought in patients with hives and, and when found, should be pursued along with other possible causes discovered during the initial evaluation.

857
Zlatich D. **An investigation of psychosomatic components of asthma in childhood and adolescence.** *Diss Abstr Int.* 1980;40:4991. (English) (unavailable at publication)

Emotions and immunity

Emotions and disease susceptibility

858

Frazier CA. **The anxious mind and disease.** *Nurs Care.* 1977;10:16-9. (English) (unavailable at publication)

859

Holmes TH. **Life situations, emotions, and disease.** *Psychosomatics.* 1978;747-54. (English)

A series of studies are described in which the author and other investigators have sought to clarify the influence of emotions, psychosocial factors, and life changes on the onset and course of disease.

860

Kronfol Z, Silva J, Greden J, Dembinski S, Carroll BJ. **Cell-mediated immunity in melancholia** (abstract). *Psychosom Med.* 1982;44:304. (English)

Mood states and immunity may be related. Clinical depression is associated with an increased risk for infection, allergy and cancer, illnesses in which deranged immune mechanisms have been postulated. Stressful life events such as bereavement impair lymphocyte function. To study the immune status of depressed patients, we compared *in vitro* lymphocytic responses to phytohemagglutinin-P (PHA), concanavalin A (Con A) and pokeweed mitogen (PWM) in three groups of subjects: 1) melancholic patients (n=14); 2) non-melancholic psychiatric controls (n=15); and 3) normal controls (n=10). The criteria for the diagnosis of melancholia included the Research Diagnostic Criteria (RDC) and the concurrent clinical diagnosis of endogenous depression. All patients were drug-free for at least two weeks prior to the study. We found a generalized and marked decrease in lymphocyte responses to mitogens in the melancholic group. Stimulation counts were lower in the melancholic group as compared to both the psychiatric control group (p<0.05, Mann-Whitney) and the normal control group (p<0.001, Mann-Whitney) for all three mitogens used. These results suggest an impairment of cell-mediated immunity in melancholia.

861

Linn BS, Linn MW, Jensen J. **Anxiety and immune responsiveness.** *Psychol Rep.* 1981;49:969-70. (English)

Assessed the association between anxiety and immune functioning in 75 chronically ill males without cancer, infection, or autoimmune disease. Ss were tested on the anxiety factor of the Hopkins Symptom Checklist and gave estimates on perceived stress and prior health. Immunological tests were performed. Stress from hospitalization was associated with depressed immunological response of lymphocytes *in vitro* but with positive reactions to skin tests of more delayed hypersensitivity. Findings suggest that psychological states of perceived stress and anxiety influence functioning of the immune system and could lead to greater vulnerability to infections and disease, including cancer.

862

Linn BS, Linn MW, Jensen J. **Degree of depression and immune responsiveness** (abstract). *Psychosom Med.* 1982;44:128-9. (English)

Several reports have suggested that stress may adversely affect immune response in animals and man. Although events like death or serious illness are likely to be perceived as stressful, degree of stress caused by these events can still vary. This study measured degree of depression after family death and/or illness and its effect on the immune response. Sixty males (mean age 54) who had experienced family deaths or serious family illness during the prior 6 months completed the Depression Factor of the Hopkins Symptom Checklist and received a battery of physical and immunological tests. Humoral immune responses were assessed by IgG, IgA and IgM. Cellular responses were measured *in vivo* by 3 delayed hypersensitivity skin tests and *in vitro* by lymphocyte response to phytohemagglutinin (PHA), concanavalin A (ConA), and pokeweed (PWM) as well as to homologous cells. Leukocyte chemotaxis was also performed. Subjects were divided by their median depression scores into high and low depression groups and immune data compared by multivariate analysis of variance. Overall, there was a multivariate difference of p<0.02 between high and low depression groups, with depressed persons having significantly less responsiveness of their own cells with that of controls (p<0.05) and less responsiveness of their lymphocytes to PHA (p<0.05). Although the IgG and IgM responses were also significantly lower in depressed patients, they were still in the normal range of responses for these variables. Data indicate that not all persons react with the same degrees of depression to stressful events and that these high and low depressed groups can be differentiated by their immune responses. Groups are being followed prospectively for occurrence of disease. If psychological states diminish biological defenses, then an individual is potentially more vulnerable to infectious disease as well as cancer.

863
Luborsky L, Mintz J, Brightman VJ, Katcher AH. **Herpes simplex virus and moods: a longitudinal study.** *J Psychosom Res.* 1976;20:543-8. (English)

The herpes simplex virus has remarkable properties (as noted by Dubois). It does not conform to the classical conception of invasion by a disease, since the organisms probably are present in certain people all of the time. A characteristic of the illness which makes it convenient for study is that it is quite common--the frequency of the population having antibodies for it is about one-third, which is about what we found in our samples. The present work is part of a series of studies on the nature of the psychological and physical context in which the virus is activated. The core of the mystery is under what conditions the virus is activated to the degree that it becomes clinically evident. A number of factors are known to play a part in activating the virus; these include colds, menstruation, sunburn, fevers (which are a concomitant of an elevation of metabolism), a scratch on the lip, and in addition there are a group of psychological factors globally referred to as "stress." "Negative affects" such as unhappiness or depression are often likely to be concomitants of stress. Anecdotal reports suggest that before academic examinations and other special stressors, cold sores are more frequent. We posed two types of questions about the role of psychological factors in the production of recurrent herpes labialis (RHL): (1) What psychological factors predict the frequency of later occurrence of RHL? (2) What psychological factors appear immediately before specific episodes of the illness? To investigate the first question, several psychological tests were administered to two classes of young women entering nurses' training (N 38), Cornell Medical Index, Clyde Mood Scale, Social Assets Scale, and the Johns Hopkins Symptom Check List. Scores on these tests were correlated with the frequency of several illnesses, including episodes of herpes labialis during the subsequent year. Among those tests with significant correlations was the Clyde Mood Scale, which correlated with episodes of herpes labialis in the subsequent year. Among those tests with significant correlations was the Clyde Mood Scale, which correlated with episodes of herpes labialis in the subsequent year--the first year of their training. Actually, the Clyde Mood Scale--a 3-to-4 min self- administered form--provides six factor scores: Friendly, Aggressive, Clear Thinking, Sleepy, Unhappy, and Dizzy. Many studies show it validly correlates with other measures in meaningful ways. Only the Unhappy factor of the Clyde Mood Scale correlated significantly with the 1-year frequency of RHL; e.g., episodes of reported herpes correlated 0.33 with Clyde Mood Scale; history of RHL correlated 0.42 with Clyde Mood Scale; documented RHL had a multiple correlation with Clyde Mood Scale, Social Assets, and Cornell Medical Index of 0.56. Social Assets correlated significantly negatively with incidence of RHL (-0.41), both in the present study and a previous one. (The Unhappy factor itself was part of a larger factor made up of the Cornell Medical Index and the main Factor 1 of the Symptom Check List. This larger factor probably reflects an inclination to complain of many illnesses.) In sum, those who judged themselves as more typically unhappy tended to have more RHL during their first year of nurses' training (and also reported a history of more illnesses in general and more psychological complaints).

864
Piccione M. **Psychosomatic aspects of anxiety: circulatory and respiratory systems.** *Clin Ter.* 1978;84:463-70. (Italian) (unavailable at publication)

865
Shanon J. **Psoriasis: psychosomatic aspects.** *Psychother Psychosom.* 1979;31:218-22. (English)

Data from studies of psoriasis patients indicate that hereditary proneness alone is not sufficient to cause psoriasis. Only when additional causes (e.g., trauma) intervene does the disease occur. The importance of stress and emotional factors in the development of the disease is discussed.

866
Thomas CB, McCabe OL. **Precursors of premature disease and death: habits of nervous tension.** *Johns Hopkins Med J.* 1980;147:137-45. (English)

Patterns of habits of nervous tension (HNT) recorded by medical students who later developed cancer, coronary occlusion, hypertension, or mental illness, or who committed suicide, were compared with those students who remained healthy 15 to 30 years later. Data came from the 25-item HNT Questionnaire previously reported. Unpaired *t* tests and two-group discriminant function analyses were the chief statistical methods used. Compared with those of the healthy group, the overall HNT patterns were significantly different for the cancer, coronary occlusion, mental illness, and suicide groups. The overall pattern for the hypertension group did not reach significance. It therefore appears that youthful reactions to stress as self-reported in checklist of habits of nervous tension reflect individual psychobiological differences that are linked with future health or disease.

867
Vendysova E, Pankova R. **Anxiety reactions in psoriatics.** *Cesk Psychol.* 1982;26:62-7. (Czech)

Observed the responses of 50 psoriatic males and a matched group of healthy controls to anxiety-inducing situations. The situations that were associated with skin disease were presented only to the psoriatics. Situations connected with psoriasis were much more stressful for the patients than situations that affected the whole population. Anxiety was caused mainly by situations of a social nature and by the somatic manifestations of the disease. The psoriatics also reported many more generalized and nonspecific manifestations of anxiety than did the healthy controls.

Emotions and cancer

868
Bageley C. **Control of the emotions, remote stress, and the emergence of breast cancer.** *Indian J Clin Psychol.* 1979;6:213-20. (English)

113 women (aged less than 70 yrs) with early cancer were studied preoperatively; Ss had been admitted to the hospital for breast tumor biopsy and had no apparent knowledge of the suspected diagnosis. After biopsies, comparisons of the 45 Ss with cancer and the 68 with benign tumors revealed significant correlations between breast cancer and (a) the occurrence of subjectively stressful events (social, psychological, and physical) up to 15 yrs before appearance of a breast tumor, and (b) a chronic behavioral pattern of abnormal emotional expression, specifically, concealment of emotions and bottling up of anger.

869

Bieliauskas L, Shekelle RB, Garron D, Maliza C, Ostfeld A, Paul O, Raynor WJ. **Psychological depression and cancer mortality** (abstract). *Psychosom Med.* 1979;41:77-8. (English)

An association between symptoms of depression and cancer has often been reported but the role of depression remains unclear. This study investigated the hypothesis that psychological depression in men without clinical evidence of cancer is associated with increased risk of death from cancer during subsequent years. Depression was measured by the MMPI D scale in 2082 employed men aged 40-55 in 1958, and cause-specific mortality was determined for the next 17 years. Up to 1974, 82 men with cancer coded on their death certificates scored an average of 2.5 points higher on the D scale than 2000 men who survived or died from other causes (p=0.035); these 2 groups did not differ significantly on the other nine MMPI clinical scales. Men with D as the highest score on the MMPI profile (n=394) had twice the odds of cancer death as compared to 1688 men with their highest score on another scale (p<0.001). The odds ratios in 3 time periods--1958-64, 1965-69, and 1970-74--were 1.7, 2.7, and 2.1 respectively. For non-cancer deaths during the same periods, the odds ratios were 1.8, 1.4 and 0.9 with an overall odds ratio of 1.3 (p=0.131). These results persisted when adjusted for age at entry, cigarette smoking, and alcohol consumption. These results support the hypothesis that psychological depression is related prospectively to increased risk of death from cancer. They do not speak directly to an etiologic role for depression in cancer though at least a concurrent role is suggested. These findings, if supported by on-going studies of cancer incidence (morbidity as well as mortality), may contribute to better identification of individuals at risk for cancer.

870

Borysenko J, Benson H, Borysenko M. **Fear, hope and cancer.** *Sci Am.* (English) (in press)

871

Borysenko J. **Behavioral-physiological factors in the development and management of cancer.** *Gen Hosp Psychiatry.* 1982;4:69-74. (English)

Recent clinical and animal model studies have demonstrated an effect of behavioral variables on the course of cancer. Unrelieved anxiety, helplessness, depression, and the inability to modulate the expression of anger have been implicated as specific predictors of poor prognosis. The endocrinological sequelae of these emotional states may affect certain parameters of cell-mediated immunity involved in host resistance neoplasia. Both corticosteroids and catecholamines are likely mediators of behavioral effects on immunological function. Hormonal variations may also affect growth of tumors directly, or through nonimmunological tissue specific mechanisms. Behavioral interventions based on elicitation of the relaxation response provide a means of influencing affective and physiological states that may have particular relevance to cancer. Practice of such interventions reduces anxiety and provides a substrate for coping that enhances the patient's sense of control. Such "immunization" against helplessness can forestall depression. Physiological effects of such behavioral interventions occur both on a direct and an indirect level. Elicitation of the relaxation response per se reduces physiological alterations consistent with decreased arousal of the sympathetic nervous system. Furthermore, by reducing fear and helplessness, physiological changes related to such dysphoric states may be minimized.

872

Brown RS. **On cancer and the emotions** (letter). *Am J Psychiatry.* 1977;134:585. (English)

873

Greer S, Morris T, Pettingale KW. **Psychological response to breast cancer: effect on outcome.** *Lancet.* 1979;2:785-7. (English)

A prospective, multidisciplinary, 5-year study of 69 consecutive female patients with early ($T_{0,1} N_{0,1} M_0$) breast cancer was conducted. Patients' psychological responses to the diagnosis of cancer was assessed 3 months postoperatively. These responses were related to outcome 5 years after operation. Recurrence-free survival was significantly common among patients who had initially reacted to cancer by denial or who had a fighting spirit than among patients who had responded with stoic acceptance or feelings of helplessness and hopelessness.

874

Greer S, Morris T. **The study of psychological factors in breast cancer: problems of method.** *Soc Sci Med.* 1978;12:129-34. (English)

160 women admitted consecutively for breast tumor biopsy were interviewed and assessed on the Hamilton Rating Scale for Depression, the Eysenck Personality Inventory, and the Hostility-Direction of Hostility Questionnaire. At operation, 69 Ss were diagnosed as having breast cancer (BC) and 91 as having benign breast disease; the latter group served as controls. A major result of statistical comparisons was a significantly correlation between the diagnosis of BC and a behavioral pattern, persisting throughout adult life, of abnormal release of anger. This abnormality was, in most cases, extreme suppression. Although major sources of bias were avoided in the present study, critical examination of its methods shows several limitations. It is suggested that further advances in this area depend on more stringent methods, and several recommendations are presented concerning such methods.

875

Levitan LJ, Levitan H, Levitan M. **The incidence of**

cancer in psychiatric patients, cancer and the emotions: a review. *Mt Sinai J Med (NY).* 1980;47:627-31. (English)

This paper will deal with the general discussion of emotions and cancer. It will be divided into a section on the historical critique of psychological states and malignancies, the incidence of major psychosis and cancer, and the various biochemical hypotheses for the correlation of schizophrenia and neoplasms. This will lead to a realization that depressive states can be shown to precede the clinical appearance of tumors and that the schizophrenic population has a decreased risk of malignancy.

876

Morris T, Greer S, Pettingale KW, Watson M. **Patterns of expression of anger and their psychological correlates in women with breast cancer.** *J Psychosom Res.* 1981; 25:111-17. (English)

Studied 71 patients (30-69 yrs old) prior to breast biopsy using structured interviews, the Eysenck Personality Questionnaire (EPQ), and the State-Trait Anxiety Inventory (STAI). Taped transcripts of interviews, independently rated with a revised anger rating scale, demonstrated a significant difference between patients with benign breast disease and those with breast cancer in expression of anger, thereby supporting previous research. Mean EPQ Neuroticism scores were significantly lower for cancer patients. STAI A-State and A-Trait scores were significantly higher than standard scores for all Ss other than young cancer patients. The pattern of correlation between variables differed for the 2 diagnostic groups, suggesting that cancer patients are more stressed by impending biopsy and that young cancer patients are more likely than other patients to use denial in the face of stress.

877

Murray JB. **Psychosomatic aspects of cancer: an overview.** *J Genet Psychol.* 1980;136:185-94. (English)

An overview of research on the psychosomatic aspects of cancer indicated that earlier psychoanalytic interpretations which focused on intrapsychic elements have given way to considerations of rehabilitation of victims of cancer and assistance with the complex emotional reactions of patients to terminal disease and of patients' families both to the disease and to death.

878

Pettingale KW, Greer S, Tee DE. **Serum IgA and emotional expression in breast cancer patients.** *J Psychosom Res.* 1977;21:395-9. (English)

As part of a multidisciplinary study of 160 women admitted consecutively for breast tumor biopsy, we measured expression of anger and serum immunoglobulins before operation, when we had no knowledge of the provisional diagnosis, and at 3, 12 and 24 months after operation. Expression of anger was not related to serum IgG, IgM or IgE levels, but IgA levels were found to be significantly higher in patients who habitually suppressed anger than in those who were able to express anger (p<0.001). This correlation was found before operation in both cancer patients and those with benign breast disease. Over the subsequent two years serum IgA levels remained consistently higher in all patients who suppressed anger, but only reached statistical significance in breast cancer patients 3 months (p<0.02) and 2 years (p<0.03) following operation. We suggest how such an association might play a part in the pathogenesis of cancer.

879

Plumb M, Holland J. **Comparative studies of pychological function in patients with advanced cancer; II--Interviewer-rated current and past psychological symptoms.** *Psychosom Med.* 1981;43:243-54. (English)

This study compared psychologic function, especially depression, in patients with advanced cancer and in sociodemographically matched, physically healthy patients who had recently attempted suicide. A companion study examined self-report of depressive symptoms; the present study relied on a semistructured interview technique. Eighty patients who were hospitalized on a research oncology ward for treatment of disseminated cancer, acute leukemia, Stage IV Hodgkins' disease, or myeloma were compared by means of the Current and Past Psychopathology Scales (CAPPS) to 80 patients hospitalized on a psychiatric unit for attempted suicide. Interviewer ratings yielded scores on eight scales characterizing each patient's psychologic adjustment during the past month and 18 scales characterizing adjustment prior to the present illness (cancer or suicide attempt). Results showed that by both self-report and observer report, cancer patients were less depressed and anxious in the past month than the psychiatric group. Approximately one-third of the cancer patients were significantly depressed, depending on the measure used; one-seventh had experienced some suicidal ideation. Cancer patients were better adjusted in the past than the comparison group; however, the cancer patients who were presently most depressed were those who had a prior history of depression and had shown a tendency to brood. Findings supported use of denial of dysphoric emotions by the cancer patients, but little denial of the diagnosis or the need to accept treatment. Despite stress of advanced illness and threat to life, cancer patients' reality testing and social role performance were superior to that of the suicide attempters, and on the average they had less disturbance of affect and cognition.

880

Plumb MM, Holland J. **Comparative studies of psychological function in patients with advanced cancer; I--Self-reported depressive symptoms.** *Psychosom Med.* 1977;39:264-76. (English)

Depressive symptoms assessed by the Beck Depression Inventory were compared in 97 cancer patients, 66 next-of-kin cancer patients, and 99 physically healthy persons who attempted suicide. Less than a fourth of the cancer patients and a fifth of their next-of-kin but over half of the psychiatric patients were moderately or severely depressed. The two patient groups were indistinguishable in somatic depressive symptoms, both scoring higher than the next-of-kin. The cancer patients and the next-of-kin were indistinguishable in nonsomatic (psychological) depressive symptoms, both scoring lower than the suicide attempters. Younger patients reported more nonsomatic symptoms than older ones. Beck scores and nearness to death were not associated in 57 cancer patients who expired. Vegetative depressive symptoms in cancer patients may reflect advanced disease, but nonsomatic symptoms should be reason for psychiatric consultation.

881
Schonfield J. **Psychological factors related to recovery from breast cancer** (abstract). *Psychosom Med.* 1977;39:51. (English)

Do psychological factors play any role in the recurrence of early carcinomas of the breast? Forty nine women with Stage I, II or III breeast cancer, who had previously undergone either a partial or radical mastectomy, were interviewed during the first week of radiation therapy. They were also asked to answer 128 items from the MMPI and a forty item disguised measure of anxiety. Two years after radiotherapy the medical status of all 49 women was obtained, and two groups were formed: (1) a group with no evidence of recurrence at that time (N=37), and (2) a group with clear evidence of recurrence who were either still alive or who had died from their disease within two years (N=12). No relationship was found between the initial stage of the disease and recurrence or non-recurrence. The group with no recurrence had significantly higher scores on an MMPI scale measuring physical well-being and significantly lower scores on the hypochondriasis scale of the MMPI. The group with a recurrence had significantly higher scores on the frustrative tension sub-scale of the anxiety measure. Just short of statistical significance (p<10) was the score on the Morale Loss (severe depression) scale of the MMPI, where the group with a recurrence scored higher than the group without. The overall picture that emerges is that the women who survived two years post breast surgery and radiotherapy without any recurrence were less anxious initially and were possibly also less depressed. All the scales with significant results in the present study (with the exception of the hypocondriasis scale) have also been found to differentiate in the same direction, cancer patients undergoing radiotherapy who do, or do not return to gainful employment one year later, when all were in remission status. It would appear that these personality scales are tapping characteristics important both in the adjustment to having had cancer, and in the length of survival from this disease.

882
Shekelle RB, Raynor WJ, Ostfeld AM, Garron DC, Bieliauskas L, Liu SC, Maliza C, Paul O. **Psychological depression and 17-year risk of death from cancer.** *Psychosom Med.* 1981;43:117-25. (English)

Psychological depression; measured in 1957-1958 by the Minnesota Multiphasic Personality Inentory at the baseline examination of 2,020 middle-aged employed men, was associated (p<0.001) with a twofold increase in odds of death from cancer during 17 years of follow-up. The association did not vary appreciably in magnitude among the early (1958-1962), middle (1963-1968), and later (1969-1974) years of follow-up, persisted after adjustment for age, cigarette smoking, use of alcohol, family history of cancer, and occupational status, and was apparently not specific to any particular site or type of cancer. This result, predicted in advance on the basis of findings by other investigators, is consistent with the hypothe-

sis that psychological depression is related to impairment of mechanisms for preventing the establishment and spread of malignant cells.

883
Spiro HM. **Depression, cancer, and guilt--what is the connection?** (editorial) *J Clin Gastroenterol.* 1979;1:297-8. (English)

884
Surawicz FG, Brightwell DR, Weltzel WD, Othmer E. **Cancer, emotions and mental illness: the present state of understanding.** *Am J Psychiatr.* 1976;133:1306-9. (English)

The authors review recent and current literature on the relationship between psychological factors and cancer. They discuss the roles of predisposing personality patterns and emotional stress in the development, site, and course of cancer; the influence of awareness of terminal illness on the behavior of cancer patients; and the management of psychiatric symptoms in these patients.

885
Surawicz FG. **Women, cancer and emotions.** *J Am Med Wom Assoc.* 1977;32:18-29. (English)

The association of emotions, mental disease, and cancer has gone through some changes throughout the centuries. The early observation of cancer in women with melancholia does not seem as striking now as it seemed to Galen. While a few researchers continue to look for a specific personality associated with cancer of the breast or cancer of the cervix, most contemporary authors focus on the reactions to the cancer, the treatment of all aspects and the potential for rehabilitation. The retrospective studies of the fifties, influenced by psychoanalysis, are giving way to an emphasis on the here and now and on the future. The view of cancer as a psychosomatic disease has changed into a "somatopsychic" disease, in which we acknowledge the influence of cancer on the patient's psychic life. Although the concepts are changing, the unity of mind and body remains, guiding the physician toward a comprehensive approach in the care of cancer patients. In the present era, we recognize that nobody lives in a vacuum. Successful treatment, therefore, should take the aspects of family, job, and social life into consideration as well in the confrontation and rehabilitation of the patient with her crisis.

886
Whitlock FA, Siskind M. **Depression and cancer: a follow-up study.** *Psychol Med.* 1979;9:747-52. (English)

Thirty-nine male and 90 female patients aged 40 and over, who had been given a primary diagnosis of depression, were followed for 2 1/3-4 years. During this period 9 male and 9 female patients died. Five male patients and 1 female died from cancer that had not been diagnosed at the time of their psychiatric admissions. The male cancer deaths are significantly higher than expected. The possible relationships of malignant neoplasm to affective disorder are discussed.

887
Wirsching M, Stierlin H, Hoffmann F, Weber G, Wirsching

B. **Psychological identification of breast cancer patients before biopsy.** *J Psychosom Res.* 1982;26:1-10. (English)

Interviewed 56 females (mean age 54 yrs) admitted consecutively for a breast biopsy on the day prior to the operation. Interviewer ratings and blind ratings (audiotapes) allowed a differentiation of Ss in whom the biopsy revealed a cancer from those whose tumor was benign. The ratings took into account characteristics assumed to be typical of the women with cancer: (1) being inaccessible or overwhelmed when interviewed, (2) emotional suppression with sudden outbursts, (3) rationalization, (4) little or no anxiety before the operation, (5) demonstration of optimism, (6) superautonomous self-sufficiency, (7) altruistic behavior, and (8) harmonization and avoidance of conflicts. On the basis of the interviews, the interviewer and a blind rater predicted the correct diagnosis in 83 and 94% of all cancer patients and in 71 and 68% of all benign cases, respectively. The identified psychological syndrome was found in all breast cancer patients but also in one-quarter to one-third of the patients with benign nodes. This may be a long-standing defensive pattern adopted in the face of extreme emotional stress. A possible etiological significance for the cancerous disease cannot be derived from the present study.

Emotions and autoimmune diseases

888
Udelman HD, Udelman DL. **Emotions and rheumatologic disorders.** *Amer J Psychother.* 1981;35:576-87. (English) (unavailable at publication)

889
Vollhardt BR, Ackerman SH, Grayzel AI, Barland P. **Psychologically distinguishable groups of rheumatoid arthritis patients: a controlled, single blind study.** *Psychosom Med.* 1982;44:353-8. (English)

Systematic measures of mood and psychological symptoms were obtained for 68 ambulatory arthritis patients on two standard questionnaires, the Brief Symptom Inventory (BSI) and the Profile of Mood States (POMS). We studied two groups of rheumatoid arthritis patients, one positive and the other negative for rheumatoid factor and erosive joint changes. A third group of patients had other forms of arthritis. All were matched for chronicity and functional impairment as well as psychosocial background variables. We found a distinct psychometric response profile that allowed us to sort patients into the three clinical groups with an accuracy ranging from 63% to 100%.

890
Vollhardt BR, Ackerman SH. **Psychologically distinguishable groups of rheumatoid arthritis patients: a controlled single blind study** (abstract). *Psychosom Med.* 1981;43:90. (English)

Patients with rheumatoid arthritis (RA) are apparently heterogenous by clinical, serologic and histocompatibility antigen criteria. We tested the hypothesis that these patients were psychologically heterogeneous as well. Thirty eight clinic patients diagnosed as having RA were evaluated blindly

with the Brief Symptom Inventory (BSI) and the Profile of Mood States (POMS). We divided the RA patients into 2 subgroups; 18 patients with positive latex factor and erosive joint changes and 20 patients lacking this combination of features. We found large and statistically significant differences between these two RA subgroups on most of the test measures. The patients with seropositive erosive RA scored significantly *lower* on measures of compulsiveness, anxiety, depression and hostility. However, these subgroups of patients were not different in chronicity of RA, functional impairment, age, sex or social class. We also studied a mixed group of 30 clinic patients with arthritis not diagnosed as RA. Scores on the BSI and POMS for this group were significantly different from the seropositive erosive RA group, but similar to the RA group without the combination of positive latex factor and erosive joint changes. Evidence from histocompatibility studies and twin studies has shown that the RA subgroup defined by the combination of positive latex factor and erosive joint changes may be genetically homogenous. Our findings now suggest that this subgroup of RA patients is also distinguishable from other RA patients by psychological measures.

Emotions and allergic disorders

891
Abramson HA. **Asthma and emotional illness in children** (editorial). *J Asthma Res.* 1977;15:VII-VIII. (English)

892
Bosse K, Hunecke P. **The pruritus of endogenous eczema patients** (author's transl). *MMW.* 1981;123:1013-6. (German)

The psychosomatic aspects of the pruritus symptom of endogenous eczema patients are presented. The phenomenon of "scratching" is analyzed descriptively from observations of the patient and his family. Psychotherapeutic approaches as a supplement to the dermatological therapy of endogenous eczema are described.

893
Buckley JM. **Asthma and depression.** *Hosp Pract.* 1980;15: 20-8. (English) (no abstract)

894
Czubalski K, Rudzki E. **Psychosomatic symptoms and disorders of bioelectrical activity of the brain in atopic dermatitis.** *Przegl Dermatol.* 1981;68:177-80. (Polish)

In 32 patients with atopic dermatitis psychosomatic investigations were carried out and in a part of these patients electroencephalographic investigations were done. Besides that, in another 40 patients the effect of short-lasting emotion on exacerbation of skin changes was studied. The obtained results show that psychic factors play a great role in the aetiology and pathogenesis of atopic dermatitis.

895
Davis DI, Offenkrantz W. **Is there a reciprocal relationship between symptoms and affect in asthma?** *J Nerv Ment Dis.* 1976;163:369-90. (English)

This is a hypothesis-seeking case study. It is the product of naturalistic research on one asthmatic patient seen 212 times in individual psychotherapy over a period of 32 months. Both retrospective and prospective data were gathered, the prospective phase beginning about halfway into the therapy. Clinical vignettes are cited from which the following hypothesis was developed: there was a reciprocal relationship between the manifestation of physical symptoms and of affective reactions in this patient. In support of the possibility of testing this hypothesis, the therapist's observations and patient's report of physical and affective reactions each independently indicated a much greater incidence of one reaction or the other occurring separately than of both together. The occasional occurrence of both together indicates that the physical and affective reactions are not mutually exclusive; therefore, the null hypothesis is also possible. A critique and synthesis of diverse literature ranging from psychoanalytic, group, and behavioral oriented clinical reports to human and animal physiological studies precede the presentation of the case study. The conclusion reached in reviewing the literature is that confirmation of the reciprocal hypothesis awaits further studies, but there is indication in the literature of support for such further study.

896

Dirks JF, Robinson SK, Dirks DL. **Alexithymia and the psychomaintenance of bronchial asthma.** *Psychother Psychosom.* 1981;36:63-71. (English)

A total of 579 adult and adolescent asthmatic patients were assessed for alexithymia while inpatients. Subsequent rehospitalization data was collected 6 months after discharge. Analyses revealed that alexithymia was related both to rehospitalization (yes-no) and to the number of days rehospitalized. These findings were seen to reinforce the concept of alexithymia as a psychomaintenance variable.

897

Gayrard P. **Should asthmatic patients laugh?** (letter). *Lancet.* 1978;2:1105-6. (English)

898

Herxheimer H. **Should asthmatic patients laugh?** (letter). *Lancet.* 1978;2:1209. (English)

899

Horton DJ, Suda WL, Kinsman RA, Souhrada J, Spector SL. **Bronchoconstrictive suggestion in asthma: a role for airways hyperreactivity and emotions.** *Am Rev Respir Dis.* 1978;117:1029-38. (English)

Using whole-body plethysmographic measurements, asthmatic patients inhaled aerosolized saline presented either as a neutral substrate (day 1) or in the guise of a bronchoconstrictor (day 2). Bronchoconstrictive suggestion resulted in increased airway resistance and decreased specific airway conductance, whereas thoracic gas volume was unchanged. The variation in the response was analyzed in relation to airways hyperreactivity, as indexed by methacholine and histamine inhalation challenges, and physiologic measures of the emotional reaction to bronchoconstrictive suggestion, as indexed by changes in blood pressure, heart rate, finger pulse ampli-

tude, and forehead electromyographic activity. It was found that the bronchoconstrictive response was significantly related to the degree of airways hyperreactivity and to the emotional response. These results suggest that asthmatic patients apt to respond to bronchoconstrictive suggestion with airways obstructions are characterized by highly hyperreactive airways. Responders also appear to be emotionally labile, although it is not yet clear whether the emotional response per se evokes airway obstruction or is merely a by-product of the occurrence of airway obstruction.

900

Kapotes C. **Emotional factors in chronic asthma.** *J Asthma Res.* 1977;15:5-14. (English) (no abstract)

901

Lebowitz MD, Thompson HC, Strunk RC. **Subjective psychological symptoms in outpatient asthmatic adolescents.** *J Behav Med.* 1981;4:439-49. (English)

The Asthma Symptom Checklist was completed by 58 outpatient adolescent asthmatics (aged 11-17 yrs). Cluster-spherical analysis indicated that Ss were similar in many respects to older institutionalized asthmatics, except that psychological symptoms were more diffuse and recognition of respiratory symptoms less severe. Further studies are needed to determine which psychological symptoms are most important in predicting prognosis in affected asthmatics or the development of "psychosomatic" asthma.

902

Meijer A. **Emotional disorders of asthmatic children.** *Child Psychiatry Hum Dev.* 1979;9:161-9. (English)

Depression, anxiety, defiance and hostility in sixty asthmatic and non-asthmatic children of school age, all with the same familial and constitutional allergic background, were measured with the mother-child questionnaire. In the sample as a whole it was found that boys were more disturbed than girls and high-dependent children were more disturbed than low-dependent children. However, asthmatic low-dependent children were significantly more disturbed than non-asthmatic low-dependent children, whereas asthmatic high-dependent children tend to be less disturbed than non-asthmatic high-dependent children. The findings show that emotional disorders in the asthmatic children are associated with pathogenic maternal family relationship patterns.

903

Moamai N. **Emotion, inhibition, asthma.** *Union Med Can.* 1979;108:48-9. (French)

After discussing the neurophysiological basis of emotion, the part played by the cortex and the hypothalamo-reticulo-limbic complex in the emotional process, the author studies the central mechanism which leads to the asthmatic crisis. The perspective of preventing psycho-physiological disorders is emphasized. Finally, on the basis of recent studies, the author reaches the conclusion that when, in a person who is predisposed to psycho-physiological disorders, the motor path of discharge is blocked, the cumulative tension is released into the visceral neuro-vegetative system, thus creating first functional disorders and finally lesions.

904

Reddihough DS, Landau L, Jones HJ, Rickards WS. **Family anxieties in childhood asthma.** *Aust Paediatr J.* 1977; 13:295-8. (English)

Forty-three asthmatic children and their parents were interviewed to define the level of understanding of the child's asthma and assess the effect that it had on the child and family. Basic misconceptions about the disease and its therapy were apparent. Fears and anxieties about death and permanent damage to heart and lungs were expressed. The disease caused a burden on all members of the family, especially the mother. The child was not able adequately to discuss his asthma with the physician. Treatment should include more time spent with the child and family to relieve many of these anxieties.

905

Soustek Z. **Role of emotional stress and allergy in the development of cholecystitis and gallbladder calculi and their treatment with antihistaminics.** *Ter Arkh.* 1981;53:75-8. (Russian)

Acute pathomorphological changes (edema, hemorrhage, necrosis) were found in 100 gallbladders removed from patients who had suffered from acute biliary colic or acute cholecystitis. The changes are consequent on a pathological angioneurotic reaction occurring in the bed of the arteria cystica during the attack. The changes in the gallbladder wall are compared with Quincke's angioneurotic edema and with Curling's ulcer. Stress is the provocative factor of an angioneurotic reaction. The formation of gallstones is a complication of the processes taking place in the wall of the gallbladder. Mental stress or allergy was detected in 40 other patients with acute biliary colic or acute cholecystitis. The successful effect of the therapy with antihistaminic drugs is described.

906

Staudenmayer H. **Parental anxiety and other psychosocial factors associated with childhood asthma.** *J Chronic Dis.* 1981;34:627-36. (English)

The effects of childhood asthma on the parents was assessed by five psychosocial factors which were empirically derived from a questionnaire administered to 159 mothers and 70 fathers. The scales were independently derived for mothers and fathers and showed good reliability. The cluster solutions for mothers and fathers were similar, and the same labels were used for the scales: Emotional Distress, Interference, Manipulation, Overprotectiveness and Family Communication. Parent anxiety, as indexed by Emotional Distress and Interference, was related to the amount of debilitation experienced by the children, as were the fathers' perceptions of Manipulation and the mothers' self-perceptions of Overprotectiveness. It was suggested that there was a relationship between the mothers' failure to acknowledge their children's manipulations and their own overprotectiveness. Good Family Communication was unrelated to debilitation, but the results were interpreted with reservations. Overall, the study indicates that parental anxiety, like the children's anxiety, analyzed in another study, was related to the medical manageability of the disease. The diagnostic instruments developed to assess this anxiety are short and easy to administer and can be readily used by physicians to aid their decisions in medical management.

907

Wulliemier F, Gueibe R. **Psychosomatic features of asthma** (author's transl). *Ther Umsch.* 1977;34:182-5. (French)

Some general psychosomatic aspects of asthma are shortly presented. Then a case study is used in order to show the importance of a real multidisciplinary approach, which correspond to the multifactorial etiology of the entity. Some crucial clinical facts, which are frequently encountered, are also discussed.

Behavioral interventions and immunity

Conditioning and the immune system

908

Ader R, Cohen N, Grota LJ. **Adrenal involvement in conditioned immunosuppression.** *Int J Immunopharmacol.* 1979;1:141-5. (English)

A taste aversion was induced in rats by pairing cyclophosphamide, an immunosuppressive drug, with the consumption of saccharin, a novel drinking solution. Three days after conditioning, animals were injected with sheep erythrocytes; hemagglutinating antibody titers were determined 6 days later. Relative to control groups, conditioned animals provided with saccharin at the time of antigen injection showed an attenuated antibody response, confirming the results of previous studies. The injection of LiCl to elicit an adrenocortical response or the exogenous administration of corticosterone in place of the conditioned stimulus (saccharin) at the time of antigen injection did not lower antibody titer significantly. The results provide no support for the hypothesis of an adrenocortical mediation of conditioned immunosuppressive effects.

909

Ader R, Cohen N. **Behaviorally conditioned immunosuppression and murine systemic lupus erythematosus** (abstract). *Psychosom Med.* 1982;44:127-8. (English)

Several converging lines of evidence implicate the central nervous system in the regulation of immune processes, including the repeated observations that behavioral conditioning techniques can be used to suppress humoral and cell-mediated immune responses. Using a taste aversion conditioning paradigm, the present experiment was designed to examine the effects of conditioned immunosuppression on the development of autoimmune disease in New Zealand hybrid mice. It was hypothesized that, in conditioned mice, the substitution of conditioned stimuli (placebo treatment) for the immunosuppressive drug would delay the progression of systemic lupus erythematosus relative to nonconditioned mice treated with the same amount of drug under the same therapeutic regimen. Beginning at 4 mo of age, females were exposed to a novel saccharin drinking solution once each week for 8 wk. Some animals were treated under a standard (traditional) chemotherapeutic regimen (Group C100%) in which each presentation of saccharin was followed by an i.p. injection of cyclophosphamide (CY). As expected, onset of disease was delayed in these mice. For Group C50%, the critical experiment group, CY followed saccharin on only half

the weekly trials. A nonconditioned group (NC50%) received the same saccharin and CY exposure as the C50% group, but these stimuli were not paired. The rate of development of proteinuria and mortality was significantly retarded in Group C50% relative to non-drug treated controls *and* NC50% mice treated with the same amount of drug. In terms of mortality, Group C50% did not differ from Group C100%--animals treated with twice the cumulative amount of drug. These results are taken as evidence of the biologic impact of conditioned immunopharmacologic responses. Further, it is hypothesized that noncontinuous schedules of pharmacologic reinforcement may be applicable in the pharmacotherapeutic control of a variety of physiological systems.

910

Ader R. **Conditioned adrenocortical steroid elevations in the rat.** *J Comp Physiol Psychol.* 1976;90:1156-63. (English)

An illness-induced taste aversion paradigm was used to condition an elevation in plasma corticosterone level. Rats were injected with cyclophosphamide 30 min after consuming a novel saccharin drinking solution. Plasma corticosterone levels were measured before conditioning to determine unconditioned steroid levels and 3 and 6 days after training when conditioned and nonconditioned animals were provided with the saccharin solution or plain water, or were left deprived. The pairing of saccharin and cyclophosphamide was effective in inducing a passive avoidance response. There were no differences between the steroid levels of conditioned and nonconditioned animals supplied with plain water or those that remained deprived, although deprivation increased corticosterone levels. Nonconditioned rats presented with saccharin had steroid levels that did not differ from control values. Conditioned animals presented wth saccharin showed an elevation in steroid level which was significantly greater than that observed in any other group. Comparable results were obtained when LiCl was used as the unconditioned stimulus.

911

Anonymous. **"Conditioning" with placebo lowers mouse drug dose** (medical news). *JAMA.* 1982;248:407. (English)

912

Bovbjerg D, Ader R, Cohen N. **Behaviorally conditioned suppression of a graft-versus-host response.** *Proc Natl*

Acad Sci. 1982;79:583-5. (English)

Cyclophosphamide (CY), previously used to condition suppression of humoral immune responses, was used to condition suppression of a graft-versus-host response (GvHR). Female (Lewis x Brown Norway) F1 rats were conditioned by pairing consumption of a saccharin solution with an intraperitoneal injection of CY at 50 mg/kg of body weight 48 days before immunization. On day 0, all animals were injected with a suspension of splenic leukocytes (2×10^7 cells per footpad) obtained from female Lewis donors. The regional GvHR was assessed on day 5 by weighing popliteal nodes. Conditioned animals given a single low-dose injection of CY and reexposed to conditioned stimuli had lymph node weights significantly lower than control groups and did not differ from animals given three injections of CY during the ongoing GvHR. The results suggest that conditioned immunosuppression, previously demonstrated in thymus-dependent and thymus-independent humoral immune responses, also affects the popliteal GvHR, a cellular immune response.

913

Cautela JR. **Toward a Pavlovian theory of cancer.** *Scand J Behav Ther.* 1977;6:117-42. (English)

Anecdotal and research data are accumulating which indicate that stress and lack of reinforcement (depression, loss) are related to the incidence and growth of cancer. Current theories of the etiology of malignant neoplasms involve cellular abnormalities. Pavlovian theorizing concerning the properties of the nervous system is also focused on cellular functioning. Observations from the Pavlovian laboratories indicate that stress (overstrain of the excitatory process and difficulty in mobility of the nervous system and excessive and/or protracted inhibition (lack of reinforcement) produce both behavioral and organic abnormalities. A current view related to the etiology of cancer that is being seriously considered is the immunocompetence theory. This is consistent with Pavlovian theory. Pavlov himself discussed the likely probability that the immune system can be conditioned. Indeed, there is preliminary research supporting Pavlov's postulation. Treatment of cancer should involve removal of stress and an increase in the level of reinforcement by behavioral means. The general postulation is that stress and/or lack of reinforcement can provide an environment in which abnormal stimulation can increase the susceptibility and growth rate of cancer.

914

Cohen N, Ader R, Green N, Bovbjerg D. **Conditioned suppression of a thymus-independent antibody response.** *Psychosom Med.* 1979;41:487-91. (English)

An illness-induced taste aversion was conditioned in mice by pairing cyclophosphamide, an immunosuppressive drug, with the consumption of saccharin, a novel drinking solution. Two weeks after conditioning, animals were injected with the hapten trinitrophenyl (TNP) coupled to the thymus-independent carrier, lipopolysaccharide. Serum antibodies to TNP were titered 6 days later by passive hemagglutination. Relative to control groups, conditioned animals provided with saccharin at the time of antigenic stimulation and, again,

3 days later showed a significant attenuation of their anti-TNP antibody response. In a second experiment, the conditioned stimulus (CS) consisted of the novel saccharin drinking solution plus the noxious internal effects of an injection of LiCl. Conditioned animals reexposed to the CS again showed the lowest antibody titers, but differed significantly from only one of the control groups. Taken together, the results of these experiments confirm previous reports of conditioned immunosuppression and suggest that the effects of conditioning on a primary humoral antibody response can be observed in response to a T-cell independent antigen in the mouse.

915

Hansen O. **A psychosomatic theory of allergic sensitization; allergy as a quasi conditioned reaction.** *Z Psychosom Med Psychoanal.* 1981;27:143-60. (German)

A psychosomatic theory concerning the sensitization process of immediate type allergy is presented. According to this theory the allergy systems form a deficient local defense function of the respiratory tract's mucous membranes. It is assumed that persons with a specific disposition and learning experiences, in certain conflict situations where emotional impulses cannot be expressed, tend to suffer an obstructive hyperfunction of the nasal and/or bronchial mucosa including hyperemia, swelling, hypersecretion (and spasms of the bronchial muscular system). These modifications of mucous function result from suppressed aggressive expressions (rage, anger, attack) in connection with avoidance tendencies. Thus the immunological reaction may also be the result of bronchial asthma and of chronic rhinitis. This theory allows [one] to regard the process of sensitization as a learning process and to consider the allergy as a classic conditioned response to the atopic allergen as a conditioned stimulus. The obstructive hyperfunction (which, of course, can also occur by stimuli other than emotional) creates critical phases. During these the immune system can be activated against atopic allergens in sufficient quantity. However, anyone is probably more sensitized against allergens found in locations where his emotional impulses are not expressed. In this context a house dust allergy, for example, refers to conflicts within the confines of the house, but does not necessarily attribute symbolic qualities to house dust itself.

916

Rogers MP, Reich P, Strom TB, Carpenter CB. **Behaviorally conditioned immunosuppression: replication of a recent study** (rapid communication). *Psychosom Med.* 1976;38:447-51. (English) (no abstract)

917

Wayner EA, Flannery GR, Singer G. **Effects of taste aversion conditioning on the primary antibody response to sheep red blood cells and Brucella abortus in the albino rat.** *Physiol Behav.* 1978;21:995-1000. (English)

It has been shown that use of the saccharin/cyclophosphamide taste aversion paradigm produced conditioned immunosuppression as well as saccharin avoidance after two postconditioning exposures to the aversive stimulus. In the present study the effects of saccharin/cyclophosphamide conditioning on the primary humoral antibody response to two antigens: sheep red blood cells (SRBC), a T-cell dependent antigen, and Brucella abortus (B. abortus), a T-cell independent antigen, were examined. In addition the effects of a third exposure to the aversive stimulus, saccharin, on conditioned immunosuppression were examined. The results indicate that the target cell of taste aversion conditioning, in relation to immune dysfunction, could be the T-lymphocyte and that conditioned immunosuppression is dependent on the presence of the behavioral response. These results constitute a replication of previous studies and provide evidence which indicates that behaviorally conditioned immunosuppression is a consequence of the parameters of taste aversion conditioning.

Hypnosis and immunity

918
Barber TX. **Hypnosis, suggestions, and psychosomatic phenomena: a new look from the standpoint of recent experimental studies.** *Amer J Clin Hypnosis.* 1978;21:13-27. (English)

A series of investigations are reviewed which indicate that suggestion (a) can block the skin reaction (dermatitis) that is produced by poison ivy-like plants, (b) can give rise to a localized skin inflammation that has the specific pattern of a previously experienced burn, (c) can be effective in the cure of warts, (d) can ameliorate congenital ichthyosiform erythrodermia ("fish skin disease"), and (e) can stimulate the enlargement of the mammary glands in adult women. Experiments are also summarized supporting the hypothesis that the aforementioned suggested phenomena may be due, in part, to localized alterations in blood flow to the skin and other organs that can occur when certain types of suggestions are accepted.

919
Gravitz MA. **The production of warts by suggestion as a cultural phenomenon.** *Am J Clin Hypnosis.* 1981;23:281-3. (English)

Describes the cultural situation in the canton of Vaud, Switzerland, early in the 20th century, in which the onset of warts (veruccae), a virus disease, could be brought about by autosuggestion based upon expectancy and practice. There are implications of this phenomenon for increased understanding of the bodily mechanisms involved in resistance to illness, immunity, and malignancy, among other vital processes. Study of the production of warts by hypnotic suggestion is indicated under appropriate ethical, professional, and experimental conditions.

920
Sheehan DV. **Influence of psychosocial factors on wart remission.** *Amer J Clin Hypnosis.* 1978;20:160-4. (English)

The effects of psychosocial events on the natural history of warts and the physiological mechanisms that mediate them are observed in two case studies. Psychosocial factors not only accelerate the remission of warts but may also reinforce their presence and proliferation as in Case No. 1. Vasomotor changes during and following nonspecific hypnotic suggestions in Case No. 2 lend confirmation to earlier speculations and hypotheses on the nature of one mediating physiological

mechanism in wart remission. The merits of an operant conditioning paradigm of so-called "hypnotic" behaviors were discussed.

921
Tasini MF, Hackett TP. **Hypnosis in the treatment of warts in immunodeficient children.** *Am J Clin Hypnosis.* 1977;19:152-4. (English)

Three patients (12- and 14-yr-old females and a 12-yr-old male) with an immunologic deficit developed multiple warts which proved refractory to all therapy. The warts disappeared in response to hypnosis in all 3 cases, and there was no recurrence after 8 mo of follow-up.

Other interventions

922
Anonymous. **Unproven methods of cancer management: O. Carl Simonton, MD.** *CA-A Cancer J for Clinicians.* 1982;32:58-61. (English)

After careful study of the literature and other information available to it, the American Cancer Society does not have evidence that treatment with O. Carl Simonton's psychotherapy method results in objective benefit in the treatment of cancer in human beings.

923
Czubalski K, Zawisza E, Borzecki M, Bochenek Z. **Acupuncture and phonostimulation in pollenosis and vasomotor rhinitis in the light of psychosomatic investigations.** *Acta Otolaryngol (Stockh)* 1977;84:446-9. (English)

Patients with vasomotor rhinitis (28) and pollenosis (23) were subjected to psychosomatic examination and treated either by acupuncture or phonostimulation exclusively. Acupuncture was performed after the classical method in 22 patients and phonostimulation in 29. Evaluation of the results was based on laryngological examinations and appraisals entered by the patients in special personal diaries. In pollenosis the condition was unchanged by the treatment. In vasomotor rhinitis, on the other hand, in which psychic factors were of importance, some of the patients usually improved temporarily at the beginning of treatment, whereas a few suffered exacerbation. These effects may be attributable to suggestion.

924
Forth MW, Jackson M. **Group psychotherapy in the management of bronchial asthma.** *Br J Med Psychol.* 1976;49:257-60. (English)

In this paper the authors present their theoretical view of the place of psychogenic factors in asthma. They review the experience they had conducting weekly analytically oriented group therapy with a group of asthmatic women for 18 months and review the difficulties they met in this work. From this experience they attempt to reconcile some of the contradictions in previously published work in this area.

925
Karasu TB. **Psychotherapy of the medically ill.** *Amer J*

Psychiat. 1979;136:1-11. (English) (unavailable at publication)

926
Knapp PH. **Free association as a biopsychosocial probe.** *Psychosom Med.* 1980;42:197-219. (English)

Free association was used as an experimental approach in a pilot study of four healthy subjects. Physiologically simultaneous measurement of respiratory minute volume showed a wide range of moment-to-moment values, possibly reflecting shifts in emotional state. Psychologically, subjects manifested classical resistance and transference attitudes. These psychological findings were confirmed in a second study using seven mild asthmatics and six healthy comparison subjects. The asthmatics showed significant constriction of verbal associative productivity and also significantly greater immaturity in drawings of two humans and of an animal, serially administered before and after three free associative sessions. A third study of associative output after stressful stimulation, using 17 asthmatics and 16 controls, confirmed the verbal constriction of the asthmatics. Free association permits study of psychosocial context and reconstruction of important self-other relationships. These factors are important in assessing the "strain" surrounding manifest expression of emotion. Verbatim associative productions from experimental subjects and from a patient in psychoanalysis are used to form a model of emotional processes in acute bronchial asthma. This is a special case of Engel's general biopsychosocial model of disease.

927
Kumar KM. **Allergy (a psychosomatic view).** *J Indian Med Assoc.* 1980;74:16-7. (English)

A case of atopic dermatitis, treated by means of psychoanalytic psychotherapy and chemotherapy, has been reported.

928
Linn MW, Linn BS, Harris R. **Effects of counseling for late stage cancer patients.** *Cancer.* 1982;49:1048-55. (English)

Much has been written about working with the dying. Few, if any, controlled studies have examined by application of principles set forth. The authors evaluate the effectiveness of working with dying cancer patients by assessing changes in quality of life, physical functioning, and survival. One-hundred twenty men with end-stage cancer were randomly assigned to experimental or control groups; the 62 exerimental groups were seen regularly by a counselor. Patients were assessed before random assignment and at one, three, six, nine, and 12 months on quality of life and functional status. Experimental group patients improved significantly more than the control group on quality of life within three months. Functional status and survival did not differ between groups. A subsample of lung cancer patients provided cross-validation of findings. Although survival was not expected to differ, it was predicted that functioning could be enhanced if quality of life improved. One interpretation is that little can be done to alter physical function and survival when intervention occurs in the late progression of a fatal disease. This in no way reduces the value of improving overall quality of life, since enhancing the quality of survival for end-stage cancer patients is a high priority medical goal.

929
Meares A. **Meditation: a psychological approach to cancer treatment.** *The Practitioner.* 1979;222:119-22. (English) (unavailable at publication)

930
Meares A. **Regression of cancer after intensive meditation (preliminary report).** *Med J Austr.* 1976;2:184. (English) (no abstract)

931
Meares A. **Regression of osteogenic sarcoma metastases associated with intensive meditation.** *Med J Aust.* 1978;2:433. (English) (unavailable at publication)

932
Overbeck G, Overbeck A. **Family dynamic perspectives in the study of psychosomatic diseases.** *Prax Kinderpsychol Kinderpsychiatr.* 1979;28:1-6. (German)

A therapy with the family of an asthmatic child is examined from three different perspectives, which generally could be applied as basic observational categories in the research of family dynamics: fusion and limited functioning; role and mission; system-regulation. The category "fusion and limited functioning" involves the mutual exchanges within a dyadic relationship-system in which the self-object boundaries are insufficient. Through reciprocal attachments and delegations on the id and ego-superego level, the autonomous cognitive and affective functioning of the individual partners is greatly hampered and distorted. Observations that pertain to "role and mission" can provide, on the one hand, an understanding of the overall context in which the limited functioning exists. Furthermore, they are particularly well suited for the description of those interactions among family members, which have their basis in the triadic relationship pattern, where self-object boundaries are more well defined. Richter's theory of roles and Stierlin's theory of delegation can be employed in this area. Observations according to the category of "system-regulation" go beyond the individual relationships among family members, to provide insights about the functioning of the family as a whole system. These insights are sought through the application of interactional and transactional theories as well as from the description of the family structure. In conclusion, this work raises the question, whether these categories, applied in the research of family dynamics, would yield relevant results in the specific area of psychosomatic medicine.

933
Piazza EU. **Comprehensive therapy of chronic asthma on a psychosomatic unit.** *Adolescence.* 1981;16:139-44. (English) (no abstract)

934
Scarf M. **Images that heal: a doubtful idea whose time has come.** *Psychol Today.* September, 1980. (English) (no abstract)

935

Simonton OC, Matthews-Simonton S, Sparks TF. **Psychological intervention in the treatment of cancer.** *Psychosomatics.* 1980;21:226-10. (English) (unavailable at publication)

936

Simonton OC, Matthews-Simonton S. **Cancer and stress: counselling the cancer patient.** *Med J Aust.* 1981;679-83. (English) (unavailable at publication)

937

Steinhausen HC. **On the psychosomatic theory of asthma bronchiale: a review** (author's transl). *Monatsschr Kinderheilkd.* 1977;125:129-36 (German)

Following a review of classical psychosomatic theory on asthma bronchiale new research findings leading to a revised formulation of an actual psychosomatic concept of this disease are reviewed. Furthermore results of different research studies in the literature using behavior modification methods and structural family therapy are presented. Finally, clinical implications of the findings reviewed are proposed.

938

Wingerson L. **Training the mind to heal.** *Discover. May,* 1982;80-5. (English) (no abstract)

Coping, social support and immunity

939
Cassel J. **The contribution of the social environment to host resistance: The fourth Wade Hampton Frost Lecture.** *Am J Epidemiol.* 1976;104:107-23. (English)

With advancing knowledge, it is perhaps not too far-reaching to imagine a preventive health service in which professionals are involved largely in the diagnostic aspects--identifying families and groups at high risk by virtue of their lack of fit with their social milieu and determining the particular nature and form of the social supports that can and should be strengthened if such people are to be protected from disease outcomes. The intervention actions then could well be undertaken by nonprofessionals, provided that adequate guidance and specific direction were given. Such an approach would not only be economically feasible, but if the notions expressed in this paper are correct, would do more to prevent a wide variety of diseases than all the efforts currently being made.

940
Cobb S, Erbe C. **Social support for the cancer patient.** *Forum on Med.* 1978;1:24-9. (English) (no abstract)

941
Cobb S. **Social support as a moderator of life stress.** *Psychosom Med.* 1976;38:300-14. (English)

Social support is defined as information leading the subject to believe that he is cared for and loved, esteemed, and a member of a network of mutual obligations. The evidence that supportive interactions among people are protective against the health consequences of life stress is reviewed. It appears that social support can protect people in crisis from a wide variety of pathological states: from low birth weight to death, from arthritis through tuberculosis to depression, alcoholism, and the social breakdown syndrome. Furthermore, social support may reduce the amount of medication required, accelerate recovery, and facilitate compliance with prescribed medical regimens.

942
Derogatis LR, Abeioff MD, Melisaratos N. **Psychological coping mechanisms and survival time in metastatic breast cancer.** *JAMA.* 1979;242:1504-8. (English) (unavailable at publication)

943
Grossarth-Maticek R. **Social psychotherapy and course of the disease.** *Psychother Psychosom.* 1980;33:129-38. (English)

This paper is designed to introduce a new therapeutic approach into the treatment of cancer patients and to give some first results of our work. The basic idea is that the development of cancer depends to a great extent on a patient's social environment and the interrelation between environment and patient. A disturbed attitude on the part of the patient towards it and towards himself can influence adversely the development of cancer. The aim of social psychotherapy is to modify such attitudes, i.e., to influence the disease by psychological means.

944
Kinsman RA, Dahlem NW, Spector SL, Staudenmayer H. **Observations on subjective symptomatology, coping behavior, and medical decisions in asthma.** *Psychosom Med.* 1977;39:102-19. (English)

The Asthma Symptom Checklist (ASC), describing the subjective symptoms reported to occur during asthmatic attacks, has been developed previously. In the present study, the ASC key cluster solution was replicated and refined within a sample of 374 asthmatic inpatients. All of the original symptom categories were reproduced, including two mood categories, panic-fear and irritability, a fatigue category, and two somatic categories, hyperventilation-hypocapnia and airway obstruction. Two refinements were notable: (1) the airway obstruction category was empirically divided into two conceptually clear components, dyspnea and congestion, and (2) three secondary mood categories, worry, loneliness, and anger, were identified, which describe a continuum of mood between the polar extremes of panic and irritability. Of the symptom categories, only panic-fear was related to the intensity of the discharge drug regimens recommended 2 to 6 months after ASC administration. Panic-fear scores were independent of pulmonary functions and panic-fear yielded the best prediction of discharge steroid regiments. Finally, those physicians rated highest in "sensitivity" to their patients by their supervisors prescribed less steroids overall, but most frequently prescribed discharge steroid regimens in relation to their patients' panic-fear scores. In contrast, physicians rated lower on sensitivity prescribed higher steroid regimens overall, but based these drug recommendations more clearly on objective pulmonary functioning, and not in relation to their patients' panic-fear scores. The results strongly suggest that the ASC panic-fear scale is associated with coping behaviors that importantly affect the patient's overall clinical picture by increasing the apparent severity of the asthma, thereby leading to intensified treatment. The findings stress the need to evaluate independently the objective medical condition and subjective symptomatology with its related coping behavior, in order to direct appropriate modes of therapy to each.

945
Kneier AW. **Repressive coping tendencies in patients with malignant melanoma: implications for the hypothesis of cancer-prone coping behavior.** *Diss Abstr Int.* 1981;42:2506. (English) (unavailable at publication)

946
Krant MJ. **Coping psychologically with breast cancer** (letter). *JAMA.* 1981;245:31-2. (English)

947
Lin N, Ensel WM, Kuo W, Simeone RS. **Social support, stressful life events, and illness: a model and empirical test.** *J Health Soc Behav.* 1979;20:108-19. (English)

The effects of social support and stressors (stressful life events) on illness (psychiatric symptoms) are examined in a model with data from a representative sample of the Chinese-American adult population in Washington, D.C. The analysis shows that, as expected, stressors are positively related to the incidence of psychiatric symptoms, and social support is negatively related to psychiatric symptoms. Further, the contribution of social support to predicting symptoms is greater in magnitude than that of stressful life events. When marital status and occupational prestige are incorporated into the model, the significant (negative) contribution of social support to symptoms is not reduced. Implications for the theoretical development of a sociomedical theory of illness are discussed.

948
Mattila VJ, Solokangas RK. **Life changes and social group in relation to illness onset.** *J Psychosom Res.* 1977;21:167-74. (English) (unavailable at publication)

949
Rogentine GN Jr, Van Kammen DP, Fox BH, Docherty JP, Rosenblatt JE, Boyd SC, Bunney WE. **Psychological factors in the prognosis of malignant melanoma: a prospective study.** *Psychosom Med.* 1979;41:647-55. (English)

Sixty-four patients with clinical Stage I or II malignant melanoma who were apparently disease free rated the amount of adjustment needed to cope with their illness on a scale of 1 to 100. The resultant figure was called the melanoma adjustment score. Twenty-nine patients who relapsed within 1 year of surgery reported a score of 53 ± 34 (mean ± SD); 35 nonrelapsers reported a score of 80 ± 20, p<0.001. Based upon analysis of individual melanoma adjustment scored in the first 34 patients, we predicted that subjects scoring <65 would stay in remission, whereas those scoring >65 would relapse. Applying this prospectively to the next 33 patients, we cor-

rectly identified 25 of 33 outcomes (76%), p<0.03. This psychological variable was independent of known biological prognostic factors, which did not predict 1 year survival. The melanoma adjustment score was also independent of the number of positive lymph nodes, which did correlate with outcome in these patients. The results suggest a role for psychological factors in the one year prognosis of this malignancy.

950
Sklar LS, Anisman H. **Stress and coping factors influence tumor growth.** *Science.* 1979;205:513-5. (English)

Growth of syngeneic P815 mastocytoma in DBA/2J male mice was evaluated as a result of various stress regimens. A single session of inescapable shock resulted in earlier tumor appearance, exaggeration of tumor size, and decreased survival time in recipient animals. Escapable shock had no such effects. The effects of the inescapable shock were mitigated if mice received long-term shock treatment.

951
Strayhorn G. **Social supports, perceived stress, and health: the black experience in medical school--a preliminary study.** *J Natl Med Assoc.* 1980;72:869-81. (English)

Black medical students perceived significantly more stressors than white medical students in a predominantly white medical school environment (p=0.001). Black medical students perceived fewer social supports than white medical students, but not significantly fewer (p=0.224). There was no significant difference between mean systolic and diastolic blood pressure levels for the low and high stress groups (p=0.302 and 0.844, respectively). The total degree of perceived stressors did not predict systolic and diastolic blood pressure when controlling for potential confounders (0.05<p<0.01). The interaction of total degree of stressors and total degree of social supports did not significantly predict systolic and diastolic blood pressures when controlling for potential confounding variables (p>0.25 and 0.1<p<0.25, respectively).

Immunopsychiatry

Immunologic aspects of mental disorder

952

Abramsky O, Litvin Y. **Autoimmune response to dopamine-receptor as a possible mechanism in the pathogenesis of Parkinson's disease and schizophrenia.** *Perspect Biol Med.* 1978;22:104-14. (English)

Clinical and neuropharmacological evidence indicates the involvement of dopaminergic mechanisms in Parkinson's disease and schizophrenia, as well as in iatrogenic Parkinsonism and drug-induced schizophrenia-like syndrome. The evidence hitherto presented stresses the existence of a reversed relationship between Parkinson's disease and schizophrenia and implicates the possibility that dysfunction of dopamine-receptors may be a central phenomenon in both diseases. In view of the recent demonstration of two separate dopamine-receptors, it is postulated that a striatal receptor blockade may cause Parkinson's disease, whereas a limbic receptor blockade may result in schizophrenia. The recent discovery that several autoimmune diseases, such as myasthenia gravis, are the result of an immunopharmacological block at receptor sites, together with several observations of immunological disorders in Parkinson's disease and schizophrenia, suggests the possibility that certain types of Parkinson's disease and schizophrenia might be the consequence of an autoimmune blockade of striatal or limbic dopamine-receptors, respectively.

953

Achterberg J, Collerain I, Craig P. **A possible relationship between cancer, mental retardation and mental disorders.** *Soc Sci Med.* 1978;12:135-9. (English)

A correlative relationship between mental disorders and low incidence of cancer has been documented in scattered incidences in the literature. The present study was conducted to more clearly define the parameters of the relationship, and to provide a detailed breakdown of diagnostic types as they relate to incidence of malignancy. The sample consisted of 3,214 client deaths reported by a state department of mental health and mental retardation over a 3.5 year period. Death from cancer in the mentally retarded and mentally disturbed constituted about 4% of all deaths, as contrasted with 18% of deaths from cancer in the general population. The findings were constant across age, sex, race, and geographical location within the state. Institutionalization also did not appear to be a contributing factor to the low incidence. Within diagnostic categories, however, differences were observed, with excep-

tionally low or absent figures in catatonics, drug abusers, personality disorders, and profoundly mentally retarded. Relatively higher rates were observed in patients diagnosed as paranoid schizophrenics and in the mildly retarded. As the clients approached normal levels of functioning, the cancer incidence also more closely approximated that of the normal population. It is concluded that regardless of whether there is a common etiology among the diverse categories of mental dysfunction, a statistical relationship between these diagnoses and low cancer incidence exists and deserves to be examined not only in a genetic investigation, but also in a biochemical study of the peculiar immunocompetencies of these groups.

954

Albrecht P, Torrey EF, Boone E, Hicks JT, Daniel N. **Raised cytomegalovirus-antibody level in cerebrospinal fluid of schizophrenic patients.** *Lancet.* 1980;2:769-72. (English)

The serum and cerebrospinal fluid (CSF) of 60 schizophrenic patients and 26 controls were analyzed for viral antibody against cytomegalovirus (CMV), vaccinia virus, herpes simplex virus type 1 (HSV), and type A influenza virus. A CSF/serum antibody ratio more than 2 standard deviations above the mean of the controls suggested local antibody production in the central nervous system. 68% of the patients had an increased CSF/serum antibody ratio for CMV antibody, 14% for vaccinia antibody, 4% for HSV antibody, and 15% for influenza virus antibody.

955

Anavi R, Baron M, Witz IP. **Serologic studies on schizophrenic patients.** *Birth Defects.* 1978;14:297-309. (English)

We studied the capacity of sera from schizophrenic patients and from normal blood bank donors to agglutinate sheep erythrocytes coated with extracts of human brain. Passive hemagglutination of coated erythrocytes was obtained with 36.4% of the assayed sera of the schizophrenia patients and with 11% of the control sera. Drug treatment did not seem to play a major role in the reactivity because the patients were either never treated before or a period of several weeks was allowed since treatment until blood was drawn. Furthermore the analysis of sera obtained by sequential bleedings of patients on drug therapy showed that drugs did not affect the serologic activity.

956
Armstrong-Esther CA, Lacey JH, Crisp AH, Bryant TN. **An investigation of the immune response of patients suffering from anorexia nervosa.** *Postgrad Med J.* 1978;54:395-9. (English)

Patients suffering from anorexia nervosa rarely appear to develop the common cold or influenza. This study examines the immunological response of 15 female anorexia nervosa patients of both the vomiting and carbohydrate-abstaining type and compares them with a control population matched for age and occupation. Both anorectics and control populations received the immune influenza vaccine. Initially both groups had similar haemagglutination inhibition titres against the three different viral antigens: A/HK; A/PC; A/ENG. However, the anorectics showed over a 2-month period a higher titre of antibody especially to the Hong Kong virus: this was significant. Cellular immune responses were measured using a tuberculin and a macrophage inhibition test; no significant difference between the two groups was observed. These results which support the clinical findings are discussed.

957
Ashkenazi A, Krasilowsky D, Levin S, Idar D, Kalian M, Or A, Ginat Y, Halperin B. **Immunologic reaction of psychotic patients to fractions of gluten.** *Am J Psychiatry.* 1979;136:1306-9. (English)

Production of a leukocyte migration inhibition factor by peripheral blood lymphocytes in response to challenge with gluten fractions was studied in hospitalized patients with schizophrenia and other psychoses compared with normal individuals and with children and adolescents with celiac disease. The schizophrenic and other psychotic patients could be subdivided into two groups, one that responded in the leukocyte migration inhibition factor test as the celiac patients did and one that responded as the normal control subjects did. The psychotic and schizophrenic patients did not show any evidence of malabsorption. The authors speculate that gluten may be involved in biological processes in the brain in certain psychotic individuals.

958
Ashkenazi A, Levin S, Krasilowsky D. **Gluten and autism** (letter). *Lancet.* 1980;1:8160. (English)

959
Aulakh GS, Kleinman JE, Aulakh HS, Albrecht P, Torrey EF, Wyatt RJ. **Search for cytomegalovirus in schizophrenic brain tissue.** *Proc Soc Exp Biol Med.* 1981;167:172-4. (English)

A human cytomegalovirus (CMV) DNA probe was developed and hybridized to DNA extracted from brain tissue of 6 patients with schizophrenia and 6 control individuals. We failed to detect any CMV-related genetic information in the DNA of these 12 individuals. These results indicate CMV is not involved in schizophrenia or that the genetic viral information, if present, is below the level of sensitivity of the present assay.

960
Ayuso Gutierrez JL, Sainz Ruiz J, Casimiro San Segundo C. **Antinuclear factors and pathological psychiatry.** *Arch Neurobiol (Madr).* 1979;42:189-98. (Spanish) (unavailable at publication)

961
Babaian NG, Bonartsev PD, Prilipko LL. **Effect of schizophrenic patients' serum on the physiological state of lymphocytes under *in vitro* conditions.** *Zh Nevropatol Psikhiatr.* 1977;77:1361-64. (Russian)

The report is concerned with the action of the serum of schizophrenic patients on the physiological state of lymphocytes in normal donors. It was established that during the early stages of incubation the action of the serum in schizophrenic patients evokes the activation of lymphocytes in normal donors, which is seen in changes of the ultrastructure and adhesive properties of these cells. On the late stages of cultivation the serum of patients destroys $13.4 + 5.9\%$ of lymphocytes of normal donors. In the remaining population 21% of lymphocytes lose their capability to react to PHA stimulation by an increase of DNA content.

962
Babaian NG, Lideman RR, Lozovskii DV, Prilipko LL, Faktor MI. **Role of serum factors in decreasing the reaction of peripheral blood lymphocytes in schizophrenia to PHA stimulation.** *Zh Nevropatol Psikhiatr.* 1978;78:80-6. (Russian)

The blood serum of schizophrenic patients and three of its studied fractions (gamma-globulins and those remaining after elimination of gamma-globulins and ultrafiltrate protein fractions) inhibit the lymphocyte response of normals and was seen only in the protein fraction. The PHA precipitating activity of the blood serum in schizophrenic patients which is mainly connected with its protein fraction is increased by 30%. However, there are no correlations between this blood serum activity and its capability to inhibit the response of lymphocytes to PHA stimulation.

963
Baldwin JA. **Schizophrenia and physical disease** (editorial). *Psychol Med.* 1979;9:611-8. (English)

964
Baron M, Stern M, Anavi R, Witz IP. **Tissue-binding factor in schizophrenic sera: a clinical and genetic study.** *Biol Psychiat.* 1977;12:199-219. (English)

The hypothesis that pathologic immune mechanisms, characterized by production of brain autoantibodies, operate in schizophrenia, was the basis for this study. Binding of serum globulin substance by human brain septal region obtained at autopsy was measured by radioimmunofixation assay in 27 schizophrenic probands, 28 first-degree relatives, 12 patients with primary affective disorder (depression), and 117 normal controls. Schizophrenic individuals tended to have higher levels of brain-serum affinity than controls. Age and sex did not appear to affect results. Within families, elevation of serum-binding activity showed intra sib-pair resemblance, distinguished healthy relatives from probands and ill relatives and relatives of probands with positive sera from relatives of probands with negative serum activity. Serum activity distinguished well relatives from normal controls and was independent of clinical state. This suggests that brain-serum affinity may be compatible with characteristics of a genetic marker of vulnerability to schizophrenia. Within sib-pairs, concordance rates for elevated serum activity and subtype diagnosis, mode, and age of illness onset were positively related. This finding supports clinico-genetic disposition in a subgroup of schizophrenic patients. To determine distribution patterns of antigenic components, selected schizophrenic and normal sera were tested against human liver and mouse brain, thymus, and liver. Wide tissue cross-reactivity was observed in schizophrenic, but not in normal sera, a finding consistent with overlap of serological reactions affecting specific tissues in autoimmune processes. The assay employed in the present study and investigation of inheritance of brain-serum affinity have not previously been reported.

965
Bell IR, Guilleminault C, Dement WC. **Hypersomnia, multiple-system symptomatology, and selective IgA deficiency.** *Biol Psychiat.* 1978;13:751-7. (English)

Individual susceptibility to specific environmental substances has long been associated with various behavioral and somatic syndromes by certain clinical observers (Hall, 1976). Selective IgA deficiency is one endogenous abnormality reported to increase the risk of systemic entry of foreign materials such as food (e.g., milk, gluten) and infectious agents (Hong and Ammann, 1972; Falchuk and Falchuk, 1975). This paper presents a patient with selective IgA deficiency whose multiple-system symptomatology, with notable sleep and gastrointestinal manifestations, was found to respond to comprehensive management of dietary and other environmental exposures. An apparently "functional" disorder had previously been diagnosed, largely through exclusion of plausible organic causes of the symptoms. In this case, however, the symptoms yielded to treatment for exposure to common foods, chemicals, and natural inhalants.

966
Bergen JR, Grinspoon L, Pyle HM, Martinez JL Jr, Pennel RB. **Immunologic studies in schizophrenic and control subjects.** *Biol Psychiat.* 1980;15:369-79. (English)

Heath and coworkers proposed that schizophrenia may be an autoimmune disorder in which antibodies are built up against specific substances in certain brain cells. Heath reports that schizophrenic patients exhibit abnormal brain waves in recordings from the caudate nucleus and septal area. These abnormal waves can also be recorded from similar sites in monkey brains after injections into the lateral ventricle cerebrospinal fluid of gamma-G-immunoglobulins (IgG) isolated from the blood of acutely ill schizophrenic patients. We prepared IgG fractions from control subjects and acutely ill schizophrenic patients and tested them in rhesus monkeys under double-blind conditions. Of 107 sera tested from 24 schizophrenic patients, 29 produced positive electroencephalographic recordings in the monkeys. From 30 control subjects we tested 80 samples and found 6 to be positive according to Heath's criteria. This amounts to more than 1 positive reaction for every 4 schizophrenic patients' fractions tested and approximately 1 positive in 13 from control subjects' serum fractions. The difference between control and patient groups is highly significant ($p<0.001$). Although our results confirm the experimental findings of the Heath group concerning abnormal EGG activity associated with an IgG fraction from schizophrenic patients, they differ from Heath's results for fractions from control persons. We found positive effects from a small number of control fractions whereas Heath claims never to have observed positive biological activity in control fractions. The autoimmune hypothesis has numerous drawbacks, the greatest of which is the inability to demonstrate the presence of circulating antibody in schizophrenic patients with the use of standard immunologic techniques.

967
Bock E. **Immunoglobulins, prealbumin, transferrin, albumin, and alpha$_2$-macroglobulin in cerebrospinal fluid and serum in schizophrenic patients.** *Birth Defects.* 1978;14:283-95. (English)

Proteins in blood of psychotic patients have been investigated frequently, whereas investigations on cerebrospinal fluid (CSF) proteins are scarce. The literature has been reviewed by Fessel, Weil-Malherbe, and Bock and Rafaelsen. The present study was undertaken in order to investigate plasma proteins in the CSF from schizophrenic patients using 3 different control groups: 1) A group of patients suffering from endogenous depression, 2) a group of demented patients that has been described previously, and 3) a control group of patients suffering from various minor psychiatric and neurologic disorders. This group has also been described previously. Immunoglobulins are not normally synthesized inside the blood-liquor barrier, but local production takes place under various pathologic conditions involving the immune apparatus. In a previous study on serum proteins in acutely psychotic patients decreased values of IgM were found in a group of schizophrenic patients. Therefore, it seemed worthwhile to determine the immunoglobulins in the present study. Prealbumin and transferrin were studied because local production inside the blood-liquor barrier of these 2 proteins takes place normally. Thus approximately 90% of CSF prealbumin and 25% of CSF transferrin are locally produced. Finally, albumin and alpha$_2$-macroglobulin were determined in order to evaluate the blood-liquor barrier permeability.

968
Bogdanova ED, Domashneva IV, Prilipko LL. **Hemolytic properties of the lymphocytes of schizophrenia patients.** *Zh Nevropatol Psikhiatr.* 1978;78:77-80. (Russian)

The authors studied the cytotoxic activity of the lymphocytes in the peripheral blood of 16 schizophrenic patients and 14 normal donors in respect to autological erthrocytes. It was demonstrated that the hemolytic activity of the lymphocytes of patients was significantly higher than in the control group. Activated cells possess cytotoxic properties.

969
Bonartsev PD, Buravlev VM. **Electron microscopic study**

of the interaction between lymphocytes of schizophrenic patients and human embryo brain cells under tissue culture conditions. *Zh Nevropatol Psikhiatr.* 1977; 77:688-92. (Russian)

The authors convened an electron microscopic study of the interaction of lymphocytes in the peripheral blood of schizophrenic patients with the brain cells of the embryo after a 24-hour joint cell incubation. It was found that in comparison with the lymphocytes of normals, the lymphocytes of schizophrenic patients much more frequently come into contact with the cells of the brain culture. The lymphocytes of the patients are characterized by an increased amount of cytoplasmatic processes. A maximum amount of lymphocytes which came into contact was seen in experiments on populations enriched in activized cells of the lymphocyte in schizophrenic patients. It is particularly the activized lymphocytes of schizophrenic patients that, when coming into contact, called forth degenerative changes in the cells of brain culture in the area of contacts.

970
Bonartsev PD. **Adhesive lymphocytes in the peripheral blood of schizophrenic patients.** *Zh Nevropatol Psikhiatr.* 1977;77:1053-57. (Russian)

The blood of schizophrenic patients compared to that of normals contain 3-4 times more adhesive lymphocytes. A blood analysis of 59 schizophrenic patients demonstrated that approximately 60% of the patients have a high content of such cells. Among the adhesive lymphocytes there are 5 times more activated, 3 times more wide plasmatic, but twice less narrow plasmatic lymphocytes compared to normals. According to the indices of adhesivity and according to ultrastructure signs it was found that the lymphocytes of schizophrenic patients react more weakly to PHA than the lymphocytes of normals. It is assumed that the blood of schizophrenic patients contains biologically active substances, which bring on an increase of adhesive properties in the lymphocytes and their physiological activation.

971
Bond PA, Cundall RL, Falloon IR. **Monoamine oxidase (MAO) of platelets, plasma, lymphocytes and granulocytes in schizophrenia.** *Br J Psychiatry.* 1979;134:360-5. (English)

Monoamine oxidase (MAO) levels in plasma, platelets, lymphocytes and granulocytes have been compared in schizophrenics and controls using three substrates. No significant difference was found between MAO levels and controls and the schizophrenic group as a whole, but platelets and lymphocytes of the latter (tyramine or benzylamine substrate) showed greater variation and in some cases higher values than controls, irrespective of treatment. Schizophrenics who experienced auditory hallucinations had significantly lower MAO levels in lymphocytes and platelets than those who did not.

972
Breier S, et al. **Contribution to the problem of the correlation between biological and psychological factors in homicide.** *Cesk Psychiat.* 1978;74:267-84. (Czech) (unavailable at publication)

973
Brown EL, Fukuhara JT, Feiguine RJ. **Alexithymic asthmatics: the miscommunication of affective and somatic states.** *Psychother Psychosom.* 1981;36:116-21. (English) (unavailable at publication)

974
Cappel R, Gregoire F, Thiry L, Sprecher S. **Antibody and cell-mediated immunity to herpes simplex virus in psychotic depression.** *J Clin Psychiatr.* 1978;39:266-8. (English)

The incidence and antibody titers to herpes simplex virus (HSV) were found significantly higher in patients with psychotic depression as compared to normal controls. Furthermore, the cell-mediated immunity (CMI) to HSV in psychotic depression was similar to that observed after acute HSV infection or recurrence. The results suggest therefore an association between HSV infection and psychotic depression.

975
Costa D, Mestes E, Coban A. **Breast and other cancer deaths in a mental hospital.** *Neoplasma.* 181;28:371-8. (English)

The neuroleptics, well known as stimulants of prolactin release, are supposed to increase breast cancer incidence. To verify this hypothesis, we selected a group of 853 deaths of female inpatients with mental disease recorded in the Dr. G. Marinescu Hospital between 1929 and 1978. Using proportionally and indirect standardization methods, we did not find any association between the incidence of breast cancer death and neuroleptic therapy, widely used in the above-mentioned hospital after 1959. Several authors reported a low cancer death incidence in mental patients. Between 1925 and 1978, 2168 deaths were recorded in this hospital. Besides death certificates, we also studied 1444 complete autopsy protocols (66.60% of all the deaths). Cancer deaths represented 1.94% of 1231 deaths recorded between 1925 and 1960. Cancer deaths represented 7.04% of 937 deaths in the period of 1961-1978, in comparison with 13.36% of the whole population of Romania ($p<0.001$). Among these 937 deaths, statistically significant lower cancer ratios than in general population were found in ten-year age groups, i.e., between 15 and 74 years in women and between 45 and 74 years in men. No case of leukemia was recorded over 1925-1978. Deaths from pneumonia, bronchopneumonia and cardio-vascular diseases are now frequent in major mental disorders. New prospective studies are required to elucidate the problem of cancer incidence in mental patients.

976
Crow TJ, Ferrier IN, Johnstone EC, MacMillan JF, Owens DGC, Parry RP, Tyrrell DAJ. **Characteristics of patients with schizophrenia or neurological disorder and virus-like agent in cerebrospinal fluid.** *Lancet.* 1979;1:842-44. (English)

A virus-like agent (V.L.A.) with a cytopathic effect on cultured cells was found in the cerebrospinal fluid of 18 of 47 patients with schizophrenia, of whom 10 had nuclear schizophrenic symptoms. In most patients with V.L.A., blood and C.S.F. protein concentrations were normal. Patients with and without V.L.A. had similar clinical characteristics but serum IgA levels were higher in those with V.L.A.. V.L.A. was also detected in the C.S.F. of 8 of 11 patients with serious or chronic neurological disease (Huntington's chorea, multiple sclerosis, and unexplained alterations of consciousness).

977
DeLisi LE, Neckers LM, Staub RA, Zaloman SJ, Wyatt RJ. **Lymphocyte monoamine oxidase activity and chronic schizophrenia.** *Psychiatr Res.* 1980;2:179-86. (English)

Lymphocyte monoamine oxidase (MAO) activity was assayed in 62 chronic schizophrenic patients, 113 normal volunteers, and 23 first-degree relatives of schizophrenic patients. Mean lymphocyte MAO activity was significantly lower ($p < 0.001$) in the chronic shcizophrenic group than in controls; first-degree relatives had a mean lymphocyte MAO activity midway between the schizophrenics and normals. No relationship was found between lymphocyte MAO activity and sex or age of subjects. When subjects were subgrouped by race, blacks had significantly lower MAO activity than whites ($p < 0.001$).

978
DeLisi LE, Weinberger DR, Potkin SG, Neckers LM, Shiling DJ, Wyatt RJ. **Quantitative determination of immunoglobulins in CSF and plasma of chronic schizophrenic patients.** *Br J Psychiatry.* 1981;139:513-8. (English)

Immunoglobulins IgG, IgA and IgM were quantified in cerebrospinal fluid (CSF) and plasma from chronic schizophrenic patients and controls using an immunofluorescent antibody technique. A generalized reduction in immunoglobulin in levels was observed in the schizophrenic patients compared with controls. While this study supports other reports of abnormal immune functioning in schizophrenia, it failed to replicate previous findings of elevations in CSF IgG and elevations in serum IgA. The aetiology and significance of these findings are hypothesized but remain elusive.

979
Deberdt R, Van Hooren J, Biesbrouck M, Amery W. **Antinuclear factor-positive mental depression: A single disease entity?** *Biol Psychiat.* 1976;11:69-74. (English)

Antinuclear factor (ANF) was present in the serum of about 30% of 53 patients newly admitted to the psychiatric hospital because of mental depression. Clinically, ANF-positive depression closely resembles manic-depressive psychosis but tends to be more resistant to treatment. It is suggested that ANF-positive depression may be a quite distinctive disease.

980
Delgado Garcia G, Garcia Landa J. **Reactivity of the intradermal test with toxoplasmosis in schizophrenic patients.** *Rev Cubana Med Trop.* 1979;31:225-31. (Spanish)

A hundred schizophrenic patients admitted to the 10 de Octubre clinical-surgical teaching hospital and 158 schizophrenic patients admitted to the psychiatric hospital, both in Havana, and 100 control healthy individuals who did not consume psychopharmacons were studied. They underwent

intradermal tests with toxoplasmin. Differences in reactor percentages between patients and healthy individuals were statistically significant as it has been reported in the foreign medical literature. The highest percentage of reactors in the group admitted to the psychiatric hospital where most advanced schizophrenics are found leads to the conclusion that the more severe the patient state the higher the frequency and intensity of test reactivity among patients. Other factors such as the dwelling conditions, age and sex were involved.

981
Delgado Garcia G, Rodriguez Perdomo E. **Reactivity of toxoplasmin intradermal test in neurotic and manic-depressive patients.** *Rev Cubana Med Trop.* 1980;32:35-9. (Spanish)

Fifty patients with manic-depressive psychosis, 120 neurotics and 100 healthy individuals were tested. They underwent the toxoplasmin intradermal test. The highest percentage of reactors was found among patients with manic-depressive psychosis (66.6%). Patients with depressive neurosis accounted for the highest number among neurotics (55.6%). The intensity of reaction was higher among patients with manic-depressive psychosis. Neurotic patients were compared to schizophrenic patients from a previous study conducted by one of the authors. It is concluded that the percentage of reactors is higher among patients with depressive mental disorders, and also that this percentage increases with mental deterioration in patients.

982
Delgado Garcia G. **Results of intradermal tests with toxoplasmin in a survey performed among mental patients admitted to the clinical surgical teaching hospital "10 de Octubre" in Havana.** *Rev Cubana Med Trop.* 1979;31:67-71. (Spanish)

Intradermal tests using toxoplasmin were performed among three hundred mentally handicapped patients admitted to the "10 de Octubre" clinical-surgical teaching hospital in Havana between 1976-1977 and 100 healthy subjects. A statistically significant difference between reactors among patients (54.7%) and reactors among healthy subjects (30.0%) was found. Results are compared to those from a similar paper performed in the psychiatric hospital of Havana in 1967. It is concluded that the higher the severity of affections the higher the percentage of reactors in the surveyed series.

983
Delgado Garcia G. **Toxoplasmosis and mental diseases.** *Rev Cubana Med Trop.* 1979;31:127-31. (Spanish)

One hundred mentally handicapped patients admitted to the 10 de Octubre clinial-surgical teaching hospital in the Havana city, 100 patients admitted to the day hospital of such institution and 100 normal subjects were studied. The first two groups had different psychiatric diseases. They underwent toxoplasmin tests. The percentage of reactors increased from 30% among healthy subjects to 45.9% among those attending the day hospital and to 60% among those admitted to wards; this is statistically significant. It is concluded that the higher the severity of the psychiatric disease, the poorer the hygienic habits and the higher the contact with the parasite phocuses.

984
Diebold K. **Leukocyte count in manics, endogenous depressive, schizophrenics and neurotics.** *Psychiatr Clin (Basel).* 1976;9:230-5. (English)

Manic, endogenous depressive, schizophrenic and neurotic patients, 80 (40 females, 40 males) in each diagnostic group, are compared with regard to the white blood count with one another and with normal controls. Significant difference of means were found (1) between some groups of patients concerning the total number of leucocytes, the number of neutrophil granulocytes, the number of eosinophil granulocytes and the number of lymphocytes, and (2) between all groups of patients and normal controls concerning the number of monocytes. The findings are discussed.

985
Domashneva IV, Bogdanova ED, Prilipko LL, Vostrikova SA. **Hemolytic properties of activated (adhesive) peripheral blood lymphocytes from schizophrenic patients.** *Zh Nevropatol Psikhiatr.* 1979;79:583-5. (Russian)

The hemolytic properties of adhesive and nonadhesive lymphocytes in the blood of schizophrenic patients and normal donors were studied. It was demonstrated that adhesive lymphocytes possess hemolytic properties. It was shown as well that the content of hemolytic active lymphocytes in the adhesive fraction of peripheral blood cells in schizophrenic patients is ten times higher than in a similar cell fraction of normal donors.

986
Domashneva IV, Maznina TP. **Clinical-immunological correlations in the study of antithymic antibodies in schizophrenia.** *Zh Nevropatol Psikhiatr.* 1976;76:78-81. (Russian)

The convened studies performed with the aid of cytotoxic reactions demonstrated that the existence of antithymic antibodies in the blood sera of schizophrenic patients is a constant sign and does not depend upon the types of development, acuity and progressivenes of the pathological process. The cytotoxic activity of the blood sera in patients with other disorders practically does not differ from the cytotoxic activity in the sera of normals.

987
Domashneva IV, Minsker EI, Panteleeva GP, Tsirkin SI. **Effect of medical treatment on the antithymic activity of schizophrenic patients' serum.** *Zh Nevropatol Psikhiatr.* 1981;81:1199-1203. (Russian)

In 16 schizophrenic patients treated with aminazin changes of the serum antithymic activity (ATA) were studied in relation to the drug pharmacokinetics and peculiarities of the patients' psychic status. It was found that in part of the patients the serum ATA level sharply fell immediately after the treatment onset; the psychopathological disturbances in these patients were reduced, and the patients developed remissions of a good quality. In another part of the patients the high serum

ATA remained unchanged throughout the whole observation period. These patients were resistant to the drug therapy and had pronounced schizophrenic defects in their status.

988
Domashneva IV. **Population of B-lymphocytes in the peripheral blood of schizophrenic patients.** *Zh Nevropatol Psikhiatr.* 1977;77:1354-57. (Russian)

With the aid of a direct immunofluorescent method the percent of the B-lymphocytes in the peripheral blood of schizophrenic patients and normals was determined. It was demonstrated that in the preparation of blood cells the portion of cells possessing superficial immunoglobulins (B-lymphocytes) significantly exceeds the portion of cells in normal donors. On the basis of achieved data it can be assumed that in the blood of schizophrenic patients there is a higher percent of B-lymphocytes than in normals and most likely lesser of T-lymphocytes.

989
Domashneva IV. *In vitro* **lysis of schizophrenic patients' erythrocytes in an autologous system.** *Zh Nevropatol Psikhiatr.* 1978;78:1347-50. (Russian)

Using the Erne method in N.N. Klemparskaya's modification the author studied peripheral blood of 59 schizophrenic patients with different types of the course and 23 normals. It is shown that in the peripheral blood preparations of schizo phrenic patients there is a reliably greater number of zones of local hemolysis of erythrocytes. This phenomenon is associated with a general immunological status of the body.

990
Dubay L, Hrbka A. **Herpes virus hominis type 1 and mental diseases** (author's transl). *Cas Lek Cesk.* 1976; 115:1614-7. (Czech)

The following appear to be evidence of aetiological connection between schizophrenia, paranoia and the so-called acute psychoses and Herpes virus hominis: (1) the frequency of positive complement fixation reactions with the antigen of Herpes virus hominis in high titres, (2) a significant difference in the strength of titres in comparison with that in healthy subjects as well as that in other diseases, e.g., neuroses and others, (3) the dynamics of antibody response in the course of the disease, (4) direct connection between the deterioration or improvement of the disease and the dynamics of antibodies. Evidence against any such aetiological connection includes the great dispersion of values of antibodies in each particular nosological group. Final proof can only be brought by systematic cultivation of investigations.

991
Dvorakova M, Jandova A, Mejsnarova B, Vinglerova M, Zvolsky P, Heyberger K, Motycka K, Coupek J. **Immunobiological examination of psychiatric patients: preliminary report** (author's transl). *Sb Lek.* 1981;83:337-41.

The authors studied cell-mediated immunity in psychiatric patients by means of inhibition of adherence of the leucocytes to sial glass. Grey matter of the frontal and temporal lobes of the brains of schizophrenics and the Riley virus were used as antigenically functional components. A positive reaction of the white blood cells to the antigen was observed in all the 40 patients examined, in contrast to 45 healthy people whose leucocytes barely reacted to these antigens. In patients with endogenous psychoses there was a high level of sensitivity toward the antigen of the temporal lobe, while those suffering from neurosis reacted more to the antigen of the frontal lobe. A positive reaction of the leucocytes to the virus antigen was observed in all the patients. All these findings were statistically significant. An immunologically active form of RNA, which was not proper to the bearer's organism, could be isolated from the cytosol of the frontal and temporal lobes of schizophrenic brains by means of a high performance gel chromatography. Further areas of diseased and healthy brains will have to be studied in order to complete these findings. The authors believe that this approach might be the means of valuable contributions to the research in the field of the etiopathogenesis of certain psychiatric diseases.

992

Dvorakova M, Zvolsky P, Herzog P. **Endogenous psychoses and T and B lymphocytes.** *Folia Haematol.* 1980;107:221-8. (English)

By means of the rosette test an increase of active T lymphocytes (AE rosettes) in percent and a decrease of B lymphocytes (EA and EAC rosettes) could be proved in 42 psychotic patients. When dividing the tested patients into the group of depressions and the group of schizophrenics, the active T lymphocytes were more numerous in the former, [while] T and also B lymphocytes were less frequent in the latter than in the sample of the population. An analysis of the entire group in response to medication indicates that administration of these drugs will probably influence these differences, too. Patients taking lithium and patients treated with phenothiazine neuroleptics more frequently showed an increased percentage of activated cells (AE rosettes) than those patients treated with other drugs (p<0.05). These changes seemed to be especially significant in patients taking both these drugs simultaneously; moreover, a high frequency of AE rosettes also produced a decrease of B lymphocytes--EA and EAC rosettes--in this patients. In all three cases p<0.001.

993

Dwyer DS. **Virus-like particles in CSF in schizophrenia** (letter). *Lancet.* 1979;1:1184-5. (English)

994

Ehrnst A, Wiesel FA, Bjerkenstedt L, Tribukait B, Jonsson J. **Failure to detect immunologic stigmata in schizophrenia.** *Neuropsychobiol.* 1982;8:169-71. (English)

The sera of 17 patients with acute or chronic schizophrenia were tested for antibodies to a human brain extract or to Molt cells, a human T-cell line, with negative results. The level of *in vivo* lymphocyte stimulation was investigated by determination of the proportion of peripheral blood lymphocytes in the G1, S or G2 + M phases of the cell cycle and by their uptake of ^{3}H-thymidine. There was no sign of increased lymphocyte mitotic activity by these two tests. Therefore, immunologic stigmata could not be detected by these methods in these schizophrenic patients.

995

Extein I, Tallman J, Smith CC, Goodwin FK. **Changes in lymphocyte beta-adrenergic receptors in depression and mania.** *Psychiatr Res.* 1979;1:191-7. (English)

The beta-adrenergic receptors were studied *in vitro* in lymphocytes obtained from patients with major affective disorders and controls. Specific L-[3H]-dihydroalprenolol binding was decreased in both depressed and manic patients compared to controls and euthymic patients. Isoproterenol-stimulated, but not prostaglandin E$_1$-stimulated, cyclic adenosine-3',5'-monophosphate production was decreased in manic and depressed patients. These results suggest decreased lymphocyte beta-receptor functioning in depression and mania. This decrease may be an index of changes in brain beta-receptors in mania and depression, or may simply reflect homeostatic regulation of peripheral beta-receptors in response to stress-induced increases in circulating catecholamines.

996

Fetisova TK. **Proliferative response of schizophrenic patient's peripheral blood lymphocytes.** *Zh Nevropatol Psikhiatr.* 1978;78:867-71. (Russian)

The author studied the proliferative abilities of lymphocytes in the peripheral blood of schizophrenic patients and normals in cultures not containing autologous plasma. The reactivity of lymphocytes in schizophrenic patients to PHA and rabbit serum to human thymocytes (ATS) appeared to be decreased. The level of their proliferative response to concanavalin A was significantly the same as in normals. The assumption is made that in schizophrenic patients there is a blocking of lymphocyte receptors, binding PHA and ATS. The possibility of a deficit of a subpopulation of T lymphocytes in the organism of patients highly sensitive to stimulation by PHA and ATS is not excluded.

997

Fontana A, Storck U, Angst J, Dubs R, Abegg A, Grob PJ. **An immunological basis of schizophrenia and affective disorders.** *Neuropsychobiology.* 1980;6:284-9. (English)

In 48 patients with schizophrenia and 32 patients with affective disorders, different immune parameters were tested. Compared to blood-donors, IgG and IgM serum concentrations were increased in both the schizophrenic and affective disorders. However, these abnormalities did not differ from hospital control populations. The patients failed to show an association of antibodies considered to be characteristic of autoimmune diseases. In addition, no increased incidence of circulating immune complexes was detected. The only substantial serologic abnormality found was an elevation of C4 levels in patients with bipolar psychosis.

998

Fox BH. **Cancer death risk in hospitalized mental patients** (letter). *Science.* 1978;201:966. (English)

999

Fuccillo DA, Kurent JE, Manne SH, Rosenthal D, Beadle E, Sever JL. **Lack of association between defective delinquents and antibody of herpesvirus hominis.** *Neurology (Minneap).* 1977;27:304-5. (English)

Several groups have reported a relation between herpesvirus hominis infection and certain psychiatric disorders. We have investigated herpes antibody levels in chronic criminal offenders who were diagnosed as defective delinquents and in criminals who were not defective delinquents. We found no difference in the frequency of titers of herpesvirus type 1 or type 2 antibody in these groups.

1000

Gastpar M, Muller W. **Auto-antibodies in affective disorders.** *Prog Neuropsychopharmacol.* 1981;5:91-7. (English)

1) One hundred depressive patients were tested for the presence of several auto-antibodies. 2) Rheumatoid factor--tested with three different techniques--antinuclear antibodies, and two other auto-antibodies (anti-mitochondrial and anti-basement membrane antibodies) could not be found in a higher frequency than in normals, whereas the occurrence of the thyroglobulin auto-antibodies was just above the upper limit of normals. 3) Factors eventually influencing the results and directions for further work are discussed on the basis of previous studies.

1001

Ghose K, Coppen A, Hurdle AD, Mcillroy I. **Antinuclear antibodies, affective disorders and lithium therapy.** *Pharmakopsychiatr Neuropsychopharmakol.* 1977;10:243-5. (English)

The prevalence of positive antinuclear antibody (ANA) was investigated in a group of patients suffering from recurrent affective disorders who had been treated for more than one year with lithium carbonate. There was no increase of ANA in these patients (8%) as compared with a group of patients suffering from affective disorders (7.5%), but untreated with lithium salts, or with the prevalence of ANA in the general population (9%) of the same age group.

1002

Goldstein AL, Rossio J, Koliaskina GI, Emory LE, Overall JB, Thurman GB, Hatcher J. **Immunological components in schizophrenia.** *In:* **Perspectives in Schizophrenia Research.** NY: Raven Press, 1980. Pp. 249-67. (English)

The results of our study indicate that a significant immunological imbalance exists in some patients with schizophrenia. The differences include abnormal lymphocyte responsiveness to selected mitogenic lectins and the presence in the serum of a cytotoxic factor directed against murine thymocytes. During a 28-day chemotherapy trial using chlorpromazine, there was an interesting tendency toward normalization of T-cell responses and a significant decrease in serum cytotoxicity. Our own studies in this area, as well as several new studies which are just appearing in the scientific literature, would suggest that there may be subtle changes in lymphocytes and serum in patients with schizophrenia related to an effect in immune regulation. Although by no means conclusive, these data certainly suggest that it would be worthwhile to take a more critical look at the role of the immune system in the etiology and progression of the schizophrenias. A few years ago it would have been almost heresy to suggest that diabetes and multiple sclerosis might have major immunological components, and yet we now know that this is indeed the case for both of these diseases. We would predict that if in-depth studies of immunological systems of schizophrenic patients were carried out, we would see similar deficiencies and correlations. Specific recommendations for new approaches to study immunologic and virologic components are presented in Table 6. Investigations of some of the questions identified in Table 6 should provide information regarding the role of viruses and the immune system in the schizophrenic process. If immunologic and/or virologic components of schizophrenia can be documented, it will provide the means to develop a whole new approach to the treatment and possible cure of this disease.

1003

Golla JA, Larson LA, Anderson CF, Lucas AR, Wilson WR, Tomasi TB Jr. **An immunological assessment of patients with anorexia nervosa.** *Am J Clin Nutr.* 1981;34:2756-62. (English)

Patients with most forms of protein-calorie malnutrition are typically more suspectible to infection. We studied the immunological consequences of a subgroup of malnourished subjects--nine patients with anorexia nervosa, who typically have a lower incidence of infection. The profiles of patients with anorexia nervosa deviated from the reported typical profile of significantly depressed cell-mediated immunity in subjects with more common forms of protein-calorie malnutrition, demonstrating normal T-lymphocyte populations and unimpaired proliferative lymphocyte responsiveness to mitogenic stimulation with phytohemagglutinin and concanavalin A. In fact, mitogen responsiveness was significantly elevated above that of controls, and with nutritional repletion, this enhanced responsiveness regressed toward control values. Since impaired cell-mediated immunity has been consistently documented in other malnourished populations, and presumably contributes to their increased propensity toward infection, the maintenance of a relatively intact cell-mediated immune system may be an important factor separating the malnourished anorexia nervosa patient from other protein-calorie malnourished patients.

1004

Goode DJ, Corbett WT, Schey HM, Suh SH, Woodie B, Morris DL, Morrisey L. **Breast cancer in hospitalized psychiatric patients.** *Am J Psychiatry.* 1981;138:804-6. (English)

Elevated serum prolactin levels caused by antipsychotic agents have been suspected of increasing the risk of breast cancer. The authors reviewed all the cases of breast cancer in 1969-1978 among the female population of a large psychiatric hospital and compared the incidence and prevalence rates of this group to expected rates. The rates of breast cancer among these psychiatric patients were not higher despite their use of antipsychotic drugs.

1005

Gotlieb-Stematsky T, Zonis J, Arlazoroff A, Mozes T, Sigal M, Szekely AG. **Antibodies to Epstein-Barr virus, herpes simplex type 1, cytomegalovirus and measles virus in psychiatric patients.** *Arch Virol.* 1981;67:333-9. (English)

Distribution of antibodies to herpes simplex type 1 (HSV1), Epstein-Barr virus (EBV), cytomegalovirus (CMV) and measles virus (MV) was studied in sera and cerebrospinal fluids (CSF) of 41 patients with schizophrenia, 27 patients with primary affective disorders and 25 control patients with neurological diseases. No significant differences in distribution and mean geometric titers (GMT) of antibodies to HSV1 between the psychiatric and control groups were found. Distribution and GMT of antibodies to EBV were highly significant in psychiatric patients as compared to controls with highest titers in the affective disorder group. Antibodies to HSV1 were present in 15 CSF specimens of psychiatric patients with reduced CSF/serum ratio in 4, and low levels of antibodies were detected in 8 control patients. Antibodies to EBV-VCA were detected in 4 CSF's of psychiatric patients. Total protein levels were determined in CSF specimens and no correlation with antibodies was found. No significant differences in distribution of antibodies to CMV or MV in the three study groups were found. No antibodies to CMV were demonstrated in CSF's and in one specimen from a patient and two controls antibodies to MV were detected.

1006

Gowdy JM. **Immunoglobulin levels in psychotic patients.** *Psychosomatics.* 1980;21:751-6. (English)

Immunoglobulin levels were measured in 77 male patients with chronic mental illness at a Veterans Administration Hospital. Immunoglobulin G (IgG) levels were found to be significantly elevated in acutely schizophrenic patients. The levels peaked at about 12 years' duration of the disease and they dropped with increased phenothiazine dosages. The author concludes that immunoglobulin levels seem related to the course of psychosis and suggests that further study be done to determine their diagnostic level.

1007

Gu TS. **Preliminary study on lymphocytic transformation test and intracutaneous tuberculin test in schizophrenias** (author's translation). *Chinese J Neurol Psychiat.* 1979; 12:193-5. (Chinese) (unavailable at publication)

1008

Herzog P, Dvorakova M, Zvolsky P. **T and B lymphocytes in psychotic patients** (author's transl). *Cesk Psychiatr.* 1979;75:153-9. (Czech)

In 42 psychotic patients the authors proved a percent increase in the active T lymphocytes (of the aE rosette) and a decrease in the lymphocytes of B population (of the EA and EAC rosettes) by rosette tests. The tested patients were divided into a group of depressives and a group of schizophrenics. In the first group active T lymphocytes were more numerous and in the latter group T and B lymphocytes were less numerous in a population sample. The analysis of the group according to the medication shows that it probably shares in these differences too. The group of patients treated with lithium and the group treated with phenothiziane neuroleptics showed an increase in the percentage of activized cells (of the aE rosettes) more frequently than patients treated by other preparations (p<0.05). The changes were particularly significant in patients taking both the drugs simultaneously: besides the high frequency of the aE rosettes, these individuals also manifested a decrease in the B lymphocytes (of the EA and EAC rosettes). All the three cases show p<0.001.

1009

Hirata-Hibi M, Higashi S, Tachibana T, Watanabe N. **Stimulated lymphocytes in schizophrenia.** *Arch Gen Psychiatry.* 1982;39:82-7. (English)

This study examines the effect of neuroleptic medication on the distribution of the reported atypical lymphocytes of schizophrenia. The predominant atypical type in schizophrenia was termed the P-type atypical lymphocyte to differentiate the cell from other types of peripheral lymphocytes. Such P cells showed stimulated features: clear cytoplasmic basophilia and an irregularly shaped nucleus with a leptochromatic structure and occasionally one or two nucleoli, but the cell size ranged from small to large. P cells were found in all 42 schizophrenic patients examined and ranged from 5% to 45% of lymphocytes. Patients receiving neuroleptic medication had a lower mean percentage of P cells (17.8%) compared with patients not receiving neuroleptic medication (28.7%). The findings indicate that neuroleptic medication is not likely to be inducing the P-cell reaction.

1010

Ishii T, Haga S. **Immuno-electron microscopic localization of immunoglobulins in amyloid fibrils of senile plaques.** *Acta Neuropathol.* 1976;36:243-9. (German)

Amyloid fibrils in senile plaques of the brain of patients with senile dementia or Alzheimer's disease combined specifically with horseradish peroxidase (HRPO)-labeled rabbit anti-human IgG. Light and electronmicroscopic immunoperoxidase technique was used to prove this. The fact may mean that immunological factors were involved in the pathogenesis of amyloid fibrils in the senile plaques, and probably also in that of senile dementia or Alzheimer's disease.

1011

Ismailov NV. **Features of the manifestations of cellular and humoral immune responses in schizophrenia of different durations.** *Zh Nevropatol Psikhiatr.* 1981;81:1353-5. (Russian)

The content of the T-lymphocytes and serum globulins A, M, and G was determined in 58 schizophrenic patients. It has been shown that in this disease both the cell and the humoral immunity systems are affected, but to a different degree depending on the morbid process duration. A functional character of the T-system insufficiency, as well as a connection between the levels of the immunoglobulins and the degree of the schizophrenia are demonstrated.

1012

Jankovic BD, Jakulic S, Horvat J. **Cell-mediated immunity and psychiatric diseases.** *Period Biol.* 1979;81:219. (English) (unavailable at publication)

1013

Jankovic BD, Jakulic S, Horvat J. **Cerebral atrophy: an immunological disorder?** *Lancet.* 1977;2:219-20. (English)

Patients with cerebral atrophy of unknown origin, patients with nuclear forms of schizophrenia or neurosis, and normal subjects were skin-tested with human brain and liver proteins. The frequency of positive delayed skin-sensitivity reactions to brain proteins was significantly higher in the cerebral-atrophy group than in other groups, thus suggesting a correlation between cerebral atrophy and cell-mediated immunity.

1014

Jankovic BD, Jakulic S, Horvat J. **Delayed skin hypersensitivity reactions to human brain S-100 protein in psychiatric patients.** *Biol Psychiat.* 1982;17:687-97. (English)

To confirm and extend previous observations concerning the correlation between cell-mediated immunity and psychiatric diseases, 511 patients with schizophrenia, cerebral atrophy, dementia, and mental retardation, and 32 control subjects and 27 control patients were skin-tested with human brain S-100 protein and human liver protein: 70.2-93.1% of tested psychiatric patients developed positive skin hypersensitivity reactions to S-100 protein, while 2.8-20.7% of patients reacted to liver protein. Of control subjects, 6.2-7.4% responded to S-100 protein, and 7.4-9.4% to liver protein. The findings indicate that cell-mediated immune processes may be involved in brain mechanisms underlying cerebral atrophy, depression, dementia, schizophrenia, and mental retardation.

1015

Jankovic BD, Jakulic S, Horvat J. **Immunopsychiatry: a new field of research in immunology.** *Immunobiol.* 1981;160:47. (English) (unavailable at publication)

1016

Jankovic BD, Jakulic S, Horvat J. **Schizophrenia and other psychiatric diseases: evidence for neurotissue hypersensitivity.** *Clin Exp Immunol.* 1980;40:515-22. (English)

Psychiatric patients (208 with cerebral atrophy, 46 with dementia, 82 with depression and 481 with schizophrenia) with control subjects (56 normal individuals and patients with neurosis) were skin-tested with human S-100 brain protein, soluble fraction from the brain and liver protein. The local Arthus and delayed hypersensitivity reactions were read at 4-6 hr and at 24 hr respectively. The great majority of tested psychiatric patients developed positive Arthus and delayed skin reactions to S-100 protein and soluble brain protein fraction. A small number of control subjects responded to those antigens. The results obtained suggest that there is a correlation between local cutaneous sensitivity to neurotissue antigens and psychiatric diseases, and that both humoral and cell-mediated immunity are involved in the pathogenesis and development of cerebral atrophy, dementia, depression and schizophrenia.

1017

Jonker C, Eikelenboom P, Tvenier P. **Immunological indices in the cerebrospinal fluid of patients with presenile dementia of the Alzheimer type.** *Br J Psychiatry.* 1982;140:44-9. (English)

In ten patients with presenile dementia of the Alzheimer type and in a control group the levels of the different immunoglobulins were determined in both serum and cerebrospinal fluid (CSF), and gel electrophoretic techniques used to determine possible oligoclonal bands in the gamma-globulin region. There is no indication that patients with Alzheimer disease produce immunoglobulins within the central nervous system.

1018

Jovicic A, Nikic SM, Miljanovic B. **Autoimmune processes in psychoses.** *Med Pregl.* 1980;33:157-60. (Polish) (no abstract)

1019

Kaplan GW, Wallace WW, Orgel HA, Miller JR. **Serum immunoglobulin E and incidence of allergy in group of enuretic children.** *Urology.* 1977;10:428-30. (English)

Serum immunoglobulin E levels were determined in 34 enuretic children and 20 age-matched controls. No differences were detected. Additionally, the incidence of allergic disorders in these enuretic children was no different from the general population.

1020

Kinnell HG, Kirkwood E, Lewis C. **Food antibodies in schizophrenia.** *Psychol Med.* 1982;12:85-9. (English) (unavailable at publication)

1021

Knight JG. **Dopamine-receptor-stimulating autoantibodies: a possible cause of schizophrenia.** *Lancet.* 1982;2:1073-6. (English)

Schizophrenia shares several genetic features with diseases known to be autoimmune and could therefore be an autoimmune disease itself. Antipsychotic drugs, which are effective in treating the psychotic symptoms of schizophrenia, have one property in common--they block dopamine receptors in the central nervous system. This observation has led to the hypothesis that overactivity of dopaminergic pathways is the cause of the psychotic symptoms, but a seeming anomaly is that the turnover of dopamine is not increased in schizophrenia. Dopamine-receptor-stimulating autoantibodies are postulated to cause the dopaminergic hyperactivity, thereby accounting for the anomaly.

1022

Kocur J, Stachowiak J, Kuklewicz C, Bialek J. **Protein content and cytotoxic activity of serum from paranoid schizophrenics.** *Psychiatr Pol.* 1977;11:1-6. (Polish)

It was found that the serum albumin fraction was lowered in patients with a history of illness longer than five years while the serum globulins were elevated regardless of duration of the disease. Serum of the majority of patients (73.7%) revealed the presence of substances cytotoxic towards leukocytes *in vitro*. A suspension of the neuroleptic treatment for 30 days did not significantly influence total serum protein level of distribution of protein reactions; it did, however, lower the number of positive cytotoxic results. The results suggest the existence of a link between duration of the disease and pharmacotherapy on the one side, and the protein metabolism and autoimmunological activity in blood, on the other.

1023

Koliaskina GI, Burbaeva GSH. **Modern approaches to the study of immunity in schizophrenia.** *Vestn Akad Med Nauk SSSR.* 1979;7:76-84. (Russian)

The paper presents some concepts significant for the understanding of currently developing research on immunity in schizophrenia. The results of studies of the humoral and cellular immunity in this disease obtained at the Institute of Psychiatry, Academy of Medical Sciences of the USSR, are described. The problems associated with a possible correction of immunopathological changes found in schizophrenia are discussed.

1024

Koliaskina GI, Tsutsul'kovskaia MIA, Domashneva IV, Maznina TP, Kil'gol'ts P. **Antithymic factor in schizophrenia patients.** *Zh Nevropatol Psikhiatr.* 1980;80:710-6. (Russian)

The paper concerns results of the studies, accomplished according to the WHO project within the framework of international collaboration in biological psychiatry. It was demonstrated that the blood sera of mental patients and normals possess antithymic activity. However, there are statistically significant differences between the groups of patients and normals with regard to the level of serum antithymic activity (0.22 ± 0.05 in normals and 0.47 ± 0.04 in patients, $p<0.05$). The medium level of antithymic activity in the group of schizophrenic patients depends upon the duration of the disease. The level of sera antithymic activity was significantly higher ($p<0.05$ in the group of patients with a duration of the disease less than 5 years and lower in patients with a duration of the process over 5 years.

1025

Koliaskina GI, Tsutsul'kovskaia MIA, Domashneva IV, Maznina TP, Kielholz P, Gastpar M, Bunney WE, Rafaelsen OJ, Heltberg J, Coppen A, Hippius H, Hoecherl B, Vartanian F. **Antithymic immune factor in schizophrenia: a World Health Organization study.** *Neuropsychobiology.* 1980;6:349-55. (English)

Six WHO collaborating centres took part in the study of the antithymic activity of blood sera of patients suffering from schizophrenia. Blood serum specimens from 118 schizophrenic patients and 62 mentally healthy donors were investigated. Statistically significant differences between schizophrenic patients and the controls were found ($p<0.05$). It is probable that as with other biological phenomena described in schizophrenia, antithymic activity is one of the biological factors, in combination with other factors, predisposing toward the development of the schizophrenic process.

1026

Koranyi EK. **Somatic illness in psychiatric patients.** *Psychosomatics.* 1980;21:887-91. (English)

The author reviews a dozen studies conducted over a period of 40 years and shows that approximately half of a total of over 4,000 psychiatric patients had major medical illnesses. Somatic conditions were directly related to the psychiatric symptoms in 9% to 42% of the cases. Approximately half of the patients' referring physicians had not diagnosed their physical illnesses. These findings and five brief case reports point up the need to follow a medical model on psychiatric services.

1027

Kovaleva ES, Bonartsev PD, Prilipko LL. **Lymphocyte reaction in schizophrenic patients to the phytomitogens, concanavalin A and phytohemagglutinin.** *Biull Eksp Biol Med.* 1977;84:182-5. (Russian)

The capability of the schizophrenic patients' lymphocytes and lymhocytes of healthy persons to respond to the stimulating action of T-mitogens-- concanavalin A and PHA--was studied. The T-cell count was determined by the method of rosette formation; the influence of adhesive cells on the lymphocyte response to mitogens was ascertained. The response to both the mitogens in the patients' lymphocyte cultures was reduced as compared to control, and the T-cell count failed to differ from normal. The removal of adhesive lymphocytes results in the disappearance of differences between the response of the patients' lymphocytes and normal lymphocytes to both the mitogens.

1028

Kovaleva ES, Lideman RR, Prilipko LL. **Resistance to osmotic shock and adhesiveness of peripheral blood lymphocytes in normal and schizophrenic patients.** *Biull Eksp Biol Med.* 1980;89:155-7. (Russian)

A study of resistance to osmotic shock of peripheral blood lymphocytes from healthy donors and schizophrenics demonstrated two lymphocyte subpopulations; a low resistant subpopulation (about 20%) and a high resistant subpopulation (about 80%). The lymphocytes from donors belonging to the former subpopulation possess increased adhesiveness. 60% of schizophrenic patients lack the subpopulation of low resistant lymphocytes. Abnormal resistance to osmotic shock is characteristic of highly adhesive lymphocytes.

1029

Kovaleva ES, Prilipko LL, Tsutsul'kovskaia MIA. **Dependence of the peripheral blood lymphocyte reaction of schizophrenia patients to concanavalin A stimulation on the clinical parameters of the pathological process.** *Zh Nevropatol Psikhiatr.* 1980;80:71-3. (Russian)

Studies were performed on an equivalent age group of schizophrenic patients and normal donors to detect the lymphocyte reaction of the peripheral blood to concanavalin A stimulation. It was demonstrated that in the blood of schizophrenic patients the part of lymphocytes capable of reaction to stimulation is 2.3 times less than in the group of normals. The studies showed that capability of cells to react to stimulation does not depend upon the duration of the disease, the duration of the postmanifest or initial periods, but differs in patients with different forms of schizophrenia. A significant negative correlation was demonstrated between the severity of positive disorders and the lymphocyte response to stimulation.

1030
Kovaleva ES, Prilipko LL. **Analysis of subpopulations of peripheral blood T-lymphocytes of schizophrenic patients.** *Zh Nevropatol Psikhiatr.* 1981;5:694-7. (Russian)

The reaction of lymphocytes to Con A and PHA and combined action of these 2 T-mitogens in the peripheral blood was studied in schizophrenic patients (25 cases) and normal donors (21 cases). It was demonstrated that the study of lymphocyte function in the peripheral blood with the aid of the 2 mitogens makes it possible to differentiate more distinctly the lymphocytes of schizophrenic patients and normals. It was established that the lymphocyte subpopulation capable of responding to both mitogens used is 4 times less in schizophrenics than in normal donors. The proportion of cells reacting only to one of these mitogens is significantly higher than in normals. The total content of mitogen-sensitive T-lymphocytes in schizophrenic patients and normal donors is approximately the same and equals about 40% of the whole lymphocyte population in the peripheral blood.

1031
Kovaleva ES, Prilipko LL. **Role of schizophrenic patients' serum in the altered osmotic resistance of their lymphocytes.** *Zh Nevropatol Psikhiatr.* 1981;81:1018-21. (Russian)

The resistance of peripheral blood lymphocytes was estimated in normal subjects and schizophrenic patients with reference to hypoosmotic effects. It was shown that in normal subjects about 20% of the lymphocytes were slightly resistant. In 60% of the schizophrenic patients the fraction of the slightly resistant lymphocytes was found to be sharply lowered. The content of those cells in the blood of patients with different forms of the disease course was different: patients with the periodic form showed the minimal, and patients with continuously progressing form the maximal deviation from normal. Patients with the schubweise form occupied an intermediate place. Incubation of the lymphocytes of the healthy donors in the serum of schizophrenic patients led to selective destruction of the donor's slightly resistant cells. A statistically significant correlation between the destructive capacity of the patients' serum and the lowering of the content of the slightly resistant lymphocytes in those patients was observed.

1032
Krachunova M, Tsoneva M, Stoikova M. **Correlation between genome mutations and the cell division types in immunological sensitization states.** *Eskp Med Morfol.* 1979;18:117-22. (Bulgarian)

The authors examined the frequency of cells with polyploidy (P), with amitotic division (AD) and with mitotic division (MD) in 25 patients with schizophrenia and proven anticerebral autoimmune sensitization by means of blast-transformation test-BS, in 20 partners of marriages with multiple spontaneous abortions and suspected isoimmunization-PCA as well as a control of 63 healthy adults and newborn infants.

Simultaneous increase of the frequency of cells with polyploidy and amitotic division was established in patients with schizophrenia--1.16% of P and 0.40% AD in 4 women with spontaneous abortions--1.5% of P and 0.80% of AD compared with the control values of 0.54% of P and 0.17% of AD. The highest percentage P--1.12, and AD--2.1, was found in BS with chronic process, in whom the blast-transformation reaction to brain antigen--34%, was mostly manifested. In the cultures of BS, treated with brain antigen, AD reached up to 1.38%. The increase of AD was accompanied with lowering of mitotic index: BS--1.2% of MD and 0.40 of AD; PSA--2.04% of MD and 0.50 of AD compared with the control values of 4% of MD and 0.17% of AD. The results showed that immunologic sensitization was accompanied by an increase of genome mutations and amitotic division and with lowering of mitotic index; they revealed polyploidy and amitotic division as compensatory mechanisms of the organisms under certain conditions.

1033
Kuritzky A, Livni E, Munitz H, Englander T, Tyano S, Wijsenbeek H, Joshua H, Kott E. **Cell-mediated immunity to human myelin basic protein in schizophrenic patients.** *J Neurol Sci.* 1976;30:369-73. (English)

Cell-mediated immune resonse to myelin human basic protein was studied by the macrophage migration inhibition test in patients suffering from schizophrenia. Eighteen out of 32 patients with chronic schizophrenia demonstrated human basic protein-induced inhibition of the migration index, while 4 out of 41 acute schizophrenics showed an inhibition of macrophage migration.

1034
Kushner SG, Maznina TP, Bunimovich LA. **Quantitative assessment of antithymocyte antibodies in schizophrenia.** *Zh Nevropatol Psikhiatr.* 1978;78:697-700. (Russian)

The use of the method of fluorescent antibodies and cytotoxic tests showed that the blood serum of schizophrenic patients and normals possess an antithymocytic activity. However, the level of this activity in patients exceeds the corresponding indices in normals ($p<0.02$). The use of indirect immunofluorescent methods permitted us to demonstrate that the antithymic antibody titres in schizophrenic patients is much higher than in normals. The amount of the cytotoxic index is in direct correlation with the level of antithymic antibodies determined by the fluorescent antibody method.

1035
Kushner SG, Maznina TP. **Classes of immunoglobulins responsible for serum antithymocyte activity in healthy subjects and mental pathology.** *Zh Nevropatol Psikhiatr.* 1981;81:1014-5. (Russian)

The antilymphocytic activity of serum was examined in schizophrenic patients and in mentally healthy donors using the method of fluorescent antibodies. It was found that the antithymocytic activity of both the schizophrenics and the healthy subjects was due to immunoglobulins G and M. The number of thymocytes showing fluorescence under the action of IgG was found to be approximately the same in both groups of persons examined. When use was made of fluorescein-labelled IgM the number of fluorescent thymocytes was found to be three times greater in the patients than in the healthy subjects. It is suggested that the differences revealed may be associated with an increased avidity of the IgM antibodies, or with disturbances of the synthesis of immunoglobulins in the patients.

1036

Kushner SG, Maznina TP. **Nature of antigens to which antibodies are detected in the serum of schizophrenic patients.** *Zh Nevropatol Psikhiatr.* 1980;80:1071-4. (Russian)

The study was conducted by the immune absorption method. The serum activity before and after absorption was studied with the cytotoxic test and the fluorescent antibody method. The studies demonstrated that antibodies, detected in the blood serum of patients and normals differ not only qualitatively but also quantitatively. It was established as well that antibodies detected in normals may be completely absorbed by the brain and thymus of mice or by similar human tissues. In absorption of antibodies in patients by tissues of mice, the activity of the sera entirely disappears. On the contrary, the brain tissue and human thymocytes only insignificantly decrease the serum titres in patients.

1037

Kushner SG, Orlova EN. **Results of a comparative study of anti-brain antibodies in the sera of healthy subjects and schizophrenic patients by the Coomb's indirect immunofluorescent method.** *Zh Nevropatol Psikhiatr.* 1977;77:1049-53. (Russian)

With the aid of the Coomb's indirect method the authors studied the blood sera of 79 patients with different forms of schizophrenia and 27 normal donors. It was demonstrated that the blood sera of schizophrenic patients and normals contain globulins capable of fixation on different components of a nervous cell. However, the character and intensity of fluorescence as well as the amount of fluorescent nerve cells in the field of vision distinguishes the examined patients from normal donors.

1038

Lederman MA, Mascio A, Shaskan EG. **Schizophrenia: biochemical and virological theories.** *Bios.* 1981;52:217-26. (English)

In this review, we have tried to establish that viruses like HSV-1 can infect the CNS and produce symptoms consistent with schizophrenia. As in all infectious diseases, however, genetic and physiological properties of the host determine pathogenetic expression. Within this realm, and in consideration of the dopamine hypothesis, is there a relationship between viruses, the immune system, and biochemical pathways in the brain? Curiously, the same virus that was associated with schizophrenia during the 1920's (Hendrick, 1928) was later associated with a proven lesion to the dopaminergic system, namely, post-encephalitic Parkinsonism (Hornykiewicz, 1966). Possibly, latent viral injection in the trigeminal nucleus could affect the function of adjacent integrative reticu-

lar nuclei with resulting hallucinations, delusions, and schizophrenic psychosis (Fissman, 1975). Conceptually, new investigations of genes modulating immune function in conjunction with expansion of our knowledge or receptors for viruses may suggest novel links between viruses and brain.

1039

Libikova H, Breier S, Kocisova M, Pogady J, Stunzner D, Ujhazyova D. **Assay of interferon and viral antibodies in the cerebrospinal fluid in clinical neurology and psychiatry.** *Acta Biol Med Ger.* 1979;38:879-93. (English)

Cerebrospinal fluids (CSF) of 245 neurological and 194 psychiatric patients were tested for viral antibodies and interferon. Complement-dependent neutralizing antibodies to herpes virus hominis 1 were found in the CSF of patients with encephalitis (50.6%), meningitis (35.4%), lesions of peripheral nerves (36.9%), sclerosis multiplex (41.2%), schizophrenia (31.9%), senile dementia (51.4%), mental retardation (11.1%) and ethylism (43.5%). Neutralizing antibodies to tick-borne encephalitis virus were found in the CSF of 38% patients with encephalitis, in 14% meningitis, 11% lesions of peripheral nerves and also in 5.6-11.8% of psychiatric patients. In encephalitis, meningitis and in lesions of peripheral nerves were found in the CSF frequently plaque-neutralizing antibodies to the tick-borne orbivirus lipovnik, complement-fixing antibodies to lymphocytic choriomeningitis virus and hemagglutination-inhibiting antibodies to measles virus. In multiple sclerosis were detected CSF antibodies to measles virus (44%), herpes virus hominis 1 (41.2%) and lipovnik virus (52.6%). In neurological patients were observed CSF antibodies simultaneously to two or three viruses in 16 to 40.6%, while in psychiatric patients in zero to 4.6%. CSF interferon was found in psychiatric patients with an equal or even higher incidence (33.7 to 51.7%) than in the neurological patients (29.6-38.6%, in multiple sclerosis only 16.7%). Non-interferon virus inhibitors were excluded. The evaluation of the ratio of serum and CSF titers of viral antibodies and of interferon indicated local synthesis of both in the central nervous system--with the exception of antibodies to herpes virus hominis 1 in CSF of some patients with very high titres in serum and probable lesions of the blood-brain barrier.

1040

Libikova H, Pogady J, Kutinova L, Breier S, Matis J. **Early and delayed skin reactivity to solubilized antigens of herpesvirus hominis 1 in psychiatric patients and guinea pigs.** *Acta Virol.* 1980;24:279-90. (Czech)

Intradermal tests with a mixture of herpesvirus hominis (HVH 1) antigens containing quantitated neutralization antigen were done in 39 schizophrenics (SCH), 42 senile demented (DS) persons, 28 alcoholics, neurotics and psychopaths (ANP) and 33 control persons. Local induration, erythema and fading as evaluated according to diameter and intensity after 15 to 30 min for anaphylactic type I reaction, after 5 hr for Arthus type III reaction and after 24 and 48 hr for delayed hypersensitivity (type IV). The diagnosed clinical forms influenced the incidence of positive reactions I, III or IV at the level alpha = 0.01. The incidence of positivity in all reactions (I, III plus IV) was significantly higher in the patients than in the control group. Type I and III reactions were most intensive in ANP and SCH, respectively. Type IV reaction was most pronounced in SCH, including the highest incidence of purple lesions, eventually with a lightly cyanotic target. In the DS group, type IV reaction surpassed the control the least of all patient groups. Unfavourable side effects of the skin tests were not observed. The importance of repeated contact with HVH 1 for a marked type IV reaction was confirmed in experimentally infected guinea pigs, which also served for safety tests and selection of antigen preparations.

1041

Libikova H, Pogady J, Rajcani J, Skodacek I, Ciampor F, Kocisova M. **Latent herpes virus hominis 1 in the central nervous system of psychotic patients.** *Acta Virol.* 1979;23:231-9. (Czech)

Cerebrospinal fluids (CSF) from 35 patients with senile or presenile dementia and from 13 patients with schizophrenia and related syndromes were examined in cell cultures with the aim to isolate herpes virus hominis 1 (HVH 1) or other viruses. Serum and CSF antibodies to HVH 1 and/or interferon in the patients indicated a recent HVH 1 antigenic or viral activity. In the CSF of two senile demented patients and of one patient with schizoaffective psychosis, agents of low virulence, causing a cytopathic effect in 3 or 4, but not more, subsequent passages were detected and identified as HVH 1 by immunofluorescence. A focus of cells containing HVH 1 antigen at the cell membrane and in cytoplasm was visualized by immunofluorescence in an explant from nucleus amygdalae from 1 of 6 patients with schizophrenia and related syndromes examined. In the original biopsy materials, various virus-like structures were found in nuclei and cytoplasm of astrocytes and neurocytes and in axons in the neuropil.

1042

Libikova H, Pogady J, Stancek D, Mucha V. **Hepatitis B and herpes viral components in the cerebrospinal fluid of chronic schizophrenic and senile demented patients.** *Acta Virol.* 1981;25:182-90. (Czech)

Cerebrospinal fluids (CSF) or sera or both from 57 chronic schizophrenics and 18 senile demented patients were examined by various tests of HBsAg. Both CSF and serum were positive in 2 schizophrenics while in six HBsAg was detected in the CSF only. Elevated values of circulating immune complexes were found in positive patients. Most CSF positive for HBsAg also contained neutralizing antibodies to herpesvirus hominis type 1. Ultramicroscopic structures similar to hepatitis B virus (HBV) components and herpesviral particles were visualized in the CSF of one patient on electron microscope EM grids coated with anti-human IgG serum. Most HBsAg positive patients appeared to be liver-symptoms-free carriers. In the CSF of a 79 years old senile demented man HBsAG was proved serologically. Several herpesviral particles complexed with globular material and spherical structures for 15 to 25 nm in diameter were visualized in the same CSF on EM grids coated with anti-human IgG serum. The findings support the importance of herpesviruses in mental illnesses. Penetration of HBsAg through the blood-brain barrier might be involved as an iatrogenic factor in the course of late psychoses.

1043

Libikova H, Pogady J, Wiedermann V, Breier S. **Presence of antibodies against herpes simplex type 1 virus in persons with psychic disturbances and among criminal population** (author's transl). *Cesk Psychiatr.* 1976;72:206-10. (Czech)

Since 1971, we have searched for a possible relationship between psychiatric disorders and latent viral infection of the central nervous system. We have chosen herpes simplex type 1 virus (HSV 1) as a model virus for this investigation. Results of the examination of 121 and 110 persons of psychiatric and criminal population, respectively, proved a significantly higher incidence of extremely high titers of HSV 1 neutralizing antibodies—1:512 and more—than in a control group of mentally healthy people from the same localities. The most pronounced results were found in patients with schizophrenia, senile dementia and in condemned felons with low IQ. The putative mechanisms are discussed, by which HSV 1 could be able to induce such microorganic changes in the CNS which would be hardly detectable but which could be implicated in the development of disorders in mental activity and behaviour.

1044

Liedeman RR, Babaian NG. **Serum humoral factors: cause of the altered physiologic state of peripheral blood lymphocytes in schizophrenic patients.** *Biull Eskp Biol Med.* 1976;82:1047-50. (Russian)

Statistically significant correlations were revealed between the following: the percentage content in the lymphocyte cultures of patients suffering from schizophrenia of cells responding to stimulation with phytohemagglutinin (PHA) by DNA synthesis, and the percentage in the white blood cell cultures of healthy donors of lymphocytes failing to respond to the PHA stimulation by the DNA synthesis as a result of cultivation of these cells in a medium containing the blood serum (20%) of schizophrenic patients. Similar correlation was revealed between the percentage content in cultures of the white blood cells of schizophrenic patients of adhesive lymphocytes and the percentage of adhesive lymphocytes in the white blood cell cultures of healthy donors in cultivation of these cells in a medium containing the blood serum (20%) of schizophrenic patients. The data obtained confirmed a supposition that the altered physiological condition of the peripheral blood lymphocytes of patients suffering from schizophrenia was caused by the factors contained in the blood serum of these patients.

1045

Liedeman RR, Prilipko LL. **The behavior of T lymphocytes in schizophrenia.** *Birth Defects.* 1978;14:365-77. (English)

The results of schizophrenic patients' peripheral blood lymphocytes will be discussed. We applied a number of methods that permitted evaluation of the general level of their functional activity and some parameters of their physiologic state. The physiologic state of the cells was tested by studying the morphology (1), the intensity of RNA synthesis (2), and adhesive properties of lymphocytes (3). To test the functional state we measured the lymphocyte response to T mitogens (PHA, Con A) in tissue culture using 80% Eagle's medium and 20% human serum (4). The studies were carried out with blood samples obtained from nontreated patients and from normal donors. The group was comprised of 68% men and 32% women with a mean age of 26.3 and 27.9 years respectively.

1046

Liedeman RR. **Some traits of the functional state of lymphocytes in cultures of the peripheral blood of schizophrenic patients.** *Zh Nevropatol Psikhiatr.* 1976;76:81-5. (Russian)

The author summarizes and discusses the results achieved in the study of some parameters characterizing the functional state of lymphocytes in the peripheral blood of schizophrenic patients in cultures: the ultrastructural organization (electron microscopy), chromatin activity (microfluorometry), the velocity of RNA synthesis (radioautography), the RNA and DNA content (cytophotometry). These studies display a high level of cell physiological activity. PGA acting on the lymphocytes of schizophrenic patients during 60 min either slightly stimulates them, or inhibits the initially high level of cell activity.

1047

Lim DT, Freel BJ, Ghani M. **Isolated IgA deficiency associated with upper airway obstruction, sleep dysrhythmia and failure to thrive: a case report.** *Ann Allergy.* 1978;41:299-302. (English) (no abstract)

1048

Livni E, Munitz H, Tyano S, Englander T, Kuritzky A, Wysenbeek H, Joshua H. **Further studies on cell-mediated immunity to myelin basic protein in schizophrenic patients.** *J Neurol Sci.* 1979;42:437-40. (English)

Cell-mediated immunity (CMI) toward myelin human basic protein (HBP) was studied in 19 chronic drug-free schizophrenic patients and in 30 patients with primary affective disorders receiving psychoactive drugs, 74% of the schizophrenics showed an inhibition of macrophage migration, whereas only one patient from the affective group showed such a response. These results indicate that drugs are not responsible for the appearance of CMI to HBP in schizophrenics. One out of 9 ECT-treated patients developed a CMI to HBP.

1049

Loseva TM. **Complementary rosette study of peripheral blood B-lymphocytes of schizophrenic patients.** *Zh Nevropatol Psikhiatr.* 1981;5:697-700. (Russian)

Examinations of the B-cell immunity system in schizophrenic patients showed that the content of B-lymphocytes in the peripheral blood exceeded normal (difference being statistically significant). The patients' lymphocyte populations had twice as much (as compared with normal) cells with increased density of immunoglobulin receptors on the superficial membrane. This points to an increase of the functional activity of B-lymphocytes in schizophrenia. The pathogenetic significance of B-cell superficial receptors was the greatest in the acute period of the schizophrenic process.

1050

Loseva TM. **Effect of thymosin on the rosette-forming capacity of peripheral blood lymphocytes in schizophrenics and healthy subjects.** *Zh Nevropatol Psikhiatr.* 1982;82:67-70. (Russian)

It has been found that the blood of schizophrenic patients contains many more thymosin-sensitive lymphocytes than the blood of healthy subjects. Thymosin produces a regulatory effect on the changed receptor activity of the T-cells revealed in the reaction of spontaneous rosette formation. The disturbances of the T-lymphocyte membrane activity that take place in schizophrenic patients can be associated with the changes of the thymus hormonal function occurring in that disease.

1051

Loseva TM. **Thymus-dependent lymphocytes in the spontaneous rosette-formation reaction in schizophrenia.** *Zh Nevropatol Psikhiatr.* 1977;77:692-5. (Russian)

The report is concerned with the capability of the peripheral blood lymphocytes in schizophrenic patients (28 cases) and normals (25 individuals) to form spontaneous rosettes with the erythrocytes of sheep. The amount of rosette forming cells in schizophrenic patients is significantly lower. Besides, part of the lymphocytes create less complete rosette forms as compared to the lymphocytes of normals. The achieved results may point to insufficiency of the immunological competency in the system of thymus-dependent cells in schizophrenic patients.

1052

Majumdar SK, Kakad PP. **Serum immunoglobulins in dementia** (letter). *Br J Psychiatry.* 1980;137:496. (English)

1053

Mascord I, Freed D, Durrant B. **Antibodies to foodstuffs in schizophrenia** (letter). *Br Med J.* 1978;1:1351. (English)

1054

Mato M, Uchiyama Y, Kurihara K, Karasawa T. **Fluorescent substance in leukocytes and platelets of psychiatric patients.** Biol Psychiatry. 1977;12:823-26. (English) (no abstract)

1055

Maznina TP, Mikhailova VA. **Dynamic study of the level of antithymocyte activity during the process of treating schizophrenic patients.** *Zh Nevropatol Psikhiatr.* 1977; 77:1194-7. (Russian)

The level of antithymocytic activity in the blood serum of schizophrenic patients (20 cases) was determined in the process of therapy by neuroleptics and neuroleptics in combination with anti-depressive drugs and tranquilizers. A drop in the anti-thymic activity was found in 4 cases. A level of the anti-thymocytic activity corresponded to the attack of the disease, while its decrease--to a remission.

1056

McGuffin P, Gardiner P, Swinburne LM. **Schizophrenia, celiac disease, and antibodies to food.** *Biol Psychiatry.*

1981;16:281-5. (English) (no abstract)

1057
Miller AE, Neighbour PA, Katzman R, Aronson M, Lipkowitz R. **Immunological studies in senile dementia of the Alzheimer type: evidence for enhanced suppressor cell activity.** *Ann Neurol.* 1981;10:506-10. (English)

To examine immunological variables in senile dementia of the Alzheimer type (SDAT), we compared SDAT patients with elderly and young controls with regard to concanavalin A (Con A)-induced suppression, lymphocyte proliferation, interferon production, and serum immunoglobulin levels. The results showed exaggerated Con A suppression and reduced lymphocyte proliferation in SDAT patients compared to elderly control subjects. Interferon production after stimulation by Con A and immunoglobulin levels did not differ between SDAT and elderly control subjects. The results suggest impaired immunoregulatory mechanisms in patients with SDAT that may be related to the cause or course of SDAT. Alternatively, these immunological changes may be secondary to pathological changes in the central nervous system.

1058
Modrzewska K, Book JA. **Schizophrenia and malignant neoplasms in a north Swedish population** (letter). *Lancet.* 1979;1:275-6.

1059
Mogilina NP, Zhirnova IG. **Indirect immunofluorescence and complement absorption test characterization of anti-brain antibodies in schizophrenia.** *Zh Nevropatol Psikhiatr.* 1981;81:397-401. (Russian)

The content and tropism of anticerebral antibodies were examined in 20 schizophrenic patients using the indirect immunofluorescence and complement fixation tests. With the aid of the latter the antibodies were revealed in 15 patients, the antibodies to the homologous brain being more frequent in patients with a more severe, continuously progressing schizophrenia, while the antibodies to a heterologous (rat) brain were more often detected in patients with slowly progressing forms of the disease. In 18 patients, the indirect immunofluorescence test showed fixation of immunoglobulins on the nervous tissue components, such as neurons, myelin, vascular walls. Rather frequently, fluorescence of the microglia cells was observed: according to literary data this is not the case with sera of neurological patients. Of attention was a selective fluorescence of the canaliculi observed in examinations of the renal tissue. The data obtained point to a participation of the immunological reactions in the schizophrenia pathogenesis, these reactions involving various morphological and functional systems.

1060
Nasr SJ, Altman EG, Meltzer HY. **Concordance of atopic and affective disorders.** *J Affective Disord.* 1981;3:291-6. (English)

The personal and family history of bronchial asthma and/or hay fever was obtained from a series of 82 psychiatric patients. We report a significantly higher incidence of atopic disorders in affective patients (16/48) than in schizophrenic patients (2/34) (chi-square = 8.754, p<0.005). There was also a significantly higher incidence of atopic disorders among the first-degree relatives of patients with affective disorders (48/356) than among the first-degree relatives of patients with schizophrenia (10/182) (chi-square 8.501, p<0.005).

1061
Noeva K, Manolova Z. **Antigamma globulin factors and IgG, IgA and IgM levels in schizophrenia, manic-depressive psychosis and disseminated sclerosis patients.** *Acta Microbiol Virol Immunol (Sofia).* 1976;4:105-12. (Bulgarian) (unavailable at publication)

1062
Nyland H, Naess A, Lunde H. **Lymphocyte subpopulations in peripheral blood from schizophrenic patients.** *Acta Psychiatr Scand.* 1980;61:313-8. (English)

Patients with acute and chronic schizophrenia were examined for T and Fc receptor-bearing lymphocytes in blood by means of rosette techniques. The patients had normal numbers of peripheral blood lymphocytes. The percentage of T lymphocytes in patients with acute schizophrenia was reduced (60 ± 2%) compared with controls (66 ± 1%) and patients with chronic schizophrenia (67 ± 3%). The total number of T lymphocytes was significantly decreased in patients with acute schizophrenia had slightly elevated numbers (1,778 ± 200 cells/mm^3, p<0.002). The percentage and total numbers of Fc receptor-bearing lymphocytes were normal in both patient groups. Both immune mechanisms and the neuroleptic drug treatment may be of importance for the observed decrease in T lymphocyte numbers in blood from patients with acute schizophrenia.

1063
Oifa AI. **Senile amyloidosis in schizophrenia.** *Neurosci Behav Physiol.* 1976;7:215-20. (English) (unavailable at publication)

1064
Oskolkova SN. **Clinical and immunological characteristics of reactive depression patients in forensic psychiatric practice.** *Sud Med Ekspert.* 1981;24:50-2. (Russian)

Immunological and allergical indexes in 53 depressive patients and in 18 psychically and somatically sane persons were confronted. A correlation between the presence of cerebral antibodies, allergical indexes and clinical features is demonstrated. The results may be an aid in early diagnosing of depressive patients, their optimal treatment and prevention of socially dangerous actions.

1065
Palmblad J, Fohlin L, Lundstrom M. **Anorexia nervosa and polymorphonuclear (PMN) granulocyte reactions.** *Scand J Haematol.* 1977;19:334-42. (English)

10 patients with anorexia nervosa were compared with controls with normal weight, regarding their peripheral blood polymorphonuclear (PMN) granulocyte reactions. The ano-

rexia patients showed a statistically significant decrease in PMN bactericidal capacity and PMN adherence. The mean chemotaxis did not differ, but in two of the anorexia patients chemotaxis was almost absent. The intracellular activity of alkaline phosphatase was below the reference values in 5 of the 6 patients in whom it was investigated. It is concluded that changes in granulocyte function may be noted in anorexia nervosa, but their clinical significance is uncertain, as no patients had recurrent or severe infectious diseases.

1066

Palmblad J, Fohlin L, Norberg R. **Plasma levels of complement factors 3 and 4, orosomucoid and opsonic functions in anorexia nervosa.** *Acta Paediatr Scand.* 1979;68:617-8. (English) (no abstract)

1067

Parfitt DN. **Lung cancer and schizophrenia** (letter). *Br J Psychiatry.* 1981;138:179-80. (English)

1068

Pert CB. **A request for serum samples from psychiatric patients with associated autoimmune disease: is some psychosis caused by an autoimmune response to neurotransmitter receptors?** (letter). *Commun Psychopharmacol.* 1977;1:307-9. (English)

1069

Pivovarova AI, Koliaskina GI. **Effect of different doses of phytomitogens on blood lymphocyte proliferation in schizophrenia.** *Biull Eksp Biol Med.* 1980;90:552-4. (Russian)

The action of various does of PHA and Con A on ^{3}H-thymidine incorporation in DNA of blood lymphocytes was studied in health and schizophrenia. The dose-response curves in schizophrenia treated with various doses of PHA and Con A lie beneath the respective curves characteristic for the cells from normal subjects. The most discriminant results with respect to the proliferative activity of lymphocytes of the two groups were obtained in the course of administering low doses of the stimulants. In schizophrenic patients, the shift of the optimal dose toward higher concentrations was seen both for PHA and Con A.

1070

Pivovarova AI, Maznina TP. **Effect of schizophrenic patients' serum on DNA synthesis in cultures of PHA stimulated lymphocytes.** *Zh Nevropatol Psikhiatr.* 1977; 77:1357-60. (Russian)

The authors studied the influence of the blood sera of schizophrenic patients on the DNA synthesis in a PHA-stimulated lymphocyte culture of normal donors. It was established that in 13 of the 15 studied patients the blood sera contained factors, inhibiting the DNA synthesis in lymphocytes in normals. The reactivity of lymphocytes on PHA was in an inverse correlation with the figure of the cytotoxic index. The assumption is being made that the inhibiting action of the serum is conditioned by the presence of antibodies to thymocytes and T-lymphocytes.

1071

Plantey F. **Antinuclear factor in affective disorders.** *Biol Psychiatry.* 1978;13:149-50. (English) (no abstract)

1072

Poletaev AB, Sherstnev VV, Dolgov ON. **Theoretical prerequisites for new methods of diagnosing and treating neuropsychic diseases of autoimmune origin.** *Vestn Akad Med Nauk SSSR.* 1982;2:53-6. (English) (unavailable at publication)

1073

Popova NN. **Investigation of brain autoantigens in the blood serum of schizophrenics.** *Neurosci Behav Physiol.* 1977;8:76-81. (English) (unavailable at publication)

1074

Prilipko LL, Kurilova II, Bogdanova ED, Vostrikova SA. **Isolation of subpopulations of activated lymphocytes from the peripheral blood of schizophrenic patients.** *Zh Nevropatol Psikhiatr.* 1977;77:78-82. (Russian)

The authors determine the physiological condition of adhesive and nonadhesive lymphocytes in the peripheral blood of schizophrenic patients. It is found that there is a subpopulation of adhesive lymphocytes in the organism of patients that possess all the signs of activation, i.e., an active state of the nucleus, cytoplasm and an increase in the synthesis of RNA.

1075

Prilipko LL, Lideman RR. **Peripheral blood lymphocytes as a biological indicator of physiologic processes in schizophrenia.** *Zh Nevropatol Psikhiatr.* 1982;82:79-86. (Russian)

The results of studying the properties of peripheral blood lymphocytes in schizophrenic patients are reviewed. Three parameters are specified in which the patients' lymphocytes differ substantially from those of healthy donors: these are the resistance to osmotic shock and responses of the cells to stimulation with phytohemagglutinin and Concanavalin A. It is shown that all the three parameters are controlled by different factors of the schizophrenic's blood serum. Two of them correlate with the clinical manifestations of the disease. It is concluded that the lymphocytes of schizophrenic patients can serve as a biological indicator of the pathophysiological processes taking place in that disease.

1076

Pulkkinen E. **Immunoglobulins, psychopathology and prognosis in schizophrenia.** *Acta Psychiatr Scand.* 1977; 56:173-82. (English)

On admission, IgA, IgG and IgM concentrations were determined in 76 schizophrenics, and the correlations of these concentrations to the variables relating to psychopathology, background and prognosis were investigated in the present study, which is a part of a more extensive unpublished study. On the basis of factorization, the highest IgM concentrations were found in withdrawn schizophrenics and the lowest in paranoid schizophrenics. Of the background variables, the patient's present age had a positive correlation and his place of birth (rural-urban) a negative correlation to IgA concentrations, both being at a statistically significant level. IgA and IgM values higher than average at the beginning of treatment predicted a short hospital stay. Earlier, these patients had also needed little hospital care in relation to the duration of the disease. A hypothesis based on the results is presented, according to which a different way of reacting to stress may explain the differences in IgM concentrations in withdrawn and paranoid schizophrenics. The connection between prognosis and immunoglobulins was considered at least partially explainable on the grounds of age at the onset of the disease.

1077
Rauscher FP, Nasrallah HA, Wyatt RJ. **Cutaneous histamine response in schizophrenia.** *J Clin Psychiatry.* 1980; 41:44-51. (English)

A diminished cutaneous response to intradermal histamine has been reported by schizophrenics in at least 12 studies over the past 50 years. This literature is reviewed and compared to the present investigation in which both the wheal and flare response to intradermal histamine is examined in chronic schizophrenic patients, their parents, and a healthy control group. Histamine insensitivity could not be demonstrated in unmedicated patients, although a diminished wheal and flare response occurred during neuroleptic treatment. A cutaneous histamine insensitivity does not appear to be a common phenomenon among chronic schizophrenic patients.

1078
Rimon R, Halonen P, Puhakka P, Laitinen L, Marttila R, Salmela L. **Immunoglobulin G antibodies to herpes simplex type 1 virus detected by radioimmunoassay in serum and cerebrospinal fluid of patients with schizophrenia.** *J Clin Psychiatry.* 1979;40:241-3. (English)

Serum and CSF specimens from 16 schizophrenic patients and 18 nonpsychiatric controls were tested by radioimmunoassay for immunoglobulin G antibody of capsid, envelope and excreted antigens of herpes simplex type 1 virus. There were no significant differences in the antibody levels between the schizophrenic patients and the controls. The etiological role of viruses and virus-like agents in schizophrenia and some methodological aspects are discussed.

1079
Rimon R, Nishmi M, Halonen P. **Serum and CSF antibody levels to herpes simplex type 1, measles and rubella viruses in patients with schizophrenia.** *Ann Clin Res.* 1978;10:291-3. (English)

Serum and CSF specimens from 12 schizophrenic patients and 10 non-psychiatric controls were tested for herpes simplex type 1 virus neutralizing antibody and for measles and rubella haemagglutination inhibiting antibodies. There were no significant differences in the distribution of virus antibody titres in serum or CSF specimens between the patients and the controls. The possible aetiological role of viruses or virus-like agents in schizophrenia and some methodological aspects are discussed.

1080
Rippere V. **Schizophrenia and antibodies to food** (letter). *Biol Psychiat.* 1982;17:955-6. (English)

1081
Roppel RM. **The cancer-schizophrenia linkage.** *Aggressologie.* 1978;19:239-45. (English) (unavailable at publication)

1082
Rudin DO. **Covert transport dysfunction in the choroid plexus as a possible cause of schizophrenia.** *Schizophr Bull.* 1979;5:623-6. (English)

Schizophrenia and certain forms of idiopathic mental retardation may result from covert immune complex disease of the basal lamina of the choroid plexus, a process already known to cause covert transport dysfunction in similar structures of, for example, skin, bowel, kidney, and endocrines. Plexial attack could lead to cerebrospinal fluid contamination and then, via an "open" ependyma, to neurotransmitter dysfunction in the periventricular limbic brain. The immune complex mechanism implies polygenic induction, direct or autoimmune, of immune sensitivity to exogenous agents and is thus compatible with the genetic picture in schizophrenia. Candidate agents include viral coat peptides and cereal grain glutens. The glutens are known to cause immune complex skin and bowel disease variants, and some empirical evidence links them to schizophrenia. Only newer immunofluorescence methods can detect the pathology, which is otherwise silent. Systemic lupus erythematosus provides a model since it is a genetic immune complex disease strongly associated with schizophreniform psychoses, exhibits choroid plexial immunofluorescence but no central nervous system pathology by ordinary methods, and may be triggered by viruses.

1083
Rudin DO. **The choroid plexus and system disease in mental illness; III--The exogenous peptide hypothesis of mental illness.** *Biol Psychiat.* 1981;16:489-512. (English)

Based on the apparent existence of a second (choroid plexial) blood-brain barrier offering a new brain attack mechanics on the periventricular primary personality brain (Rudin, 1980) and which may be breached to produce the schizophreniform psychosis characteristic of systemic lupus erythematosus (Rudin, 1981), we here assess the evidence that viruses and exogenous peptides, including especially the glutens of cereal grains, may be the primary triggers for schizophrenia. Schizophrenia would then be supposed to result as one expression of gene-determined combined transport organ dysfunction with underlying basal laminar immunopathy at the tissue level and possibly a prostaglandin disorder at the chemical and membrane level in turn, finally disrupting neurotransmission in the periventricular limbic system. We conclude that the evidence warrants test of the hypothesis, including a clinical trial under national auspices employing an elemental diet, plasmapheresis, immunosuppression together with an antiviral regimen.

1084
Rudin DO. **The choroid plexus and system disease in**

mental illness; I--A new brain attack mechanism via the second blood-brain barrier. *Biol Psychiat.* 1980;15:517-39. (English)

Schizophrenia and certain idiopathic neuroses and retardations may be caused by polygenic sensitization to exogeneous peptide antigens or viruses causing a covert immune complex basal lamina disease of the choroid plexus. This organ has the general structure and disease susceptibility of many other transport organs but acts as a second blood-brain barrier putting at risk to contamination and dysfunction the periventricular primary personality (limbic) brain now thought to be centrally involved in schizophrenia. Genetic variability selects different antigens and different target organs so that a complex statistical structure of disease expression can result over the transport organ group as well as between this group and the endocrines and exocrines. This leads to the concept of intra- and intercombined system diseases all of which may have a covert biphasic (hyper-hypo) time course. To this extrinsic combinatorial complexity may be added an intrinsic or neural combinatorial complexity resulting from the fact that the choroid plexus is threaded throughout the limbic system and subject to spotty disease characteristic of many immunopathies. In this way a wide range of behavioral disorders may arise as well as mental retardations if the process occurs during development. In this paper we discuss basic mechanisms. In the next paper of the series we examine systemic lupus erythematosus, the prototypical "combined transport" dysfunction, as a model for schizophrenia. In the last paper we search for specific exogenous peptide triggers for schizophrenia viewed as one expression of combined transport organ dysfunction. We conclude that immunofluorescent and virological surveys should be conducted in all mental illnesses as well as clinical trials of interferon therapy and elemental diets.

1085
Rudin DO. **The choroid plexus and system disease in mental illness; II-- Systemic lupus erythematosus: a combined transport dysfunction model for schizophrenia.** *Biol Psychiat.* 1981;16:373-97. (English)

Carr *et al.* (1978) and Rudin (1979) independently suggested that systemic lupus erythematosus (SLE) might provide a model for schizophrenia since SLE is strongly associated with schizophreniform psychoses and exhibits only a covert CNS pathology revealed by immunofluorescent immune complex deposits in the choroid plexus. To carry the concept forward we here examine SLE employing the ideas developed in the preceding paper (Rudin, 1980) indicating that the choroid plexus is part of a second blood-brain barrier guarding the periventricular primary personality brain, the limbic system, and that the choroid plexus is also but one of a set of "transport organs" sharing common vulnerability to covert basal lamina immune complex pathology. In this context both SLE and schizophrenia are viewed as expressions of combined transport dysfunction syndromes, resulting from polygenic-induced sensitivity to exogenous peptides or viruses causing basal laminar immune complex disease, but exhibiting differing statistical expressions over the transport organ group due to differences in genes which elicit different transport organ sensitivities to different exogenous viruses or peptide antigens. Immune disease processes are briefly reviewed.

1086
Saillant C, Fontaine C, Maunoury R, Delpech B, Vedrenne C. **Psychoses, immunity and neurospecific antigens: current knowledge and perspectives.** *Encephale.* 1979; 5:61-69. (French)

Investigations performed by various workers during the last ten years suggest that some forms of mental illness are associated with a variety of immunological reactions. Significant variations in immunoglobulin ratios have been observed in patients with psychotic illness, and cellular and humoral cytotoxic activities against cerebral tissue have been demonstrated *in vitro*. At the molecular level, several subjects can be proposed for investigation into immunological phenomena in neuropatholgy. Thus, the neurospecific antigens, which have been isolated by biochemical methods, but the physiological role of which is largely unknown, open new ways to the experimental exploration of psychopathology.

1087
Schayer RW, Pilc A, Zaborwski A, Kazimierczak W, Maslinski C. **The histamine-induced skin reaction in schizophrenic and normal subjects.** *J Clin Psychiatry.* 1982; 43:7-9. (English)

Most published data on histamine skin tests on schizophrenic patients show them to be insensitive relative to normals or other psychotic patients. However, experimental conditions have varied and in most cases only a single dose of histamine was used. We have compared 13 volunteer controls and 16 paranoid schizophrenics; each subject was injected intradermally with histamine, 10, 20, and 50 microgram, doses predetermined in volunteers to give a dose-response curve. Wheal and flare were measured at 10 and 20 minutes, intervals near the time of maximum flare. We found no statistically significant differences between normal controls and schizophrenic patients.

1088
Semenov SF, Pashutova EK. **Fate of immunopathologic principles in patients whose schizophrenia commenced after childbirth.** *Zh Nevropatol Psikhiatr.* 1977;77:72-8. (Russian)

On the basis of comprehensive immuno-biological studies of schizophrenia where the disease manifests itself after delivery, the authors come to the conclusion that a certain role is played in the development of the disease by immuno-allergic processes. Facts confirming this supposition are detection of brain antigens and the expressiveness of sensitization even during the initial stage of the disease, a sufficiently high frequency of revealed autoantibodies, and their correlation with the quality of remissions. Besides these facts, the authors were able to distinguish individually different types of antibody formation in recurrent and attack-like-progressive forms of schizophrenia, a fall in the complement activity in the blood serum of patients as well as a certain connection between the indices of organospecific immunity and the dynamics of the morbid process.

1089
Shaposhnikov VS, Oleinik AV, Vifrenko AE, Korotonozhkii

VG, Savchenko VP. **Assessment of cellular and humoral immunity of affective psychosis patients.** *Vrach Delo.* 1981;7:80-3. (Russian) (unavailable at publication)

1090
Shaposhnikov VS. **Clinico-immunological study of psychoses in old age.** *Vrach Delo.* 1980;6:96-8. (Russian) (unavailable at publication)

1091
Singh MM, Kay SR. **Wheat gluten as a pathogenic factor in schizophrenia.** *Science.* 1976;191:401-2. (English)

Schizophrenics maintained on a cereal grain free and milk-free diet and receiving optimal treatment with neuroleptics showed an interruption or reversal of their therapeutic progress during a period of "blind" wheat gluten challenge. The exacerbation of the disease process was not due to variations in neuroleptic doses. After termination of the gluten challenge, the course of improvement was reinstated. The observed effects seemed to be due to a primary schizophrenia-promoting effect of wheat gluten.

1092
Sisenbaev SK, Melkumov GA, Budnevich RI. **Tuberculin sensitivity in various mental disorders.** *Probl Tuberk.* 1981;2:13-5. (Russian) (unavailable at publication)

1093
Solntseva EI, Faktor MI. **Effect of schizophrenic patients' serum immunoglobulins on nerve cell potentials.** *Zh Nevropatol Psikhiatr.* 1979;79:206-12. (Russian)

With the aid of the microelectrode method, the influence of different protein fractions isolated from the blood serum of schizophrenic patients and normals on an edible snail was studied. The fractions were isolated by means of ion exchange chromatography and contained immunoglobulins (IgG, IgA, IgM). It was established that the fraction of the blood serum in schizophrenic patients, containing IgM is significantly stronger than the respective fraction in normals, depolarizing and inactivating the neuron membrane. It is suggested that there is an increased content of tropic to the nervous tissue antibodies of this class in the blood serum of schizophrenic patients.

1094
Solntseva EI, Korobtsov GN. **Changes in responses of neurons to serotonin produced by blood serum from schizophrenics.** *Neurosci Behav Physiol.* 1979;9:329-31. (English) (unavailable at publication)

1095
Solomon JG, Solomon S. **Psychotic depression and bronchogenic carcinoma.** *Am J Psychiatry.* 1978;135:859-60. (English) (no abstract)

1096
Stefanis C, Issidorides MR. **Histochemical changes in the blood cells of schizophrenic patients under pimozide treatment.** *Biol Psychiat.* 1976;11:53-68. (English)

Chromatin structure and nucleohistone pattern were investigated histochemically in the neutrophils of 11 schizophrenics and 16 healthy controls. Compared to controls, all schizophrenic patients prior to medication showed a distinctly different histochemical pattern consisting of increased concentration and abnormal distribution of nucleohistones. This pattern has been attributed to an increase of arginine-rich histones in schizophrenics. Pimozide administration exerted a normalizing effect on the nucleohistone distribution pattern. These findings further support our view that genomic expression abnormalities may be related to schizophrenic illness.

1097
Stevens FM, Lloyd RS, Geraghty SM, Reynolds MT, Sarsfield MJ, McNicholl B, Fottrell PF, Wright R, McCarthy CF. **Schizophrenia and coeliac disease--the nature of the relationship.** *Psychol Med.* 1977;7:259-63. (English)

To test the hypothesis of an association between schizophrenia and coeliac disease, the sera of 380 chronic schizophrenic in-patients in two mental hospitals in the west of Ireland have been screened for the presence of reticulin antibodies. Antibodies were found in 26 patients. Twenty-one of these patients were further studied by proximal duodenal mucosal biopsy. None of the biopsies showed the morphological and histological features found in untreated coeliac disease. The incidence of reticulin antibodies found in schizophrenic patients and controls is similar. The findings of this study lead to the rejection of the hypothesis of a positive genetic relationship between schizophrenia and coeliac disease.

1098
Strahilevitz M. **Possible utilization of extracorporeal immunoadsorption and other immunologic methods in the treatment of schizophrenia.** *Birth Defects.* 1978; 14;261-76. (English) (no abstract)

1099
Strahilevitz M. **Virus-like agents, IgA, and schizophrenia** (letter). *Lancet.* 1979;2:145-6. (English)

1100
Stubbs EG, Crawford ML. **Depressed lymphocyte responsiveness in autistic children.** *J Autism Child Schizo.* 1977;7:49-55. (English)

Although there are associations linking autism with prenatal rubella, cytomegalovirus, syphilis, and varicella, the etiology of the autistic state remains obscure. Host defense against the etiologic agents postulated to be responsible for the autism-associated syndromes is believed to be primarily of the cell-mediated type. In this preliminary study, cellular immune function was assessed *in vitro* by phytohemagglutinin (PHA) stimulation of lymphocyte cultures. Twelve autistic children and thirteen control subjects were compared. The autistic group exhibited a depressed lymphocyte transformation response to PHA when compared to the control subjects ($p<0.01$).

1101
Stubbs EG. **Autistic children exhibit undetectable hemag-**

glutination-inhibition antibody titers despite previous rubella vaccination. *J Autism Child Schizo.* 1976;6:269-74. (English)

The etiology of autism is unknown, but autism has been associated with a number of diseases, including prenatal rubella. Rubella vaccine challenge was used in an attempt to retrospectively diagnose prenatal rubella in autistic children. This test was selected because unresponsiveness of antibody titer has been reported as helpful in retrospective diagnosing of prenatal rubella. Fifteen autistic children and eight controls matched for age were challenged with rubella vaccine. Rubella vaccine challenge did not differentiate autistic children from the control subjects. However, 5 of 13 autistic children had undetectable titers despite previous vaccine; all control subjects had detectable titers. This finding of undetectable titers in autistic children suggests these children may have an altered immune response.

1102
Sugerman AA, Southern DL, Curran JF. **A study of antibody levels in alcoholic, depressive and schizophrenic patients.** *Ann Allergy.* 1982;48:166-71. (English)

A study was undertaken to compare IgG, IgA, IgM, IgE and IgD antibodies in adult alcoholic,depressive and schizophrenic patients with healthy, adult controls. Total IgG, IgA, IgM, IgE, and IgD and specific-IgE antibodies were assessed using 33 allergens: 12 inhalant and 21 foods. There was no significant difference observed in the total immunoglobulin results between the patients and controls. There were, however, significant differences between the groups for allergen specific-IgE with the depressive patients exhibiting the greatest number of positive test results. The depressives had an overall t-test value of 10.080 (5% = 1.960), the alcoholics t = 6.800 and the schizophrenics t = 6.015. The allergens most often positive were those from the perennial/mold group, although the most frequently positive single allergen was egg white and 100% of the depressives were sensitive to it. The data in this investigation suggest that psychiatric patients with alcohol dependence, depression and schizophrenia be studied further so that information on a causal relationship between allergen specific-IgE antibodies and these mental disoders can be evaluated.

1103
Swartz C. **Hormonal influence on viruses in psychiatric illness** (letter). *Lancet.* 1980;2:1035. (English)

1104
Sylvester-Jrgensen O, Vejlsgaard-Goldschmidt V, Faber-Vestergaard B. **Herpes simplex virus (HSV) antibodies in child psychiatric patients and normal children.** *Acta Psychiatr Scand.* 1982;66:42-9. (English)

The prevalence of herpes simplex virus (HSV) antibodies has been investigated in 123 child psychiatric patiets and 86 normal children. HSV antibodies were measured by ELISA technique. The prevalence of HSV antibodies in different diagnostic groups (conduct disorder, emotional disorder, hyperkinetic syndrome, anorexia nervosa, infantile autism and borderline schizophrenia in childhood) was compared

with age-matched normal children, but no significant differences were found.

1105
Tachibana T, Watanabe N, Masuko K, Hirata-Hibi M, Shohmori T, Kohsaka M, Nagao T, Akiyama K, Otsuki S. **Immunological study of blood of schizophrenia: atypical lymphocytes and quantitative analyses of various immunological measures** (author's transl). *Seishin Shinkeigaku Zasshi.* 1981;83:406-17. (Japanese) (unavailable at publication)

1106
Tantam D, Kalucy R, Brown DG. **Sleep, scratching and dreams in eczema: a new approach to alexithymia.** *Psychother Psychosom.* 1982;37:26-35. (English)

6 patients with itching due to skin disorder and 6 student controls were studied in the sleep laboratory. It was found that some of the patients had personality characteristics consistent with Sifneos' concept of alexithymia and that these were associated with a trend towards less REM sleep and with a significant lack of involvement in dreams collected under standardised sleep laboratory conditions. It is suggested that dreams collections in a sleep laboratory may be a valuable new method in the study of the link between emotional life and psychosomatic disorders.

1107
Tavolato B, Argentiero V. **Immunogical indices in presenile Alzheimer's disease.** *J Neurol Sci.* 1980;46:325-31. (English)

Immunological indices, both T- and B-dependent, were studied in 11 patients affected by presenile Alzheimer's disease. The data obtained were compared with those from a group of normal adults of similar age and from a group of normal young subjects. Furthermore, antisera were produced in rabbits against Alzheimer's serum and compared to antisera against normal human serum. The following results were obtained: decrease of serum IgM levels; no monoclonal aspects or auto-antibodies were detected in our patients. The kappa/lambda ratio was also normal. The T cell system was functionally normal, but with a slight decrease of the T cell number and with an increase of the null lymphocytes. No specific serum proteins were found in the anti-Alzheimer antisera. The data are discussed in correlation to the possible genesis of senile plaques.

1108
Taylor WM. **Schizophrenia, rheumatoid arthritis and tryptophan metabolism.** *J Clin Psychiatry.* 1978;39:499-503. (English)

Rheumatoid arthritis and schizophrenia have been described in early surveys as mutually exclusive disorders. Such claims are seen as especially interesting in view of: (1) indications that both illnesses often follow prodromes of severe psychological stress, (2) theories regarding hypermethylation of indoleamines producing endogenous psychotogens in schizophrenia, and (3) studies of rheumatoid arthritis reporting excessive binding of L-tryptophan to plasma protein, abnormalities of urinary tryptophan metabolites, decreased serotonin binding capacity of thrombocytes, and decreased MAO activity in joint fluid. Further comparative studies of tryptophan metabolism in schizophrenia and rheumatoid arthritis might enhance knowledge of pathogenesis in either or both diseases.

1109
Torack RM, Lynch RG. **Cytochemistry of brain amyloid in adult dementia.** *Acta Neuropathol (Berl).* 1981;53:189-96. (English)

A cytochemical study of 14 cases of adult dementia revealed the presence of gamma globulin in the amyloid of three cases of congophilic angiopathy by means of immunofluorescence microscopy. In these cases, the additional identification of human albumin is regarded to indicate a non-specific macromolecular leak in the blood-brain barrier. Both reactions are inhibited by prior absorption with the appropriate serum protein. Twelve of the 14 cases had congophilic amyloid deposits which were not affected by permanganate pretreatment, so that immunoglobulin content remains a possibility, despite the negative immune reaction. Alcianophilia was studied at a varying pH and electrolyte concentration, but these findings do not appear to have nosologic significance. The three positive cases are characterized by a rapid terminal decline. The heterogeneity of amyloid and the significance of immunoamyloid in the pathologenesis of adult dementia is discussed.

1110
Torrey EF, Peterson MR, Brannon WL, Carpenter WT, Post RM, Van Kammen DP. **Immunoglobulins and viral antibodies in psychiatric patients.** *Br J Psychiatry.* 1978; 132:342-8. (English)

The serum and CSF of 66 patients with functional psychoses were tested for immunoglobulins and antibodies to measles, HSV-1, CMV, and rubella viruses. Ten surgical and 80 neurological patients were controls. There were no significant findings in the serum, consistent with most previous studies. In the CSF 6 of 17 multiple admission schizophrenic patients had definite elevations of IgG or measles antibody and differed significantly from the surgical controls. Immunologically this group resembled the seriously ill neurological patients. No previous study has been made of immunoglobulins or viral antibodies in the CSF of psychiatric patients. It is concluded that further work is warranted in a search for biological subgroups of schizophrenia.

1111
Torrey EF, Peterson MR. **The viral hypothesis of schizophrenia.** *Schizophr Bull.* 1976;2:136-46. (English) (unavailable at publication)

1112
Torrey EF, Yolken RH, Winfrey CJ. **Cytomegalovirus antibody in cerebrospinal fluid of schizophrenic patients detected by enzyme immunoassay.** *Science.* 1982:21:892-4. (English)

By means of enzyme immunoassay techniques to detect the presence of antibody to cytomegalovirus, the cerebrospinal fluid of 178 patients with schizophrenia, 17 patients with bipolar disorders, and 11 other psychiatric patients was compared with that of 78 neurological patients and 41 normal control subjects. The cerebrospinal fluid of 20 of the schizophrenic patients and 3 of the patients with bipolar disorders showed significant increases in immunoglobulin M antibody to cytomegalovirus; no difference was found in patients on or off psychotropic medication.

1113
Torrey EF. **CSF better than serum in study of immunology in mental patients.** *Clin Psychiatr News.* 1977;5. (English) (no abstract)

1114
Tyrrell DAJ. **Schizophrenia and virus infection.** *Trends Neurosci.* 1981;4:VII-IX. (English) (no abstract)

1115
Vartanian ME, Burbaeva GSH, Ignatov SA, Nazarian KB. **Organ specific water-soluble cerebral cortex proteins; possible participation in physiological functions and pathologic manifestations.** *Vopr Biokhim Mozga.* 1978; 13:144-51. (Russian)

The spectre of activer antigens in brain is studied. The presence of 3 protein and 3 glycoprotein brain specific antigens is demonstrated. The possible participation of brain specific antigens in increased antibody formation in schizophrenics, multiple sclerosis and lateral amyotrophic sclerosi is studied. The data obtained indicate the role of brain specific antigens to autoimmunity on those patients. The possible participation of one of the specific antigens of the brain, sialoglcyoprotein GP-350, in physiological processes connected with the mechanism of memory is also studied. In experiments of inbred trained rats an activation of the synthesis of GP-350 is observed.

1116
Vilkov GA, Siletskii OIA, Gul'iants ES, Siziakina LP, Mezhova LI. **Detection of the neurotropic properties of the serum of schizophrenia patients.** *Zh Nevropatol Psikhiatr.* 1980;80:67-70. (Russian)

A method of testing neurotropic properties of the serum of schizophrenic patients is proposed. This method was tested on 27 schizophrenic patients and was based on experimental data. In all cases there was a narrowing of the width of the glomerular zone in the adrenal glands of rats administered the serum of schizophrenic patients intravenously. There was a significant difference in the width of the zone depending upon the stage of the disease and exacerbation, while in experiments, depending upon the presence of antibodies to brain subcommissural organs.

1117
Vilkov GA, Siletskii OIA, Mezhova LI, Volcho LS. **Kinin system components and immune complexes in schizophrenia.** *Zh Nevropatol Psikhiatr.* 1979;79:581-3. (Russian)

The sera of schizophrenic patients showed existence of immune complexes and increased activity of kallikrein, as well as relationship between these indices and the phase of the process. Their totality may be recommended for evaluating the activity of the process and efficacy of the treatment.

1118
Vuia O. **Paraproteinosis and amyloidosis of the cerebral vessels and senile plaques.** *J Neurol Sci.* 1978;39:37-46. (English)

A case is reported of progressive dementia and a terminal picture of generalized tetaniform contractures. The relationship of the generalized tetaniform contractures to the stiff-man syndrome is discussed. Morphologically, diffuse amyloid deposition was found in the pial and cortical vessels, accompanied by amyloid deposition in the senile plaques in the cortical and cerebellar cortex. Apart from the typical staining and ultrastructural aspects of amyloid, a deposition of material was observed, corresponding in optical and electron microscopy to a paraprotein. This case demonstrated not only the relationship between the deposition of amyloid and the formation of senile plaques, but also sustains the direct connection between amyloid in senile plaques and the paraprotein substances deriving from the blood. The probable relationship between the unusual deposition of paraproteins in the vessels and nervous system and the treatment with immunoglobulins is discussed.

1119
Watanabe M, Funahashi T, Suzuki T, Nomura S, Nakazawa T, Noguchi T, Tsukada Y. **Antithymic antibodies in schizophrenic sera.** *Biol Psychiat.* 1982;17:699-710. (English)

Sera from normal controls and schizophrenics were examined for antithymic activity, employing a cytotoxicity test with C3H mouse thymocytes. The average level of antithymic activity in schizophrenics was considerably higher than that of controls, i.e., 50.3 ± 27.1 (n = 54) and 35.3 ± 19.5 (n = 33), respectively (p<0.01), in a fourfold serum dilution. The antithymic activity in newly admitted unmedicated patients was not statistically different from that of hospitalized medical patients. There was no difference in antithymic activity within the subdivisions of schizophrenia, such as hebephrenic, catatonic, and paranoid types. The antithymic titer also did not correlate with the psychopathological status as assessed by the BPRS total score. The antithymic activity against C3H mouse thymocytes in both the schizophrenic and control sera was completely adsorbed with mouse brain tissue homogenate (where Thy-1 antigen was present) and liver homogenate (where Thy-1 was absent), but not with human brain and liver. It seems unlikely therefore that antithymic factor in human sera contains antibodies against Thy-1 (brain-associated thymic) antigen. Antithymic activity is not considered specific for schizophrenic illness, and the high antithymic activity found in schizophrenics might be produced against unknown xenoantigens, probably as a result of a nonspecific dysfunction of the immunological system in such patients.

1120
Witz IP, Anavi R, Weisenbeck H. **A tissue-binding factor in the serum of schizophrenic patients.** *In: The Impact of Biology on Modern Psychiatry.* ES Gershon et al. (eds.). New York: Plenum Press, 1977. Pp.113-24. (English)

Studies using an indirect radioimmunofixation assay, have revealed the presence of a serum factor (or factors) in schizophrenic patients with the capacity to bind to human brain tissue, as well as to other human and mouse tissues. The tissue binding property is detected in the serum of 50%-60% of schizophrenic patients, and in the serum of about 10% or less of blood-bank donors. The serum factor precipitates with 33% saturated ammonium sulfate but does not seem to be IgG. It is unknown whether or not this tissue-binding property of schizophrenic serum is an immunological reaction.

1121
Young JG, Caparulo BK, Shaywitz BA, Johnson WT, Cohen DJ. **Childhood autism: cerebrospinal fluid examination and immunoglobulin levels.** *J Am Acad Child Psychiatry.* 1977;16:174-9. (English)

The cerebrospinal fluid (CSF) of 15 children afflicted with primary childhood autism was examined. There were no abnormalities of glucose, protein, cells, or folate. There is evidence that slow viral infections may underlie a variety of chronic neurological diseases and it has been hypothesized that slow viruses may play a role in the etiology of adult schizophrenia. We have evaluated this viewpoint in relation to childhood autism. Preliminary studies of CSF immunoglobulin levels in children with autism offer no support to the hypothesis.

Immunogenetics of mental disorder

1122

Gattaz WF, Beckmann H. **HLA system in psychiatric research** (author's transl). *Fortschr Neurol Psychiatr.* 1981; 49:145-51. (German)

The production of the human leucocyte antigens (HLA) is controlled by a gene complex which is localised on the chromosome 6. These HLA are important above all in the organ transplantation as it provides the best possible histocompatibility conditions. Various diseases with a noticeable autoimmune component and frequent occurrence within the family showed a statistically significant correlation with specific HLA. This correlation was also shown in the studies of HLA in some psychiatric disorders, namely the endogenous psychoses. Nevertheless, results obtained until the present moment are contradictory. In 8 studies of HLA in manic-depressive patients, 17 antigens were being recognised, which occurred with a different frequency in patients when compared with controls (16 of these antigens showed statistically significant differences). In 9 researches of HLA in schizophrenic patients, 28 antigens showed a different frequency in patients when compared with controls (23 of these antigens showed statistically significant differences). Contrasting to the studies in manic-depressive patients, the HLA studies in schizophrenic patients showed a relatively greater homogeneity, e.g., the HLA-A1 appeared with an increased frequency in patients in 6 out of 9 studies; an increased frequency of HLA-A9 was found in 5 out of 9 studies; the HLA-B27 frequency was decreased in 3 studies. Nevertheless, contradictory results were being found as well, e.g., the HLA-A10 had a decreased frequency in 3 studies and increased in the 4th; HLA-Bw17 appeared with a higher incidence in 2 works and lower in the results of another author. Some circumstances could be responsible for this heterogeneity among the findings. Besides the possibility of the non-existence of associations between HLA and endogenous psychoses, methodological bias should also be considered, e.g., the use of different diagnostic criteria (or in some cases the absence of them), ethnic difference among the compared groups, small patients and control groups, the use of different serological procedures, *et cetera*. Only the observation of these strict conditions could bring further studies to more accurate results.

1123

Sasazuki T, McDevitt HO, Grumet FC. **The association between genes in the major histocompatibility complex and disease susceptibility.** *Annu Rev Med.* 1977;28:425-52. (English) (no abstract)

HLA and affective illness

1124

Campillo F, Duque del Rio M, Fuentenebro de Diego F, Llorente L, Mendez Barroso JR. **Evaluation of the HLA system in a sample of patients with endogenous depression.** *Actas Luso Esp Neurol Psiquiatr.* 1981;9:363-6. (Spanish) (unavailable at publication)

1125

Del Vecchio M, Farzati B, Maj M, Minucci P, Guida L, Kemali D. **Cell membrane predictors of response to lithium prophylaxis of affective disorders.** *Neuropsychobiology.* 1981;7:243-7. (English)

HLA antigens and RBC/plasma lithium ratio were studied in a sample of 49 patients, diagnosed as bipolar affective psychotics (n=22), unipolar depressive psychotics (n=18) and cycloid psychotics (n=9), receiving prophylactic lithium for 1-4 years and maintained at lithium plasma levels of 0.6-1.2 mEq/l. Mean values of the ratio were found to be significantly higher in patients who responded to treatment when compared with nonresponders, whereas the frequency of the HLA-A3 antigen was significantly higher in non-responders. The only 6 patients with a lithium ratio above the median and the absence of the HLA-A3 antigen coexistent with bipolarity and a family history of the illness were all good responders to treatment. Further research in this field will probably bring about the isolation of a subgroup of lithium-responsive patients with well-defined clinical and biological features. When patients were divided into two subgroups according to their lithium ratios (above and below the median), the HLA-A3 and Aw26 antigens were found to be significantly more frequent in those with ratios below the median. It can be hypothesized that these antigens disturb transport in some way, leading to low lithium ratio values.

1126

Faber R. **Depressive disorders and HLA** (letter). *N Engl J Med.* 1982;306:1238-9. (English)

1127

Govaerts A, Mendlewicz J, Verbanck P. **Manic-depressive illness and HLA.** *Tissue Antigens.* 1977;10:60-2. (English)

One hundred and eighteen cases of manic-depressive illness, subclassified into 68 unipolars and 50 bipolars, were typed for

HLA-A and B. Both groups showed the same antigen frequencies, with the exception of a slight increase of HLA-B15 in bipolar patients. The incidence of HLA-Bw15 was reduced in affectively ill patients as compared to controls.

1128
James NM, Smouse PE, Carroll BJ, Haines RF. **Affective illness and HLA frequencies: no compelling association.** *Neuropsychobiology.* 1980;6:208-16. (English)

114 patients suffering from an endogenomorphic affective illness were typed for HLA antigens at the A and B loci, and the frequencies were compared with those of a control panel numbering 439 individuals. Using new analytical procedures, a large number of tests were conducted, but no convincing evidence for an association of HLA types with affective disorders was obtained. A reanalysis of the same data, where patients are classified according to Danish diagnostic criteria, yields a marginally significant association of the B locus alleles. The sample sizes for this latter analysis were small, the test criteria are undoubtedly inflated, and no compelling case can be made for a useful association.

1129
Johnson GF, Hunt GE, Robertson S, Doran TJ. **A linkage study of manic- depressive disorder with HLA antigens, blood groups, serum proteins and red cell enzymes.** *J Affect Disord.* 1981;3:43-58. (English)

Families with a two-generational history of affective disorder and well and ill sibs were selected from a population of bipolar manic-depressive patients and typed for HLA antigens, blood groups, serum proteins and red cell enzymes. Segregation of specific HLA alleles was not associated with affective illness across family pedigrees. Further, no significant associations were found between affective disorder and ABO, Rh, MNSs blood groups or Hp EsD, C3, Gc or PGM. Using the lod score method of Morton (1955) for determining linkage, these data indicated that close linkage is unlikely for affective disorder and HLA alleles, haptoglobin, Rh factor, or ABO blood groups.

1130
Johnson GF. **HLA antigens and manic-depressive disorders.** *Biol Psychiat.* 1978;13:409-12. (English) (no abstract)

1131
Majsky A, Dvorakova M, Zvolsky P. **Modifications of lymphocyte HL-A antigens as a consequence of therapy in patients with manic-depressive psychosis.** *Folia Haematol (Leipz).* 1978;105:509-17. (German)

In 54 (=46.9%) of 115 patients with manic-depressive psychosis an HLA modification could be identified. This modification turned out to be temporary and from a serological point of view it revealed a different character. In 29 cases a loss of HLA antigens could be observed, in 3 cases there was a decrease, in 14 cases a combination of both changes, twice a polyreactivity was observed and 6 times a change of the antigen HLA-A in A28 could be determined. These serological modifications appeared after therapy with lithium as well as with various antidepressive and neuroleptic medications.

The connection between therapy and development of HLA modification could be ensured statistically. The modifications of HLA antigens A10 and B7 developed after administering neuroleptic medications, those of HLA antigens A9, A11, B12, and B13 after therapy with antidepressive medications. HLA antigens B27 and B40 showed a relative resistance towards therapy. The significance of these findings for the possibility of mistakes in HLA typing and from the standpoint of therapy efficiency in connection with the patient's HLA phenotype is discussed.

1132
Matthysse S, Kidd KK. **Evidence of HLA linkage in depressive disorders** (editorial). *N Engl J Med.* 1981; 305:1340-1. (English)

1133
Perris C, Strandman E. **Genetic identification of a subgroup of depressed patients.** *Psychiatr Clin.* 1980;13:13-24. (English)

HLA antigens, blood groups and red cell enzyme polymorphisms were studied in patients with different types of affective disorders and in patients suffering from cycloid psychoses. Several statistically significant results were found. In particular, a sub-group of depressed patients characterized by a very extreme distribution of haptoglobin groups was identified. The implications of this last finding for the definition of a particular sub-group of depressed patients is discussed.

1134
Psychochemistry Institute (Department of Psychiatry, Copenhagen, Denmark). **HLA antigens and manic-depressive disorders: further evidence of an association.** *Psychol Med.* 1977;7:387-96. (English)

One hundred and seven unrelated Danish patients considered to be manic-depressive according to strict diagnostic, symptomatic and course criteria were typed for antigens of the HLA system, the major histocompatibility system in man. Preliminary results from the first 47 patients had previously been reported to suggest a positive association between manic-depressive disorders and HLA-A3, HLA-B7, and HLA-Bw16 and a negative association between such disorders and HLA-B8. Results from the extended series provide confirmatory evidence that there is a positive association between manic-depressive disorders and HLA-Bw16 and also strongly suggest a positive association between HLA-B7 and such disorders. HLA typing may prove to be a useful way of identifying sub-groups of manic-depressive patients for other biological studies. The associations described provide a potential lead for formulating hypotheses about the nature of biological mechanisms which predispose to manic-depressive disorders.

1135
Shapiro RW, Bock E, Rafaelsen OJ, Ryder LP, Svejgaard A. **Histocompatibility antigens and manic-depressive disorders.** *Arch GenJ Psychiatry.* 1976;33:823-5. (English)

Forty-seven unrelated Danish patients considered to be manic-depressive, according to strict diagnostic, symptomatic, and course criteria, were typed for histocompatibility (HLA) antigens. Significantly more manic-depressive patients than controls were found to have HLA-A3, HLA-B7, and HLA-Bw16, while significantly fewer manic-depressives than controls had HLA-B8. All eight of the patients with HLA-Bw16 were bipolar patients, and none were unipolar depressive patients. We emphasize the need to consider the results with caution in view of the large number of antigens considered and the relatively small number of patients involved. When statistical corrections are made for the large number of antigens investigated, only the difference between bipolar patients and controls remains significant. The best way to determine if our findings are really significant is to attempt to confirm them in other series of patients. The importance of utilizing strict symptomatic and course criteria for the selection and polarization of probands is stressed.

1136
Smeraldi E, Bellodi L. **Possible linkage between primary affective disorder susceptibility locus and HLA haplotypes.** *Am J Psychiatry.* 1981;138:1232-4. (English)

The authors analyzed the concordance of sib pairs of HLA typing in cases where both sibs had affective illness and where the sibs were discordant. They detected an excess of HLA similarities in doubly affected sibs and a lack of similarities in discordant sibs. Therefore, the authors hypothesize that HLA may be linked with a primary affective disorder susceptibility locus or it may be associated with such a locus in some other way.

1137
Smeraldi E, Negri F, Melica AM, Scorza-Smeraldi R, Fabio G, Bonara P, Bellodi L, Sacchetti E, Sabbadini-Villa MG, Cazzullo CL, Zanussi C. **HLA typing and affective disorders: a study in the Italian population.** *Neuropsychobiology.* 1978;4:344-52. (English)

HLA phenotype distribution was investigated in 91 affective patients. Significant increases over those of the control population were found in HLA-A29 and in Bw22 frequencies, while A10 and A30 were decreased. No significant difference was shown between the two clinical subgroups (41 unipolar patients and 50 bipolar ones). On comparing our data with those from other authors, Bw16 was significantly increased. However, a high degree of heterogeneity was also shown for this antigen. Of some interest is the finding that relapsed and non-relapsed patients during long-term lithium therapy display diverging HLA phenotype distributions, with B5 increased among the non-relapsed subjects.

1138
Stein G, Holmes J, Bradford JW, Kennedy L. **HLA antigens and affective disorder: a family case report.** *Psychol Med.* 1980;10:677-81. (English)

A family of 6 affectively ill siblings is described. Two suffered from bipolar illnesses, two from recurrent unipolar illness, and the remainder showed alcoholism, depression and schizoaffective disorder. HLA typing revealed that all the tested members shared the antigens A3 and B7. Because only ill members were available for testing, there was insufficient

information in the family to draw any definite conclusion as to whether these antigens were linked to the illness. However, the observation is of some interest in the light of other recent reports which have suggested that these 2 antigens are associated with affective disorder.

1139
Stember RH, Fieve RR. **Histocompatibility antigens in affective disorders.** *Clin Immunol Immunopathol.* 1977; 7:10-14. (English)

Primary affective (manic-depressive) illness has hereditary factors which have yet to be clarified. The histocompatibility antigens (HLA) of 50 patients were determined by a standard lymphocyte cytotoxicity test. HLA A13 was present in 12% of affective disorder patients contrasted to 2.4% of controls, HLA A5 was present in 24% of patients compared to 12% in controls, HLA A12 was present in 10% of patients and 24% of controls, and HLA Aw5 was found in 34% of patients versus 22.8% of controls. The frequency distribution in the affective disorder population of 24 other HLA antigens did not show any significant difference from controls. The findings of altered frequency of three HLA antigens and a marginal altered frequency of a fourth HLA antigen in this population may suggest the possibility that primary affective disorders have an association with the major histocompatibility complex.

1140
Targum SD, Gershon ES, Van Eerdewegh M, Rogentine N. **Human leukocyte antigen system not closely linked to or associated with bipolar manic-depressive illness.** *Biol Psychiat.* 1979;14:615-36. (English)

An association and linkage study of the HLA system and bipolar affective illness is reported. HLA B14 showed an increased frequency and HLA Bw27 a decreased frequency in 92 bipolar patients compared to 210 controls, but significance is not reached when appropriate statistical corrections are made. It is shown that ethnological differences can lead to sampling biases; a purported increased frequency of HLA Bw16 in Ashkenazi Jewish bipolar patients is negated when ethnologically similar controls are used. The transmission of HLA alleles in nine families with at least two generations of affective illness revealed independent assortment, and non-linkage to either locus A or B was demonstrated using a multigenerational method of linkage analysis. The nonreplicability of the HLA association studies, and the failure to demonstrate linkage of the HLA loci with development of affective illness, although further analyses are necessary.

1141
Turner WJ, King S. **Two genetically distinct forms of bipolar affective disorder?** *Biol Psychiat.* 1981;16:417-39. (English)

In five pedigrees in which bipolar affective illness (BPD) can be traced through three generations with no father-son transmission, no linkage to HLA could be established. This group was evidently dependent on a single dominant gene (X-linked?), for which the noncommittal designation BPD1 was proposed. Two pedigrees of BPD, in which father-son transmission occurred at least twice, showed highly suggestive linkage to HLA (lod = 2.61 at theta = 0.15). BPD2 was proposed as the designation for this gene. Loss of BPD in one HLA-A/B cross-over suggests that a single dominant gene in this group has a locus in p2-pter region of chromosome 6.

1142
Turner WJ. **Blood types and affective disorders** (letter). *Am J Psychiatry.* 1977;134:1053-4. (English)

1143
Weitkamp LR, Stancer HC, Persad E, Flood C, Guttormsen S. **Depressive disorders and HLA--a gene on chromosome 6 that can affect behavior.** *N Engl J Med.* 1981; 305:1301-6. (English)

To determine whether HLA-linked genes on chromosome 6 influence susceptibility to depressive disorders, we tested hypotheses concerning the distribution of HLA haplotypes among specific constellations of affected and unaffected family members. HLA haplotype identity among pairs of affected siblings in families with two affected siblings and among pairs of older unaffected siblings in families with one or two affected siblings was increased over random expectation (p<0.005). There was no increase in HLA haplotype identity among affected siblings in sibships with more than two affected members. When parents had a relative difference in estimated load of genes for susceptibility, HLA haplotypes were randomly transmitted to unaffected or affected children from the affected, "high load" parent, but not from the unaffected, "low-load" parent (p<0.001). These results locate a gene contributing to suseptibility to depressive illness on chromosome 6 and provide a second example of the value of the hypotheses in defining the genetic bases of nonmendelian, familial diseases.

1144
Wentzel J, Roberts DF, Whalley LJ. **HLA in manic-depressive psychosis.** *Psychol Med.* 1982;12:275-8. (English) (no abstract)

1145
Whalley LJ, Roberts DF, Wentzel J, Wright AF. **Genetic factors in puerperal affective psychoses.** *Acta Psychiatr Scand.* 1982;65:180-93. (English)

The hypothesis that puerperal affective psychosis (PAP) is genetically related to manic-depressive disorder was tested by comparing the morbidity risks for puerperal and non-puerperal affective disorders in the relatives of 17 PAP subjects and 20 parous manic-depressives (PMD) with no history of puerperal illness. The risk for affective disorder (manic-depression or suicide) and puerperal affective disorder was the same in the two groups of relatives and the test hypothesis was accepted, although the sample size was small. The frequencies of HLA-A, B and C locus antigens, nine blood group antigens and 10 red blood cell isoenzymes were not significantly different in the PAP and PMD subjects, showing that in this series genetic markers do not distinguish puerperal from non-puerperal affective psychoses.

1146
Zemek P, Zvolsky P, Soucek K, Dvorzhakova M. **Chief**

histocompatibility system in cyclophrenia and its relationship to lithium therapy. *Zh Nevropatol Psikhiatr.* 1977;77:1199-1200. (Russian)

The peripheral blood lymphocytes in 46 patients with cyclophrenia and endogenous depressions who were treated by lithium for a long period of time, were typed to HLA-system antigens. The results of these studies did not detect any connection between the prognosis of lithium treatment on the basis of a study of the HLA system.

1147
Zvolsky P, Dvorakova M, Majsky A, Soucek K. **Histocompatibility antigens in primary affective disorders.** *Arch Psychiatr Nervenkr.* 1978;225:159-62. (Czech)

We determined 27 histocompatibility antigens of A, B, and C locus with a standard lymphocyte cytotoxicity test in 125 patients suffering from primary affective disorders, 77 of bipolar type, 24 of unipolar type, and 24 with schizo-affective psychosis. Comparison with a normal control group showed significant increases in the frequencies of antigens Bw40 and Cw4 in unipolar patients and a significantly decreased frequency of antigen Cw3 in bipolar patients. The statistical significances which were at the 5% level disappeared when the p values were corrected for the number of antigens investigated. Our results failed to confirm previous findings of significantly altered antigen frequencies among patients with primary affective disorders.

1148
Zvolsky P, Majsky A, Dvorakova M, Soucek K, Zemek P, Vinarova E. **Histocompatibility antigens in lithium treated manic-depressive patients.** *Act Nerv Super.* 1978;20:72. (English) (no abstract)

HLA and schizophrenia

1149
Asaka A, Okazaki Y, Namura I, Juji T, Miyamoto M, Ishikawa B. **Study of HLA antigens among Japanese schizophrenics.** *Br J Psychiatry.* 1981;138:498-500. (English)

HLA antigens were typed among 136 Japanese schizophrenics. Increased frequencies were seen in A9 (Aw24), A10 (A26) and Bw54, and decreased frequency in B40 antigens when compared to 187 Japanese controls. It is suggested that there may be an association between A9 (Aw24) and schizophrenia with a chronic-progressive course and also an association between A10 (A26) and hebephrenia.

1150
Barocci S, Roccatagliata G, Maffini M, Costantini M. **Schizophrenia and HLA antigens.** *Schweiz Arch Neurol Neurochir Psychiatr.* 1981;129:31-5. (German)

38 schizophrenic patients (21 hebephrenics and 17 paranoids) and 124 healthy subjects were matched for HLA antigens. HLA typing was determined by the microdroplet lymphocyte toxicity method developed by Terasaki of UCLA. In order to detect 47 HLA antigens as many as 118 antisera were used.

No significant differences in HLA typing were found between the two groups. However, the separate evaluation of HLA antigens of hebephrenic schizophrenics did not give any statistical significance as well. The authors discuss these findings in the light of previous studies on the topic.

1151
Beckmann H, Gattaz WF, Moises HW, Haas S, Ewald RW. **HLA antigens and schizophrenia** (author's transl). *Arzneimittelforsch.* 1980;30:1211-12. (English) (no abstract)

1152
Crowe RR, Thompson JS, Flink R, Weinberger B. **HLA antigens and schizophrenia.** *Arch Gen Psychiatry.* 1979; 36:231-3. (English)

We typed 45 schizophrenic patients for 35 HLA antigens and compared their frequencies with 1,263 population controls. No significant differences between schizophrenics and controls were found. When the schizophrenics were subtyped, a significant (p<0.05) excess of Aw26 was found among the hebephrenics, compared with the population controls. When the published literature on schizophrenia-HLA associations was surveyed, none of the reported associations were found to be consistent across studies. Some possible explanations for the heterogeneity among studies are discussed and it is concluded that an association between schizophrenia and any of the HLA antigens has not yet been demonstrated.

1153
Domashneva IV, Shapiro IUA, Gindilis VM. **Genetic analysis of serum antilymphocytic activity in schizophrenia.** *Zh Nevropatol Psikhiatr.* 1981;81:394-6. (Russian)

A genetic analysis of the immunological disturbances observed in patients with schizophrenic psychoses and registered from the level of the serum antilymphocytic activity was carried out. The analysis has shown that the contribution of genetic factors to the determination of interindividual differences in that feature exceeds more than twice the contribution of environmental factors. The close correlation between the serum antilymphocytic activity and the genetic component of the predisposition to the disease gives one grounds to regard a rise of the serum antilymphocytic activity as a pathogenetic marker of hereditary predisposition to schizophrenia. The results obtained, if taken together with literary data, may be of interest for studies concerned with the multicomponent structure of the hereditary predisposition to schizophrenic psychoses and their pathogenesis.

1154
Frangos E, Renieri-Livieratou N, Athanassenas G, Stavropoulou-Ghioka E, Kourkoubas A. **HLA antigens in schizophrenia: no difference between patients with and without evidence of brain atrophy.** *Br J Psychiat.* 1982; 140:607-10. (English)

The HLA antigens distribution was studied in 56 chronic schizophrenic in-patients with or without brain atrophy determined by CAT examination, and compared with that of 200 controls. There was no difference in the incidence of HLA-A2 in the whole sample, and an increase in those with-out brain atrophy (by comparison with normal controls) failed to reach statistical significance. A decrease of Bw35 in the whole sample, more prominent in those without brain atrophy, again failed to be significant after multiplying the probability by the number of antigens studied.

1155
Gattaz WF, Beckmann H, Mendlewicz J. **HLA antigens and schizophrenia: a pool of 2 studies.** *Psychiatr Res.* 1981; 5:123-8. (English)

Results from two studies on HLA antigens in schizophrenic patients were pooled and analyzed. A statistically significant difference appeared in the frequency for HLA-B27, which was increased in the patient group (n=164) as compared to the controls (n=585). The strong correlation between this antigen and some forms of arthropathies and the fact that arthropathies and schizophrenia very seldom occur in the same individual suggest that HLA-B27 could serve as a genetic marker for both diseases. The development of either one or the other may depend upon the interplay between the genetic marker (HLA-B27) and other biological and environmental factors. In addition to the potential value of HLA-B27 as a market for vulnerability to schizophrenia, the human leucocyte antigens may also serve to differentiate between various subtypes of the illness.

1156
Gattaz WF, Beckmann H. **HLA antigens and schizophrenia** (letter). *Lancet.* 1980;1:98-9. (English)

1157
Gattaz WF, Ewald RW, Beckmann H. **The HLA system and schizophrenia: a study in a German population.** *Arch Psychiatr Nervenkr.* 1980;228:205-11. (English)

Various diseases with a noticeable autoimmune component and frequent occurrence within one family show a statistically significant correlation with specific human leukocyte antigens (HLA). This correlation was also shown in studies of HLA in psychiatric disorders. However, results have been contradictory. The phenotype frequencies of HLA specificities were investigated in 400 schizophrenic patients and 472 controls from the same geographic area in Germany. The frequency of HLA B27 was significantly increased in the patient group as a whole (p=0.017) and in the subgroups of paranoid patients (p=0.005), chronic schizophrenics (p<0.001), patients with poor prognosis (p<0.001), and in patients with onset of the disease before the age of 20 years (p=0.004). In the latter three groups an elevated incidence of HLA A9 was also found. The combination A9-B27 was detected in 0.63% of our control group and in 7% of the patients (p<0.001). Of these patients 85.7% were chronic paranoid patients with poor prognostic features. This study gives support to the possibility of using HLA typing in genetic studies of schizophrenia as well as in the differential diagnosis and prognosis.

1158
Gattaz WF, Kasper S, Beckmann H. **HL-A antigens, schizophrenia and brain atrophy** (letter). *Br J Psychiatry.* 1980;137:398-9. (English)

1159

Gattaz WF, Kasper S, Ewald RW, Beckmann H. **HLA, schizophrenias, and arthropathies.** *Psychiatr Clin (Basel).* 1981;14:49-55. (German)

Significantly more individuals with human leucocyte antigens (HLA) A9 and B27 have been identified in the group of chronic paranoid schizophrenics with early onset of the disease. It is known that individuals with HLA B27 have a markedly increased risk to fall ill from arthropathies (i.e., Bechterew's disease). Generally, it seems extremely rare that arthropathies and schizophrenia occur together in the same person. In 16 chronic paranoid schizophrenics with HLA B27 no form of arthropathy and in 288 arthropathic patients no case of schizophrenia could be detected (evidenced in a psychiatric case register). Furthermore in 131 arthropathic patients with HLA B27 no psychiatric disease (except one feeble-minded and one with alcohol problems) could be identified. On the other hand, in the group of arthropathic patients without HLA B27 the incidence of psychiatric diseases was 5 times higher than in the group with HLA B27 and so comparable to the morbidity of the normal population. It is conceivable that HLA B27 is a "genetic marker" for arthropathy as well as for a defined subgroup of schizophrenia. These data agree with the hypothesis that schizophrenia and arthropathies are mutually exclusive in one individual.

1160

Golse B, Debray-Ritzen P, Dausset J, Lipinski M, Hors J. **HLA groups in the infantile psychoses during development, and hypothesis for an enzyme defect.** *C R Acad Sci D (Paris).* 1977;284:1733-5. (French)

The HLA typing (loci A and B) of a series of fifteen psychotic children has shown an increase of the frequency of both HLA-A9 and B5 antigens. These preliminary data and previous biochemical findings in psychotic patients lead the authors to postulate the hypothesis of a qualitative or quantitative anomaly of the superoxide dismutase (SOD-2), the gene of which is situated on the same chromosome (sixth) as the HLA complex.

1161

Goudemand M, Goudemand J, Goudemand-Joubert C, Parquet PJ. **Heredity and childhood psychoses: histocompatibility antigens (HLA A and B) and early onset of childhood psychoses.** *Acta Psychiatr Belg.* 1981; 81:57-71. (French)

We first consider current arguments in favor of a genetic etiology of childhood psychoses. These psychoses have to be separated into early psychoses (before age 5) and late onset ones (between 5 years and adolescence). These late onset psychoses appear to be genetically determined and related to schizophrenia, while early psychoses may be in part genetically related and subject to environmental factors. We also report a study on HLA in early onset psychoses in the North of France, which could not show any association between the HLA system and the psychoses.

1162

Goudemand M, Goudemand J, Parquet PJ, Fontan M.

Schizophrenic psychoses and HLA antigens: personal data and review of the literature. *Encephale.* 181;7:609-22. (French)

Genetic factors play probably an important part in the development of schizophrenic psychoses. As a consequence the use of a genetic marker [such] as the HLA system appears to be interesting in determining the disease susceptibility gene of these psychoses. Methods and results of an investigation about the frequencies of 33 HLA alleles observed in 51 patients considered as paranoid schizophrenics are presented. The frequency of HLA-A29 was diminished while the one of HLA-B15 was increased but the differences were no longer significant when p was corrected. However when all the results published from 1974 to 1980 were pooled in a combined statistical analysis, some associations became significant. It seems that schizophrenia as a whole and paranoid and hebephrenic sub-types have to be distinguished. It may be concluded from these data that correlations between schizophrenia and HLA antigens which remain doubtful could be explained with a biological genetic heterogeneity of schizophrenic disorders. Review of literature concerning the identification of HLA haplotypes in schizophrenics pedigrees and about the HLA system as a genetic marker for the clinical response to neuroleptics in schizophrenic patients or *in vitro*, is also discussed.

1163

Goudemand M, Goudemand J, Parquet PJ, Goudemand-Joubert C, Letallec-Duytschaever F, Fontan M. **Histocompatibility antigens in early and late onset childhood psychoses.** *J Genet Hum.* 1981;29:419-29. (French)

Childhood psychoses could have a genetic etiology, but early and late onset psychoses have to be separated. Genetic factors are certainly implicated in the development of late onset psychoses and appear to overlap with those of adult schizophrenia. Evidence implicating genetics in early onset psychoses is likely, as twin studies have supported this hypothesis. HLA system is a particularly suitable genetic marker. We report the results of an investigation on HLA A and B antigens we have performed on 57 psychotics (30 early onset psychotics, 27 late onset psychotics). No genetic association appears in the whole population, as well as in the early and late onset psychosis series. These results have to be compared with Golse's et al. (1977, 1980), Stebbs and Magenis' (1980) and adult schizophrenia data. Further researches with population and family pedigrees are required with other major histocompatibility complex markers.

1164

Goudemand M, Goudemand-Joubert C, Parquet PJ, Goudemand J. **Histocompatibility antigens (HLA A and B) in early child psychoses** (letter). *Nouv Presse Med.* 1980; 9:3278. (French)

1165

Ivanyi P, Ivanyi D, Zemek P. **HLA-Cw4 in paranoid schizophrenia.** *Tissue Antigens.* 1977;9:41-4. (English)

On a group of 40 paranoid schizophrenic patients HLA serotypes for HLA-A, B, C antigens a significant increase of

Cw4 was observed. It is argued that this finding represents the common denominator for previous data reporting increased A9 and A28 antigen in SCH because these antigens are frequently present on haplotypes bearing Cw4. The possible role of the HLA "central" parts, i.e., the chromosomal segment between HLA-A and HLA-B locus in the pathogenesis of schizophrenia was stressed.

1166

Julien RA, Mercier P, Chouraqui P, Sutter JM. **Schizophrenia and histocompatibility antigens.** *Encephale.* 1978; 4:99-113. (French)

Schizophrenias have a genetical support as it is now proved by the study of twins born from schizophrenic parents and of the adopted children of schizophrenics. The HLA typing brings an additional argument in favour of this hypothesis. After a recall of data concerning the system of tissue histocompatibility, the results are given of the HLA typing of a population of 65 schizophrenics (59 men, 6 women) including 27 hebephrenics and 38 paranoids. The paranoid group is clearly individualized from a genetic point of view. If 40% of the schizophrenics carry the A9 antigen versus 21.2% found in the normal population, 47.4% of the paranoid schizophrenics present this antigen ($X_2 = 12.16$, $p<0.001$). The association of the two antigens A9 and Cw4 is even more significant: 414.3% of the total population ($X_2 = 13.3$, $p<0.0005$). The paranoid group reached a rate of 24.3% ($X_2 = 27.3$, $p<0.0005$). A subject carrier of both antigens A9 + Cw4 has 11.5 times the risk of being a paranoid schizophrenic than a subject not possessing these two antigens.

1167

Kyner WT, Bennahum DA, Troup GM, Rada RT, Kellner R. **The HLA-SD antigens and schizophrenia--a statistical analysis.** *Birth Defects.* 1978;14:185-90. (English)

The purpose of this paper is to present some statistical data obtained in a study of a distribution of HLA-SD antigens in white schizophrenic patients and those of a white control group. The patients and the controls were non-Spanish-American residents of New Mexico. The diagnosis for each patient was established by the same psychiatrist using the criteria recommended by Feighner and his co-workers. The HLA typing was performed by the standard NIH technique. The data were first analyzed by means of contingency tables and the chi-square test with Yates correction. Then discriminant analysis was used to investigate patterns that might have polyantigenic interpretation.

1168

Lange V. **Genetic markers of atypical phasic psychoses.** *Psychiatr Clin.* 1980;13:38-56. (German)

The 93 patients of the present study resemble each other in their psychosis by phasic course and complete recovery. Frequently the attacks showed an anxious and paranoid syndrome in monopolar repetition or in bipolar change with ecstatic systems. Rarely an incoherent state of agitation or stupor could be observed. Considering the distribution of simple inherited serum groups, there is a significant increase of GC1-1 and HP 2-2 in the patient collective. Evidently these serum groups are risk components in a multifactorial hereditary system system possessing with GC 1-1 a marker of the schizophrenic disposition and with HP 2-2 A determinating trait for affective psychoses. A selective interaction is discussed for both serum groups regarding the vitamin D transport of the GC fraction with their relation to neuronal function and the possible role of HP 2-2 in a transport or regulatory system.

1169

Lange V. **Genetics of psychoses under a new aspect.** *Psychiatr Clin.* 1976;9:32-44. (German)

The analysis of the biological pathways of the genetic activity in psychoses is growing more and more to an important goal. The research in this field should be started on the assumption of a multifactorial hereditary system controlling the somatic base of mental illness in a specific way as can be argued from twin and family studies. Screening the present data, there is strong evidence that the metabolism of affective psychoses is characterized by quantitative deviations only concerning the 5-hydroxytryptamine and norepinephrine turnover particularly. The biochemical findings in schizophrenic psychoses are suspicious for qualitative abnormalities too. There are some indications of toxic products in the catecholamine metabolism and of antibodies against brain substances. All these disturbances could be caused by structural gene mutants or by mutations of the genetical regulatory system changing the sensitivity for the environmental stimulus. The simultaneous investigation of simple inherited serum groups is described as a useful tool for biological marking of the responsible genotypes.

1170

Luchins DJ, Torrey EF, Weinberger DR, Zaloman S, DeLisi LE, Johnson A, Rogentine N, Wyatt RJ. **HLA antigens in schizophrenia: differences between patients with and without evidence of brain atrophy.** *Br J Psychiatry.* 1980;136:243-8. (English)

A survey of 14 published studies found no consistent association between specific HLA antigens and schizophrenia. Since these studies lacked diagnostic or biological criteria, an investigation was undertaken using recognized diagnostic criteria and CT scan findings. Typing for HLA antigens at loci A, B and C was carried out on 130 patients. Among 92 black schizophrenic patients there was an increase of HLA-A2 which remained significant even after correcting for the number of antigens studied. When the patients for whom CT scans were available were divided according to the presence or absence of evidence of brain atrophy, there was an increase of A2 in the black schizophrenic patients without evidence of atrophy, which remained significant after multiplying by the number of antigens studied. However, there was no significant increase of A2 in those with evidence of atrophy. Similar trends held for the white population but they failed to reach significance. The need for HLA studies on biologically defined groups of schizophrenic patients is stressed.

1171

Luchins DJ, Weinberger DR, Kleinman JE, Neckers LM, Rosenblatt JE, Bigelow LB, Wyatt RJ. **Human leukocyte**

antigen A2 and psychopathology in chronic schizophrenia. *Am J Psychiatry.* 1980;137:499-500. (English)

Several diseases have been shown to be associated with specific human leukocyte antigens (HLA). Although schizophrenia may be genetically linked to the HLA systems, there is no clear association between the disease and any specific HLA. We addressed this issue and reported that the prevalence of HLA-A2 was increased in a sample of schizophrenic patients. The increase was concentrated in the subgroup of patients who had no morphologic abnormalities suggestive of brain atrophy on computed tomography (CT) scan. Because the patients studied had chronic courses and because A2 and morphologic abnormalities appeared to be segregated, we hypothesized that either characteristic might be a factor contributing to chronicity. Subsequently, Weinberger and associates reported that lateral ventricular enlargement on CT scan was associated with a poor clinical response to neuroleptics. We were interested, therefore, in examining the relationship between A2 and response to neuroleptic treatment. To investigate this relationship we examined in patients with and without A2: 1) clinical response to neuroleptics, 2) serum neuroleptic-like concentrations as measured by dopamine receptor binding, and 3) *in vitro* haloperidol binding. Our hypothesis was that differences in clinical responses would be explained by differences in the pharmacokinetics or binding of neuroleptics in patients with A2.

1172
Luchins DJ, Weinberger DR, Torrey EF, Johnson A, Rogentine N, Wyatt RJ. **HLA-A2 antigen in schizophrenic patients with reversed cerebral asymmetry.** *Br J Psychiatry.* 1981;138:240-3. (English)

The frequency of HLA-A2 was examined in 32 black and 22 white schizophrenic patients separated into two groups according to whether they had normal or reversed cerebral hemisphere asymmetries as determined by computed tomography. The black patients with reversed asymmetry had a significantly greater frequency of HLA-A2 as compared to black patients with normal asymmetry and a black normal control group. There were no significant differences for any other A,B or C antigens. These findings also held when only the 22 black patients without evidence of brain atrophy were studied. The results for the white patients were in the same direction but did not reach statistical significance. These findings suggest that, at least for schizophrenic patients, reversed cerebral asymmetry is associated with an increased frequency of HLA-A2.

1173
McGuffin P, Farmer AE, Rajah SM. **Histocompatability antigens and schizophrenia.** *Br J Psychiatry.* 1978; 132:149-51. (English)

The HLA (human leucocyte antigen) types A and B were studied in 80 patients diagnosed as schizophrenic. There was an increased incidence of HLA-Bw5 and a decrease in HLA-Aw29 and HLA-Bw17 as compared with healthy controls. In the subgroup of patients exhibiting Schneider's first-rank symptoms there was an increased incidence of HLA-A1 with a decrease in HLA-A2 and HLA-Bw17.

1174
McGuffin P, Farmer AE, Yonace AH. **HLA antigens and subtypes of schizophrenia.** *Psychiatr Res.* 1981;5:115-22.

Studies on HLA antigens in schizophrenia have produced conflicting results, but there has been greater agreement when clinical subtypes of the disorder have been separated. In view of this, we reassessed 68 previously studied patients with hospital diagnoses of schizophrenia and, while blind to their HLA types, used operational criteria to define clinical subtypes. We compared and combined the results with those from all available similar studies. Those of our patients who fulfilled operational criteria for paranoid schizophrenia showed a nonsignificant increase in HLA A9 as compared with controls. The magnitude of the increase was similar to that from all previous reports, and when data from all sources were combined, the evidence for an association between HLA A9 and paranoid schizophrenia was consistent and highly significant. Patients who were diagnosed as suffering from hebephrenic schizophrenia showed significant increases in HLA A1 and B8 compared with controls. An association between hebephrenia and A1, but not B8, remained on combining the results with those of other studies.

1175
McGuffin P. **Is schizophrenia an HLA-associated disease?** *Psychol Med.* 1979;9:721-8. (English)

Certain specificities of the human leukocyte antigen (HLA) system have been shown to be associated with particular diseases. A review of recent studies in schizophrenia shows inconsistent results for schizophrenia as a whole, although a significant increase in HLA A28 remains on combining the data. There are more consistent findings for disease subtypes. In particular, HLA A9 and HLA Cw4 are increased in paranoid schizophrenics, while HLA A1 and the A1-B8 haplotype are increased in nuclear forms. It is postulated that the relationship between the schizophrenias and certain HLA types could be due to an influence of the latter upon neuronal post-synaptic membrane sensitivity to central neurotransmitters such as dopamine.

1176
McGuffin P. **What have transplant antigens got to do with psychosis?** *Br J Psychiatry.* 1980;136:510-2. (English) (no abstract)

1177
Mendlewicz J, Linkowski P. **HLA antigens and schizophrenia** (letter) *Lancet.* 1980;1:765. (English)

1178
Mendlewicz J, Verbanck P, Linkowski P, Govaerts A. **HLA antigens in affective disorders and schizophrenia.** *J Affective Disord.* 1981;3:17-24. (English)

The distribution of HLA antigen frequencies has been studied in patients with affective disorders. There were no significant differences between bipolar patients, unipolar patients, or controls. Preliminary data on HLA antigen distribution in schizophrenic patients are reported. Our negative results in affective disorders are discussed in relation to HLA studies reported from other laboratories, with special reference to some potential methodological problems.

1179

Mitkevich SP. **HLA antigens and schizophrenia.** *Zh Nevropatol Psikhiatr.* 1981;81:1076-8. (Russian)

The distribution of HLA-system antigens was examined in 87 schizophrenic patients with various forms of the disease course, and in 130 healthy donors. An increase of the number of persons with HLA-A10 antigen among patients with continuous schizophrenia, and of persons with HLA-B12 antigen among patients with paroxysmal form of the disease was revealed. At the same time no differences in the distribution of HLA antigens were noted on comparing healthy donors with the total group of the patients.

1180

Perris C, Roman G, Wahlby L. **HLA antigens in patients with schizophrenic syndromes.** *Neuropsychobiology.* 1979; 5:290-3. (English)

HLA antigens were studied in 50 patients, 40 males, 10 females and two brothers of patients, all suffering from schizophrenic syndromes. The average duration of illness for the whole group was 18 ± 1.5 years. The frequency of A10 antigen was increased in the schizophrenic patients as compared with 449 healthy individuals. None of the findings concerning HLA and schizophrenia reported in the literature could be verified in the present study. Two ill brothers comprised in the study proved to have the same HLA phenotype as their respective ill sibling. So far there is no conclusive evidence for association between any HLA antigen and "schizophrenia." Further investigations should be concerned with families and not with single patients.

1181

Roberts DF, Kinnell HG. **Immunogenetics and schizophrenia.** *Psychol Med.* 1981;11:441-7. (English) (unavailable at publication)

1182

Singer L, Mayer S, Tongio MM, Hauptmann G, Roos M, Danion JM, Bernard H, Leclercq P, Mander P. **HLA-A, B, C antigens, Bf antigen and schizophrenia.** *J Genet Hum.* 1981;29:555-63. (English) (unavailable at publication)

1183

Singer L, Mayer S, Tongio MM, Roos M, Danion JM, Bernard H, Leclercq P, Hauptmann G, Kapfer MT, Bindler J, Mandel P. **Frequencies of HLA-A, C and Bf antigens in schizophrenic patients originated from Alsace** (author's translation). *Encephale.* 1982;8:9-15. (French)

A comparison of the frequency of HLA-A, B, C and Bf antigens observed in a group of 75 chronic schizophrenics and in a control group of 184, all strictly from Alsace, does not carry any argument in favour of a strong genetic association between schizophrenia and the antigens studied. In effect, the modifications observed in the schizophrenic sample--decrease in the frequency of A10 and B5 antigens, and increase of A29 and BfF-- are not statistically significant when the probabili-

ties are multiplied by the number of tested antigens. These preliminary results however do not permit one to exclude the possibility of an association between schizophrenia and the tested antigens.

1184

Smeraldi E, Bellodi L, Sacchetti E, Cazzullo CL. **The HLA system and the clinical response to treatment with chlorpromazine.** *Br J Psychiatry.* 1976;129:486-9. (English)

A group of 33 schizophrenic patients were typed for HLA-SD antigens and their qualitative clinical responses to chlorpromazine therapy determined. A highly significant positive correlation was found between response to chlorpromazine and HLA-A1 positive, while HLA-A2 positive subjects showed a significant negative correlation to chlorpromazine treatment. In a second group of 17 patients the clinical response to chlorpromazine was evaluated quantitatively, by WPRS, in HLA-A1 positive and HLA-A1 negative patients. There were no pre-treatment differences in the scores. After treatment the scores of positive patients were significantly lower, indicating that they responded to a greater degree. Since the frequency of HLA-A1 in hebephrenic patients is higher than that in other schizophrenics this may explain our earlier finding that hebephrenics, as a group, respond better to chlorpromazine than do other schizophrenics.

1185

Smeraldi E, Bellodi L, Scorza-Smeraldi R, Fabio G, Sacchetti E. **HLA-SD antigens and schizophrenia: statistical and genetical considerations.** *Tissue Antigens.* 1976; 8:191-6. (English)

The HLA-SD phenotype distributions of hebephrenic and paranoid schizophrenics, and of the two groups combined, in an Italian population and in a combined group from the Swedish population have been analyzed statistically. There is a significantly decreased frequency of HLA-A10 in all of these. There are some preliminary indications of an increased frequency (a positive association) for some of the other antigens of the HLA-SD series, but there is insufficient data at present for evaluating the significance of these findings. Differences between hebephrenic and paranoid schizophrenics have been detected.

1186

Solntseva EI, Lideman RR, Trubnikov VI, Gindilis VM. **Possible role of genetic factors in increasing the serum neurotropic activity of schizophrenic patients.** *Zh Nevropatol Psikhiatr.* 1978;78:707-11. (Russian)

The authors studied the accumulation of individuals with an increased neurotropic blood serum activity among the relatives of schizophrenic patients. In order to evaluate the degree and character of the genetical determination of the biological indices 2 independent approaches were used: the method of a sequential search of genetical significant threshold values of signs (within the framework of a polygenic Falkoner-Edwards model) and the method of a partition of the total phenotypic variance into main compounds on the basis of intrafamilial correlations. It was demonstrated that the studied signs are characterized by a very high degree of a genetical determination. It is assumed that the small amount of specific loci (major genes) with the effect of intraloci dominance or intraloci epistatic interaction are responsible for the given biological marker.

1187

Stubbs G. **Shared parental HLA antigens and autism** (letter). *Lancet.* 1981;2:534. (English)

1188

Zaretskyaya IUM. **Biological role and the clinical significance of the HLA histocompatibility system.** *Vestn Akad Med Nauk SSSR.* 1979;7:71-6. (Russian)

The clinical importance of HLA antigens (the main histocompatibility system of man) was analyzed from the point of view of (i) HLA and kidney allograft survival and (ii) HLA and diseases. The longevity of the graft was shown to increase with an increase in the extent of compatibility between the donor and the recipient. Positive and negative associations between HLA antigens and rheumatoid, neuropsychic, dermatoid, carcinogensis, and endocrine diseases (data of the WHO Reference Center) were developed.

1189

Zemek P. **HL-A antigens and their possible relationship to schizophrenia** (author's transl). *Cesk Psychiatr.* 1977; 73:184-7. (Czech)

HL-A antigen distribution was tested in 200 male patients with schizophrenia. An increase in haplotypes HL-A A10 and HL-A B18 was found. There was also a higher frequency of HL-A A28 and HL-A Cw4 antigens in paranoid schizophrenia while in patients with the hebephrenic form of the disease of a significant increase in antigen HL-A A1 was detected. Some hypotheses are presented on the significance of such findings for the development of schizophrenia.

HLA and organic mental disorder

1190

Cohen D, Eisdorfer C, Walford RL. **Histocompatibility antigens (HLA) and patterns of cognitive loss in dementia of the Alzheimer type.** *Neurobiol Aging.* 1981;2:277-80. (English)

Recent data suggest that a proportion of patients with primary neuronal degeneration of the Alzheimer type have the HLA-B7 antigen. However, the possibility that other differences might exist between patients with and without the marker has not been examined. We tested a range of cognitive skills in Alzheimer patients with and without the HLA-B7 to examine whether those individuals with the HLA marker would exhibit a profile of cognitive loss different from those without it. Our results indicate that patients with HLA-B7 antigens had selective attentional scores that were significantly lower than Alzheimer patients without the antigen. Neither group was signficantly different in either memory capacity or retrieval from short-term and long-term memory. The data support the hypothesis that there may be more than one disorder in what is now referred to as dementia of the Alzheimer type.

1191

Eicher W, Spoljar M, Cleve H, Murken JD, Richter K, Stangel-Rutkowski S. **H-Y antigen in trans-sexuality** (letter). *Lancet.* 1979;2:ll37-8. (English)

1192

Henschke PJ, Bell DA, Cape RD. **Alzheimer's disease and HLA.** *Tissue Antigens.* 1978;12:132-5. (English)

Thirty-four unrelated patients with Alzheimer's disease were typed for HLA-A, -B and -C serological determinants. HLA-Cw3 was increased over control antigen frequencies. This difference lost significance when corrected for the number of antigens tested.

1193

Lange V. **Genetic markers in delusional diseases in middle age.** *Psychiatr Clin.* 1981;14:23-34. (German)

In the distribution of their serum groups the totality of 48 patients with paranoid psychoses of late onset is characterized by failure of the well-known markers of manic-depressive or schizophrenic illness. However, when differentiated psychopathologically, the haptoglobin (HP) type 2-2 as a risk factor of cyclothymic psychoses is found to be significantly overrepresented in the patient group with a cyclic axis syndrome. On the other hand, an excess of HP 1-1 can be observed and statistically confirmed in comparison with the population level among the patients offering a schizophrenic axis syndrome or resting unclassified. Possibly, the HP serum groups play a role in the bioregulation of emotionality. The "noncyclic" group does not show the marker traits of process psychoses, but in this sampling there is, in contrast to the "cyclics," a higher concentration of the immunoglobulin G serum level on the statistical border line, which perhaps is caused by destructive factors. The results correspond with the special state of the examined psychoses basing on biological determinants of different origin.

1194

Majsky A, Dvorakova M, Zvolsky P. **Binding of lithium and neuroleptics on lymphocyte HLA antigens *In vitro*.** *Folia Haematol.* 1980;107:74-80. (German)

The effect of lithium and five neuroleptics (melleril, chlorprotixen, chlorpromazine, tisercin, haloperidol) on cytotoxic reactivity and absorption capacity of lymphocyte HLA antigens A1,2,3,9,10,11, B5,7,8,12,13 *in vitro* was studied. Depending on the preparation, solution concentration, period of treatment and some not-yet-recognized individual properties of the lymphocytes, the cytotoxic reactivity of HLA antigens in treated lymphocytes remained unchanged or exceptionally became lost; rather frequently the preparations tended to kill the blood cells which later showed as polyreactive. The treated lymphocytes which had been demonstrated to lose cytotoxic reactivity or polyreactivity simultaneously showed the inhibition of absorption capacity. This phenomenon was sometimes observed even in the lymphocytes which on the day of treatment showed unchanged cytotoxic reactivity; in this case they became polyreactive following 24 hours of storing. The results confirm the necessity to perform both tests for evaluating the drug effects on lymphocyte HLA antigens *in vitro*. The present results demonstrate the binding of neuroleptics and lithium on HLA antigens, and support the hypothesis of Svejgaard and Ryder on the interaction of HLA molecules with non-immunological ligands.

1195

Mehne P, Grunwald P, Gerner-Beurle E. **A serogenetic approach to the study of Alzheimer's disease** (author's transl). *Aktuel Gerontol.* 1976;6:259-66. (German)

The analysis of 15 hereditarily-controlled blood characteristics in 57 Alzheimer patients revealed abnormalities in the distribution of ABO blood-groups and phenotypes in the third component of complement system. These data indicate that the phenogenesis of the Alzheimer syndrome is multiconditional and is obviously influenced by selective processes of immuno-genetic factors. This selective vulnerability offers a lead into the elucidation of amyloid deposition in Alzheimer's disease.

1196

Renvoize EB, Hambling MH, Pepper MD, Rajah SM. **Possible association of Alzheimer's disease with HLA-Bw15 and cytomegalovirus infection** (letter). *Lancet.* 1979;1:1238. (English)

1197

Snowden PR, Woodrow JC, Copeland JR. **HLA antigens in senile dementia and multiple infarct dementia.** *Age Ageing.* 1981;10:259-63. (English)

HLA A and B antigens were determined in 50 patients with senile dementia, in 50 patients with multiple infarct dementia and in 550 healthy controls. No significant associations with any HLA antigen were found in either group of patient and previous claims for an association are not supported.

1198

Sulkava R, Koskimies S, Wikstrom J, Palo J. **HLA antigens in Alzheimer's disease.** *Tissue Antigens.* 1980;16:191-4. (English)

The histocompatibility antigens of the A, B and C loci were typed for 32 patients with Alzheimer's disease and 5 controls of the same age. The results were also compared to the distribution of HLA antigens in a series of 900 healthy blood donors. No statistically significant differences were found between the Alzheimer patients and the controls. HLA-Cw1 was found significantly less frequently in the group comprising the patients with Alzheimer's disease and their controls together, than in the younger blood group. This leads us to suggest that an age-matched control group may be needed, at least when the patients are elderly.

1199

Whalley LJ, Urbaniak SJ, Darg C, Peutherer JF, Christie JE. **Histocompatibility antigens and antibodies to viral and other antigens in Alzheimer pre-senile dementia.** *Acta Psychiatr Scand.* 1980;61:1-7. (English)

Alzheimer's disease may arise from an interaction between a conventional infective agent and a particular disease suscep-tibility (related to the HLA-A or B locus). HLA antigens and antibodies to conventional infective agents were examined in 14 patients with pre-senile dementia. Most of the sample probably suffered Alzheimer's disease, though one subject may have had Pick's disease. No particular HLA type or antibody was associated with the sample.

1200

Whitsett C, Turner WJ, Lee TD, Dupont B. **HLA antigen frequencies in paralytic dementia.** *J Neurol Sci.* 1976; 30:417-20 (English)

HLA typing was performed on 75 caucasian and 58 black patients with paralytic dementia hospitalized at 2 state mental institutions in New York. Serological testing was performed to confirm previous infection with *T. pallidum*. The caucasian patients showed an increase in B18 (18.7% vs. 9.6% in controls). The black patients showed an increase in A2 (48.3% vs. 28.7% in controls) and an increase in B7 (27.6% vs. 15.7% in controls).

1201

Wilcox CB, Caspary EA, Behan PO. **Histocompatibility antigens in Alzheimer's disease. A preliminary study.** *Eur Neurol.* 1981;20:25-8. (English)

A preliminary study of Alzheimer's disease showed an apparent excess of the antigen A2 in patients who presented the disease before the age of 60, whereas those with onset after 64 showed different frequencies of the antigens A1 and A3 when compared with the local population. There was no abnormality in the distribution of B locus antigens. The findings are briefly discussed.

Interactions between the immune system and psychiatric functioning or behavior

1202

Bresnihan B. **CNS lupus** (review). *Clin Rheum Dis.* 1982; 8:183-95. (English)

1203

Cadie M, Nye FJ, Storey P. **Anxiety and depression after infectious mononucleosis.** *Br J Psychiatry.* 1976;128:559-61. (English)

Thirty-six patients who had had infectious mononucleosis (IM) were followed up a year later and assessed by the Middlesex Hospital Questionnaire and by interview or (in five cases) by postal questionnaire. The results support the view that IM leads to depression in a considerable number of cases, but in this series only women were so affected.

1204

Cantell K, Pulkkinen E, Elosuo R, Suominen J. **Effect of interferon on severe psychiatric diseases.** *Ann Clin Res.* 1980;12:131-2. (English) (no abstract)

1205

Carr RI, Shucard DW, Hoffman SA, Hoffman A, Bardana EJ, Harbeck R. **Neuropsychiatric involvement in systemic lupus erythematosus.** *Birth Defects.* 1978;14:209-35. (English)

Central nervous system involvement in SLE may produce a variety of behavioral abnormalities, a number of which are seen in schizophrenic non-SLE patients. Thus, the possibility exists that at least some pathogenic mechanisms in classic schizophrenia may be similar to those suspected to be involved in the development of CNS-SLE. Currently, a number of such pathogenic mechanisms are under investigation in SLE. These include immune complex mediated phenomena, lymphocyte antibodies which cross react with brain antigens, specific antineuronal antibodies, and a direct or indirect effect of a viral agent. It is as yet unclear which, if any, of these mechanisms are involved in the development of the CNS disturbances seen in SLE. In addition, more than one such mechanism may be involved (including others as yet unsuspected) acting individually or together to produce CNS disturbances. Figure 2 outlines some of the possible interactions which may occur in the development of autoimmune CNS disease. The degree to which these mechanisms and interactions actually play a role in CNS disease is now under intensive investigation in our laboratories.

1206

Copperman SM. **"Alice in Wonderland" syndrome as a presenting symptom of infectious mononucleosis in children: a description of three affected young people.** *Clin Pediatr (Phila).* 1977;16:143-6. (English)

Three cases of "Alice in Wonderland" syndrome (metamorphosia) are presented and described as a presenting symptom of infectious mononucleosis in a preadolescent male and in two late teenage females. In each instance, the classical infectious mononucleosis symptoms and diagnosis followed the onset of visual aberration. Thorough physical and blood examination of patients who present with such a syndrome must be undertaken before these symptoms are ascribed to psychiatric abnormalities. It is emphasized that infectious mononucleosis is a diffuse disorder, often associated with encephalopathies, which may include visual imbalance symptoms.

1207

Crook WG. **Adverse reactions to food can cause hyperkinesis** (letter). *Am J Dis Child.* 1978;132:819-20. (English)

1208

Dunleavy RA. **Neuropsychological correlates of asthma: effect of hypoxia or drugs.** *J Consult Clin Psychol.* 1981;49:137. (English)

The neuropsychological deficits seen in asthmatic children are thought by Suess and Chai to be possibly a function of certain antiasthma medication. Recent work by Dunleavy and Baade on neuropsychological adaptive behavior patterns of asthmatic children does not provide support for this hypothesis.

1209

Gale AE. **Food additives and hyperactivity** (letter). *Med J Aust.* 1976;2:546-7. (English)

1210

Goetz CG, Klawans HL. **Chronic agonist-induced hypersensitivity and on-off hyperkinesis.** *Ann Neurol.* 1979; 6:277-8. (English) (no abstract)

1211

Goldney RD, Temme PB. **Case report: manic depressive psychosis following infectious mononucleosis.** *J Clin Psychiatry.* 1980;41:322-3. (English)

The onset of manic depressive psychosis following infectious mononucleosis is reported. The patient appeared to be predisposed to develop such an illness, and it is postulated that the initial hypomanic episode may have been precipitated by an alteration in cerebral biogenic amines due to the infectious mononucleosis.

1212

Hendler N, Leahy W. **Psychiatric and neurologic sequelae of infectious mononucleosis.** *Am J Psychiatry.* 1978; 135:842-4. (English)

Infectious mononucleosis is usually thought to be a benign disease with occasional neurologic sequelae. Depression, incoordination, a reduction in intellectual ability, and altered

EEG patterns were found in two patients; one recovered and the other seemed to have permanent residual effects. The possibility of tranylcypromine as a treatment for the depression and appropriate counseling of patient and family are discussed.

1213

Hughes EC, Oettinger L Jr, Johnson F, Gottschalk GH. **Case report: a chemically defined diet in diagnosis and management of food sensitivity in minimal brain dysfunction.** *Ann Allergy.* 1979;42:174-6. (English) (no abstract)

1214

Kamenskii AA, Antonova LV, Samoilova NA, Galkin OM, Andreev SM. **Excitatory effect of tuftsin tetrapeptide on the activity of white rats.** *Biull Eksp Biol Med.* 1980;89:43-5. (Russian)

Studies on male white rats have shown that tuftsin (trelys-pro-arg) enhances the locomotion in animals as disclosed by a series of behavioral tests. The effect is dose-dependent: a dose of 50 microgram/kg did not change any of the test parameters, while that of 150 microgram/kg induced short-term elevation of locomotion measured with "animeks". Administration of tuftsin in a dose of 300 microgram/kg led to the enhancement of the animals' locomotion as measured with the "animeks", to the increased "open field" running time and to the reduced latent period of the reaction during the training in a t-shaped maze. Also this dose of the peptide relaxed the reactions associated with fear. It is assumed that the effects observed are consequent on the stimulant action of tuftsin on the body of white rats.

1215

King DS. **Can allergic exposure provoke psychological symptoms? A double-blind test.** *Biol Psychiat.* 1981;16:3-19. (English)

Clinical ecologists report that exposure to allergens can induce cognitive and emotional symptoms as well as somatic symptoms in susceptible individuals, but controlled tests are meager. In a test of the hypothesis that sublingual exposure to allergens would produce cognitive-emotional symptoms in allergy patients, double-blind provocative testing was conducted at an allergy clinic; 30 allergy patients complaining of at least one psychological symptom were selected. Self-report, heart-rate, and several mood and psychological performance measures were obtained. MMPI scores indicated a pathological sample. Reported cognitive-emotional symptoms were greater for allergens than for placebos (p = 0.001), while placebo symptoms were equal to base rate. Greater variability of heart rate changes was found for allergens than for placebos (p = 0.008). Severe reactions occurred more frequently to allergens (p = 0.02). Other dependent measures were not affected by the allergens or the placebos. It is concluded that allergens may contribute to psychopathology in some individuals.

1216

Levine PM, Silberfarb PM, Lipowski ZJ. **Mental disorders in cancer patients.** *Cancer.* 1978;42:1385-91. (English) (unavailable at publication)

1217

Mayron LW. **Allergy, learning, and behavior problems.** *J Learn Disabl.* 1979;12:32-42. (English) (unavailable at publication)

1218

Mitsuya H. **Toxic psychosis due to ephedrine-containing antiasthmatics-- report of three cases** (author's transl). *Seishin Shinkeigaku Zasshi.* 1978;80:155-68. (Japanese) (unavailable at publication)

1219

O'Shea JA, Porter SF. **Double-blind study of children with hyperkinetic syndrome treated with multi-allergen extract sublingually.** *J Learn Disabl.* 1981;14:189-91. (English) (unavailable at publication)

1220

Rapp DJ. **Food allergy treatment for hyperkinesis.** *J Learn Disabl.* 1979;12:608-16. (English) (unavailable at publication)

1221

Robinson LA. **Pediatric drug information: food allergies, food additives, and the Feingold diet.** *Pediatr Nurse.* 1980;6:38-9. (English) (unavailable at publication)

1222

Roppel RM. **Cancer and mental illness** (letter). *Science.* 1978;201:398. (English)

1223

Rubin RL. **Adolescent infectious mononucleosis with psychosis.** *J Clin Psychiatry.* 1978;39:773-5. (English)

This report describes an adolescent with an acute catatonic schizophrenic illness associated with infectious mononucleosis. The literature and clinical evience supporting a diagnosis of infectious mononucleosis encephalopathy are reviewed. Diagnostic questions in such cases are discussed from a clinical psychiatric perspective. Therapeutic and developmental issues in managing adolescent psychosis of uncertain etiology are explored.

1224

Sinanan K, Hillary I. **Post-influenzal depression.** *Br J Psychiatry.* 1981;138:131-3. (English)

A prospective study was carried out on post-influenzal depression. Four hundred patients presenting with psychiatric illness for the first time took part. The results show that there is no correlation between depressive illness and the demonstration of influenza antibody titres, an indication of recent influenza infection.

1225

South MA, Crowley B. **School problems and hypersensitivities.** *Cutis.* 1980;26:545, 548, 561. (English) (no abstract)

1226

Suess WM, Chai H. **Neuropsychological correlates of asthma: brain damage or drug effects.** *J Consult Clin Psychol.* 1981;49:135-6. (English)

Dunleavy and Baade's conclusions regarding hypoxic-induced neuropsychological deficit in asthmatic children seem somewhat premature until the possibility of similar deficits as a function of certain antiasthma medication can be taken into account.

1227
Taylor E. **Food additives, allergy and hyperkinesis.** *J Child Psychol Psychiatry.* 1979;20:357-63. (English) (no abstract)

1228
Traxel WL. **Hyperactivity and the Feingold diet** (letter). *Arch Gen Psychiat.* 1982;39:624. (English)

1229
Tryphonas H, Trites R. **Food allergy in children with hyperactivity, learning disabilities and/or minimal brain dysfunction.** *Ann Allergy.* 1979;42:22-7. (English)

Ninety hyperactive children, 22 children with learning disability and eight emotional-inattentive children were tested for allergy to 43 food extracts using the *in vitro* radioallergosorbent test (RAST). Fifty-two percent of all childen exhibited allergy to one or more of the foods tested. Within the hyperactive group a statistically significant association was found between the number of allergies and teachers' (Conners) scores of hyperactivity. This association was statistically significant only in those hyperactive children who also had learning disability and minimal brain dysfunction. A statistically weak association was also found between a small number of children clinically diagnosable as hyperactive and the number of allergies or total allergy scores. A causal relationship between food allergy and a small subgroup of children with a primary diagnosis of hyperactivity is suspected.

1230
Vievskaia GA, Baida NA, Vievskii AN. **Mental disorders in persons with chemical allergoses.** *Zh Nevropatol Psikhiatr.* 1977;77:908-11. (Russian)

In 83 patients with chronic chemical allergoses the authors observed depressive, hypochondriacal, apathical variants of a pathological personality development. The studies demonstrated a changed content of biogenic amines in this group of patients which confirmed the chemical nature of the process.

Aging and Immunity

Aging and Immunity

1231

Abrass IB, Scarpace PJ. **Human lymphocyte beta-adrenergic receptors are unaltered with age.** *J Gerontol.* 1981;36:298-301. (English)

To investigate the mechanism of receptor changes associated with aging, we developed a beta-adrenergic receptor assay in whole human lymphocytes which fulfills strict affinity, stereospecificity, and specificity criteria. Lymphocyte beta-adrenergic receptors were quantified in 54 (36 males and 18 females) healthy subjects on no medications divided into two age groups, 18 to 30 years (mean: 24) and 60 to 72 years (mean: 64). Using this assay, we report no change in the number of lymphocyte beta-adrenergic receptors in elderly (mean ± SE: 801 + 114 sites/cell) compared to young individuals (680 ± 47). When the values are examined separately for males and females there again is no significant difference between younger and older groups. We, therefore, suggest that further investigation is necessary before decreased hormonal responsiveness in the elderly is ascribed to decreased hormone receptor number on the basis of lymphocyte beta-adrenergic receptors.

1232

Alexianu M, Arsene A, Brasla N, Dragutoiu N, Grigoriu M, Lazar C, Lucaciu B, Nedelcu A, Roman E, Simionescu N, Stefanescu E, Talaban I, Tudor S, Tudorache B, Dumitrescu A. **Serum immunoglobulins in middle and old age dementia.** *Neurol Psychiatr (Bucur).* 1979;17:269-76. (English) (unavailable at publication)

1233

Anisimov VN, Khavinson VK, Morozov VG. **Carcinogenesis and aging; IV--Effect of low-molecular-weight factors of thymus, pineal gland and anterior hypothalamus on immunity, tumor incidence and life span of C3H/Sn mice.** *Mech Ageing Dev.* 1982;19:245-58. (English)

The low-molecular-weight polypeptide factors were obtained from bovine thymus (TF), pineal gland (PF) and anterior hypothalamus (AHF). Both TF and PF administration enhanced the rejection of skin allograft and stimulated the immunological response to sheep erythrocytes in adult CBA mice. Treatment of CBA mice with AHF increased the graft survival and inhibited antibody formation to sheep erythrocytes. Chronic TF or PF administration decreased spontaneous tumor development and prolonged the life span of female

C3H/Sn mice. Administration of AHF failed to influence the life span and the tumor incidence of female C3H/Sn mice. The role of immunity and hormonometabolic shifts in mechanisms of both aging and the age-associated increase in cancer incidence are discussed.

1234

Antel JP, Weinrick M, Arnason BG. **Circulating suppressor cells in man as a function of age.** *Clin Immunol Immunopathol.* 1978;9:134-41. (English)

Concanavalin A (Con A) was used to activate suppressor cells derived from the peripheral blood of human donors. Activated suppressor cells reduced the mitogenic response of autologous peripheral blood lymphocytes (PBLs) more markedly in elderly than in young adults (72.2 ± 5.0 vs. 41.8 ± 7.2%, p<0.02). The baseline mitogenic response of PBLs from elderly adults was significantly lower than that of PBLs from normal young adults (9497 ± 2609 vs. 28,068 ± 3973 cpm, p<0.01). A group of young multiple sclerosis patients showed poor mitogenic responsiveness (11,017 ± 2679 cpm) and low suppressor activity (36.0 ± 3.0%) suggesting that suppressor influence need not depend on the activity of responder cells. Unconcentrated supernatants from Con A-activated cells did not suppress a human lymphoblast cell line (Raji).

1235

Beregi E, Lengyel E, Biro J. **Autoantibodies in aged individuals.** *Aktuel Gerontol.* 1978;8:77-80. (English)

Authors determined in 282 individuals autoantibodies in 132 T and B lymphocytes. Their results were as follows: 1) The frequency of the presence of autoantibodies increases with age. 2) In the presence of autoantibodies the absolute T and B lymphocyte counts of aged persons markedly decrease; the absolute T and B lymphocyte counts of young adult people do not change by existing autoantibodies. 3) There is a significant difference between the absolute T cell counts of aged and young adult age groups, both age groups having autoantibodies. 4) Comparing the frequency of occurrence of autoantibodies in aged healthy persons and in aged ones with cardiovascular changes and being in the habit of smoking and consuming alcohol, respectively, a significant difference could be demonstrated; in the latter group the frequency was much higher.

1236

Bianchi C, Bartoli M, Brollo A, D'Osualdo E. **Amyloid senile plaques in late senility.** *Pathologica.* 1977;69:993-4. (Italian)

75 of 100 subjects (aged 80 to 103) showed amyloid senile plaques in cerebral cortex. A significantly higher frequency of plaques in the females was found. No significant correlation between occurrence of plaques and age was observed.

1237

Bianchi C, Berti N, Grandi G. **Cerebral and extracerebral amyloidosis in senile dementia of the Alzheimer type.** *Pathologica.* 1980;72:67-70. (English)

Sections of brain and extracerebral tissues were examined for amyloid, using Congo red staining and polarization in 13 post-mortem cases of senile dementia of the Alzheimer type. Amyloid senile plaques and cerebrovascular amyloidosis were seen in all cases. Extracerebral amyloid deposits were found in two cases, in myocardium. The results of the present study suggest that cerebral amyloidosis is a specific form of amyloidosis.

1238

Bilder GE, Denckla WD. **Restoration of ability to reject xenografts and clear carbon after hypophysectomy of adult rats.** *Mech Ageing Dev.* 1977;6:153-63. (English)

Earlier work suggested that a new pituitary function might account for the decline of minimal O_2 consumption with age by decreasing peripheral tissue responsiveness to thyroxine and triiodothyronine. It was of interest to see if removal of the pituitary from adult rats could restore juvenile competence in other systems of the body by reversing the postulated age-associated end-organ hypothyroidism. Four and 64 week old intact rats reject xenografts in 6 and 13.8 days, respectively. After hypophysectomy and thyroxine replacement, 64 week old rats reject xenografts in 6.5 days. Four and 64 week old intact rats have a V_{max} of colloidal carbon clearance of 18.9 and 2.5 mg/kg fat free body weight, respectively. After hypophysectomy and thyroxine replacement 60 week old rats have a V_{max} of 15.5 mg. Corticosterone was the only other hormone given to the hypophysectomized rats and at the various doses tested it did not appear to affect the rates of the two functions studied.

1239

Blichert-Toft M, Christensen V, Engquist A, Fog-Moller F, Kehlet H, Madsen SN, Skovsted L, Thode J, Olgaard K. **Influence of age on the endocrine metabolic response to surgery.** *Ann Surg.* 1979;190:761-70. (English)

The pathogenesis of the increased operative risk in elderly patients is unknown. From a theoretical point of view, a change in endocrine-metabolic response might be involved. A battery of hormonal and metabolic variables were measured in eight young and eight elderly healthy males undergoing elective inguinal hernial repair under general anesthesia. Blood was drawn before induction of anesthesia, at skin incision, and 1, 2, and 6 h after skin incision. Plasma cortisol increase was significantly higher in elderly than in young controls. Plasma renin level was lower in old age, but renin-aldosterone and electrolyte response patterns were alike in the 2 groups. Thyroid parameters, in terms of serum T_4, serum T_3, serum rT_3, and T_3-resin uptake, responded normally to surgery and showed no age-related differences. The hyperglycemic response was not significantly influenced by age indicating unchanged glycoregulatory mechanisms also verified by determinations of plasma catecholamines, c(cyclic) AMP, and insulin. Blood lymphocyte count was constantly lower in elderly than in young and decreased with time, but the age-related difference was not significant. Blood polymorphonuclear leukocytes showed an increase of the same magnitude in both age groups, although at a significantly slower rate in the elderly. Age affects some aspects of the initial endocrine-metabolic response to surgery.

1240

Blichert-Toft M, Hummer L. **Immunoreactive corticotrophin reserve in old age in man during and after surgical stress.** *J Gerontol.* 1976;31:539. (English)

Attempts have been made to establish whether the immunoreactive corticotrophin (IR-ACTH) reserve was impaired in old age during surgical stress and whether an exhaustion of the IR-ACTH reserve could be traced postoperatively. Recognition of the degenerative changes of the senescent adenohypophysis has made this investigation essential in an effort to analyze factors responsible for the high risk involved in surgery on the aged. In the study, 18 young and 14 elderly patients were subjected to elective abdominal or thoracic surgery, and the IR-ACTH response was determined. No significant age-related difference in response to surgery was found. On the fifth day after operation an intravenous metyrapone test was carried out, and the IR-ACTH response in plasma determined. In the elderly, the IR-ACTH response to metyrapone was not found to be inferior to that in young patients. It was concluded that the IR-ACTH reserve was unimpaired during surgery in old age and that exhaustion was not in evidence based on unimpaired IR-ACTH response during repeated stress in the postoperative period. Therefore, decreased ACTH reserve seems not to be a factor involved in the higher surgical risk in the elderly.

1241

Busse E, Helmholz M, Magdon R. **Age-related changes of cAMP and prostaglandin content in the brain and lymphocytes of spontaneously tumor-producing C3H mice.** *Onkologie.* 181;4:328-30. (German)

Age-caused concurrent changes in the activation of the adenylate-cyclase activity by dopamine in the diencephalon and the stimulation of the basal level of cAMP by isoproterenol in the lymphocytes were demonstrated in the spontaneously tumor producing C3H mice. These changes may be related to the occurrence of tumors in these animals. The above-mentioned changes in the cAMP system were not found in AB mice. By treating the adult C3H mice with substances which increase the cAMP level, it was possible to achieve a renewed stimulation of the cAMP system as seen in young mice. With this treatment the spontaneous tumor-induction rate was also reduced. In the adenocarcinomas of the C3H mice a decrease in the level of prostaglandin E and an increase in the level of prostaglandin F_2 alpha was observed.

1242

Cohen D, Eisdorfer C, Vitaliano PP, Bloom V. **The relationship of age, anxiety, and serum immunoglobulins with crystallized and fluid intelligence.** *Biol Psychiat.* 1980; 15:699-709. (English)

Serum immunoglobulin concentrations (IgG, IgA, and IgM), cognitive performance (crystallized and fluid intelligence), and self-reports of anxiety were evaluated in 24 men and women 60-75 years, and 50 men and women, 30-45 years. Trait anxiety was an important factor relating to performance differences between the young and old on crystallized and fluid subtests. IgM was inversely related to performance in the older age groups. Anxiety was not related to serum immunoglobulin levels.

1243

Cohen D, Eisdorfer C. **Antinuclear antibodies in the cognitively impaired elderly.** *J Nerv Ment Dis.* 1980;168:179-80. (English)

The frequency of antinuclear antibodies was evaluated in older men and women aged 60 to 100 years with presumptive diagnoses of chronic brain syndrome or dementing illness. Thirteen percent of the women and none of the men with organic brain syndrome had positive titers, compared to 3% for older men and women aged 60 to 89 years evaluated in a medical clinic population. It would appear to be valuable to evaluate the significance of antinuclear antibodies and other autoantibodies in the pathogenesis of dementing illness in the elderly.

1244

Cohen D, Eisdorfer C. **Behavioral immunologic relationships in older men and women.** *Experimental Aging Res.* 1977;3:225-9. (English)

Serum immunoglobulin levels (IgG, IgA and IgM) and intellectual performance were examined in a group of fourteen elderly men (mean age 74.2) and twenty-three women (mean age 73.2) who reported that they were in good health. Significant negative Pearson product-moment correlations between performance and IgG and IgA emerged for men. Among women the relationship was not significant.

1245

Cohen D, Eisdorfer C. **Serum immunoglobulins and cognitive status in the elderly; 1--A population study.** *Br J Psychiatry.* 1980;136:33-9. (English)

Fifty-seven cognitively impaired elderly had significantly elevated serum IgG (p<0.005) and IgA (p<0.01) levels and similar IgM levels, compared to a population of 65 elderly matched for age and sex, who did not manifest cognitive impairment. These findings are compatible with a current hypothesis that immunological factors may be important in the cognitive disorders observed with increased frequency among the aged.

1246

Crapper DR, Deboni U. **Brain aging and Alzheimer's disease.** *Can Psychiatr Assoc J.* 1978;23:229-33. (English)

The most common cause of senile dementia appears to be a pathological process indistinguishable from that found in presenile dementia of the Alzheimer type. Consideration of the neuropathological changes suggest that this disease may involve an interaction of at least three processes: a viral-like infection, a disorder in the immune system and the neurotoxic effect of an environmental agent. The evidence in support of this hypothesis is reviewed.

1247

Denckla WD. **Interactions between age and the neuroendocrine and immune systems.** *Fed Proc, Fed Am Soc Exp Biol.* 1978;37:1263-7. (English)

Three conclusions are suggested by some of the recent work on aging, immunology and the neuroendocrine system. 1) There appears to be sufficient data to implicate the neuroendocrine system in both the maturation and the senescence of at least some components of the immune system. 2) The thymus by its presence or its absence appears to influence certain functions of the pituitary; thus, there appears to be a possible reciprocal relationship between the pituitary and the thymus. 3) Changes in the levels of pituitary hormones or hormones that are controlled by the pituitary can restore in older rats and mice certain functions that are generally considered as part of the immune surveillance and defense system. Consequently, it can be hoped that further studies of neuroendocrine-immune relationships might lead to an understanding of some of the causes for the decline in immune competence with age in mammals.

1248

Dilman VM. **Ageing, metabolic immunodepression and carcinogenesis.** *Mech Ageing Dev.* 1978;8:153-73. (English) (no abstract)

1249

Eisdorfer C, Cohen D. **Serum immunoglobulins and cognitive status in the elderly; II--An immunological-behavioral relationship.** *Br J Psychiatry.* 1980;136:40-5. (English)

In 42 patients with cognitive dysfunction (senile dementia) significant correlations between immunoglobulins and various tests of intelligence were observed. Serum IgG emerged as the single best predictor of behavioural status. There is need for further research in this field.

1250

Garfinkel R. **Treatment of a psychosomatic ailment in an elderly woman.** *Psychosomatics.* 1980;21:1015-6. (English)

Because of their physical vulnerability, the elderly under stress are particularly susceptible to physical breakdown. The following case report illustrates the success of relaxation training in conjunction with psychotherapy in treating a debilitating psychosomatic condition, bronchial asthma.

1251

Haaijman JJ, Hijmans W. **Influence of age on the immunological activity and capacity of the CBA mouse.** *Mech Ageing Dev.* 1978;7:375-98. (English)

The immunological activity and capacity were studied in the CBA mouse as a function of its age. The activity was determined by the number of immunoglobulin containing (C-Ig) cells in different lymphoid organs and the immunoglobulin levels of the serum in non-artificially stimulated animals. It was confirmed that in older age the bone marrow takes over from the spleen the role of the major site of immunoglobulin production. A clear decrease in the number of C-Ig cells was observed in the mesenteric lymph nodes and the Peyer's patches. The Ig serum levels remained constant after the sixth month of age, with the exception of IgG_1 and IgG_{2b}. There was a striking increase in variation between the individual animals with advancing age. From these data it can be concluded that the B-cell system of old animals is as active as that of young animals. The immunological capacity of CBA mice of various ages was assessed by measuring the levels of specific antibodies after the administration of human serum albumin in complete Freund's adjuvant. A severe decline of the primary and the secondary response was observed on ageing. The reaction of three-year-old animals was negligible. The discrepancy between the declining immunological capacity and the constant or increasing immunological activity is explained by an age-related deficiency of the T-cell compartment in the spleen.

1252

Kay MMB. **Effect of age on T cell differentiation.** *Fed Proc, Fed Am Soc Exp Biol.* 1978;37:1241-4. (English)

A brief overview of the area of T cell aging is presented by first discussing the age-related changes in T cell activities, and then by focusing attention on the possible mechanisms that may be responsible for the decline. Present evidence indicates that thymic involution precedes and therefore may be responsible for the age-dependent decline in the ability of the immune system to generate functional T cells. At this time, it appears that the primary effect of thymic involution is on a T cell differentiation pathway affecting the more mature T cells first with time, and then the less mature T cells. Thus, the thymus may be the aging clock for the immune system. Further studies should be centered around processes regulating growth and atrophy of the thymus.

1253

Kent S. **Can normal aging be explained by the immunologic theory?** *Geriatrics.* 1977;32:111-21. (English) (no abstract)

1254

Kishimoto S, Tomino S, Mitsuya H, Fugiwara H. **Age-related changes in suppressor functions of human T cells.** *J Immunol.* 1979;123:1586-93. (English)

Functions of both naturally-occurring suppressor and Con A-activated suppressor cells were compared among newborns, young adults, and aged subjects. When T cells were irradiated to remove suppressor activity and added to PWM-stimulated allogeneic B cell cultures, an enhanced Ig production resulted. This irradiation-induced enhancement for IgG production was significantly lower in aged group than in newborns or young adults (p<0.01). With regard to IgM production, the enhancement was significantly depressed in aged subjects as compared with newborns (p = 0.05). The radiation dose for the generation of T cells capable of exerting the greatest enhancement was between 900 and 1200 rads in both young adults and aged subjects, but as high as 1600 rads in newborns. Furthermore, newborns were shown to be enriched for T suppressor activity by co-culturing of allogeneic PBL with T cells in the presence of PWM as compared with young adults. T cells isolated from young adults, but not from aged subjects, enhanced IgM and IgG production by allogeneic B cells beyond the synergy obtained by control T cells when pretreated with mitomycin and then co-cultured with B cells and PWM. The means of maximal enhancements were significantly greater in young adults than in the aged (p = 0.02 for IgG, p<0.05 for IgM). The study on the kinetics of generation of Con A-activated suppressor cells revealed that T cells isolated from young adults mediated maximal suppression of Ig production when activated by incubation with Con A for 2 days and added to PWM-stimulated PBL cultures. By contrast, T cells from aged humans required 1 or 2 more days of incubation with Con A to be activated to obtain the maximal suppressor activity. In addition, the means of maximal suppression of IgM and IgG production mediated by Con A-activated T cells were significantly greater in young adults than in the aged (p = 0.02 for IgG and p = 0.05 for IgM). Impaired function of both naturally-occurring suppressor and Con A-activated suppressor cells is discussed in relation to altered immunocompetence seen in aged humans.

1255

Krall JF, Connelly M, Weisbart R, Tuck ML. **Age-related elevation of plasma catecholamine concentration and reduced responsiveness of lymphocyte adenylate cyclase.** *J Clin Endocrinol Metab.* 1981;52:863-7. (English)

Plasma catecholamine (norepinephrine) concentration during upright posture and lymphocyte adenylate cyclase response to the beta-adrenergic catecholamine isoproterenol were compared in two age groups of healthy subjects. Compared to subjects between the ages of 19-39 yr, those between 65-88 yr had higher plasma norepinephrine concentrations (353 ± 42 vs. 577 ± 65 pg/ml) and reduced lymphocyte adenylate cyclase responsiveness to NaF, isoproterenol, guanyl nucleotide, and isoproterenol in the presence of guanylyl nucleotide. There were important differences between the properties of adenylate cyclase in cells from the aged subjects and those from younger subjects pretreated with norepinephrine *in vitro*. Pretreated cells had diminished responsiveness to isoproterenol (desensitization), but not to guanylyl nucleotide. Moreover, guanylyl nucleotide restored isoproterenol responsiveness to the desensitized enzyme. Thus, reduced responsiveness of lymphocyte adenylate cyclase from aged subjects was not attributable solely to acutely elevated plasma catecholamine levels. The interactions between the guanylyl nucleotide-requiring coupling factors and the catalytic subunits of adenylate cyclase were similar in the two age groups, as evidenced by similar K_m values of activation by the nonhydrolyzable GTP analog Gpp[NH]p (guanyl-5'-yl imidodiphosphate) and by Hill coefficients of activation near unity. The initial velocity of product formation by adenylate cyclase from the older group was only about half that from the younger group in the presence of Gpp[NH]p. These differences could not be attributed to age-related changes in the distribution of cell types in the leukocyte population. The results suggest that decreases in the concentration of either the guanylyl nucleotide-requiring coupling factors or the catalytic subunits of adenylate cyclase may accompany aging and contribute to the diminished responsiveness of the lymphocyte enzyme. Similar decreases could occur in less accessible catecholamine target tissues as a consequence of human aging.

1256

Lord A, Sutton RN, Baker AA, Hussein SA. **Serological studies in the elderly.** *Age Ageing.* 1978;7:116-22. (English)

Sera from 108 elderly patients in psychiatric and general hospitals were tested for antibodies to seven viruses. Measles virus antibody levels were significantly higher in patients from the psychiatric hospital, regardless of diagnosis, than in those from other hospitals. Demented patients, regardless of their hospital, had significantly higher levels of antibody to adenovirus than control patients.

1257

Macdonald SM, Goldstone AH, Morris JE, Exton-Smith AN, Callard RE. **Immunological parameters in the aged and in Alzheimer's disease.** *Clin Exp Immunol.* 1982; 49:123-8. (English)

Peripheral blood from patients with Alzheimer's disease, elderly normal subjects and young (normal subjects) was examined with respect to leucocyte phenotypes and proliferative responses to lectins. Whole blood cell analysis showed that the neutrophil count was similar in all three groups. However, the lymphocyte count was depressed in the Alzheimer group. The monocyte count was reduced in the healthy aged and further reduced in the Alzheimer group. Analysis of peripheral blood mononuclear cells showed no change in the proportion of E+ cells, total T determined with the monoclonal antibody UCHT1 (similar to OKT3) and the T cell subsets: active E and T dot (discrete esterase staining). However, the proportion of T cells bearing the antigen detected by UCHT3 monoclonal antibody (similar to Leu 1 and OKT1) was reduced in the healthy aged and further reduced in the Alzheimer group. Proliferative responses to PHA, Con A, PA, and PWM were similarly depressed in both the aged and Alzheimer groups.

1258

Makinodan T. **Immunobiology of aging.** *J Am Geriatr Soc.* 1976;24:249-52. (English)

Normal immune functions can begin to decline shortly after an individual reaches sexual maturity. Although changes in cellular environment are partially responsible, the decline is due primarily to changes within the cells, especially the T cells and to some extent the stem cells. This is reflected in their inability to proliferate and differentiate efficiently. What needs to be resolved is whether the altered properties of T cells and stem cells are permanent or reversible and, if permanent, whether they are due to a stochastic or a genetically programmed event. The decline with age in certain normal immune functions is associated with an increase in the frequency of autoimmune and immune complex diseases,

certain types of cancer, and viral and fungal infections. These diseases compromise normal immune functions in short-lived strains of mice. In long-lived mice and in humans, however, the decline in immune functions to threshold levels seems to predispose individuals to illness. Three general approaches recently have been used to improve the immune system of aging mice: a) dietary manipulation, b) drug therapy, and c) cellular therapy. Preliminary results of ongoing studies have been most encouraging. Future immunopathogenic studies of aging mice with such an improved immune system should clarify the role of fidelity of the immune system in diseases of the aged. The immune system continues to serve as an excellent model for: a) the etiology of aging at the cellular and molecular levels, b) the pathogenesis of aging, and c) effective approaches to improve the quality of life for the aged.

1259

Makinodan T. **Mechanism of senescence of immune response.** *Fed Proc, Fed Am Soc Exp Biol.* 1978;37:1239-69. (English) (no abstract)

1260

Martin JM, Kellett JM, Kahn J. **Aneuploidy in cultured human lymphocytes; II--A comparison between senescence and dementia.** *Age Ageing.* 1981;10:24-8. (English)

A study has been made of aneuploidy in the cultured lymphocytes of senile dements (46 females and 8 males), arteriosclerotic dements (10 females and 8 males) and normal geriatric controls (55 females and 18 males). Contrary to previous reports of senile dements having a higher degree of hypodiploidy (chromosome loss) than age-matched controls, there were no significant differences between any of the diagnostic groups. The association between individual subjects' age and hypodiploidy is positive, though not significant, with a high degree of individual variation. The reasons for the discrepancies between this and previous studies are discussed as are possible future lines of research in this field.

1261

Mayer PP, Chughtai MA, Cape RD. **An immunological approach to dementia in the elderly.** *Age Ageing.* 1976; 5:164-70. (English)

A study into the relationship of immune change in the serum and the presence of senile dementia is reported. Three groups were studied, senile dementia, cerebrovascular disease and subjects without evidence of brain disease. All were aged 65 years and over. The immunofluorescent studies showed an excess of antineuronal reactivity and a fall in antinuclear antibody in females with senile dementia. There was no significant difference between the groups with respect to immunoglobulins, slide latex and a complement fixation test, against a variety of tissues. The significance of the findings in relation to other published results is discussed.

1262

Palmblad J, Haak A. **Ageing does not change blood granulocyte bactericidal capacity and levels of complement factors 3 and 4.** *Gerontology.* 1978;24:381-5. (English)

The bactericidal capacity of blood polymorphonuclear granulcoytes and the plasma levels of complement factors 3 and 4 did not differ between 15 aged patients and 15 control subjects, nor did these important antimicrobial functions predict morbidity and mortality in the next six months.

1263
Platt R. **Infectious disease in the elderly: assessment of risk factors** (abstract). *The Gerontologist.* 1982;22:203. (English)

There is ample evidence that the aged have a higher than average risk of acquiring infections of many types. For some infections this excess risk appears not to be a direct consequence of the physiological events of aging. Instead, age is a marker for other non-age dependent conditions which are more closely associated with infection and are more likely to be causes of the infection. The recognition of this phenomenon has implications both for the understanding of the pathogenesis of infection and for the design of measures to prevent infection. These concepts will be illustrated by analysis of age and other risk factors for urinary tract infection.

1264
Popp DM. **Qualitative changes in immunocompetent cells with age: reduced sensitivity to cortisone acetate.** *Mech Ageing Dev.* 1977;6:355-62. (English)

Recent studies suggest that immunocompetent cells that respond to a primary antigenic stimulus in old mice are different cell types from those that respond in young mice. This hypothesis was tested by determining the cortisone acetate sensitivity of antigen-sensitive lymphocytes from young and old donors. It was found that antigen-reactive lymph node lymphocytes from young donors are cortisone-acetate sensitive whereas the antigen-reactive lymph node lymphocytes from old donors are cortisone-acetate resistant.

1265
Singhal SK, Roder JC, Duwe AK. **Suppressor cells in immunosenescence.** *Fed Proc, Fed Am Soc Exp Biol.* 1978;37:1245-52. (English)

The antibody, cell-mediated and mitogen responses of many, if not all, murine strains decline markedly with age. In general, thymic-dependent responses to antigens and mitogens decline earlier and at a faster rate than thymic-independent responses, whereas the mitogenic response to the precursor B cell mitogen, dextran sulfate, does not decline until much later in life. In addition, the immune response of old spleen cells can be restored by cells or agents (activated thymocytes, lipopolysaccharide, 2-mercaptoethanol) that act directly on B cells or replace T cell function, thereby suggesting that a) early stages in stem cell differentiation are not deficient in old mice and b) immunosenescence may result from an active block in some later maturation stage such as T or B cell activation by antigen or mitogen. Recent observations suggest that depressed immune function is accompanied by an age-dependent increase in suppressor B cell activity. B cell suppression is nonspecific and acts by preventing lymphocyte activation and differentiation. Age-related immunodepression is accompanied by a) an increased suppressive activity of bone marrow

cells *in vitro*, b) the appearance of B suppressor cells in the spleen which release soluble mediators and prevent early activation events in the immune response when added to young syngeneic spleen cells *in vitro*, and c) an increased suppression of both plaque forming cell and mitogen responses by B cell-derived factors in normal mouse serum.

1266
Von Gaudeceker B. **Ultrastructure of the age-involuted adult human thymus.** *Cell Tissue Res.* 1978;186:507-25. (English)

Age-involuted thymus tissue from a middle aged (33 years) and an old (63 years) man have been examined by electron microscopy and compared with thymus tissue from children. Biopsies had been taken during surgical correction of congenital heart defects. The fine structural architecture of cortex, medulla and connective tissue in the remaining lymphatic islands in the adult thymus investigated was not different to the thymus of children. We were surprised to find vigorous lymphocytopoiesis in the cortical regions and to recognize extended areas of medulla with a cellular composition which obviously provides the same microenvironment for T-cell maturation as the medulla of the non-involuted thymus. Our findings are discussed in relation to the increasing arguments that the human thymus serves an immunological function throughout life.

1267
Yunis EJ, Fernandes G, Greenberg LJ. **Tumor immunology, autoimmunity and aging.** *J Am Geriatr Soc.* 1976; 24:258-63. (English)

Cell-mediated immune function declines with aging, and may be associated with autoimmunity and malignancy. Humoral immune responses also decline with aging. The chief age-related effect on the immune system is a decrease in T-cell function. The "thymus clock" and immunogenesis are discussed in relation to aging. In animals, attempts at immunologic rejuvenation by cellular or hormonal means have not been as successful as the results attained by genetic manipulation.

Nutritional Influences
on Immunity

Nutritional influences on immunity

1268

Alderson MR. **Nutrition and cancer: evidence from epidemiology.** *Proc Nutr Soc.* 1981;40:1-6. (English)

This paper begins by commenting on trends in cancer and some of the major known causes of cancer in the world. Though there have been many suggestions that diet may influence the risk of malignant disease, the evidence is somewhat diffuse. The paper indicates two different ways of studying the problem: (1) looking for variation in incidence or mortality from the disease, including collation studies relating variation in incidence or mortality to variation at various environmental indices, and (2) specific studies on patients or subjects, collecting detailed results in order to identify variation in risk of cancer. Due to limitations of space, no consideration is given to agents added to food in manufacture, preparation, or cooking. Contamination, such as by mycotoxins, is also not covered.

1269

Anonymous. **Oral zinc and immunoregulation: a nutritional or pharmacological effect of zinc supplementation?** (review) *Nutr Rev.* 1982;40:72-4. (English)

1270

Beisel WR, Edelman R, Nauss K, Suskind RM. **Single-nutrient effects on immunologic functions: report of a workshop sponsored by the department of Food and Nutrition and its Nutrition Advisory Group of the AMA.** *JAMA.* 1981;245:53-8. (English)

Immune system dysfunction can result from single-nutrient deficiencies or excesses, alone or in combination with generalized protein-energy malnutrition. Acquired immune dysfunctions in man occur with deficiencies of iron, zinc, vitamins A and B_{12}, pyridoxine, and folic acid and with excesses of essential fatty acids and vitamin E. Additional micronutrients are important for maintaining immunologic competence in animals. Deficits or excesses of many trace elements and single nutrients thus have potential for causing immune dysfunctions in man. Since nutritionally induced immune dysfunction is generally reversible, it is important to recognize and identify clinical illnesses in which immunologic dysfunctions are of nutritional origin. Correction of malnutrition should lead to prompt reversal of acquired immune dysfunctions.

1271

Bistrian BR. **Interaction of nutrition and infection in the hospital setting.** *Am J Clin Nutr.* 1977;30:1228-35. (English)

A substantial portion of hospitalized patients suffer from protein-calorie malnutrition acquired as a result of their illness, their semi-starvation dietary regimens, or the combination of both insults together. When energy needs are not met by the diet, the deficient calories must come from body stores, muscle, or visceral proteins and fat. The status of these stores can be assessed clinically by easily performed measurements. In adult kwashiorkor-like syndromes, the insulin response to the combined stimulus of catabolic stress and carbohydrate feedings reduces the mobilization of fat and protein stores. In adult marasmus there is hypoaminoacidemia and loss of skeletal muscle. Both forms of malnutrition have a profound impact on immune function. Nutritional support should be given preeminent consideration as an additional necessary form of therapy in these patients.

1272

Bonfils S, Rougier P. **Dietary behavior and digestive diseases.** *Ann Nutr Aliment.* 1976;30:243-53. (French)

The influence of alimentation on the digestive pathology is very important. In this report the authors review the principal results of epidemiologic studies and animal experimentations. According to this survey of the literature it can be stated that some presumptions exist for: -- the responsibility of diet without vegetal fibers in the frequency of constipation, colonic diverticular disease, piles and hiatal hernia. The comparison of the alimentary habits in the western Europe with rural Africa is very instructive on that matter; -- the responsibility of alcohol consumption, use of hypercaloric regimen and hyperlipidic ingestants as causative factors for chronic pancreatitis; -- the importance of an hypercaloric, hyperlipidic and low residue regimen as etiologic actors in biliary gallstones; -- the role of denutrition and alcoholism in liver steatosis and cirrhosis in developed country; -- more important, perhaps, is the suspicion of the role of nutrition in the development of digestive cancer: alcohol will facilitate oesophageal cancer, alimentary nitrites gastric cancer meanwhile fiberless regimen and biles salts will promote colonic cancer. Impairments of nutrition observed after digestive resections in case of inappropriate alimentation are also analyzed as well as the principal alimentary disturbances related to allergy or enzymatic deficiency.

1273

Chavapil M, Stankova L, Weldy P, Bernhard D, Campbell J, Carlson EC, Cox T, Peacock J, Bartos Z, Zukoski C. **The role of zinc in the function of some inflammatory cells.** *Prog Clin Biol Res.* 1977;14:103-27. (English) (no abstract)

1274

Dianzani MU, Torrielli MV, Canuto RA, Garcea R, Feo F. **The influence of enrichment with cholesterol on the phagocytic activity.** *J Pathol.* 1976;118:193-9. (English)

Prolonged treatment of rats with a cholesterol-rich diet induced hypercholesterolaemia and increased free cholesterol content of peritoneal macrophages. A 2.2 times increase in plasma membrane cholesterol was demonstrated in cholesterol-enriched macrophages. These cells showed a significant inhibition of phagocytosis. The inhibition was 37.0 percent and 91.7 per cent for latex particles or lipid droplets, respectively.

1275

Enstrom JE. **Assessing human epidemiologic data on diet as an etiologic factor in cancer development** (review). *Bull NY Acad Med.* 1982;58:313-22. (English)

1276

Good RA, Fernandes G, Yunis EJ, Cooper WC, Jose DC, Cramer RT, Hansen MA. **Nutritional deficiency, immunologic function and disease.** *Am J Pathol.* 1976;84:599-614. (English)

Several experiments conducted by our group over a period of 6 years have shown that nutritional stress, especially protein and/or calorie deprivation, leads to many, often dramatic, changes in the immune responses of mice, rats, and guinea pigs. Chronic protein deprivation (CPD) has been shown to create an enhancing effect on the cell-mediated immune responses of these animals. Humoral responses under CPD conditions were most often found to be depressed, but sometimes were unaffected, depending on the nature of the antigen employed. Chronic protein deprivation, consistent with the pattern just mentioned, improved tumor immunity by depressing production of B-cell blocking factors, and, in at least one instance, resistance to development of mammary adenocarcinoma in C3H mice was associated with evidence of increased numbers of T suppressor cells. Profound nutritional deficits (less than 5% protein per total daily food intake) depressed both cellular and humoral immunity. Early, though temporary, protein deprivation caused a long-term depression of both cellular and humoral immunity also, with the humoral component being the first to recover. Manipulation of protein and calories was found to have a profound effect on certain autoimmune conditions. Diets high in fat and low in protein favored reproduction but shortened the life of NZB mice, whereas diets high in protein and low in fat inhibited development of autoimmunity and prolonged life. Chronic moderate protein restriction permitted NZB mice to maintain their normally waning immunologic functions much longer than mice fed a normal protein intake. Further, the low-protein diet was associated with a delay in development of manifestations of autoimmunity. Decreasing dietary calories by a reduction of fats, carbohydrates, and proteins more than doubled the average life span of $(NZBxNZW)F_1$

mice, a strain prone to early death from autoimmune disease. Histopathologic studies using immunofluorescent microscopy revealed that the development of the renal lesions caused by the deposition of antigen-antibody complexes, which is so characteristic of these mice, was markedly delayed.

1277

Gross RL, Newberne PM. **Role of nutrition in immunologic function.** *Physiol Rev.* 1980;60:188-302. (English) (no abstract)

1278

Hirata F, Axelrod J. **Phospholipid methylation and biological signal transmission.** *Science.* 1980;209:1082-90. (English)

Many types of cells methylate phospholipids using 2 methyltransferase enzymes that are asymmetrically distributed in membranes. As the phospholipids are successively methylated, they are translocated from the inside to the outside of the membrane. When catecholamine neurotransmitters, lectins, immunoglobulins or chemotaxic peptides bind to the cell surface, they stimulate the methyltransferase enzymes and reduce membrane viscosity. The methylation of phospholipids is coupled to Ca^{2+} influx and the release of arachidonic acid, lysophosphatidylcholine and prostaglandins. These closely associated biochemical changes facilitate the transmission of many signals through membranes, resulting in the generation of cAMP in many cell types, release of histamine in mast cells and basophils, mitogenesis in lymphocytes and chemotaxis in neutrophils.

1279

Holm G, Palmblad J. **Acute energy deprivation in man: effect on cell-mediated immunological reactions.** *Clin Exp Immunol.* 1976;25:207-11. (English)

The effects of 10 days of total energy deprivation on lymphocyte functions and cell-mediated immunity was evaluated in fourteen healthy, normal-weighted males. Lymphocytes from seven of the subjects were tested *in vitro*. A significant depression was noted of the DNA synthesis after stimulation with pokeweed mitogen and PPD while there was no effect on the response to concanavalin A. No change was noted in the percentages and total numbers of circulating B and T lymphocytes and monocytes. The delayed skin reactivity following intracutaneous PPD and mumps antigen was not different from non-starving control subjects.

1280

Horrobin DF, Manku MS, Oka M, Morgan RO, Cunnane SC, Ally AI, Ghayur T, Schweitzer M, Karmali RA. **The nutritional regulation of T lymphocyte function.** *Med Hypotheses.* 1979;5:969-85. (English)

Prostaglandin (PG) E_1 plays a major role in the regulation of thymus development and T lymphocyte function and the evidence for this is reviewed. The production of PGE_1 is dependent on nutritional factors with linoleic acid, gamma-linolenic acid, pyridoxine, zinc and vitamin C playing key roles. Inadequate intake of any one of these will lead to inadequate PGE_1 formation and defective T lymphocyte function. Megadoses of any one are likely to be only minimally effective in the absence of adequate intakes of the others. By careful attention to diet it should be possible to activate T lymphocyte function in the large number of diseases including rheumatoid arthritis, various auto-immune diseases, multiple sclerosis, and cancer in which such function is defective. It is possible that T lymphocytes may require both endogenous and exogenous PGE_1 in order to function adequately. It is therefore of particular interest that many cancer cells and virally infected cells are unable to make PGE_1 because they cannot convert linoleic acid to gamma-linolenic acid. The direct provision of gamma-linolenic or dihomo-gammalinolenic acids in these situations is worthy of full investigation.

1281

Juhlin L. **Incidence of intolerance to food additives.** *Int J Dermatol.*Dermatol 1980;19:548-51. (English) (no abstract)

1282

Kaiser N, Edelman JS. **Calcium dependence of glucocorticoid-induced lymphocytolysis.** *Proc Natl Acad Sci.* 1977; 74:638-42. (English)

A potent glucocorticoid, triamcinolone acetonide (9-alpha-fluoro-11-beta,16-alpha,17-alpha,21-tetrahydroxypregna-1,4-diene -3,20-dione-16,17-acetonide) and a divalent cation ionophore (A23187) had similar effects *in vitro* on [^{3}H]uridine uptake and on lysis of thymocytes of adrenalectomized rats. Removal of Ca^{2+} from the medium blunted the cytolytic action of triamcinolone acetonide and virtually eliminated that of A23187. In Ca^{2+}-free media, treatment of the thymocytes for 15 hr with triamcinolone acetonide or A23187 followed by re-introduction of Ca^{2+} resulted in a rapid decrease in cell survival. Based on the time courses of the responses, triamcinolone acetonide and A23187 evoked proportionate increases in ^{45}Ca uptake and lysis of the thymocytes. These findings implicate enhanced Ca^{2+} uptake in glucocorticoid-dependent lymphocytolysis.

1283

Latham MC. **Needed research on the interactions of certain parasitic diseases and nutrition in humans.** *Rev Infect Dis.* 1982;4:896-900. (English)

For the purpose of assigning priorities for research, each of the following parasitic diseases is examined in regard to its effect on the nutritional status of the host: schistosomiasis, malaria, amebiasis, giardiasis, ascariasis, and hookworm. The epidemiology, diagnosis, immune response to, and available therapies for these diseases are discussed. It is suggested tha highest priority be given to three diseases: hookworm, ascariasis, and schistosomiasis, because they can be treated successfully, diagnosed easily, and have a high prevalence.

1284

Mackarness R. **Can the food we eat drive us mad?** *J Psychosom Res.* 1978;22:355. (English)

Psychosomatic research has come to be regarded by most people as being concerned with psyche influencing soma, not the other way round, but in my work at the Clinical Ecology

Research Unit at Basingstoke and in the Out-patient department connected with it, I study the effects of changes in the body affecting the mind. The subject is known as Clinical Ecology and this is concerned with the effects of hypersensitivity in certain susceptible people to specific factors in the non-living physical environment. In practice this means that an attempt is made to identify the foods and chemicals which may be causing adverse reactions in the brain. If it can be commonly accepted that certain tissues can become the target organs of an unsuspected allergy to a food or chemical, then, if the central nervous system becomes involved, the resulting signs and symptoms may be neurological or psychiatric. In this way, a person may actually appear to be mad after eating a certain food. The methods of identifying the causative foods and chemicals are described with illustrative case histories which brings out the important points in the book *Not all in the mind.* A short film was shown on the subject.

1285

Mann GV. **Food intake and resistance to disease.** *Lancet.* 1980;1:1238-9. (English)

Food and health are a persistent pair in biomedical discussions. Almost everyone thinks that a sick plump individual is healthier than one with a lean and hungry look; and chicken soup is a well-known remedy. But there are still some enigmas. For example, why do people lose their appetites when they become feverish? Why is vomiting so often associated with a febrile illness? Could anorexia be a protective device? The role of food and feeding in resistance to disease is an important matter with many facets.

1286

McFarlane H. **Malnutrition and impaired response to infection.** *Proc Nutr Soc.* 1976;35:263-72. (English)

The cycle of events which leads to an impairment of the immune response in the malnourished child includes poverty, food deprivation and frequent infections. It is of great significance, however, that the marked suppression of the immune response can be repaired reasonably promptly, if the disease commences after the child has attained 1 year of age. Prenatal infection not only generates growth retardation but also a higher maternal to foetal IgG ratio, higher IgM in the neonate and a sustained immune depression. Passive cutaneous anaphylaxis measurements in the baboon skin and specific IgE in PEM is due to parasitic infestation and common allergens and has little or no relationship with decreased T-cell function.

1287

Morosco GJ, Goeringer GC. **Lifestyle factors and cancer of the pancreas: a hypothetical mechanism.** *Med Hypotheses.* 1980;6:971-85. (English)

The interaction of a genetically determined protease inhibitor, the enzymes whose functions are modified by that inhibitor and lifestyle factors, such as cigarette smoking, high lipid diet and alcohol consumption, are considered key factors in a proposed protease-antiprotease imbalance mechanism for pancreatic oncogenesis. Epidemiologic and experimental laboratory evidence in support of the mechanism is presented along with a discussion of suggested research initiatives to further test the hypothesis.

1288
Murray MJ, Murray AB. **Starvation suppression and refeeding activation of infection: an ecological necessity?** *Lancet.* 1977;1:123-6. (English)

The hypothesis is advanced that starvation suppresses and refeeding activates certain infections as an essential part of an ecological balance between man, his animals, and his environment. During famine, then, man fails to thrive, but his ultimate extinction is prevented in part by the parallel decline in fecundity of his "micropredators." In times of plenty the parallel increase in the same predators is a check against his excessive multiplication.

1289
Palmblad J, Cantell K, Holm G, Norberg R, Strander H, Sunblad L. **Acute energy deprivation in man: effect on serum immunoglobulins antibody response, complement factors 3 and 4, acute phase reactants and interferon-producing capacity of blood lymphocytes.** *Clin Exp Immunol.* 1977;30:50-5. (English)

The effects of ten days of total energy deprivation on serum levels of immunoglobulins, antibodies, acute phase reactants and on interferon production were evaluated in fourteen healthy, normal-weight males. A significant depression was noted of the serum levels of complement factor 3, haptoglobin and orosomucoid. The titres of mercaptoethanol-sensitive specific antibodies to flagellin were higher in the subjects inoculated at the end of the starvation period than in controls and those inoculated at the start of the period. The serum levels of IgG, IgM, IgA, IgE, alpha₁-antitrypsin and complement factor 4, and the interferon-producing capacity of blood lymphocytes, were not changed. Thus, 10 days of total energy deprivation depresses the serum levels of several acute phase reactants and re-feeding may enhance antibody production.

1290
Palmblad J, Halberg D, Rossner S. **Obesity, plasma lipids and polymorphonuclear (PMN) granulocyte functions.** *Scand J Haematol.* 1977;19:293-303. (English)

20 obese subjects were compared with 20 controls with normal weight regarding their polymorphonuclear (PMN) granulocyte functions, and plasma lipids. The obese subjects showed a significantly decreased PMN bactericidal capacity, and increased PMN adherence. No differences were found in their mean PMN chemotaxis and opsonic capacity of plasma. The values of plasma triglycerides and free fatty acids were higher in the obese, while plasma cholesterol and phospholipids corresponded to the control values. The changes in granulocyte function did not correlate significantly to plasma lipid levels or to body weight and Broca's index in either group. It is concluded that changes in granulocyte function occur in obesity, but are not related to plasma lipids or degree of overweight.

1291
Palmblad J. **Fasting (acute energy deprivation) in man:**

effect on polymorphonuclear granulocyte functions, plasma iron and serum transferrin. *Scand J Haematol.* 1976;17:217-26. (English)

The effect of 10 days of total fasting (energy deprivation) on blood polymorphonuclar granulocyte functions, leukocyte numbers, iron and transferrin levels was evaluated in 14 healthy, normal-weight males. Granulocytes from 7 of the subjects were tested *in vitro*. A statistically significant depression was noted in their bactericidal capacity against Staph. aureus. The 14 subjects showed a marked decrease in the stainable activity of granulocyte alkaline phosphatase and decreases were noted in the plasma iron and serum transferrin levels. The iron saturation of serum transferrin was unchanged. Thus, impairment of granulocyte bactericidal functions may occur secondarily to short-term total energy deprivation, in the absence of iron deficiency.

1292
Pertschuk MJ, Crosby LO, Barot L, Mullen JL. **Immunocompetency in anorexia nervosa.** *Am J Clin Nutr.* 1982;35:968-72. (English)

Twenty-two consecutively admitted patients diagnosed for anorexia nervosa were evaluated for cellular immune functioning by means of an anergy panel to test delayed hypersensitivity. The panel included candida, streptokinase-streptodornase, and mumps antigen administered by a standard protocol. A standard nutritional profile including current weight, usual weight, total protein, albumin, total iron-binding capacity, white blood cell count, total lymphocyte count, triceps skinfold, and arm muscle circumference was concurrently compiled on these subjects. Six of 22 patients studied were anergic. Visceral protein measures were generally within normal limits even in the most depleted patients. Malnutrition as measured by severity of weight loss and triceps skinfolds was significantly related to anergy, whereas visceral protein indicators (serum albumin, total iron binding capacity, transferrin) were not correlated with anergy. Anergy appeared to be related more strongly to anthropometric indices of malnutrition than to visceral protein values. Cellular immunity was generally preserved until weight loss was far advanced.

1293
Phillips JL. **Uptake of transferrin-bound zinc by human lymphocytes.** *Cell Immunol.* 1978;35:318-29. (English)

Uptake of transferrin-bound zinc was stimulated in phytohemagglutinin-treated human lymphocytes as compared to untreated lymphocytes. Stimulation of zinc uptake depended on the concentration of phytohemagglutinin to lymphocyte cultures. Thereafter, increased zinc uptake declined until approximately basal levels were reached 5 hr after addition of phytohemagglutinin. Stimulation of zinc uptake was insensitive to sulfhydryl reagents, but was decreased by KCN, actinomycin D, aurin tricarboxylic acid, and by lowering the incubation temperature. Two compounds, NaF and poly-L-ornithine, were found to markedly increase zinc uptake over that seen with only phytohemagglutinin. Additionally, compounds known to increase cellular levels of cyclic AMP, such as epinephrine, histamine, serotonin, glucagon, and prostaglandin E$_1$, as well as 8-bromo-cyclic AMP and dibutyryl-cyclic AMP, also increased uptake of transferrin-bound zinc by phytohemagglutinin-stimulated lymphchocytes.

1294
Ross-Smith P, Jenner FA. **Diet (gluten) and schizophrenia.** *J Hum Nutr.* 1980;34:107-12. (English)

Four aspects of clinical evidence for an association between gluten and schizophrenia are examined. The scientific evidence for the role of gluten is set out. Finally, reference is made to other dietary approaches.

1295
Sullivan JL, Ochs HD. **Copper deficiency and the immune system** (letter). *Lancet.* 1978;2:686. (English)

1296
Tengerdy RP. (et al.) **Vitamin E, immunity and disease resistance.** *Adv Exp Med Biol.* 1981;135:27-42. (English) (no abstract)

1297
Uden AM, Trang L, Venizelos N, Palmblad J. **Neutrophil functions and clinical performance after total fasting in patients with rheumatoid arthritis** (abstract). *Int Symp. of Infections in the Immunocompromised Host.* The Netherlands: Veldhofen, 1980. P. 55. (English) (unavailable at publication)

1298
Valverde E, Vich JM, Garcia-Calderon JV, Garcia-Calderon PA. **In vitro response of lymphocytes in patients with allergic tension-fatigue syndrome.** *Ann Allergy.* 1980; 45:185-8. (English)

The authors studied the stimulation of lymphocytes in 44 patients with histories of allergic tension-fatigue syndrome using a series of food extracts and additives. Of a total of 44 patients studied, 42 produced a positive response (RI), 18.1% produced a positive response to additives, 40.9% to food and 36.6% to both. The elimination diets prescribed in accordance with the *in vitro* results obtained produced a total remission of the tension-fatigue syndrome in 38 patients (86.3%), partial remission in two (4.5%) and no change in four (9.0%).

1299
Waddell CC, Taunton OD, Twomey JJ. **Inhibition of lymphoproliferation by hyperlipoproteinemic plasma.** *J Clin Invest.* 1976;58:950-4. (English)

Plasma from patients with primary type IV or V hyperlipo-proteinemia inhibited [^{3}H]thymidine incorporation by cultured mononuclear leukocytes. This previously unreported abnormality affected mononuclear leukocytes from patients with type IV or V hyperlipoproteinemia and from normal subjects. Patient cells incorporated [^{3}H]thymidine normally when washed and incubated in medium containing normal plasma. Both spontaneous incorporation and stimulated incorporation in response to various mitogens and antigens were inhibited. The inhibitory effect was identified with the chylomicron and very low density lipoprotein fractions iso-

lated from plasma and was concentration-dependent. Lectin used to stimulate cultured cells and [^{3}H]thymidine used to measure responses were not bound to the lipoproteins in appreciable amounts. [^{3}H]Thymidine incorporation correlated well with morphologic evidence of lymphoproliferation. The mechanism of the inhibitory effect of type IV or V hyperlipoproteinemic plasma upon the response tested was not identified but may be related to interaction between lipoproteins and the cell membranes. We suggest that these lipoproteins may also interfere with the function of other cells.

1300
Wynder EL, Reddy BS, McCoy GD, Weisburger JH, Williams GM. **Diet and gastrointestinal cancer.** *Clin Gastroenterol.* 1976;5:463-82. (English) (no abstract)

1301
Wynder EL, Reddy BS, McCoy GD, Weisburger JH, Williams GM. **Diet and cancer of the gastrointestinal tract.** *Adv Inter Med.* 1977;22:397-419. (English) (no abstract)

1302
Wynder EL. **Dietary habits and cancer epidemiology.** *Cancer.* 1979;43:1955-61. (English)

Data indicate that most cancers appear to be related to environmental factors and that diet is one of these factors which appears to play a vital role. Epidemiologic evidence has increasingly implicated nutritional factors in the etiology of several forms of cancer in man. The effect of specific nutritional deficiencies, as well as unbalanced metabolism from dietary excesses, is discussed in relation to colon and breast cancer development. The possibility that excessive alcohol consumption among smokers, with its associated nutritional deficiencies, could act as a tumor promoter is discussed. It is timely to integrate the work of related specialties in cancer research, for cancer can no longer be viewed as a single disease with a single etiology.

1303
Yunis EJ, Watson ALM, Shankariah K, Halberg F. **Dietary restriction and aging** (abstract). *The Gerontologist.* 1982; 22:203-4. (English)

Diets low in fat and high in protein and fiber content lead to delayed development of autoimmunity and prolonged life span of (male and female) NZB mice. The restriction of protein intake alone does not produce the same effect, though it apparently benefits T-cell functions. B/W mice fed a usual diet in restricted amounts (10 cal/day) lived at least twice as long as mice fed the same diet freely (20 cal/day). Extensive nutritional studies reveal that reduction in total food intake is responsible for inhibiting the development of autoimmune disease in B/W mice. In C$_3$H mice, which develop spontaneous mammary tumors, 2 methods have been successful in prevention or delay of tumor development: daily calorie restrictions or alternate day feeding. A difference of 16 cal/day vs. 10 cal/day showed a reduction of mortality from 71% (16 cal/day) to 0% (10 cal/day) at 500 days of age. Alternate-day feeding also reduces the mammary tumor incidence of C$_3$H female mice. Mice fed *ad libitum* had a tumor incidence of

83%, whereas mice on the alternate-day feeding schedule had only a 53% incidence of mammary tumors (p<0.005).

1304
Zumoff B. **Influence of obesity and malnutrition on the metabolism of some cancer-related hormones.** *Cancer Res.* 1981;41:3805-7. (English)

It has been suggested that the well-documented relationship of dietary composition to the incidence of human breast cancer is mediated by the effects of dietary constituents on hormone levels. There is fairly good evidence for diet-hormone relationships in animals, but the evidence in humans is unconvincing. In this paper, we describe three of our findings relating nutrition to hormone levels: (a) that obesity causes retention of a tracer of estradiol in women but not in men, a finding we attribute to the presence of specific estrogen receptor in the adipose tissue of women but not men; (b) that obese men have elevated plasma estrone and estradiol levels but obese women do not, a finding we attribute to greater androstenedione-to-estrone conversion in the adipose tissue of men than in that of women; and (c) that cachectic girls with anorexia nervosa fail to have the normal nocturnal surge of prolactin secretion, a finding that we attribute to deficiency of tryptophan, which is an adequate stimulus for prolactin secretion. These findings give support to the concept that dietary factors affect hormone secretion and/or metabolism in humans.

Appendix

Review articles

1305

Ader R. **Presidential address, 1980: Psychosomatic and psychoimmunologic research.** *Psychosom Med.* 1980; 42:307-21. (English) (no abstract)

1306

Blackwell B. **Current psychiatric research: psycho-immunology.** *Psychiatric Opinion.* 1980;17:4. (English) (no abstract)

1307

Cox T, Mackay C. **Psychosocial factors and psychophysiological mechanisms in the aetiology and development of cancers.** *Soc Sci Med.* 1982;16:381-96. (English)

Socio-cultural factors which may play a contributory role in the aetiology of cancer have been extensively investigated and it is well established that the incidence rates of different forms and sites of the disease are not equally distributed throughout the population. Social class, occupational, environmental and "life-style" differences, amongst others, have been found to be associated with an excess risk of cancer, although the argument concerning the relative importance of these various factors remains a controversial one. It seems increasingly clear however, that there are large behavioural components which govern exposure to potential carcinogens and there is growing interest in the extent to which social and psychological demands may be associated with these agents or may operate as contributory factors in their own right. A number of early studies of psychological approaches to the study of cancer aetiology are reviewed from a methodological perspective. Much of the early work suffered from the problem that psychological characteristics of individuals who already had cancer were used to construct models concerned with aetiological factors. A number of the more recent studies which have attempted to overcome these difficulties are discussed. Tentatively, these later investigations suggest that two main groups of factors are related to an increased risk of cancer. First, the loss of, or lack of closeness or attachment to an important relation (often a parent) early in life, and second, the inability to express hostile feelings or more generally the abnormal release of emotion. Several psychophysiological mechanisms are reviewed which have attempted to account for the relationship between psychological disturbances and the onset of cancer, particularly the growing evidence which implicated a role for the immune system as a link between the central nervous system and disease processes.

1308

Engel GL. **The clinical application of the biopsychosocial model.** *Am J Psychiatr.* 1980;137:535-44. (English) (unavailable at publication)

1309

Martin MJ. **Psychosomatic medicine: a brief history.** *Psychosomatics.* 1978;19:697-700. (English) (no abstract)

1310

McKegney FP. **Psychoneuroimmunology: what lies ahead.** *Drug Therapy.* 1982;August:61-71. (English) (no abstract)

1311

Murray JB. **New trends in psychosomatic research.** *Genetic Psychology Monographs.* 1977;96:3-74. (English)

Advances in physiological psychology and neuroendocrinology, together with epidemiological studies, have added new dimensions to psychosomatic research. Psychological influences still are accepted as exacerbators or trigger mechanisms, if less often as causes. Theories of psychosomatics which connected specific personality profiles with specific psychosomatic illnesses have lost favor, and multifactorial explanations, which include heredity, environment, social class, life stress, endocrines, brain areas, neurohormones, and immunological mechanisms, are new areas of research. Research methods have become more sophisticated scientifically, particularly in the selection and size of samples tested and the variety of situations investigated. Psychological reactions to illness in general, terminal disease, and death, and psychological experiences of pain, in addition to variable effects of psychotherapeutic methods and psychotherapists' personality, are identifiable but unquantified influences which seem acceptable as contributors to, if not causes of, psychophysiological disorders.

1312

Rogers MP, Dubey D, Reich P. **The influence of the psyche and the brain on immunity and disease susceptibility: a critical review.** *Psychosom Med.* 1979;41:147-64. (English)

In critically reviewing the sources of evidence connecting psyche and brain with the immune system, the authors include a brief review of current knowledge of the immune system, its interactions with the neuroendocrine system, and other factors influencing its regulation. These include developmental stages, aging, rhythmicity, and a variety of exogenous influences. The need for developing further information about normal base lines is emphasized. Against that background, many sources of data demonstrating connections between the central nervous system and the immune system are presented: indirect evidence from clinical and experimental illnesses involving the immune system, and direct changes in either humoral or cellular immunity after natural or experimental stress, conditioning, hypnosis, and direct brain stimulation. Possible mechanisms are discussed, as well as some important methodological issues for further research.

1313
Solomon GF, Amkraut AA. **Psychoneuroendocrinological effects on the immune response** (review). *Annu Rev Microbiol.* 1981;35:155-84. (English) (unavailable at publication)

1314
Stein M. **A biopsychosocial approach to immune function and medical disorders.** *Psychiatr Clin N Am.* 1981; 4:203-21. (English)

This review suggests that an extensive network of central nervous system, neurotransmitter, endocrine, and other biological processes may be involved in the modulation of the immune system. In addition, considerable evidence demonstrating a relationship between psychosocial factors and immune functions is accumulating. Psychosocial processes may be reflected in changes in central nervous system activity, and pathways linking limbic and higher cortical areas with the hypothalamus may be involved in the effects of psychosocial processes on visceral, endocrine, and immune functions. The interaction of biopsychosocial phenomena with the immune system may, in turn, alter the development, onset, and course of a range of medical diseases. This article has emphasized that there is no single specific factor involved in illness. A long chain of relevant biopsychosocial processes appear to be involved. As pointed out by Weiner, the general approach has given way to a consideration of smaller subgroups of the various entities because of many newly discovered mechanisms. As we acquire increasing knowledge of biologic control mechanisms, the processes underlying syndromes appear to be quite complex and continuous rather than discrete. The notion of specificity persists, but there has been a shift from the specificity associated with a disorder to a specificity within the individual. As knowledge is unfolding, predisposing risk factors are being elucidated which may provide a means for studying individuals prior to the onset of an illness and enable us to ascertain whether biopsychosocial systems are involved antecedent to a disease, at its onset, or as a consequence of an illness. The conceptualization and utilization of a biopsychosocial model in medicine does not limit its application to only a specific group of disorders, but rather provides a comprehensive approach to all aspects of health and illness.

1315
Weiner H. **The illusion of simplicity: the medical model revisited.** *Am J Psychiat.* 1978;135:27-33. (English)

Traditional medical models have been found to be linear, restrictive, and oversimplified. Only a truly biological model, encompassing evolutionary as well as molecular and cellular biology, can account for the complex origins, forms, and effects of disease. These are illustrated by a discussion of hepatitis B and slow virus disease. An updated biological model of disease takes into account predisposition to disease, the timing and route of infection, multiple disease forms, variable adaptive response, and the role of social and cultural factors and views disease as a failure of adaptation in one or more systems. Its application to psychiatry is shown in a discussion of stress, bereavement, and separation.

Books and book chapters

1316
Achterberg J, Simonton OC, Matthews-Simonton S. **Stress: Psychological Factors and Cancer.** Fort Worth, Texas: New Medicine Press, 1976.

1317
Ader R, Cohen N. **Conditioned immunopharmacologic responses.** In: *Psychoneuroimmunology.* R Ader (ed.). NY: Academic Press, 1981. Pp. 281-319. (English)

1318
Ader R. **A historical account of conditioned immunobiologic responses.** In: *Psychoneuroimmunology.* R Ader (ed.). NY: Academic Press, 1981. Pp. 321-52. (English)

1319
Ader R. **Animal models in the study of brain, behavior and bodily disease.** In: *Brain, Behavior and Bodily Disease.* Research Publications: Association fnr Research in Nervous and Mental Disease, Vol. 59. H Weiner, M A Hofer, A J Stunkard (eds.). NY: Raven Press, 1981. Pp. 11-26. (English)

1320
Ader R. **Behavioral influences on immune responses.** In: *Perspectives on Behavioral Medicine.* S M Weiss, J A Herd, B H Fox (eds.). NY: Academic Press, 1981. Pp. 163-81. (English)

1321
Ader R. (ed.) **Psychoneuroimmunology.** NY: Academic Press, 1981. (English)

1322
Ahlqvist J. **Hormonal influences on immunologic and related phenomena.** In: *Psychoneuroimmunology.* R Ader (ed.). NY: Academic Press, 1981. Pp. 355-403. (English)

1323
Anisman H, Sklar LS. **Stress provoked neurochemical changes in relation to neoplasia.** In: *Biological Mediators of Behavior and Disease: Neoplasia.* S M Levy (ed.). NY: Elsevier Biomedical, 1982. Pp. 123-45. (English)

1324
Anonymous. **Lithium effects on granulopoiesis and immune function.** In: *Adv Exp Med Biol.* 1980;127:1-475. (English)

1325

Antonovsky A. **Health, Stress and Coping.** San Francisco: Jossey-Bass, 1981. (English)

1326

Bach JF, Bach MA, Carnaud C, Dardenne M, Monier JC. **Thymic hormones and autoimmunity.** In: *Autoimmunity: Genetic, Immunologic, Virologic and Clinical Aspects.* N Talal (ed.). NY: Academic Press, 1977. Pp. 207-30. (English)

1327

Bahnson CB. **Emotional and personality characteristics of cancer patients.** In: *Oncologic Medicine: Clinical Topics and Practical Management.* A I Sutnick, P F Engstrom (eds.). Baltimore: University Park Press, 1976. (English)

1328

Bahnson CB. **Psychosomatic issues in cancer.** In: *The Psychosomatic Approach to Illness.* R L Gallon (ed.). NY: Elsevier Biomedical, 1982. Pp. 53-87. (English)

1329

Bakal DA. **Psychology and Medicine: Psychobiological Dimensions of Health and Illness.** NY: Springer Publ. Co., 1979. (English)

1330

Bakshi K, Brusick D, Bullock L, Bardin CW. **Hormonal regulation of carcinogen metabolism in mouse kidney.** In: *Origins of Human Cancer.* Book B. H H Hiatt, J D Watson, J A Winsten (eds.). Cold Spring Harbor, NY: Cold Spring Harbor Laboratory, 1977. Pp. 683-95. (English)

1331

Bammer K, Newberry BH. (eds.) **Impact of Stress on Immunity and Cancer.** Toronto: C.J. Hogrefe, Inc., 1982. (English)

1332

Bammer K, Newberry BH. (eds.) **Stress and Cancer.** Toronto: C.J. Hogrefe, Inc., 1982. (English)

1333

Bell IR. **Clinical Ecology: A New Medical Approach to Environmental Illness.** Bolinas, CA: Common Knowledge Press, 1982. (English)

1334

Besedovsky HO, Sorkin E. **Immunologic-neuroendocrine circuits: physiological approaches.** In: *Psychoneuroimmunology.* R Ader (ed.). NY: Academic Press, 1981. Pp. 545-74. (English)

1335

Bieliauskas L. **Stress and its relationship to health and illness.** Boulder, CO: Westview Press, 1982. (English)

1336

Bloom JR, Ross RD. **Measurement of the psychological aspects of cancer: sources of bias.** In: *Psychosocial Aspects of Cancer.* J Cohen et al. (eds). NY: Raven Press, 1982. Pp. 255-74. (English)

1337

Bloom JR. **Social support systems and cancer: a conceptual view.** In: *Psychosocial Aspects of Cancer.* J Cohen, J W Cullen, L R Martin (eds.). NY: Raven Press, 1982. Pp. 129-50. (English)

1338

Bock E. **Plasma and CSF proteins in schizophrenia.** In: *Neurochemical and Immunologic Components in Schizophrenia.* D Bergsma, A L Goldstein (eds.). NY: Alan R. Liss, Inc., 1978. Pp. 283-95. (English)

1339

Borysenko J. **Higher cortical function and neoplasia: psychoneuroimmunology.** In: *Biological Mediators of Behavior and Disease: Neoplasia.* S M Levy (ed.). NY: Elsevier Biomedical, 1982. Pp. 29-53. (English)

1340

Boushey HA. **Neural mechanisms in asthma.** In: *Brain, Behavior and Bodily Disease.* Research Publications: Association for Research in Nervous and Mental Disease, Vol. 59. H Weiner, M A Hofer, A J Stunkard (eds.). NY: Raven Press, 1981. Pp. 27-44. (English)

1341

Bunney W Jr, Shapiro A, Ader R, Davis J, Herd A, Kopin IJ Jr, Krieger D, Matthysse S, Stunkard A, Weissman M, Wyatt RJ. **Panel report on stress and illness.** In: *Stress and Human Health: Analysis and Implications of Research.* G R Elliott, C Eisdorfer (eds.). NY: Springer Publishing Co., 1982. Pp. 255-337. (English)

1342

Byron JW. **Cyclic nucleotides and the cell growth of the hematopoietic stem cell.** In: *Cylic Nucleotides and the Regulation of Cell Growth.* M Abou-Sabe (ed.). Stroudsburg: Dowden, Hutchinson & Ross, Inc., 1976. Pp. 81-93. (English)

1343

Chandra RK. **Immunology of Nutritional Disorders.** London: Edward Arnold, Ltd., 1980. (English)

1344

Chebotariov VF. **Endocrinal Regulation of Immunogenesis.** Kiev, 1979. (Russian)

1345

Ciaranello R, Lipton M, Barchas J, Barchas PR, Bonica J, Ferrario C, Levine S, Stein M. **Panel report on biological substrates of stress.** In: *Stress and Human Health: Analysis and Implications of Research.* G R Elliott, C Eisdorfer (eds.). NY: Springer Publishing Co., 1982. Pp. 189-254. (English)

1346

Cohen J, Cullen JW, Martin LR. (eds.) **Psychosocial Aspects of Cancer.** NY: Raven Press, 1982. (English)

1347

Cohen MM. **Psychosocial morbidity in cancer: a clinical perspective.** In: *Psychosocial Aspects of Cancer.* J Cohen, J

W Cullen, L R Martin (eds.). NY: Raven Press, 1982. Pp. 117-28. (English)

1348
Cohen SI, Ross RD. **Progress in Psychoimmunology.** (in press) (English)

1349
Cohen SI. **Some implications of current neuropeptide studies for clinical psychophysiology of the future.** In: *Neuropeptide Influences on the Brain and Behavior.* L H Miller, C A Sandman, A J Kastin (eds.). NY: Raven Press, 1977. Pp. 269-91. (English)

1350
Cullen JW. **Coping and health: a clinician's perspective.** In: *Coping and Health.* S Levine, H Ursin (eds.). NY: Plenum Press, 1980. Pp. 295-322. (English)

1351
Cullen JW. **Role of the social and behavioral sciences in cancer prevention.** In: *Psychosocial Aspects of Cancer.* J Cohen, J W Cullen, L R Martin (eds.). NY: Raven Press, 1982. Pp. 33-38. (English)

1352
Cunningham AJ. **Mind, body and immune response.** In: *Psychoneuroimmunology.* R Ader (ed.). NY: Academic Press, 1981. Pp. 609-17. (English)

1353
Cunningham AJ. **Should we investigate psychotherapy for physical disease, especially cancer?** In: *Biological Mediators of Behavior and Disease: Neoplasia.* S M Levy (ed.). NY: Elsevier Biomedical, 1982. Pp. 83-100. (English)

1354
Curtis GC. **Psychoendocrine stress response: steroid and peptide hormones.** In: *Mind and Cancer Prognosis.* BA Stoll (ed.). London: Wiley, 1979. (English)

1335
D'Onofrio CN. **Psychosocial research needed to improve the use and evaluation of cancer screening techniques.** In: *Psychosocial Aspects of Cancer.* J Cohen, J W Cullen, L R Martin (eds.). NY: Raven Press, 1982. Pp. 57-72. (English)

1356
Daleva M, Piperova D, Nakasheva E, Tsaneva N. **Changes in circadian rhythm of catecholamine excretion in shift workers under neuroemotional stress.** In: *Catecholamines and Stress: Recent Advances.* Usdin, Kvetnansky, Kopin (eds.) Amsterdam: Elsevier North Holland, 1980. Pp. 471-6. (English)

1357
Fabris N. **Hormones and aging.** In: *Immunology and Aging* . T Makinodan, E Yunis (eds.). New York: Plenum Press, 1977. Pp. 73-89. (English)

1358
Faulk WP, Cockrell JR. **Nutrition and immunity: possible new approaches to research in schizophrenia.** In: *The Biological Basis of Schizophrenia.* G Hemmings, W A Hemmings (eds.). Baltimore: University Park Press, 1978. Pp. 231-8. (English)

1359
Fobair P, Cordoba CS. **Scope and magnitude of the cancer problem in psychosocial research.** In: *Psychosocial Aspects of Cancer.* J Cohen, J W Cullen, L R Martin (eds.). NY: Raven Press, 1982. Pp. 9-31. (English)

1360
Fox BH, Boyd S, Van Kammen DP, Rogentine GN Jr. **Further analysis of psychological variables in predicting relapse after stage II melanoma surgery.** In: *Proc Third Int Symp Psychobiol Psychophysiol Psychosom Sociosom Aspects Neoplastic Dis.* Bohinj, Yugoslavia, 1978. (English) (in press, 1980)

1361
Fox BH. **A psychological measure as a predictor in cancer.** In: *Psychosocial Aspects of Cancer.* J Cohen, J W Cullen, L R Martin (eds.). New York: Raven Press, 1982. Pp. 275-95. (English)

1362
Fox BH. **Behavioral issues in cancer.** In: *Perspectives on Behavioral Medicine.* S M Weiss, J A Herd, B H Fox (eds.). NY: Academic Press, 1981. Pp. 101-133. (English)

1363
Fox BH. **Endogenous psychosocial factors in cross-national cancer incidence.** In: *Social Psychology and Behavioral Medicine.* J R Eiser (ed.). London: Wiley, 1982. Pp. 101-41. (English)

1364
Fox BH. **Psychological factors and cancer.** In: *Psychological Dimensions of Cancer.* J Cohen, J W Cullen, L R Martin (eds.). NY: Raven Press, 1981. (English)

1365
Fox BH. **Psychosocial factors and the immune system in human cancer.** In: *Psychoneuroimmunology.* R Ader (ed.). NY: Academic Press, 1981. Pp. 103-57. (English)

1366
Gajdusek DC. **The possible role of slow virus infection in chronic schizophrenia dementia.** In: *Neurochemical and Immunologic Components in Schizophrenia.* D Bergsma, A L Goldstein (eds.). NY: Alan R. Liss, Inc., 1978. Pp. 81-7. (English)

1367
Goldstein AL, Cohen GH, Thurman GB, Hooper JA, Rossio JL. **Regulation of immune balance of thymosin: potential role in the development of suppressor T cells.** In: *Immune Reactivity of Lymphocytes.* M Feldman, A Globerson (eds.). NY: Plenum Press, 1976. Pp. 221-8. (English)

1368
Green LW, Rimer B, Elwood TW. **Biobehavioral ap-**

proaches to cancer prevention and detection. In: *Perspectives on Behavioral Medicine*. S M Weiss, J A Herd, B H Fox (eds.). NY: Academic Press, 1981. Pp. 215-33. (English)

1369
Hall NR, Goldstein AL. **Neurotransmitters and the immune system.** In: *Psychoneuroimmmunology*. R Ader (ed.). NY: Academic Press, 1981. Pp. 521-43. (English)

1370
Hall NR, McGillis JP, Spangelo B, Palaxzynski E, Moody T, Goldstein AL. **Evidence for a neuroendocrine-thymus axis mediated by thymosin polypeptide.** In: *Human Cancer Immunology*. Vol. 2. B Serrou (ed.). NY: Elsevier North-Holland, 1981.

1371
Hall NR. **Neuroendocrine interactions with immunogenesis.** In: *Molecular and Behavioral Neuroendocrinology*. C B Nemeroff, A J Dunn (eds.). NY: Spectrum, in press. (English)

1372
Hekkens WTJM. **Antibodies to gliadin in serum of normals, coeliac patients and schizophrenics.** In: *Biological Basis of Schizophrenia*. G Hemmings, A Hemmings (eds.). Baltimore: University Park, 1978. Pp. 259-61. (English)

1373
Henry JP, Stephens PM. **Stress, Health, and the Social Environment.** New York:Springer-Verlag, 1977. (English)

1374
Herberman RB. **Possible effects of central nervous system on natural killer (NK) cell activity.** In: *Biological Mediators of Behavior and Disease: Neoplasia*. S M Levy (ed.). NY: Elsevier Biomedical, 1982. Pp. 235-48. (English)

1375
Holland JC, Rowland JH. **Psychiatric, psychosocial and behavioral interventions in the treatment of cancer: an historical overview.** In: *Perspectives on Behavioral Medicine*. S M Weiss, J A Herd, B H Fox (eds.). NY: Academic Press, 1981. Pp. 235-59. (English)

1376
Joseph JG, Syme SL. **Social connection and the etiology of cancer: an epidemiological review and discussion.** In: *Psychosocial Aspects of Cancer*. J Cohen, J W Cullen, L R Martin (eds.). NY: Raven Press, 1982. Pp. 151-62. (English)

1377
Kalisnik M, Vraspir-Porenta C, Logonder-Mlinsek M, Zorc M, Pajntar M. **Interaction of stress and transplanted Ehrlich ascitic tumor in mice.** In: *Proc Third Int Symp Psychobiol Psychophysiol Psychosom Sociosom Aspects Neoplastic Dis*. Bohinj, Yugoslavia, 1978. (English) (in press, 1980)

1378
Karush A, Daniels GE, Flood C, O'Connor JF. **Psychotherapy in chronic ulcerative colitis.** Philadelphia: W.B. Saunders Co., 1977. (English)

1379
Keirns JJ, Birnbaum JE, Moore JB. **Cyclic nucleotides in proliferation and immunological diseases.** In: *Cyclic 3',5'-Nucleotides: Mechanisms of Action*. H Cramer, J Schultz (eds.). NY: John Wiley and Sons, 1977. Pp. 415-33. (English)

1380
Keller RH, Calvanico NJ, Tomasi TB Jr. **Immunosuppressive properties of AFP: role of estrogens.** In: *Onco-Developmental Gene Expression*. W H Fishman, S Sell (eds.). NY: Academic Press, 1976. Pp. 287-95. (English)

1381
Korneva EA, Klimenko VM, Shkhinek EK. **Neurohumoral Maintenance of Immune Homeostasis.** Leningrad: Nauka, 1978. (Russian) (English translation in preparation: U. of Chicago Press)

1382
Kujalova V, Komarek L, Sperlingova I, Zeleny A. **Work strain evaluation by catecholamine excretion.** In: *Catecholamines and Stress: Recent Advances*. Usdin, Kvetnansky, Kopin (eds.). Amsterdam: Elsevier North Holland, 1980. Pp. 467-70. (English)

1383
Lanning M. **Spontaneous, PPD Tuberculin and Phytohaemmaggluninin (PHA)-induced Transformation of Blood Lymphocytes in Man from Birth to Old Age.** Oulu, Finland: Acta Univ Ouluensis, 1978. (English)

1384
Lazarus RS. **Psychological stress and coping in adaptation and illness.** In: *Psychosomatic Medicine: Current Trends and Clinical Applications*. Z J Lipowski, D R Lipsitt, P C Whybrow (eds.). NY: Oxford Univ. Press, 1977. (English)

1385
Lazarus RS. **Stress and coping as factors in health and illness.** In: *Psychosocial Aspects of Cancer*. J Cohen, J W Cullen, L R Martin (eds.). NY: Raven Press, 1982. Pp. 163-90. (English)

1386
Levy SM. (ed.) **Biological Mediators of Behavior and Disease: Neoplasia.** NY: Elsevier Biomedical, 1982. (English)

1387
Lichtenstein LM. **Hormone receptor modulation of cAMP in the control of allergic and inflammatory responses.** In: *The Role of Immunologic Factors in Infectious, Allergic, and Autoimmune Processes*. R F Beers Jr, E G Bassett (eds.). NY: Raven Press, 1976. Pp. 339-54. (English)

1388
Lippman M. **Interactions of psychic and endocrine factors with progression of neoplastic diseases.** In: *Biological Mediators of Behavior and Disease: Neoplasia*. S M Levy (ed.). NY: Elsevier Biomedical, 1982. Pp. 55-82. (English)

1389
Locke SE, Ader R, Besedovsky H, Hall N, Solomon GF, Strom T. (eds.) **Classics in Psychoneuroimmunology.** NY: Aldine Publishing Co., in press. (English)

1390
Locke SE, Kraus LJ. **Modulation of natural killer cell activity by life stress and coping ability.** In: *Biological Mediators of Behavior and Disease: Neoplasia.* S M Levy (ed.). NY: Elsevier North-Holland, 1982. Pp.3-28. (English)

1391
Lundberg U. **Catecholamine and cortisol excretion under psychologically different laboratory conditions.** In: *Catecholamines and Stress: Recent Advances.* Usdin, Kvetnansky, Kopin (eds.). Amsterdam: Elsevier North Holland, 1980. Pp. 455-66. (English)

1392
Maccalla TA. **Sociocultural dimensions relevant to preventing cancer.** In: *Psychosocial Aspects of Cancer.* J Cohen, J W Cullen, L R Martin (eds.). NY: Raven Press, 1982. Pp. 103-110. (English)

1393
Maclean D, Reichlin S. **Neuroendocrinology and the immune process.** In: *Psychoneuroimmunology.* R Ader (ed.). NY: Academic Press, 1981. Pp. 475-520. (English)

1394
Maestroni GJ, Pierpaoli W. **Pharmacologic control of the hormonally mediated immune response.** In: *Psychoneuroimmunology.* R Ader (ed.). NY: Academic Press, 1981. Pp. 405-28. (English)

1395
Makinodan T, Yunis EJ. (eds.) **Immunology and Aging.** NY: Plenum Press, 1977. (English)

1396
Mantell JE. **Sexuality and cancer.** In: *Psychosocial Aspects of Cancer.* J Cohen, J W Cullen, L R Martin (eds.). NY: Raven Press, 1982. Pp. 235-48. (English)

1397
Martin LR. **Overview of the psychosocial aspects of cancer.** In: *Psychosocial Aspects of Cancer.* J Cohen, J W Cullen, L R Martin (eds.) NY: Raven Press, 1982. Pp. (English)

1398
Miller NE. **A perspective on the effects of stress and coping on disease and health.** In: *Coping and Health.* S Levine, H Ursin (eds.). NY: Plenum Press, 1980. Pp. 323-53. (English)

1399
Miller NE. **An overview of behavioral medicine: opportunities and dangers.** In: *Perspectives on Behavioral Medicine.* S M Weiss, J A Herd, B H Fox (eds.). NY: Academic Press, 1981. Pp. (English)

1400
Miller NE. **Some behavioral factors relevant to cancer.** In: *Biological Mediators of Behavior and Disease: Neoplasia.* S M Levy (ed.). NY: Elsevier Biomedical, 1982. Pp. 113-22. (English)

1401
Miller T, Spratt JS Jr. **Critical review of reported psychological correlates of cancer prognosis and growth.** In: *Mind and Cancer Prognosis.* B A Stoll (ed.). London: Wiley, 1979. (English)

1402
Monjan AA. **Stress and immunologic competence: studies in animals.** In: *Psychoneuroimmunology.* R Ader (ed.). NY: Academic Press, 1981. Pp. 185-228. (English)

1403
Morrison FR, Paffenbarger RA Jr. **Epidemiologic aspects of biobehavior in the etiology of cancer: a critical review.** In: *Perspectives on Behavioral Medicine.* S M Weiss, J A Herd, B H Fox (eds.). NY: Academic Press, 1981. Pp. 135-61. (English)

1404
Nemeth G. **Prospective psychologic and somatic examinations of patients who later developed carcinoma.** In: *Proc Third Int Symp Psychobiol Psychophysiol Psychosom Sociosom Aspects Neoplastic Dis.* Bohinj, Yugoslavia, 1978. (English) (in press, 1980)

1405
Newberry BH. **Effects of presumably stressful stimulation (PSS) on the development of animal tumors: some issues.** In: *Perspectives on Behavioral Medicine.* S M Weiss, J A Herd, B H Fox (eds.). New York: Academic Press, 1981. Pp. 329-49. (English)

1406
Newberry BH. **Stress and mammary cancer.** In: *Stress and Cancer.* K Bammer, B H Newberry (eds.). Toronto: C.J. Hogrefe, 1981. Pp. 233-64. (English)

1407
Paffenbarger RS. **Psychosocial Factors in Students Predictive of Cancer.** *Grant No. 1R01CA225 74-01, National Cancer Institute, Bethesda MD.* 1977. (English)

1408
Palmblad J. **Stress and immunologic competence: studies in man.** In: *Psychoneuroimmunology.* R Ader (ed.). NY: Academic Press, 1981. Pp. 229-57. (English)

1409
Panagis DM. **Psychological factors and cancer outcome.** In: *Psychosocial Aspects of Cancer.* J Cohen, J W Cullen, L R Martin (eds.). NY: Raven Press, 1982. Pp. 209-20. (English)

1410
Parker CW. **The role of intracellular mediators in the immune response.** In: *Biology of the Lymphokines.* S Cohen, E Pick, J J Oppenheim (eds.). NY: Academic Press, 1979. Pp 541-83. (English)

Cohen, E Pick, J J Oppenheim (eds.). NY: Academic Press, 1979. Pp. 541-83. (English)

1411
Pelletier K R. **Mind as Healer: Mind as Slayer.** San Francisco: Delacorte Press, 1977. (English)

1412
Peters LJ, Mason KA. **Influence of stress on experimental cancer.** In: *Mind and Cancer Prognosis.* BA Stoll (ed.). London: Wiley, 1979. (English)

1413
Pierpaoli W, Haemmerli M, Sorkin E, Hurni H. **Role of thymus and hypothalamus in ageing.** In: *European Symposium on Basic Research in Gerontology.* 1977. Pp. 141-50. (English)

1414
Pierpaoli W. **Integrated phylogenetic and ontogenetic evolution of neuroendocrine and identity-defense, immune functions.** In: *Psychoneuroimmunology.* R Ader (ed.). NY: Academic Press, 1981. Pp. 575-606. (English)

1415
Plaut SM, Friedman SB. **Psychosocial factors in infectious disease.** In: *Psychoneuroimmunology.* R Ader (ed). NY: Academic Press, 1981. Pp. 3-30. (English)

1416
Ponten J. **Abnormal cell growth (neoplasia) and aging.** In: *Handbook of the Biology of Aging.* C E Finch, L Hayflick (eds.). Princeton: Van Nostrand-Reinold, 1977. Pp. 536-60. (English)

1417
Riley V, Fitzmaurice MA, Spackman DH. **Animal models in biobehavioral research: effects of anxiety stress on immunocompetence and neoplasia.** In: *Perspectives on Behavioral Medicine.* S M Weiss, J A Herd, B H Fox (eds.). NY: Academic Press, 1981. (English)

1418
Riley V, Fitzmaurice MA, Spackman DH. **Biobehavioral factors in animal work on tumorigenesis.** In: *Perspectives on Behavioral Medicine.* S M Weiss, J A Herd, B H Fox (eds.). NY: Academic Press, 1981. Pp. 183-213. (English)

1419
Riley V, Fitzmaurice MA, Spackman DH. **Immunocompetence and neoplasia: role of anxiety stress.** In: *Biological Mediators of Behavior and Disease: Neoplasia.* S M Levy (ed.). NY: Elsevier Biomedical, 1982. Pp. 175-217. (English)

1420
Riley V, Fitzmaurice MA, Spackman DH. **Psychoneuroimmunologic factors in neoplasia: studies in animals.** In: *Psychoneuroimmunology.* R Ader (ed) NY: Academic Press, 1981. Pp. 31-102. (English)

1421
Riley V. **Stress and cancer: fresh perspectives.** In: *Proc*

Int Symp Detect Prev Cancer, 3rd. NY: Marcel Dekker Inc., 1978. Pp. 1769-76. (English)

1422
Rimon R, Halonen P. **Antibody levels to viruses in psychiatric illness.** In: *The Impact of Biology on Modern Psychiatry.* Gershon ES, et al. (eds.) New York: Plenum Press, 1977. Pp. 105-12. (English)

1423
Rose RM. **Endocrine responses to stressful psychological events.** In: *Advances in Psychoneuroendocrinology.* The Psychiatric Clinics of North America (Vol. 3, No. 2). E J Sachar (ed.). Philadelphia: W.B. Saunders Co., 1980. Pp. 251-76. (English)

1424
Schmale AH. **Discussion of "Stress and coping as factors in health and illness" by Lazarus.** In: *Psychosocial Aspects of Cancer.* J Cohen, J W Cullen, L R Martin (eds.). NY: Raven Press, 1982. Pp. 191-8. (English)

1425
Sharkis SJ, Ahmed A, Sensenbrenner LL, Jedrzecjzak WW, Goldstein AL, Sell KW. **The regulation of hematopoiesis: effect of thymosin or thymocytes in a diffusion chamber.** In: *Experimental Hematology jToday. Vol 2.* S J Baum, G D Ledney (eds.). New York: Springer Verlag, 1979. Pp. 17-22. (English)

1426
Shaskan EG, Oreland L, Wadel G. **Is there functional significance for dopamine antagonist binding sites upon lymphoid cells?** In: *Research on Viral Hypothesis of Mental Disorders.* PV Morozov (ed.). Basel, Switzerland: S Karger AG, Medical and Scientific Publishers, in press. (English)

1427
Simonton OC, Matthews-Simonton S, Creighton J. **Getting Well Again.** Los Angeles: J.P. Tarcher, Inc., 1978. (English)

1428
Solomon GF, Amkraut AA, Rubin R. **Stress and psychoimmunological response.** In: *Mind and Cancer Prognosis.* B A Stoll (ed.). London: Wiley, 1979. (English)

1429
Solomon GF, Amkraut AA, Rubin RT. **Stress and psychoimmunological response.** In: *Proc Acad Behav Med Res.* S Weiss (ed.). NY: Academic Press, 1980. (English)

1430
Solomon GF. **Emotional and personality factors in rheumatoid arthritis and other autoimmune disease.** In: *Psychoneuroimmunology.* R Ader (ed.). NY: Press, 1981. Pp. 159-82. (English)

1431
Solomon GF. **Immunologic abnormalities in mental illness.** In: *Psychoneuroimmunology.* R Ader (ed.). NY: Academic Press, 1981. Pp. 259-78. (English)

1432

Spector NH, Korneva EA. **Neurophysiology, immuno-physiology and immunomodulation.** In: *Psychoneuro-immunology*. R Ader (ed.). NY: Academic Press, 1981. Pp. 449-73. (English)

1433

Spinetta JJ. **A guide to psychosocial field research in cancer.** In: *Psychosocial Aspects of Cancer*. J Cohen, J W Cullen, L R Martin (eds.). NY: Raven Press, 1982. Pp. 249-54. (English)

1434

Stein M, Keller SE, Schleifer SJ. **Role of the hypothalamus in mediating stress effects on the immune system.** In: *Mind and Cancer Prognosis*. B A Stoll (ed.). London: Wiley, 1979. (English)

1435

Stein M, Keller SE, Schleifer SJ. **The hypothalamus and the immune response.** In: *Brain, Behavior and Bodily Disease*. Research Publications: Association for Research in Nervous and Mental Disease, Vol. 59. H Weiner, M A Hofer, A J Stunkard (eds.). NY: Raven Press, 1981. Pp. 45-66. (English)

1436

Stein M, Keller SE, Schleifer SJ. **The roles of brain and the neuroendocrine system in immune regulation: potential links to neoplastic disease.** In: *Biological Mediators of Behavior and Disease: Neoplasia*. S M Levy (ed.). NY: Elsevier Biomedical, 1982. Pp. 147-74. (English)

1437

Stein M, Schleifer SJ, Keller SE. **Hypothalamic influences on immune responses.** In: *Psychoneuroimmunology*. R Ader (ed.). NY: Academic Press, 1981. Pp. 429-47. (English)

1438

Stein M. **Biopsychosocial factors in bronchial asthma.** In: *Critical Issues in Behavioral Medicine*. L J West, M Stein (eds.). Philadelphia: J.B. Lippincott Co., 1982. (English)

1439

Stoll BA. (ed.) **Mind and Cancer Prognosis.** London: Wiley, 1979. (English)

1440

Tache J, Selye H, Day SB. **Cancer, Stress and Death.** NY: Plenum Medical Book Co., 1979. (English)

1441

Vartanian ME, Koliaskina GI, Lozovskii DV, Burbaeva GSH, Ignatov SA. **Aspects of humoral and cellular immunity in schizophrenia.** In: *Birth Defects*. 1978;14:339-64. (English)

1442

Wayner L, Cox T, Mackay C. **Stress, immunity and cancer.** In: *Research in Psychology and Medicine*. Vol 1. D J Osbourne, M M Gruenberg, J R Eiser (eds.) NY: Academic Press, 1979. Pp. 108-16. (English)

1443

Weiner H. **Brain, behavior and bodily disease: a summary.** In: *Brain, Behavior and Bodily Disease*. Research Publications: Association for Research in Nervous and Mental Disease, Vol. 59. H Weiner, M A Hofer, A J Stunkard (eds.). NY: Raven Press, 1981. Pp. 335-369. (English)

1444

Weiner H. **Bronchial asthma.** In: *Psychobiology and Human Disease*. NY: Elsevier, 1977. Pp. 219-317. (English)

1445

Weiner H. **Graves' disease.** In: *Psychobiology and Human Disease*. H Weiner. NY: Elsevier, 1977. Pp. 319-413. (English)

1446

Weiner H. **Rheumatoid arthritis.** In: *Psychobiology and Human Disease*. H Weiner. NY: Elsevier, 1977. Pp. 415-493. (English)

1447

Weiner H. **Ulcerative colitis: with a note on Crohn's disease.** In: *Psychobiology and Human Disease*. NY: Elsevier, 1977. Pp. 495-573. (English)

1448

Whitlock FA. **Mental illness and skin disorder.** In: *Psychophysiological Aspects of Skin Disease*. F A Whitlock. London: W.B. Saunders Co., Ltd., 1976. Pp. 211-19. (English)

1449

hitlock FA. **Hypnosis and the skin.** In: *Psychophysiological Aspects of Skin Disease*. F A Whitlock. London: W.B. Saunders Co., Ltd., 1976. Pp. 69-89. (English)

1450

Whitlock FA. **Psychophysiological phenomena in the skin.** In: *Psychophysiological Aspects of Skin Disease*. F A Whitlock. London: W.B. Saunders Co., Ltd., 1976. Pp. 37-57. (English)

1451

Wolf SG. **Introduction: the role of the brain in bodily disease.** In: *Brain, Behavior and Bodily Disease*. Research Publications: Association for Research in Nervous and Mental Disease, Vol. 59. H Weiner, M A Hofer, A J Stunkard (eds.). NY: Raven Press, 1981. Pp. 1-9. (English)

1452

Wunderlich J. **Behavioral regulation of immunity: implications for human cancer.** In: *Biological Mediators of Behavior and Disease: Neoplasia*. S M Levy (ed.). NY: Elsevier Biomedical, 1982. Pp. 219-34. (English)

1453

Zatz MM. **Effects of cortisone on lymphocyte homing.** In: *Lymphocytes and Their Cell Membranes*. M Schlesinger (ed.). NY: Academic Press, 1976. Pp. 140-7. (English)

Acknowledgements to Publishers

The following abstracts are reprinted with permission of the American Psychological Association, publishers of **Psychological Abstracts** and the PsycINFO Database (Copyright (c) by the American Psychological Association) and may not be reproduced without its prior permission:

Achterberg J, Collerain I, Craig P. A possible relationship between cancer, mental retardation and mental disorders. *Soc Sci Med.* 1978;12:135-9. (English)

Achterberg J, Lawlis GF, Simonton OC, Matthews-Simonton S. Psychological factors, blood factors and blood chemistries as disease outcome predictors for cancer patients. *Multivar Exp Clin Res.* 1977;3:107-22. (English)

Achterberg J, Lawlis GF. A canonical analysis of blood chemistry variables related to psychological measures of cancer patients. *Multivar Exp Clin Res.* 1979;4:1-10. (English)

Bageley C. Control of the emotions, remote stress, and the emergence of breast cancer. *Indian J Clin Psychol.* 1979;6:213-20. (English)

Burchfield SR, Woods SC, Elich MS. Effects of cold stress on tumor growth. *Physiol Behav.* 1978;21:537-40. (English)

Chauhan NS, Dhar U. A psychodynamic study of children suffering from leprosy: a preliminary communication. *Indian J Clin Psychol.* 1980;7:75-6. (English)

Chobotova Z. Psychological factors in asthma. *Psychol Patopsychol Dietata.* 1980;15:421-31. (Czech)

Conti C, Biondi M, Pancheri P. A statistical evaluation of stressful events in 144 neoplastic and psychiatric patients. *Riv Psichiat.* 1981;16:357-77. (Italian)

Dyregrov A. Psychological factors in the development of cancer: a critical evaluation. *Tidsskrift Norsk, Psykologforening.* 1981;18:257-65. (Norwegian)

Fickova E. Personality profile of asthmatics in Cattell's 16 inventory. *Studia Psychol.* 1980;22:306-10. (Russsian)

Greer S, Morris T. The study of psychological factors in breast cancer: problems of method. *Soc Sci Med.* 1978;12:129-34. (English)

Grossarth-Maticek R. Synergetic effects of cigarette smoking, systolic blood pressure, and psychosocial risk factors for lung cancer, cardiac infarct and apoplexy cerebri. *Psychother Psychosom.* 1980;34:267-72. (English)

Hara C, Manabe K, Ogawa N. Influence of activity stress on thymus, spleen and adrenal weight of rats: possibility for an immunodeficiency model. *Physiol Behav.* 1981;27:243-8. (English)

Hara C, Ogawa N, Imada Y. The activity-stress ulcer and antibody production in rats. *Physiol Behav.* 1981;27:609-13. (English)

Jenner C. The psyche of the stomach cancer patient: cancer-releasing agent--a carcinogenic development. *Z Psychosom Med Psychoanal.* (German)

Jones NF, Kinsman RA, Schum R, Resnikoff P. Personality profiles in asthma. *J Clin Psychol.* 1976;32:285-91. (English)

Lambert PL, Harrell EH, Achterberg J. Medial hypothalamic stimulation decreases the phagocytic activity of the reticuloendothelial system. *Physiol Psychol.* 1981;9:193-6. (English)

Linn BS, Linn MW, Jensen J. Anxiety and immune responsiveness. *Psychol Rep.* 1981;49:969-70. (English)

Margarey CJ, Todd PB, Blizard PJ. Psycho-social factors influencing delay and breast self-examination in women with symptoms of breast cancer. *Soc Sci Med.* 1977;11:229-32. (English)

Michaut R-J, et al. Influence of early maternal deprivation on adult humoral immune response in mice. *Physiol Behav.* 1981;26:189-91. (English)

Morris T, Greer S, Pettingale KW, Watson M. Patterns of expression of anger and their psychological correlates in women with breast cancer. *Psychosom Res.* 1981;25:111-17. (English)

Pfitzner R. The psychodynamics of psoriasis vulgaris as revealed in the Rorschach test. *Z Psychosom Med Psychoanal.* 1976;22:190-7. (English)

Rees WL. Etiological factors in asthma. *Psychiatr J Univ Ottawa.* 1980;5:250-4.(English)

Seth M, Saksena NK. Personality characteristics of lung cancer patients. *Indian J Clin Psychol.* 1978;5:43-8. (English)

Seth M, Saksena NK. Personality differences between male and female cancer patients. *Indian J Clin Psychol.* 1978;5:155-60. (English)

Seth M, Saksena NK. Personality of patients suffering from cancer, cardiovascular disorders, tuberculosis and minor ailments. *Indian J Clin Psychol.* 1977;4:135-40. (English)

Shanon J. Psoriasis: psychosomatic aspects. *Psychother Psychosom.* 1979;31:218-22. (English)

Sheldrake P. Predispositions to illness: patterns in the reporting of psychosomatic illness. *J Psychosom Res.* 1977;21:225-30. (English)

Staudenmayer H, Kinsman RA, Jones NF. Attitudes toward respiratory illness and hospitalization in asthma: relationships with personality, symptomatology, and treatment response. *J Nerv Ment Dis.* 1978;166:624-34. (English)

Syvalahti E, Lammintausta R, Pekkarinen A. Effect of psychic stress of examination on serum growth hormone, serum insulin and plasma renin activity. *Acta Pharmac Tox.* 1976;38:344-52. (English)

Teiramaa E. Psychosocial and psychic factors and age at onset of asthma. *J Psychosom Res.* 1979;23:27-37. (English)

Teiramaa E. Psychosocial factors in the onset and course of asthma: a clinical study on 100 patients. *Acta Univ Ouluensis.* 1977;D-14:135.

Teiramaa E. Psychosocial factors in the onset and course *Acta Univ Ouluensis.* 1977;D-14:135. (English)

Totman R, Kiff J, Reed SE, Craig JW. Predicting experimental colds in volunteers from early measures of recent life stress. *J Psychosom Res* 1980;24:155-63. (English)

Tsuda A, et al. Effects of divided feeding on activity-stress ulcer and the thymus weight in the rat. *Physiol Behav.* 1981;27:349-53. (English)

Vendysova E, Pankova R. Anxiety reactions in psoriatics. *Cesk Psychol.* (Czech)

Vogel PG. Psychodynamic aspects of psoriasis vulgaris. *Z Psychosom Med Psychoanal.* 1976;22:177-89. (English)

Voth HM. Cancer and personality. *Percept Mot Skills.* 1976:42:1131-7. (English)

Weiss JH, Lyness J, Molk L, Riley J. Induced respiratory change in asthmatic children. *J Psychosom Res.* 1976;20:115-23. (English)

Wirsching M, Stierlin H, Hoffmann F, Weber G, Wirsching B. Psychological indentification of breast cancer patients before biopsy. *J Psychosom Res.* 1982;26:1-10. (English)

The following dissertation titles and abstracts are published with permission of University Microfilms International, publishers of Dissertation Abstracts International ((c) Copyright 1981 by University Microfilms International), and may not be reproduced without their prior permission:

Bulloch K. Neuroendocrine-immune circuitry: pathways involved with the induction and persistence of humoral immunity. *Diss Abstr Int.* 1981;41:4447-B. (English)

Morrison FR. Psychosocial factors in the etiology of cancer. *Diss Abstr Int.* 1981;42:155B. (English)

The following abstract is reprinted with permission of CA--A Cancer Journal for Clinicians, (c) American Cancer Society, Inc., 1982, from the following source:

Anonymous. Unproven methods of cancer management: O. Carl Simonton, MD. *CA-A Cancer J for Clinicians.* 1982;32:58-61. (English)

The following abstracts are reprinted with permission of W. B. Saunders Co., from the following sources:

Makinodan T. Immunobiology of aging. *J Am Geriatr Soc.* 1976;24:249-52. (English)

Petrich J, Holmes TH. Life change and onset of illness. *Med Clinics N Am.* 1977;61:825-38. (English)

Rose RM. Endocrine responses to stressful psychological events. *Psychiat Clin N Amer.* 1980;3:251-76. (English)

Stein M. A biopsychosocial approach to immune function and medical disorders. *Psychiatr Clin N Am.* 1981;4:203-21. (English)

Yunis EJ, Fernandes G, Greenberg LJ. Tumor immunology, autoimmunity and aging. *J Am Geriatr Soc.* 1976;24:258-63. (English)

The following abstract is reprinted with permission of the New York Academy of Sciences, from the following source:

DiSorbo D, Rosen F, McPartland RP, Millolland RJ. Glucocorticoid activity of various progesterone analogs: correlation between specific binding in thymus and liver and biologic activity. *Ann NY Acad Sci.* 1977;286:355-66. (English)

The following abstracts are reprinted by permission of PJD Publications Ltd., Post Office Box 966, Westbury, NY 11590, from the following sources:

Bidart JM, Assicot M, Bohuon C. Catechol-O-methyl transferase activity in human mononuclear cells. *Res Commun Chem Pathol Pharmacol.* 1981;34:47-54. (English)

Johnson DL, Gordon MA. Effect of chronic beta-adrenergic therapy on the human lymphocyte response to concanavalin A. *Res Commun Chem Pathol Pharmacol.* 1981;32:377-80. (English)

Kasahara K, Tanaka S, Hamashima Y. Suppression of the primary immune response by chemical sympathectomy. *Res Commun Chem Pathol Pharmacol.* 1977;16:687-94. (English)

Shaskan EG, Lovett EJ III. Effects of haloperidol, a dopamine receptor antagonist, on a delayed-type hypersensitivity reaction to 1-chloro, 2,4-dinitrobenzene in mice. *Res Commun Psychol Psychiat Behav.* 1980;5:241-54. (English)

The following abstract is reprinted with permission of the American Sociological Association, (c) Copyright 1979, from the following sources:

Lin N, Ensel WM, Kuo W, Simeone RS. Social support, stressful life events, and illness: a model and empirical test. *J Health Soc Behav.* 1979;20:108-19. (English)

The following abstract is reprinted with permission of the American Sociological Association, (c) Copyright 1980, from the following sources:

McFarlane AH, Norman GR, Streiner DL, Roy R, Scott DJ. A longitudinal study of the influence of the psychosocial environment on health status; a preliminary report. *J Health Soc Behav.* 1980;21:124-33. (English)

The following abstract is reprinted by permission of the Johns Hopkins University Press, from the following source:

Thomas CB, McCabe OL. Precursors of premature disease and death: habits of nervous tension. *Johns Hopkins Med J.* 1980;147:137-45. (English)

The following abstracts are reprinted by permission of the Southern Medical Journal from the following sources:

Erwin WJ, Granacher RP Jr. New behavioral data concerning the auto-erythrocyte sensitization syndrome. *South Med J.* 1977;70:876-8. (English)

Hanna WT, Fitzpatrick R, Krauss S, Machado E, Dunn CD. Psychogenic purpura (autoerythrocyte sensitization). *South Med J.* 1981;74:538-42. (English)

The following abstract is reprinted by permission of the University of Chicago Press as publishers, (c) Copyright 1978, Perspectives in Biology and Medicine, from the following source:

Abramsky O, Litvin Y. Autoimmune response to dopamine-receptor as a possible mechanism in the pathogenesis of Parkinson's disease and schizophrenia. *Perspect Biol Med.* 1978;22:104-14. (English)

The following abstract is reprinted by permission of the University of Chicago Press as publishers, (c) Copyright 1980, Journal of Infectious Disease, from the following source:

Bryson YJ, Monahan C, Pollack M, Shields WD. A prospective double-blind study of side effects associated with the administration of amantadine for influenza A virus prophylaxis. *J Infect Dis.* 1980;141:543-7. (English)

The following abstracts are reprinted by permission of Psychological Reports, from the following source:

Kinsman RA, Dirks JF, Dahlem NW, Heller AS. Anxiety in asthma: panic-fear symptomatology and personality in relation to manifest anxiety. *Psychol Rep.* 1980;46:196-8. (English)

Mehrabian A, Ross M. Quality of life change and individual differences in stimulus screening in relation to incidence of illness. *Psychol Rep.* 1977;41:367-78. (English)

*The following abstract is reprinted with permission of **Perceptual and Motor Skills**, from the following source:*

Dahlem NW, Kinsman RA. Panic-fear in asthma: a divergence between subjective report and behavioral patterns. *Percept Mot Skills.* 1978;46:95-8. (English)

The following abstract is reprinted with permission of the American Academy of Pediatrics, (c) Copyright American Academy of Pediatrics 1981, from the following source:

Gunn T, Reece ER, Metrakos K, Colle E. Depressed T cells following neonatal steroid treatment. *Pediatrics.* 1981;67:61-7. (English)

*The following abstract is reprinted by permission of the **International Journal of Psychiatry in Medicine**, (c) Copyright 1979, from the following source:*

Scurry MT, Levin EM. Psychosocial factors related to the incidence of cancer. *Int J Psychiatry Med.* 1978-79;9:159-77. (English)

The following abstracts are reprinted with permission of Munksgaard International Publishers, Ltd. (c) Copyright 1976 Munksgaard International Publishers, Ltd., Copenhagen, Denmark, from the following sources:

Palmblad J. Fasting (acute energy deprivation) in man: effect on polymorphonuclear granulocyte functions, plasma iron and serum transferrin. *Scand J Haematol.* 1976;17:217-26. (English)

Smeraldi E, Bellodi L, Scorza-Smeraldi R, Fabio G, Sacchetti E. HLA-SD antigens and schizophrenia: statistical and genetical considerations. *Tissue Antigens.* 1976;8:191-6. (English)

The following abstracts are reprinted with permission of Munksgaard International Publishers, Ltd. (c) Copyright 1977 Munksgaard International Publishers, Ltd., Copenhagen, Denmark, from the following sources:

Eriksson B, Hedfors E. The effect of adrenalin, insulin and hydrocortisone on human peripheral blood lymphocytes studied by cell surface markers. *Scand J Haematol.* 1977;18:121-8. (English)

Gerritsen SM, Akkerman JW, Nijmeijer B, Sixma JJ, Witkop CJ, White J. The Hermansky-Pudlak syndrome: evidence for a lowered 5-hydroxytryptamine content in platelets of heterozygotes. *Scand J Haematol.* 1977;18:249-56. (English)

Govaerts A, Mendlewicz J, Verbanck P. Manic-depressive illness and HLA. *Tissue Antigens.* 1977;10:60-2. (English)

Ivanyi P, Ivanyi D, Zemek P. HLA-Cw4 in paranoid schizophrenia. *Tissue Antigens.* 1977;9:41-4. (English)

Palmblad J, Fohlin L, Lundstrom M. Anorexia nervosa and polymorphonuclear (PMN) granulocyte reactions. *Scand J Haematol.* 1977;19:334-42. (English)

Palmblad J, Halberg D, Rossner S. Obesity, plasma lipids and polymorphonuclear (PMN) granulocyte functions. *Scand J Haematol.* 1977;19:293-303. (English)

Pulkkinen E. Immunoglobulins, psychopathology and prognosis in schizophrenia. *Acta Psychiatr Scand.* 1977;56:173-82. (English)

The following abstract is reprinted with permission of Munksgaard International Publishers, Ltd. (c) Copyright 1978 Munksgaard International Publishers, Ltd., Copenhagen, Denmark, from the following source:

Henschke PJ, Bell DA, Cape RD. Alzheimer's disease and HLA. *Tissue Antigens.* 1978;12:132-5. (English)

The following abstracts are reprinted with permission of Munksgaard International Publishers, Ltd. (c) Copyright 1980 Munksgaard International Publishers, Ltd., Copenhagen, Denmark, from the following sources:

Fernandez LA, MacSween JM. Lithium and T cell colonies. *Scand J Haemotol.* 1980;25:382-4. (English)

Nyland H, Naess A, Lunde H. Lymphocyte subpopulations in peripheral blood from schizophrenic patients. *Acta Psychiatr Scand.* 1980;61:313-8. (English)

Sharma S, Nandkumar VK. Personality structure and adjustment pattern in bronchial asthma. *Acta Psychiatr Scand.* 1980;61:81-8. (English)

Sulkava R, Koskimies S, Wikstrom J, Palo J. HLA antigens in Alzheimer's disease. *Tissue Antigens.* 1980;16:191-4. (English)

Whalley LJ, Urbaniak SJ, Darg C, Peutherer JF, Christie JE. Histocompatibility antigens and antibodies to viral and other antigens in Alzheimer pre-senile dementia. *Acta Psychiatr Scand.* 1980;61:1-7. (English)

The following abstracts are reprinted with permission of Munksgaard International Publishers, Ltd. (c) Copyright 1982 Munksgaard International Publishers, Ltd., Copenhagen, Denmark, from the following sources:

Sylvester-Jrgensen O, Vejlsgaard-Goldschmidt V, Faber-Vestergaard B. Herpes simplex virus (HSV) antibodies in child psychiatric patients and normal children. *Acta Psychiatr Scand.* 1982;66:42-9. (English)

Whalley LJ, Roberts DF, Wentzel J, Wright AF. Genetic factors in puerperal affective psychoses. *Acta Psychiatr Scand.* 1982;65:180-93. (English)

*The following abstract is reprinted by permission of **Excerpta Medica**. from the following source:*

Besedovsky HO, Sorkin E. Hormonal control of immune processes. *Proc 5th Int Congr Endocrinol, Excerpta Medica.* Vol. 2. V H T James (ed.). Amsterdam: Oxford U. Press, 1977. Pp. 504-13. (English)

*The following abstract is reprinted by permission of **Ciba Foundation Symposia**, from the following source:*

Allison AC, Hovi T, Watts RW, Webster AD. The role of *de novo* purine synthesis in lymphocyte transformation. *Ciba Found Symp.* 1977;48:207-24. (English)

*The following abstract is reprinted with permission of The American Society for Clinical Nutrition, (c) Copyright **American Journal of Clinical Nutrition**, American Society for Clinical Nutrition, from the following sources:*

Bistrian BR. Interaction of nutrition and infection in the hospital setting. *Am J Clin Nutr.* 1977;30:1228-35. (English)

Golla JA, Larson LA, Anderson CF, Lucas AR, Wilson WR, Tomasi TB Jr. An immunological assessment of patients with anorexia nervosa. *Am J Clin Nutr.* 1981;34:2756-62. (English)

Pertschuk MJ, Crosby LO, Barot L, Mullen JL. Immunocompetency in anorexia nervosa. *Am J Clin Nutr.* 1982;35:968-72. (English)

*The following abstract is reprinted by permission of **American Review of Respiratory Disease**, from the following source:*

Horton DJ, Suda WL, Kinsman RA, Souhrada J, Spector SL. Bronchoconstrictive suggestion in asthma: a role for airways hyperreactivity and emotions. *Am Rev Respir Dis.* 1978;117:1029-38. (English)

*The following abstracts are reprinted by permission of **British Medical Journal**, from the following sources:*

Corenblum B, Whitaker M. Inhibition of stress-induced hyperprolactinemia. *Br Med J.* 1977;2:1328. (English)

Cove-Smith JR, Kabler P, Pownall R, Knapp MS. Circadian variation in an immune response in man. *Brit Med J.* 1978;2:253-4. (English)

Pankaskie MC, Abdel-Monem MM, Raina A, Wang T, Foker JE. Inhibitors of polyamine biosynthesis; 9--Effects of S-adenosyl-L-methionine analogues on mammalian aminopropyltransferases *in vitro* and polyamine biosynthesis in transformed lymphocytes. *J Med Chem.* 1981;24:549-53. (English)

Presley AP, Kahn A, Williamson N. Antinuclear antibodies in patients on lithium carbonate. *Br Med J.* 1976;2:280-1. (English)

Pullan PT, Clement-Jones V, Corder R, Lowry PJ, Rees GM, Rees LH, Besser GM, Macedo MM, Galvao-Teles A. Ectopic production of methionine enkephalin and beta-endorphin. *Brit Med J.* 1980;280:758-9. (English)

Runge LA, Pinals RS, Tomar RH. Treatment of rheumatoid arthritis with levamisole: long-term results and immune changes. *Ann Rheum Dis.* 1979;38:122-7. (English)

The following abstract is reprinted by permission of **Grune & Stratton, Inc.** *and the author, from the following source:*

Wagner H, Hengst K, Zierden E, Gerlach U. Investigations of the antiproliferative effect of somatostatin in man and rats. *Clin Exp Metab.* 1979;27:1381-6. (English)

The following abstract is reprinted permission of M.I.T. Press, (c) Copyright M.I.T. Press 1980, from the following source:

Shinefeld LA, Sato JL, Rosenberg NE. Monoclonal rat anti-mouse brain antibody detects Abelson murine leukemia virus target cells in mouse bone marrow. *Cell.* 1980;20:11-17. (English)

The following abstracts are reprinted by permission of **Clinical Research,** *from the following sources:*

Osband M, Gallison D, Miller B, Agarawel RP, McCaffrey R. Concanavalin A activation of suppressor cells mediated by histamine and blocked by cimetidine (abstract). *Clin Res.* 1980;28:356A. (English)

Rogers MP, Trentham DE, Dynesius RA, Reich P, David JR. Exacerbation of type II collagen-induced arthritis by auditory stress (abstract). *Clin Res.* 1980;28:508A. (English)

The following abstract is reprinted by permission of **Pediatric Annals,** *from the following source:*

Weston WL, Huff JC. Atopic dermatitis: etiology and pathogenesis. *Pediatr Ann.* 1976;5:759-62. (English)

The following abstract is reprinted by permission of **Cutis,** *from the following source:*

Meister MM, Bodner AC. Autoerythrocyte sensitization--a psychogenic purpura. *Cutis.* 1977;19:221-4. (English)

The following abstract is reproduced with permission from the American Diabetes Association, Inc., from the following source:

Gozes Y, Caruso J, Strom TB. The absence of cryptic insulin receptors on resting lymphocytes. *Diabetes.* 1981;30:314-6. (English)

The following abstracts are reprinted by permission of **Federation Proceedings,** *from the following sources:*

Blecha F, Barry RA, Kelly KW. Stress-induced alterations in cell-mediated immunity of mice *in vivo* (abstract). *Fed Proc, Fed Am Soc Exp Biol.* 1980;39:479. (English)

Bursztajn S, Askenase PW, Gershon RK, Gershon MD. Role of vasoactive amines during early stages of delayed-type hypersensitivity skin reactions. *Fed Proc, Fed Am Soc Exp Biol.* 1978;37:590. (English)

Crary B, Borysenko M, Borysenko J, Benson H. Release of granular lymphocytes into peripheral blood after epinephrine administration in humans: correlation with T_G lymphocytes and suppression of mitogen-responsiveness (abstract). *Fed Proc, Fed Am Soc Exp Biol.* 1982;41:591. (English)

Cross RJ, Markesbery WR, Brooks WH, Roszman TL. The acute effect of hypothalamic lesions on the immune response (abstract). *Fed Proc, Fed Am Soc Exp Biol.* 1980;39:1162. (English)

Denckla WD. Interactions between age and the neuroendocrine and immune systems. *Fed Proc, Fed Am Soc Exp Biol.* 1978;37:1263-7. (English)

Eskra JD, Stevens JS, Carty TJ. Beta$_2$-adrenergic receptors in thymocytes (abstract). *Fed Proc, Fed Am Soc Exp Biol.* 1978;37:687. (English)

Kay MMB. Effect of age on T cell differentiation. *Fed Proc, Fed Am Soc Exp Biol.* 1978;37:1241-4. (English)

Levy JA, Munson AE. Suppression of antibody-mediated primary hemolytic plaque-forming cells (PFC) by haloperidol (abstract). *Fed Proc, Fed Am Soc Exp Biol.* 1976;35:333. (English)

Nagy E, Berczi I. Immunodeficiency in hypophysectomized rats (abstract). *Fed Proc, Fed Am Soc Exp Biol.* 1979;38:1355. (English)

Shaskan EG, Peszke MA, Niederman JC, Kasl SV. Monoamine oxidase activity (MAOA) as a screen for host-resistance to infectious disease. *Fed Proc.* 1978;37:878. (English)

Singhal SK, Roder JC, Duwe AK. Suppressor cells in immunosenescence. *Fed Proc, Fed Am Soc Exp Biol.* 1978;37:1245-52. (English)

Spackman DH, Riley V. Modification of cancer by stress: effects of plasma corticosterone elevations on immunological system components in mice (abstract). *Fed Proc, Fed Am Soc Exp Biol.* 1976;35:1693. (English)

Stutman O, Shen FW. Post-thymic precursor cells are sensitive to steroids and belong to the Ly 1,2,3+, subset (abstract). *Fed Proc, Fed Am Soc Exp Biol.* 1977;36:1301. (English)

Warejcka DJ, Levy NL. Central nervous system (CNS) control of the immune response: effect of hypothalamic lesions on PHA responsiveness in rats (abstract). *Fed Proc, Fed Am Soc Exp Biol.* 1980;39:914. (English)

The following abstracts are reprinted by permission of J. B. Lippincott, from the following sources:

Blichert-Toft M, Christensen V, Engquist A, Fog-Moller F, Kehlet H, Madsen SN, Skovsted L, Thode J, Olgaard K. Influence of age on the endocrine metabolic response to surgery. *Ann Surg.* 1979;190:761-70. (English)

Copperman SM. "Alice in Wonderland" syndrome as a presenting symptom of infectious mononucleosis in children: a description of three affected young people. *Clin Pediatr (Phila).* 1977;16:143-6. (English)

Fritz GK. Psychological aspects of atopic dermatitis: a viewpoint. *Clin Pediatr (Phila).* 1979;18:360-4. (English)

Linn MW, Linn BS, Harris R. Effects of counseling for late stage cancer patients. *Cancer.* 1982;49:1048-55. (English)

Mehta RG, Fricks CM, Moon RC. Androgen receptors in chemically-induced colon carcinogenesis. *Cancer.* 1980;45:1085-9. (English)

Morillo E, Gardner LI. Activation of latent Graves' disease in children: review of possible psychosomatic mechanisms. *Clin Pediatr.* 1980;19:160-3. (English)

Peters LJ, Kelly H. The influence of stress and stress hormones on the transplantability of a non-immunogenic syngeneic murine tumor. *Cancer.* 1977;39:1482-8. (English)

Wynder EL. Dietary habits and cancer epidemiology. *Cancer.* 1979;43:1955-61. (English)

*The following abstract is reprinted by permission of **Annals of Internal Medicine**, from the following sources:*

Follansbee SE, Busch DF, Wofsy CB, Coleman DL, Gullet J, Aurigenna GP, Ross T, Hadley WK, Drew WL. An outbreak of *Pneumocystic carinii* pneumonia in homosexual men. *Ann Intern Med.* 1982;96:705-13. (English)

Friedman-Kien AE, Laubenstein LJ, Rubinstein P, Buimovici-Klein E, Marmor M, Stahl R, Spigland I, Kim KS, Zolla-Pazner S. Disseminated Kaposi's sarcoma in homosexual men. *Ann Intern Med.* 1982;96:693-700. (English)

MacGregor RR. Granulocyte adherence changes induced by hemodialysis, endotoxin, epinephrine, and glucocorticoids. *Ann Intern Med.* 1977;86:35-9. (English)

Mildvan D, Mathur U, Enlow RW, Romain PL, Winchester RJ, Colp C, Singman H, Adelsberg BR, Spigland I. Opportunistic infections and immune deficiency in homosexual men. *Ann Intern Med.* 1982;96:700-4. (English)

Morris L, Distenfeld A, Amorosi E, Karpatkin S. Autoimmune thrombocytopenic purpura in homosexual men. *Ann Intern Med.* 1982;96:714-7. (English)

Thomas CB. Precursors of premature disease and death: the predictive potential of habits and family attitudes. *Ann Intern Med.* 1976;85:653-8. (English)

Volpe R. The role of autoimmunity in hypoendocrine and hyperendocrine function: with special emphasis on autoimmune thyroid disease. *Ann Intern Med.* 1977;87:86-99. (English)

Zarrabi MH, Zucker S, Miller F, Derman RM, Romano GS, Hartnett JA, Varma AO. Immunologic and coagulation disorders in chlorpromazine-treated patients. *Ann Intern Med.* 1979;91:194-9. (English)

The following abstracts are reprinted by permission of the British Psychological Society, from the following sources:

Dirks JF, Kinsman RA, Jones NF, Fross KH. New developments in panic-fear research in asthma: validity and stability of the MMPI Panic-Fear scale. *Br J Med Psychol.* 1978;51:119-26. (English)

Dirks JF, Paley A, Fross KH. Panic-fear research in asthma and the nuclear conflict theory of asthma; similarities, differences and clinical implications. *Br J Med Psychol.* 1979;52:71-6. (English)

Dirks JF, Schraa JC, Brown EL, Kinsman RA. Psycho-maintenance in asthma: hospitalization rates and financial impact. *Br J Med Psychol.* 1980;53:349-54. (English)

Fava GA, Perini GI, Santonastaso P, Fornasa CV. Life events and psychological distress in dermatologic disorders: psoriasis, chronic urticaria and fungal infections. *Br J Med Psychol.* 1980;53:277-82. (English)

Forth MW, Jackson M. Group psychotherapy in the management of bronchial asthma. *Br J Med Psychol.* 1976;49:257-60. (English)

Jackson M. Psychopathology and psychotherapy in bronchial asthma. *Br J Med Psychol.* 1976;49:249-55. (English)

*The following abstracts are reprinted by permission of **Science**, (c) Copyright 1976 by the American Association for the Advancement of Science, from the following sources:*

Becker B, Shier DH, Palmberg PF, Waltman SR. HLA antigens and corticosteroid response. *Science.*1976;194:1427-8. (English)

Rabkin JG, Struening EL. Life events, stress and illness. *Science.* 1976;194:1013-20. (English)

Seifter E, Cohen MH, Riley V. Of stress, vitamin A, and tumors (letter). *Science.* 1976;193:74-5. (English)

Singh MM, Kay SR. Wheat gluten as a pathogenic factor in schizophrenia. *Science.* 1976;191:401-2. (English)

Stein M, Schiavi RC, Camerino MS. Influence of brain and behavior on the immune system. *Science.* 1976;191:435-40. (English)

*The following abstracts are reprinted by permission of **Science**, (c) Copyright 1977 by the American Association for the Advancement of Science, from the following sources:*

Cotzias CG, Tang LC. An adenylate cyclase of brain reflects propensity for breast cancer in mice. *Science.* 1977;197:1094-6. (English)

Greenberg JH, Saunders ME, Mellors A. Inhibition of a lymphocyte membrane enzyme by delta-9-tetrahydrocannabinol *in vitro. Science.* 1977;197:475-6. (English)

Herman JJ, Brenner JK, Colten HR. Inhibition of histaminase release from human granulocytes by production of histaminase activity. *Science.* 1977;2206:77-8. (English)

Lattime EC, Strausser HR. Arteriosclerosis: is stress-induced immune suppression a risk factor? *Science.* 1977;198:302-3. (English)

Monjan AA, Collector MI. Stress-induced modulation of the immune response. *Science.* 1977;197:307-8. (English)

Roskowski W, Plaut M, Lichtenstein LM. Selective display of histamine receptors on lymphocytes. *Science.* 1977;195:683-5. (English)

*The following abstract is reprinted by permission of **Science**, (c) Copyright 1978 by the American Association for the Advancement of Science, from the following sources:*

Wang T, Sheppard JR, Foker JE. Rise and fall of cyclic AMP required for onset of lymphocyte DNA synthesis. *Science.* 1978;201:155-7. (English)

*The following abstracts are reprinted by permission of **Science**, (c) Copyright 1979 by the American Association for the Advancement of Science, from the following sources:*

Gelfand EW, Dosch HM, Hastings D, Shore A. Lithium: a modulator of cyclic AMP-dependent events in lymphocytes? *Science.* 1979;203:365-7. (English)

Hazum E, Chang KJ, Cuatrecasas P. Specific nonopiate receptors for beta-endorphin. *Science.* 1979;205:1033-5. (English)

Martin TW, Lagunoff D. Inhibition of mast cell histamine secretion by N-substituted derivatives of phosphatidylserine. *Science.* 1979;204:631-3. (English)

Sklar LS, Anisman H. Stress and coping factors influence tumor growth. *Science.* 1979;205:513-5. (English)

*The following abstracts are reprinted by permission of **Science**, (c) Copyright 1980 by the American Association for the Advancement of Science, from the following sources:*

Harden TK, Cotton CU, Waldo GL, Lutton JK, Perkins JP. Catecholamine- induced alteration in sedimentation behavior of membrane-bound beta-adrenergic receptors. *Science.* 1980;210:441-3. (English)

Hirata F, Axelrod J. Phospholipid methylation and biological signal transmission. *Science.* 1980;209:1082-90. (English)

Kuehl FA Jr, Egan RW. Prostaglandins, arachidonic acid and inflammation. *Science.* 1980;210:978-84. (English)

Santoro MG, Benedetto A, Carruba G, Garaci E, Jaffe BM. Prostaglandin A compounds as antiviral agents. *Science.* 1980;209:1032-4. (English)

Simon RH, Lovett EJ III, Tomaszek D, Lundy J. Electrical stimulation of the midbrain mediates metastatic tumor growth. *Science.* 1980;209:1132-3. (English)

*The following abstracts are reprinted by permission of **Science**, (c) Copyright 1981 by the American Association for the Advancement of Science, from the following sources:*

Keller SE, Weiss J, Schleifer SJ, Miller NE, Stein M. Suppression of immunity by stress: effect of a graded series of stressors on lymphocyte stimulation in the rat. *Science.* 1981;213:1397-1400. (English)

Moody TW, Pert CB, Gazdar AF, Carney DN, Minna JD. High levels of intracellular bombesin characterize human small-cell lung carcinoma. *Science.* 1981;214:1246-8. (English)

Riley V. Psychoneuroendocrine influences on immunocompetence and neoplasia. *Science.* 1981;212:1100-9. (English)

*The following abstracts are reprinted by permission of **Science**, (c) Copyright 1982 by the American Association for the Advancement of Science, from the following sources:*

Torrey EF, Yolken RH, Winfrey CJ. Cytomegalovirus antibody in cerebrospinal fluid of schizophrenic patients detected by enzyme immunoassay. *Science.* 1982;21:892-4. (English)

Visintainer MA, Volpicelli JR, Seligman ME. Tumor rejection in rats after inescapable or escapable shock. *Science.* 1982;216:437-9. (English)

*The following abstracts are reprinted by permission of **Psychosomatics**, from the following sources:*

Bahnson CB. Stress and cancer: the state of the art, part 1. *Psychosomatics.* 1980;21:975-81. (English)

Bahnson CB. Stress and cancer: the state of the art, part 2. *Psychosomatics.* 1981;22:207-20. (English).

Garfinkel R. Treatment of a psychosomatic ailment in an elderly woman. *Psychosomatics.* 1980;21:1015-6. (English)

Gowdy JM. Immunoglobulin levels in psychotic patients. *Psychosomatics.* 1980;21:751-6. (English)

Holmes TH. Life situations, emotions, and disease. *Psychosomatics.* 1978: 747-54. (English)

Keegan DL. Chronic urticaria: clinical psychophysiological and therapeutic aspects. *Psychosomatics.* 1976;17:160-3. (English)

Koranyi EK. Somatic illness in psychiatric patients. *Psychosomatics.* 1980;21:887-91. (English)

Meijer A. Sources of dependence in asthmatic children. *Psychosomatics.* 1978;19:351-5. (English)

Minter RE, Kimball CP. Life events and illness onset: a review. *Psychosomatics.* 1978;19:334-9. (English)

Zeitlin DJ. Psychological issues in the management of rheumatoid arthritis. *Psychosomatics.* 1977;18:7-14. (English)

*The following abstracts are reprinted by permission of the **New England Journal of Medicine**, from the following sources:*

Claman HN. Corticosteroids and lymphoid cells. *N Engl J Med.* 1972; 287:388-97. (English)

Colucci WS, Alexander RW, Williams GH, Rude RE, Holman BL, Konstam MA, Wynne J, Mudge GH Jr, Braunwald E. Decreased lymphocyte beta-adrenergic receptor density in patients with heart failure and tolerance to the beta-adrenergic agonist pirbuterol. *N Engl J Med.* 1981;305:185-90. (English)

Fraser CM, Venter JC, Kaliner M. Autonomic abnomalties and autoantibodies to beta-adrenergic receptors. *N Engl J Med.* 1981:305:1165-70. (English)

Glasser L, Heustis DW, Jones JF. Functional capabilities of steroid-recruited neutrophils harvested for clinical transfusion. *N Engl J Med.* 1977;297:1033-36. (English)

Kirtland HH, Mohler DN, Horwitz DA. Methyldopa inhibition of suppressor- lymphocyte function: a proposed cause of autoimmune hemolytic anemia. *N Engl J Med.* 1980;302:825-32. (English)

Lyman GH, Williams CC, Preston D. The use of lithium carbonate to reduce infectious leukopenia during systematic chemotherapy. *N Engl J Med.* 1980;302:257-60. (English)

Motulsky HJ, Insel PA. Adrenergic receptors in man. *N Engl J Med.* 1982;307:18-29. (English)

Vaillant GE. Natural history of male psychological health: effects of mental health on physical health. *N Engl J Med.* 1979;301:1249-54.

Weitkamp LR, Stancer HC, Persad E, Flood C, Guttormsen S. Depressive disorders and HLA—a gene on chromosome 6 that can affect behavior. *N Engl J Med.* 1981;305:1301-6. (English)

The following abstracts are reprinted by permission of Cambridge University Press, from the following sources:

Alderson MR. Nutrition and cancer: evidence from epidemiology. *Proc Nutr Soc.* 1981;40:1-6. (English)

Davis JB. Neurotic illness in the families of children with asthma and wheezy bronchitis: a general practice population study. *Psychol Med.* 1977;7:305-10. (English)

Gardiner BM. Psychological aspects of rheumatoid arthritis. *Psychol Med.* 1980;10:159-63. (English)

Greer S. Psychological enquiry: a contribution to cancer research. *Psychol Med.* 1979;9:81-9. (English)

Lazarus JH, John R, Bennie EH, Chalmers RJ, Crockett G. Lithium therapy and thyroid function: a long-term study. *Psychol Med.* 198l;11:85-92. (English)

McFarlane H. Malnutrition and impaired response to infection. *Proc Nutr Soc.* 1976;35:263-72. (English)

McGuffin P. Is schizophrenia an HLA-associated disease? *Psychol Med.* 1979;9:721-8. (English)

Psychochemistry Institute (Department of Psychiatry, Copenhagen, Denmark). HLA antigens and manic-depressive disorders: further evidence of an association. *Psychol Med.* 1977;7:387-96. (English)

Reid AH, Martin KW, Ballinger BR, Heather BB. The possible relationship of herpes simplex virus infection to cause of retardation in severe mental handicap. *Psychol Med.* 1980;10:555-7. (English)

Singh U. Effect of catecholamines on lymphopoiesis in fetal mouse thymic explants. *J Anat.* 1979:279-92. (English)

Stein G, Holmes J, Bradford JW, Kennedy L. HLA antigens and affective disorder: a family case report. *Psychol Med.* 1980;10:677-81. (English)

Stevens FM, Lloyd RS, Geraghty SM, Reynolds MT, Sarsfield MJ, McNicholl B, Fottrell PF, Wright R, McCarthy CF. Schizophrenia and coeliac disease--the nature of the relationship. *Psychol Med.* 1977;7:259-63. (English)

Whitlock FA, Siskind M. Depression and cancer: a followup study. *Psychol* 1979;9:747-52. (English)

The following abstract is reprinted by permission of the American Institute of Biological Sciences, (c) Copyright 1981 by the American Institute of Biological Sciences, from the following source:

Lederman MA, Mascio A, Shaskan EG. Schizophrenia: biochemical and virological theories. *Bios.* 1981;52:217-26. (English)

The following abstracts are reprinted by permission of Elsevier Biomedical Press B.V., from the following sources:

Anisimov VN, Khavinson VK, Morozov VG. Carcinogenesis and aging; IV--Effect of low-molecular-weight factors of thymus, pineal gland and anterior hypothalamus on immunity, tumor incidence and life span of C3H/Sn mice. *Mech Ageing Dev.* 1982;19:245-58. (English)

Bardos P, Biziere K, De Genne D, Renoux G. Regulation of natural killer activity by the cerebral neocortex. In: Natural Killers: Fundamental Aspects and Role in Cancer. *Human Cancer Immunology*, Vol 6. B Serron, R B Herberman (eds.). Amsterdam: Elsevier/North Holland, in press. (English)

Bilder GE, Denckla WD. Restoration of ability to reject xenografts and clear carbon after hypophysectomy of adult rats. *Mech Ageing Dev.* 1977;6:153-63. (English)

Borysenko J. Behavioral-physiological factors in the development and management of cancer. *Gen Hosp Psychiatry.* 1982;4:69-74. (English)

Borysenko M, Borysenko J. Stress, behavior and immunity: animal models and mediating mechanisms. *Gen Hosp Psychiat.* 1982;4:59-67. (English) (unavailable at publication)

Cross RJ, Markesbery WR, Brooks WH, Roszman TL. Hypothalamic-immune interactions; I--The acute effect of anterior hypothalamic lesions on the immune response. *Br Res.* 1980;196:79-87. (English)

DeLisi LE, Neckers LM, Staub RA, Zaloman SJ, Wyatt RJ. Lymphocyte monoamine oxidase activity and chronic schizophrenia. *Psychiatr Res.* 1980;2:179-86. (English)

Depelchin A, Letesson JJ. Adrenaline influence on the immune response; II--Its effects through action on the suppressor T-cells. *Immunol Lett.* 1981;3:207-13. (English)

Depelchin A, Letesson JJ. Adrenaline influence on the immune response; I--Accelerating or suppressor effects according to the time of application. *Immunol Lett.* 1981;3:199-205. (English)

Extein I, Tallman J, Smith CC, Goodwin FK. Changes in lymphocyte beta-adrenergic receptors in depression and mania. *Psychiatr Res.* 1979; 1:191-7. (English)

Gattaz WF, Beckmann H, Mendlewicz J. HLA antigens and schizophrenia: a pool of 2 studies. *Psychiatr Res.* 1981;5:123-8. (English)

Haaijman JJ, Hijmans W. Influence of age on the immunological activity and capacity of the CBA mouse. *Mech Ageing Dev.* 1978;7:375-98. (English)

Johnson GF, Hunt GE, Robertson S, Doran TJ. A linkage study of manic-depressive disorder with HLA antigens, blood groups, serum proteins and red cell enzymes. *J Affect Disord.* 1981;3:43-58. (English)

Locke SE. Stress, adaptation, and immunity: studies in humans. *Gen Hosp Psychiatry.* 1982;4:49-58. (English)

Maslinski W, Grabczewska E, Ryzewski J. Acetylcholine receptors of rat lymphocytes. *Biochim Biophys Acta.* 1980;633:269-73. (English)

McGuffin P, Farmer AE, Yonace AH. HLA antigens and subtypes of schizophrenia. *Psychiatr Res.* 1981;5:115-22.

Mendlewicz J, Verbanck P, Linkowski P, Govaerts A. HLA antigens in affective disorders and schizophrenia. *J Affective Disord.* 1981;3:17-24. (English)

Miles K, Quint'ans J, Chelmicka-Schorr E, Arnason BG. The sympathetic nervous system modulates antibody response to thymus-independent antigens. *J Neuroimmunol.* 1981;1:101-5. (English)

Morris RJ, Gower S, Pfeiffer SE. Thy-1 cell surface antigen on cloned cell lines of the rat and mouse: stimulation by cAMP and by butyrate. *Br Res.* 1980;183:145-59. (English)

Nasr SJ, Altman EG, Meltzer HY. Concordance of atopic and affective disorders. *J Affective Disord.* 1981;3:291-6. (English)

Peterson CS, Herlin T, Esmann V. Effects of catecholamines and glucagon on glycogen metabolism in human polymorphonuclear leukocytes. *Biochim Biophys Acta.* 1978;542:77-87. (English)

Popp DM. Qualitative changes in immunocompetent cells with age: reduced sensitivity to cortisone acetate. *Mech Ageing Dev.* 1977;6:355-62. (English)

Shaskan EG, Lovett EJ III. Effects of psychotropic drugs on delayed hypersensitivity reactions in mice: relevant sites of action. In: *Proc of the 3rd World Congr of Biol Psychiatry.* C Perris, G Struwe, B Jansson (eds.). Amsterdam: Elsevier Biomedical Press, 1981. Pp. 73-84. (English)

Shenkman L, Wadler S, Borkowsky W, Shopsin B. Adjuvant effects of lithium chloride on human mononuclear cells in suppressor-enriched and suppressor-depleted systems. *Immunopharmacology.* 1981;3:1-8. (English)

Stolc V. Control of adenylate cyclase EC-4.6.1.1 by divalent cations and agonists: analysis of interactions by the Hill equation. *Biochim Biophys Acta.* 1979;569:267-76. (English)

Watts H, Kennedy PG, Thomas M. The significance of anti-neuronal antibodies in Alzheimer's disease. *J Neuroimmunol.* 1981;1:107-16. (English)

Weinstein Y. Impairment of the hypothalamo-pituitary-ovarian axis of the athymic "nude" mouse. *Mech Ageing Dev.* 1978;8:63-8. (English)

Whalley LJ, Roberts DF, Wentzel J, Watson KC. Antinuclear antibodies and histocompatibility antigens in patients on long-term lithium therapy. *J Affective Disord.* 1981;3:123-30. (English)

Williams JM, Peterson RG, Shea PA, Schmedtje JF, Bauer DC, Felten DL. Sympathetic innervation of murine thymus and spleen: evidence for a functional link between the nervous and immune systems. *Br Res Bull.* 1981;6:83-94. (English)

The following abstract is reprinted by permission of **Nature,** (c) Copyright 1976, Macmillan Journals Limited, from the following source:

Shyamala G, Dickson C. Relationship between receptor and mammary tumor virus production after stimulation of glucocorticoid. *Nature.* 1976; 262:107-12. (English)

The following abstracts are reprinted by permission of **Nature,** (c) Copyright 1979, Macmillan Journals Limited, from the following sources:

Hazum E, Chang KJ, Cuatrecasas P. Role of disulphide and sulphhydryl groups in clustering of enkephalin receptors in neuroblastoma cells. *Nature.* 1979;282:626-8. (English)

Huddlestone JR, Merigan TC Jr, Oldstone MBA. Induction and kinetics of natural killer cells in humans following interferon therapy. *Nature.* 1979; 282:417-9. (English)

The following abstracts are reprinted by permission of Churchill Livingstone, Inc., from the following sources:

Boyd GW. Stress and disease, the missing link: a vasospastic theory; III--Stress, vasospasm and general disease. *Med Hypotheses.* 1978;4:432-44. (English)

Cunnane SC, Manku MS, Horrobin DF. The pineal and regulation of fibrosis: pinealectomy as a model of primary biliary cirrhosis. Roles of melatonin and prostaglandins in fibrosis and regulation of T lymphocytes. *Med Hypotheses.* 1979;5:403-14. (English)

Horrobin DF, Lieb J. A biochemical basis for the actions of lithium on behavior and on immunity: relapsing and remitting disorders of inflammation and immunity such as multiple sclerosis or recurrent herpes as manic-depression of the immune system. *Med Hypotheses* 1981;7:891-905. (English)

Horrobin DF, Manku MS, Oka M, Morgan RO, Cunnane SC, Ally AI, Ghayur T, Schweitzer M, Karmali RA. The nutritional regulation of T lymphocyte function. *Med Hypotheses.* 1979;5:969-85. (English)

Lieb J. Immunopotentiation and inhibition of herpes virus activation during therapy with lithium chloride. *Med Hypotheses.* 1981;7:885-90. (English)

Morosco GJ, Goeringer GC. Lifestyle factors and cancer of the pancreas: a hypothetical mechanism. *Med Hypotheses.* 1980;6:971-85. (English)

Shenkman L, Borkowsky W, Shopsin B. Lithium as an immunological adjuvant. *Med Hypotheses.* 1980;6:1-6. (English)

*The following abstract is reprinted by permission of **Tissue & Cell**, from the following source:*

Reilly FD, McCuskey PA, Miller ML, McCuskey RS, Meineke HA. Innervation of the periarteriolar lymphatic sheath of the spleen. *Tissue Cell.* 1979;11:121-6. (English)

*The following abstract is reprinted by permission of **Journal of Pathology**, from the following source:*

Dianzani MU, Torrielli MV, Canuto RA, Garcea R, Feo F. The influence of enrichment with cholesterol on the phagocytic activity. *J Pathol.* 1976; 118:193-9. (English)

*The following abstracts are reprinted by permission of **Annals of Allergy**, from the following sources:*

Ben-Zvi A, Russel A, Shneyour A, Trainin N. Changes in intra cellular cyclic AMP levels of human peripheral blood lymphocytes in bronchial asthma. *Ann Allergy.* 1979;43:223-4. (English)

Filipp G, Szentivanyi A. Anaphylaxis and the nervous system. *Ann Allergy.* 1958;16:306-11. (English)

Mue S, Ohmi T, Tamura G, Ishihara T, Fujimoto S, Takishima T. The effect of sympathomimetic drugs on immediate skin reactions and metabolic responses in asthmatic patients. *Ann Allergy.* 1979;43:302-9. (English)

Sugerman AA, Southern DL, Curran JF. A study of antibody levels in alcoholic, depressive and schizophrenic patients. *Ann Allergy.* 1982;48:166-71. (English)

Tryphonas H, Trites R. Food allergy in children with hyperactivity, learning disabilities and/or minimal brain dysfunction. *Ann Allergy.* 1979;42:22-7. (English)

Valverde E, Vich JM, Garcia-Calderon JV, Garcia-Calderon PA. *In vitro* response of lymphocytes in patients with allergic tension-fatigue syndrome. *Ann Allergy.* 1980;45:185-8. (English)

The following abstract is reprinted by permission of the American Psychiatric Association, (c) Copyright 1976, the American Psychiatric Association, from the following source:

Surawicz FG, Brightwell DR, Weltzel WD, Othmer E. Cancer, emotions and mental illness: the present state of understanding. *Am J Psychiatr.* 1976;133:1306-9. (English)

The following abstract is reprinted by permission of the American Psychiatric Association, (c) Copyright 1977, the American Psychiatric Association, from the following source:

Nasr SJ, Atkins RW. Coincidental improvement in asthma during lithium treatment. *Am J Psychiatry.* 1977, from the following sources:

The following abstracts are reprinted by permission of the American Psychiatric, Association, (c) Copyright 1978, the American Psychiatric Association, from the following sources:

Hendler N, Leahy W. Psychiatric and neurologic sequelae of infectious mononucleosis. *Am J Psychiatry.* 1978;135:842-4. (English)

Weiner H. The illusion of simplicity: the medical model revisited. *Am J Psychiat.* 1978;135:27-33. (English)

The following abstract is reprinted by permission of the American Psychiatric Association, (c) Copyright 1979, the American Psychiatric Association, from the following source:

Ashkenazi A, Krasilowsky D, Levin S, Idar D, Kalian M, Or A, Ginat Y, Halperin B. Immunologic reaction of psychotic patients to fractions of gluten. *Am J Psychiatry.* 1979;136:1306-9. (English)

The following abstract is reprinted by permission of the American Psychiatric Association, (c) Copyright 1980, the American Psychiatric Association, from the following source:

Luchins DJ, Weinberger DR, Kleinman JE, Neckers LM, Rosenblatt JE, Bigelow LB, Wyatt RJ. Human leukocyte antigen A2 and psychopathology in chronic schizophrenia. *Am J Psychiatry.* 1980;137:499-500. (English)

The following abstracts are reprinted by permission of the American Psychiatric Association, (c) Copyright 1981, the American Psychiatric Association, from the following sources:

Goode DJ, Corbett WT, Schey HM, Suh SH, Woodie B, Morris DL, Morrisey L. Breast cancer in hospitalized psychiatric patients. *Am J Psychiatry.* 1981;138:804-6. (English)

Smeraldi E, Bellodi L. Possible linkage between primary affective disorder susceptibility locus and HLA haplotypes. *Am J Psychiatry.* 1981;138:1232-4. (English)

The following abstracts are reprinted with permission of Pergamon Press, Ltd., (c) Copyright 1977, Pergamon Press, Ltd., from the following sources:

Benjamin S. Is asthma a psychosomatic illness? I--A retrospective study of mental illness and social adjustment. *J Psychosom Res.* 1977;21:463-9. (English)

Benjamin S. Is asthma a psychosomatic illness? II--A comparative study of respiratory impairment and mental health. *J Psychosom Res.* 1977;21:471-81. (English)

Frederick JF. Grief as a disease process. *Omega:Journal of Death and Dying.* 1976-7;7:297-305. (English)

Haney CA. Illness behavior and psychosocial correlates of cancer. *Soc Sci Med.* 1977;11:223-8. (English)

Haynes SG, McMichael AJ, Tyroler HA. The relationship of normal, involuntary retirement to early mortality among U.S. rubber workers. *Soc Sci Med.* 1977;11:105-14. (English)

Pettingale KW, Greer S, Tee DE. Serum IgA and emotional expression in breast cancer patients. *J Psychosom Res.* 1977;21:395-9. (English)

The following abstracts are reprinted with permission of Pergamon Press, Ltd., (c) Copyright 1978, Pergamon Press, Ltd., from the following sources:

Dirks JF, Fross KH, Paley A. Panic-fear in asthma: state-trait relationship and rehospitalization. *J Chronic Dis.* 1978;31:605-9. (English)

Jankovic BD, Isakovic K, Kuezeivic A. Ontogeny of the immuno-neuro-endocrine relationship. Changes in lymphoid tissues of chick embryos surgically decapitated at 33-38 hours of incubation. *Dev Comp Immunol.* 1978;2:479-91. (English)

Mackarness R. Can the food we eat drive us mad? *J Psychosom Res.* 1978;22:355. (English)

Mellett P. The birth of asthma. *J Psychosom Res.* 1978;22:239-46. (English)

Niemi T, Jaaskelainen J. Cancer morbidity in depressive persons. *J Psychosom Res.* 1978;22:117-20. (English)

Plutchik R, Williams MH Jr, Jerrett I, Karasu TB, Kane C. Emotions, personality and life stresses in asthma. *J Psychosom Res.* 1978;22:425-31. (English)

Reichman ME, Villee CA. Estradiol binding by rat thymus cytosol. *J Steroid Biochem.* 1978;9:5637-41. (English)

Teiramaa E. Psychic disturbances and duration of asthma. *J Psychosom Res.* 1978;22:127-32. (English)

Teiramaa E. Psychic disturbances and severity of asthma. *J Psychosom Res.* 1978;22:401-8. (English)

Wayner EA, Flannery GR, Singer G. Effects of taste aversion conditioning on the primary antibody response to sheep red blood cells and Brucella abortus in the albino rat. *Physiol Behav.* 1978;21:995-1000. (English)

The following abstracts are reprinted with permission of Pergamon Press, Ltd., (c) Copyright 1979, Pergamon Press, Ltd., from the following sources:

Ader R, Cohen N, Grota LJ. Adrenal involvement in conditioned immuno-suppression. *Int J Immunopharmacol.* 1979;1:141-5. (English)

Bonnyns M, McKenzie JM. Interactions of stress and endocrine status on rat peripheral lymphocyte responsiveness to phytomitogens. *Psychoneuroendrocrinology.* 1979;4:67-73. (English)

Grossman CJ, Sholiton LJ, Blaha GC, Nathan P. Rat thymic estrogen receptor; II--Physiological properties. *J Steroid Biochem.* 1979;11:1241-6. (English)

Kater L, Oosterom R, McClure JE, Goldstein AL. Presence of thymosin-like factors in human thymic epithelial conditioned medium. *Int J Immunopharmacol.* 1979;1:273-84. (English)

Teiramaa E. Asthma, psychic disturbances and family history of atopic disorders. *J Psychosom Res.* 1979;23:209-17. (English)

Teiramaa E. Psychic factors and the inception of asthma. *J Psychosom Res.* 1979;23:253-62. (English)

The following abstract is reprinted with permission of Pergamon Press, Ltd., (c) Copyright 1980, Pergamon Press, Ltd., from the following source:

Pedernera E, Romano M, Aguilar MC. Influence of early surgical bursectomy on the Leydig cells in the chick embryo testis. *J Steroid Biochem.* 1980;12:517-9. (English)

The following abstracts are reprinted with permission of Pergamon Press, Ltd., (c) Copyright 1981, Pergamon Press, Ltd., from the following sources:

Brodde O-E, Engel G, Hoyer D, Bock KD, Weber F. The beta-adrenergic receptor in human lymphocytes: subclassification by the use of a new radioligand, $(\pm)$-^{125}iodocyanopindolol. *Life Sci.* 1981;29:2189-98. (English)

Gastpar M, Muller W. Auto-antibodies in affective disorders. *Prog Neuropsychopharmacol.* 1981;5:91-7. (English)

Montecucco C, Ballardin S, Zaccolin GP, Pozzan T. Effect of local anesthetics on lymphocyte capping and energy metabolism. *Biochem Pharmacol.* 1981;30:2989-92. (English)

Pettingale KW, Philalithis A, Tee DE, Greer HS. The biological correlates of psychological responses to breast cancer. *J Psychosom Res.* 1981;25:453-8. (English)

Reite M, Harbeck R, Hoffman A. Altered cellular immune response following peer separation. *Life Sci.* 1981;29:1133-6. (English)

Rothschild AM. Plasma kallikrein-generating activity evoked by rat peritoneal fluid mast cells following treatment with epinephrine, 8-bromo-cyclic GMP or compound 48-80. *Biochem Pharmacol.* 1981;30:481-8. (English)

Staudenmayer H. Parental anxiety and other psychosocial factors associated with childhood asthma. *J Chronic Dis.* 1981;34:627-36. (English)

Teiramaa E. Psychosocial factors, personality and acute-insidious asthma. *J Psychosom Res.* 1981;25:43-50. (English)

The following abstracts are reprinted with permission of Pergamon Press, Ltd., (c) Copyright 1982, Pergamon Press, Ltd., from the following sources:

Cox T, Mackay C. Psychosocial factors and psychophysiological mechanisms in the aetiology and development of cancers. *Soc Sci Med.* 1982; 16:381-96. (English)

Krall JF, Connelly M, Tuck ML. *In vitro* desensitization of human lymphocytes by epinephrine. *Biochem Pharmacol.* 1982;31:117-9. (English)

Silverman AY, Darnell BJ, Montiel MM, Smith CG, Asch RH. Response of rhesus monkey lymphocytes to short-term administration of THC. *Life Sci.* 1982;30:107-15. (English)

The following abstract is reprinted by permission of the American Psychological Association, (c) Copyright 1977 by the American Psychological Association, from the following source:

Watson CG, Schuld D. Psychosomatic factors in the etiology of neoplasms. *J Consult Clin Psychol.* 1977;45:455-561. (English)

The following abstracts are reprinted by permission of the American Psychological Association, (c) Copyright 1978 by the American Psychological Association, from the following sources:

Kellerman J. A note on psychosomatic factors in the etiology of neoplasms. *J Consult Clin Psychol.* 1978;46:1522-3. (English)

Watson CG, Schuld D. Psychosomatic etiological factors in neoplasms: a response to Kellerman. *J Consult Clin Psychol.* 1978;46:1524-5. (English)

The following abstract is reprinted by permission of the American Psychological Association, (c) Copyright 1979 by the American Psychological Association, from the following source:

Kobasa SC. Stressful life events, personality and health: an inquiry into hardiness. *J Pers Soc Psych.* 1979;37:1-11. (English)

The following abstract is reprinted by permission of the American Psychological Association, (c) Copyright 1980 by the American Psychological Association, from the following source:

Dattore PJ, Shontz FC, Coyne L. Premorbid personality differentiation of cancer and noncancer groups: a test of the hypothesis of cancer proneness. *J Consult Clin Psychol.* 1980;48:388-94. (English)

The following abstracts are reprinted by permission of the American Psychological Association, (c) Copyright 1981 by the American Psychological Association, from the following sources:

Dunleavy RA. Neuropsychological correlates of asthma: effect of hypoxia or drugs. *J Consult Clin Psychol.* 1981;49:137. (English)

Sklar LS, Anisman H. Stress and cancer. *Psychol Bull.* 1981;89:369-406. (English)

Suess WM, Chai H. Neuropsychological correlates of asthma: brain damage or drug effects. *J Consult Clin Psychol.* 1981;49:135-6. (English)

The following abstract is reprinted by permission of the American Psychological Association, (c) Copyright 1982 by the American Psychological Association, from the following source:

McClelland DC, Alexander C, Marks E. The need for power, stress, immune function, and illness among male prisoners. *J Abnormal Psychol.* 1982; 91:61-70. (English)

The following abstracts are reprinted by courtesy of Marcel Dekker, Inc., from the following sources:

Fauci AS. Mechanisms of the immunosuppressive and anti-inflammatory effects of glucocorticosteroids. *J Immunopharmacol.* 1978-9;1:1-25. (English)

Levy JA, Heppner GH. Alterations of immune reactivity by haloperidol and delta-9-tetrahydrocannabinol. *J Immunopharmacol.* 1981;3:93-109. (English)

Newberry BH, Sengbusch L. Inhibitory effects of stress on experimental mammary tumors. *Cancer Detect Prev.* 1979;2:225-33. (English)

Nieburgs HE, Weiss J, Navarrete M, Strax P, Teirstein A, Grillione G, Siedlecki B. The role of stress in human and experimental oncogenesis. *Cancer Detect Prev.* 1979;2:307-36. (English)

Renoux G, Renoux M. Immunopotentiation and anabolism induced by sodium diethyldithiocarbamate. *J Immunopharmacol.* 1979;1:247-67. (English)

Riley V, Spackman DH, McClanahan H, Santisteban GA. The role of stress in malignancy. *Cancer Detect Prev.* 1979;2:235-55. (English)

Riley V. Cancer and stress: overview and critique. *Cancer Detect Prev.* 1979;2:163-95. (English)

Riley V. Introduction: stress-cancer contradictions--a continuing puzzlement. *Cancer Detect Prev.* 1979;2:159-62. (English)

Riley V. Stress and cancer: fresh perspectives. In: *Proc Int Symp Detect Prev Cancer, 3rd.* NY: Marcel Dekker Inc., 1978. Pp. 1769-76. (English)

Solomon GF, Amkraut AA. Neuroendocrine aspects of the immune response and their implications for stress effects on tumor immunity. *Cancer Detect Prev.* 1979;2:197-224. (English)

Weinstein Y, Melmon KL. Control of immune responses by cyclic AMP and lymphocytes that adhere to histamine columns. *Immunol Commun.* 1976;5:401-16. (English)

The following abstracts are reprinted by permission of **The Gerontologist,** *from the following sources:*

Kraus LJ. Augmentation of human natural killer cell activity by catecholamines (abstract). *The Gerontologist.* 1982;22:204. (English)

Locke SE. Looking ahead: possible mechanisms of stress effects on immunity (abstract). *The Gerontologist.* 1982;22:204. (English)

Platt R. Infectious disease in the elderly: assessment of risk factors (abstract). *The Gerontologist.* 1982;22:203. (English)

Stein M. Stress, brain and immune function (abstract). *The Gerontologist.* 1982;22:203. (English)

Strom TB. Neuroendocrine influences on immunity: immunoregulation via second messenger systems (abstract). *The Gerontologist.* 1982;22:204. (English)

Yunis EJ, Watson ALM, Shankariah K, Halberg F. Dietary restriction and aging (abstract). *The Gerontologist.* 1982;22:203-4. (English)

The following abstracts are reprinted by permission of the **Journal of Gerontology,** *from the following sources:*

Abrass IB, Scarpace PJ. Human lymphocyte beta-adrenergic receptors are unaltered with age. *J Gerontol.* 1981;36:298-301. (English)

Blichert-Toft M, Hummer L. Immunoreactive corticotrophin reserve in old age in man during and after surgical stress. *J Gerontol.* 1976;31:539. (English)

The following abstracts are reprinted by permission of Plenum Press, from the following sources:

Anonymous. Lithium effects on granulopoiesis and immune function. In: *Adv Exp Med Biol.* 1980;127:1-475. (English)

Baker GA, Santalo R, Blumenstein J. Effect of psychotropic agents upon the blastogenic response of human T-lymphocytes. *Biol Psychiat.* 1977;12:159-69. (English)

Baron M, Stern M, Anavi R, Witz IP. Tissue-binding factor in schizophrenic sera: a clinical and genetic study. *Biol Psychiat.* 1977;12:199-219. (English)

Bell IR, Guilleminault C, Dement WC. Hypersomnia, multiple-system symptomatology, and selective IgA deficiency. *Biol Psychiat.* 1978;13:751-7. (English)

Bergen JR, Grinspoon L, Pyle HM, Martinez JL Jr, Pennel RB. Immunologic studies in schizophrenic and control subjects. *Biol Psychiat.* 1980;15:369-79. (English)

Borysenko M, Turesky S, Borysenko J, Quimby F, Benson H. Stress and dental caries in the rat. *J Behav Med.* 1980;3:233-43. (English)

Cohen D, Eisdorfer C, Vitaliano PP, Bloom V. The relationship of age, anxiety, and serum immunoglobulins with crystallized and fluid intelligence. *Biol Psychiat.* 1980;15:699-709. (English)

Deberdt R, Van Hooren J, Biesbrouck M, Amery W. Antinuclear factor-positive mental depression: A single disease entity? *Biol Psychiat.* 1976;11:69-74. (English)

Fox BH. Premorbid psychological factors as related to cancer incidence. *J Behav Med.* 1978;1:45-134. (English)

Friedenberg WR, Marx JJ. The bactericidal defect of neutrophil function with lithium therapy. *Adv Exp Med Biol.* 1980;127:389-99. (English)

Gelfand EW, Cheung R, Hastings D, Dosch HM. Characterization of lithium effects on two aspects of T cell function. *Adv Exp Med Biol.* 1980;127:429-46. (English)

Jankovic BD, Jakulic S, Horvat J. Delayed skin hypersensitivity reactions to human brain S-100 protein in psychiatric patients. *Biol Psychiat.* 1982;17:687-97. (English)

Johnson SB. Psychosocial factors in juvenile diabetes: a review. *J Behav Med.* 1980;3:95-116. (English)

King DS. Can allergic exposure provoke psychological symptoms? A double-blind test. *Biol Psychiat.* 1981;16:3-19. (English)

Lebowitz MD, Thompson HC, Strunk RC. Subjective psychological symptoms in outpatient asthmatic adolescents. *J Behav Med.* 1981;4:439-49. (English)

Locke SE, Heisel JS. The influence of stress and emotions on the human immune response (abstract). *Biofeedback Self-Regul.* 1977;2:320. (English)

McMahon CE, Hastrup JL. The role of imagination in the disease process: post-Cartesian history. *J Behav Med.* 1980;3:205-17. (English)

Pohl RB, Berchou R, Gupta BK. Lithium-induced hypothyroidism and thyroiditis. *Biol Psychiat.* 1979;14:835-7. (English)

Rudin DO. The choroid plexus and system disease in mental illness; III--The exogenous peptide hypothesis of mental illness. *Biol Psychiat.* 1981;16:489-512. (English)

Rudin DO. The choroid plexus and system disease in mental illness; I--A new brain attack mechanism via the second blood-brain barrier. *Biol Psychiat.* 1980;15:517-39. (English)

Rudin DO. The choroid plexus and system disease in mental illness; II--Systemic lupus erythematosus: a combined transport dysfunction model for schizophrenia. *Biol Psychiat.* 1981;16:373-97. (English)

Seegmiller JE, Watanabe T, Shreier MH, Waldmann TA. Immunological aspects of purine metabolism. *Adv Exp Med Biol.* 1977;76A:412-33. (English)

Stefanis C, Issidorides MR. Histochemical changes in the blood cells of schizophrenic patients under pimozide treatment. *Biol Psychiat.* 1976;11:53-68. (English)

Stubbs EG, Crawford ML. Depressed lymphocyte responsiveness in autistic children. *J Autism Child Schizo.* 1977;7:49-55. (English)

Stubbs EG. Autistic children exhibit undetectable hemagglutination-inhibition antibody titers despite previous rubella vaccination. *J Autism Child Schizo.* 1976;6:269-74. (English)

Targum SD, Gershon ES, Van Eerdewegh M, Rogentine N. Human leukocyte antigen system not closely linked to or associated with bipolar manic-depressive illness. Biol Psychiat. 1979;14:615-36. (English)

Turner WJ, King S. Two genetically distinct forms of bipolar affective disorder? *Biol Psychiat.* 1981;16:417-39. (English)

Watanabe M, Funahashi T, Suzuki T, Nomura S, Nakazawa T, Noguchi T, Tsukada Y. Antithymic antibodies in schizophrenic sera. *Biol Psychiat.* 1982;17:699-710. (English)

Watanabe M, Noguchi T, Tsukada Y. Regional, cellular, and subcellular distribution of Thy-1 antigen in rat nervous tissues. *Neurochem Res.* 1981;6:507-19. (English)

The following abstracts are reproduced by permission of Williams and Wilkins Co., (c) Copyright 1976, The Williams & Wilkins Co., from the following sources:

Brouet JC, Toben H. Characterization of a subpopulation of human T lymphocytes reactive with an heteroantiserum to human brain. *J Immunol.* 1976;116:1041. (English)

Davis DI, Offenkrantz W. Is there a reciprocal relationship between symptoms and affect in asthma? *J Nerv Ment Dis.* 1976;163:369-90. (English)

Ferguson RM, Schmidtke JR, Simmons RL. Inhibition of mitogen-induced lymphocyte transformation by local anesthetics. *J Immunol.* 1976;116:627-34. (English)

Fernandes G, Halberg F, Yunis EJ, Good RA. Circadian rhythmic plaque-forming cell response of spleens from mice immunized with SRBC. *J Immunol.* 1976;117:962-6. (English)

Foon KA, Wahl SM, Oppenheim JJ, Rosenstreich DL. Serotonin-induced production of a monocyte chemotactic factor by human peripheral blood leukocytes. *J Immunol.* 1976;117:1545-52. (English)

Galant SP, Lundak RL, Eaton L. Enhancement of early human E rosette formation by cholinergic stimuli. *J Immunol.* 1976;117:48-51. (English)

McMillan R, Longmire R, Yelenosky R. The effects of corticosteroids on human IgG synthesis. *J Immunol.* 1976;116:1592-5. (English)

Miyabo S, Hisada T, Asato T, Mizushima N, Ueno K. Growth hormone and cortisol responses to psychological stress: comparison of normal and neurotic subjects. *J Clin Endocrinol Metab.* 1976;42:1158-62. (English)

Patterson R, Suszko IM, Metzger WJ, Roberts M. *In vitro* production of IgE by human peripheral blood lymphocytes: effect of cholera toxin and beta-adrenergic stimulation. *J Immunol.* 1976;117:97-101. (English)

Reed CE, Busse WW, Lee TP. Adrenergic mechanisms and the adenyl cyclase system in atopic dermatitis. *J Invest Dermatol.* 1976;67:333-8. (English)

Sullivan TJ, Parker KL, Kulczycki A Jr, Parker CW. Modulation of cyclic AMP in purified rat mast cells; III—Studies on the effects of concanavalin A and anti-IgE on cyclic AMP during histamine release. *J Immunol.* 1976;117:713-6. (English)

Swierenga SHH, MacManus JP, Braceland BM, Youdale T. Regulation of the primary immune response *in vivo* by parathyroid hormone. *J Immunol.* 1976;117:1608-11. (English)

The following abstracts are reproduced by permission of Williams and Wilkins Co., (c) Copyright 1977, The Williams & Wilkins Co., from the following sources:

Coffey RG, Hadden EM, Hadden JW. Evidence for cyclic GMP and calcium mediation of lymphocyte activation by mitogens. *J Immunol.* 1977;119:1387-94. (English)

Fauci AS, Pratt KR, Whalen G. Activation of human B lymphocytes; IV—Regulatory effects of corticosteroids on the triggering signal in the plaque-forming cell response of human peripheral blood B lymphocytes to polyclonal activation. *J Immunol.* 1977;119:598-603. (English)

Hunninghake GW, Fauci AS. Immunologic reactivity of the lung; III—Effects of corticosteroids on alveolar macrophage cytotoxic effector cell function. *J Immunol.* 1977;118:146-50. (English)

Lee K-C. Cortisone as a probe for cell interactions in the generation of cytotoxic T cells; I—Effect on helper cells, cytotoxic T cell precursors, and accessory cells. *J Immunol.* 1977;119:1836-45. (English)

Lesniak MA, Gorden P, Roth J. Reactivity of non-primate growth hormones and prolactins with human growth hormone receptors on cultured human lymphocytes. *J Clin Endocrinol Metab.* 1977;44:838-99. (English)

Mishell RI, Lucas A, Mishell BB. The role of activated accessory cells in preventing immunosuppression by hydrocortisone. *J Immunol.* 1977;119:118-22. (English)

Miyabo S, Asato T, Mizushima N. Prolactin and growth hormone responses to psychological stress in normal and neurotic subjects. *J Clin Endocrinol Metab.* 1977;44:947-51. (English)

Parker CW, Kennedy S, Eisen AZ. Leukocyte and lymphocyte cyclic AMP responses in atopic eczema. *J Invest Dermatol.* 1977;68:302-6. (English)

Schwartz A, Askenase PW, Gershon RK. The effect of locally injected vasoactive amines on the elicitation of delayed-type hypersensitivity. *J Immunol.* 1977;118:159-65. (English)

Straker N, Bieber J. Asthma and the vicissitudes of aggression: two case reports of childhood asthma. *J Am Acad Child Psychiatry.* 1977;16:132-9. (English)

Weinstein Y. 20-alpha-hydroxysteroid dehydrogenase: a T lymphocyte-associated enzyme. *J Immunol.* 1977;119:1223-9. (English)

Young JG, Caparulo BK, Shaywitz BA, Johnson WT, Cohen DJ. Childhood autism: cerebrospinal fluid examination and immunoglobulin levels. *J Am Acad Child Psychiatry.* 1977;16:174-9. (English)

The following abstracts are reproduced by permission of Williams and Wilkins Co., (c) Copyright 1978, The Williams & Wilkins Co., from the following sources:

Gallin JI, Sandler JA, Clyman RI, Manganiello VC, Vaughan M. Agents that increase cyclic AMP inhibit accumulation of cGMP and depress human monocyte locomotion. *J Immunol.* 1978;120:492-6. (English)

Ohara J, Kishimoto T, Yamamura Y. *In vitro* immune response of human peripheral lymphocytes; III—Effect of anti-mu or anti-gamma antibody on PWM-induced increase of cyclic nucleotides in human B lymphocytes. *J Immunol.* 1978;121:2058-96. (English)

Pierpaoli W, Maestroni GJ. Pharmacologic control of the hormonally modulated immune response; III—Prolongation of allogeneic skin graft rejection and prevention of runt disease by a combination of drugs acting on neuroendocrine functions. *J Immunol.* 1978;120:1600-3. (English)

Rosenberg JC, Lysz K. Suppression of human cytotoxic lymphocytes by methylprednisolone. *Transplantation.* 1978;25:115-20. (English)

Theoharides TC, Douglas WW. Somatostatin induces histamine secretion from rat peritoneal mast cells. *Endocrinology.* 1978;102:1637-40. (English)

The following abstracts are reproduced by permission of Williams and Wilkins Co., (c) Copyright 1979, The Williams & Wilkins Co., from the following sources:

Beck-Nielsen H, Kuhl C, Pedersen O, Bjerre-Christensen C, Nielsen TT, Klebe JG. Decreased insulin binding to monocytes from normal pregnant women. *J Clin Endocrinol Metab.* 1979;49:810-4. (English)

Dann JA, Wachtel SS, Rubin AL. Possible involvement of the central nervous system in graft rejection. *Transplantation.* 1979;27:223-6. (English)

Dirks JF, Kinsman RA, Staudenmayer H, Kleiger JH. Panic-fear in asthma: symptomatology as an index of signal anxiety and personality as an index of ego resources. *J Nerv Ment Dis.* 1979;167:615-9. (English)

Gillis B, Crabtree GR, Smith KA. Glucocorticoid-inhibition of T cell growth factor production; I—The effect of mitogen-induced lymphocyte proliferation. *J Immunol.* 1979;123:1624-31. (English)

Gillis S, Crabtree GR, Smith KA. Glucocorticoid-induced inhibition of T cell growth factor production; II—The effect on the *in vitro* generation of cytolytic T cells. *J Immunol.* 1979;123:1632-8. (English)

Hong KM, Hopwood MA, Wirt RD, Yellin AM. Psychological attributes, patterns of life change, and illness susceptibility. *J Nerv Ment Dis.* 1979;167:275-81. (English)

Kishimoto S, Tomino S, Mitsuya H, Fugiwara H. Age-related changes in suppressor functions of human T cells. *J Immunol.* 1979;123:1586-93. (English)

Sullivan TJ, Parker CW. Possible role of arachidonic acid and its metabolites in mediator release from rat mast cells. *J Immunol.* 1979;122:431-6. (English)

Williams RS, Guthrow CE, Lefkowitz RJ. Beta-adrenergic receptors of human lymphocytes are unaltered by hyperthyroidism. *J Clin Endocrinol Metab.* 1979;48:503-5. (English)

Wybran J, Appelboom T, Famacy J-P, Govaerts A. Suggestive evidence for receptors for morphine and methionine-enkephalin on normal human blood T-lymphocytes. *J Immunol.* 1979;123:1068-70. (English)

The following abstracts are reproduced by permission of Williams and Wilkins Co., (c) Copyright 1980, The Williams & Wilkins Co., from the following sources:

Cohen D, Eisdorfer C. Antinuclear antibodies in the cognitively impaired elderly. *J Nerv Ment Dis.* 1980;168:179-80. (English)

Davies AO, Lefkowitz RJ. Corticosteroid-induced differential regulation of beta-adrenergic receptors in circulating human polymorphonuclear leukocytes and mononuclear leukocytes. *J Clin Endocrinol Metab.* 1980;51:599-605. (English)

Krall JF, Connelly M, Tuck ML. Acute regulation of beta-adrenergic catecholamine sensitivity in human lymphocytes. *J Pharmacol Exp Ther.* 1980;214:554-60. (English)

McDonough RJ, Madden JJ, Falek A, Shafer DA, Pline M, Gordon D, Bokos P, Kuehnle JC, Mendelson J. Alteration of T and null lymphocyte frequencies in the peripheral blood of human opiate addicts: *in vivo* evidence for opiate receptor sites on T lymphocytes. *J Immunol.* 1980;125:2539-43. (English)

Tuck ML, Fittingoff D, Connelly M, Krall JF. Beta-adrenergic catecholamine regulation of lymphocyte sensitivity heterologous desensitization to prostaglandin E$_2$ by isoproterenol. *J Clin Endocrinol Metab.* 1980; 51:1-6. (English)

The following abstracts are reproduced by permission of Williams and Wilkins Co., (c) Copyright 1981, The Williams & Wilkins Co., from the following sources:

Goodwin JS, Bromberg S, Staszak C, Kaszubowski PA, Messner RP, Neal JF, Effect on physical stress on sensitivity of lymphocytes to inhibition by prostaglandin E$_2$. *J Immunol.* 1981;127:518-22. (English)

Jacobs S, Cuatrecasas P. Insulin receptor: structure and function. *Endocrinol Rev.* 1981;2:251-63. (English)

Krall JF, Connelly M, Weisbart R, Tuck ML. Age-related elevation of plasma catecholamine concentration and reduced responsiveness of lymphocyte adenylate cyclase. *J Clin Endocrinol Metab.* 1981;52:863-7. (English)

Strom TB, Lane MA, George K. The parallel, time-dependent, bimodal change in lymphocyte cholinergic binding activity and cholinergic influence upon lymphocyte-mediated cytotoxicity after lymphocyte activation. *J Immunol.* 1981;127:705-10. (English)

The following abstracts are reproduced by permission of Williams and Wilkins Co., (c) Copyright 1982, The Williams & Wilkins Co., from the following sources:

Stephens CG, Snyderman R. Cyclic nucleotides regulate the morphologic alterations required for chemotaxis in monocytes. *J Immunol.* 1982; 128:1192-7. (English)

Strom TB, Bangs JD. Human serum-free mixed lymphocytes: the stereospecific effect of insulin and its potentiation by transferrin. *J Immunol.* 1982;128:1555-9. (English)

Vanley GT, Huberman R, Lufkin RB. Atypical pneumocystis carinii pneumonia in homosexual men with unusual immunodeficiency. *AJR.* 1982;138: 1037-41. (English)

The following abstract is reproduced by permission of Williams and Wilkins Co., (c) Copyright 1983, The Williams & Wilkins Co., from the following source:

Crary B, Borysenko M, Sutherland DC, Kutz I, Borysenko J, Benson H. Decrease in mitogen responsiveness of mononuclear cells from peripheral blood after epinephrine administration in humans. *J Immunol.* 1983; 130:694-7. (English)

The following abstract is reprinted by permission of the American Medical Association, (c) Copyright 1976, American Medical Association, from the following source:

Shapiro RW, Bock E, Rafaelsen OJ, Ryder LP, Svejgaard A. Histocompatibility antigens and manic-depressive disorders. *Arch Gen Psychiatry.* 1976;33:823-5. (English)

The following abstracts are reprinted by permission of the American Medical Association, (c) Copyright 1977, American Medical Association, from the following sources:

Fu T-K, Jarvik LF, Yen F-S, Matsuyama SS. *In vitro* effects of imipramine on proliferation of human leukocytes. *Arch Gen Psychiatry.* 1977;34:728-30. (English)

Monroe EW, Jones EH. Urticaria: an updated review. *Arch Dermatol.* 1977;113:80-90. (English)

The following abstracts are reprinted by permission of the American Medical Association, (c) Copyright 1979, American Medical Association, from the following sources:

Crowe RR, Thompson JS, Flink R, Weinberger B. HLA antigens and schizophrenia. *Arch Gen Psychiatry.* 1979;36:231-3. (English)

Monto AS, Gunn RA, Bandyk MG, King CL. Prevention of Russian influenza by amantadine. *JAMA.* 1979;241:1003-7. (English)

Skoven I, Thormann J. Lithium compound treatment and psoriasis. *Arch Dermatol.* 1979;115:1185-7. (English)

The following abstract is reprinted by permission of the American Medical Association, (c) Copyright 1980, American Medical Association, from the following source:

Dimsdale JE, Moss J. Plasma catecholamine in stress and exercise. *JAMA.* 1980;243:340-2. (English)

The following abstract is reprinted by permission of the American Medical Association, (c) Copyright 1981, American Medical Association, from the following source:

Beisel WR, Edelman R, Nauss K, Suskind RM. Single-nutrient effects on immunologic functions: report of a workshop sponsored by the department of Food and Nutrition and its Nutrition Advisory Group of the AMA. *JAMA.* 1981;245:53-8. (English)

The following abstract is reprinted by permission of the American Medical Association, (c) Copyright 1982, American Medical Association, from the following source:

Hirata-Hibi M, Higashi S, Tachibana T, Watanabe N. Stimulated lymphocytes in schizophrenia. *Arch Gen Psychiatry.* 1982;39:82-7. (English)

The following abstracts are reprinted by permission of C. V. Mosby Co., from the following sources:

Bishopric NJ, Cohen HJ, Lefkowitz RJ. Beta-adrenergic receptors in lymphocyte subpopulations. *J Allergy Clin Immunol.* 1980;65:29-33. (English)

Busse WW, Anderson CL, Hanson PG, Folts JD. The effect of exercise on the granulocyte response to isoproterenol in the trained athlete and unconditioned individual. *J Allergy Clin Immunol.* 1980;65:358-64. (English)

Busse WW, Lee TP. Decreased adrenergic responses in lymphocytes and granulocytes in atopic eczema. *J Allergy Clin Immunol.* 1976;58:586-96. (English)

Dahlem NW, Kinsman RA, Horton DJ. Panic-fear in asthma: Requests for as-needed medications in relation to pulmonary function measurements. *J Allergy Clin Immunol.* 1977;60:295-300. (English)

Friedman E, Katcher AH, Brightman VJ. Incidence of recurrent herpes labialis and upper respiratory infection: a prospective study of the influence of biologic, social and psychologic predictors. *Oral Surg.* 1977;43:873-8. (English)

Galant SP, Allred SJ, Demonstration of beta$_2$-adrenergic receptors of high coupling efficiency in human neutrophil sonicates. *J Lab Clin Med.* 1980;96:15-23. (English)

Galant SP, Underwood S, Duriseti L, Insel PA. characterization of high-affinity beta$_2$-adrenergic receptor binding of (-)[^{3}H]dihydroalprenolol to human polymorphonuclear cell particulates. *J Lab Clin Med.* 1978;92:613-8. (English)

Grieco MH, Siegel I, Goel Z. Modulation of human T lymphocyte rosette formation by autonomic agonists and cyclic nucleotides. *J Allergy Clin Immunol.* 1976;58:149-59. (English)

Hanifin JM. Atopic dermatitis. *J Am Acad Dermatol.* 1982;6:1-13. (English)

Keller AJ, Irvine WJ, Jordan J, Loudon NB. Phytohemagglutinin-induced lymphocyte transformation in oral contraceptive users. *Obstet Gynecol.* 1977;49:83-91. (English)

Kim SP, Ferrara A, Chess S. Temperament of asthmatic children: a preliminary study. *J Pediatr.* 1980;97:483-6. (English)

Kohn BA, Twarog FJ, Geha RS. Differential effects of pharmacologic agents on EAC3 rosette formation by lymphocytes from normal and asthmatic subjects. *J Allergy Clin Immunol.* 1979;64:182-8. (English)

Lee TP, Busse WW, Reed CE. Effect of beta-adrenergic agonist, prostaglandins, and cortisol on lymphocyte levels of cyclic adenosine monophosphate and glycogen: abnormal lymphocytic metabolism in asthma. *J Allergy Clin Immunol.* 1977;59:408-13. (English)

Lee TP. Effects of histamine-sensitizing factor and cortisol on lymphocyte adenyl cyclase responses. *J Allergy Clin Immunol.* 1977;59:79-82. (English)

Makino S, Ikemori K, Kashima T, Fukuda T. Comparison of cyclic adenosine monophosphate response of lymphocytes in normal and asthmatic subjects to norepinephrine and salbutamol. *J Allergy Clin Immunol.* 1977;59:348-52. (English)

Marone G, Lichtenstein LM. Adenosine-adenosine deaminase modulation of histamine release. *J Allergy Clin Immunol.* 1978;61:131. (English)

Mori T, Kobayashi H, Nishimoto H, Suzuki A, Nishimura T, Mori T. Inhibitory effect of progesterone and 20-alpha-hydroxypregn-4-en-3-one on the phytohaemagglutinin-induced transformation of human lymphocytes. *Am J Obstet Gynecol.* 1977;127:1512-7. (English)

Morito T, Bankhurst AD, Williams RC Jr. Studies on the pharmacologic manipulation of suppressor cells associated with impaired immunoglobulin production. *J Lab Clin Med.* 1980;96:232-7. (English)

Morris HG, Rusnak SA, Barzens K. Leukocyte cyclic adenosine monophosphate in asthmatic children: effects of adrenergic therapy. *Clin Pharmacol Therap.* 1977;22:352-7. (English)

Pattillo RA, Shalaby MR, Hussa RO, Bahl OMP, Mattingly RF. Effect of crude and purified hCG on lymphocyte blastogenesis. *Obstet Gynecol.* 1976;47:557-61. (English)

Rasmussen EO, Cooper KD, Kang K, White CR Jr, Regan DH, Hanifin JM. Immunosuppression in a homosexual man with Kaposi's sarcoma. *J Am Acad Dermatol.* 1982;6:870-9. (English)

The following abstracts are reprinted by permission of Blackwell Scientific Publications Limited, from the following sources:

Ahmar H, Kurban AK. Psychological profile of patients with atopic dermatitis. *Br J Dermatol.* 1976;95:373-7. (English)

Bardos P, Degenne D, Lebranchu Y, Biziere K, Renoux G. Neocortical lateralization of NK activity in mice. *Scand J Immunol.* 1981;13:609-11. (English)

Berenbaum MC, Cope WA, Bundick RV. Synergistic effect of cortisol and prostaglandin E on the PHA response. *Clin Exp Immunol.* 1976;26:534-41. (English)

Berenbaum MC, Purves EC, Allison IE. Intercellular immunological controls and modulation of cyclic AMP levels: some doubts. *Immunology.* 1976;30:815-23. (English)

Besedovsky HO, Del Rey A, Sorkin E. Antigenic competition between horse and sheep red blood cells as a hormone-dependent phenomenon. *Clin Exp Immunol.* 1979;37:106-13. (English)

Besedovsky HO, Sorkin E. Network of immune-neuroendocrine interactions. *Clin Exp Immunol.* 1977;27:1-12. (English)

Cooper DA, Duckett M, Petts V, Penny R. Corticosteroid enhancement of immunoglobulin synthesis by pokeweed mitogen-stimulated human lymphocytes. *Clin Exp Immunol.* 1979;37:145-51. (English)

Fauci AS. Mechanisms of corticosteroid action on lymphocyte subpopulations; II—Differential effects of *in vivo* hydrocortisone, prednisone and dexamethasone on *in vitro* expression of lymphocyte function. *Clin Exp Immunol.* 1976;24:54-62. (English)

Fernandez LA, Fox RA. Perturbation of the human immune system by lithium. *Clin Exp Immunol.* 1980;41:527-32. (English)

Holm G, Palmblad J. Acute energy deprivation in man: effect on cell-mediated immunological reactions. *Clin Exp Immunol.* 1976;25:207-11. (English)

Jankovic BD, Jakulic S, Horvat J. Schizophrenia and other psychiatric diseases: evidence for neurotissue hypersensitivity. *Clin Exp Immunol.* 1980;40:515-22. (English)

Macdonald SM, Goldstone AH, Morris JE, Exton-Smith AN, Callard RE. Immunological parameters in the aged and in Alzheimer's disease. *Clin Exp Immunol.* 1982;49:123-8. (English)

Mendelsohn J, Multer MM, Bernheim JL. Inhibition of human lymphocyte stimulation by steroid hormones: cytokinetic mechanisms. *Clin Exp Immunol.* 1977;27:127-34. (English)

Palmblad J, Cantell K, Holm G, Norberg R, Strander H, Sunblad L. Acute energy deprivation in man: effect on serum immunoglobulins antibody response, complement factors 3 and 4, acute phase reactants and interferon-producing capacity of blood lymphocytes. *Clin Exp Immunol.* 1977;30:50-5. (English)

Pedersen EB, Morgensen CE, Selling K, Amdisen A, Darling S. Urinary excretion of albumin beta$_2$-microglobulin and free light chains during lithium treatment. *Scand J Clin Lab Invest.* 1978;38:269-72. (English)

Pierpaoli W, Kopp HG, Bianchi E. Interdependence of thymic and neuroendocrine functions in ontogeny. *Clin Exp Immunol.* 1976;24:501-6. (English)

Pierpaoli W, Maestroni GJ. Pharmacologic control of the hormonally modulated immune response; II—Blockade of antibody production by a combination of drugs acting on neuroendocrine function—its prevention by gonadotropins and corticotropin. *Immunol.* 1978;34:419-30. (English)

Pochet R, Delespesse G, Gausset PW, Collet H. Distribution of beta-adrenergic receptors on human lymphocyte sub-populations. *Clin Exp Immunol.* 1979;38:578-84. (English)

Ritter M. Embryonic mouse thymocyte development enhancing effect of corticosterone at physiological levels. *Immunol.* 1977;33:241-6. (English)

Roszman TL, Cross RJ, Brooks WH, Markesbery WR. Hypothalamic-immune interactions; I--The effect of hypothalamic lesions on the ability of adherent spleen cells to limit lymphocyte blastogenesis. *Immunology.* 1982;45:737-42. (English)

Ryzewski J, Roszkowski-Sliz W, Krzystyniak K. The action of thiols on lymphocyte membranes. *Immunology.* 1976;31:145-9. (English)

Singh U. *In vitro* lymphopoiesis in foetal thymic organ cultures: effect of various agents. *Clin Exp Immunol.* 1980;41:150-5. (English)

Teng CS, Smith BR, Clayton B. Thyroid stimulating antibodies to the immunoglobulins in opthalmic Graves' disease. *Clin Endocrinol.* 1977;6:207-11. (English)

Wyle FA, Kent JR. Immunosuppression by sex hormones; I--The effect upon PHA- and PPD-stimulated lymphocytes. *Clin Exp Immunol.* 1977;27:407-15. (English)

Yu DT, Clements PJ. Human lymphocyte subpopulations: effect of epinephrine. *Clin Exp Immunol.* 1976;25:472-9. (English)

Zucker S, Zarrabi MH, Romano GS, Miller F. IgM inhibitors of the contact activation phase of coagulation in chlorpromazine-treated patients. *Br J Haematol.* 1978;40:447-57. (English)

The following abstracts are reprinted by permission of Springer-Verlag, (c) Copyright 1976, from the following sources:

Ader R. Conditioned adrenocortical steroid elevations in the rat. *J Comp Physiol Psychol.* 1976;90:1156-63. (English)

Ishii T, Haga S. Immuno-electron microscopic localization of immunoglobulins in amyloid fibrils of senile plaques. *Acta Neuropathol.* 1976;36:243-9. (German)

Tutton PJM, Barkla DH. A comparison of cell proliferation in normal and neoplastic intestinal epithelia following either biogenic amine depletion or monoamine oxidase inhibition. *Virchows Arch B Cell Path.* 1976;21:161-8. (English)

The following abstract is reprinted by permission of Springer-Verlag, (c) Copyright 1978, from the following source:

Von Gaudecker B. Ultrastructure of the age-involuted adult human thymus. *Cell Tissue Res.* 1978;186:507-25. (English)

The following abstracts are reprinted by permission of Springer-Verlag, (c) Copyright 1979, from the following sources:

Ago Y, Teshima H, Nagata S, Inoue S, Ikemi Y. Psychosomatic studies of allergic disorders. *Psychother Psychosom.* 1979;31:197-204. (English)

Becker H. Psychodynamic aspects of breast cancer--differences in younger and older patients. *Psychother Psychosom.* 1979;32:287-96. (English)

Groen JJ. The psychosomatic theory of bronchial asthma. *Psychother Psychosom.* 1979;31:38-48. (English)

Pierloot RA. Psychogenesis of somatic disorders. *Psychother Psychosom.* 1979;32:27-40. (English)

The following abstracts are reprinted by permission of Springer-Verlag, (c) Copyright 1980, from the following sources:

Grossarth-Maticek R. Psychosocial predictors of cancer and internal diseases: an overview. *Psychother Psychosom.* 1980;33:122-8. (English)

Grossarth-Maticek R. Social psychotherapy and course of the disease. *Psychother Psychosom.* 1980;33:129-38. (English)

Madle S, Obe G, Schroeter H, Herha J, Pietzcker A. Possible mutagenicity of the psychoactive phenathiazine derivative perazine *in vivo* and *in vitro.* *Hum Genet.* 1980;53:357-61. (English)

Quay WB, Gorray KC. Pineal effects on metabolism and glucose homeostasis: evidence for lines of humoral mediation of pineal influences on tumor growth. *J Neural Transm.* 1980;47:107-20. (English)

Skinner GR, Harley C, Buchan A, Harper L, Gallimore P. The effect of lithium chloride on the replication of herpes simplex virus. *Med Microbiol Immunol (Berl).* 1980;168:139-148. (English)

Smeraldi E, Scorza-Smeraldi R, Fabio G, Negri F. Interference between anti-HLA antibodies and chlorpromazine metabolites. *Psychopharmacol (Berl).* 1980;67:87-9. (English)

The following abstracts are reprinted by permission of Springer-Verlag, (c) Copyright 1981, from the following sources:

Dirks JF, Robinson SK, Dirks DL. Alexithymia and the psychomaintenance of bronchial asthma. *Psychother Psychosom.* 1981;36:63-71. (English)

Gotlieb-Stematsky T, Zonis J, Arlazoroff A, Mozes T, Sigal M, Szekely AG. Antibodies to Epstein-Barr virus, herpes simplex type 1, cytomegalovirus and measles virus in psychiatric patients. *Arch Virol.* 1981;67:333-9. (English)

Krakowka S, Wallace AL, Koestner A. Shared antigenic determinants between brain and thymus-derived lymphocytes in dogs. *Acta Neuropathol.* 1981;54:75-82. (English)

Siadak AW, Nowinski RC. Thy-2: a murine thymocyte-brain alloantigen controlled by a gene linked to the major histocompatibility complex. *Immunogenetics.* 1981;12:45-58. (English)

Spoljar M, Eicher W, Eiermann W, Cleve H. H-Y antigen expression in different tissues from transsexuals. *Hum Genet.* 1981;57:52-7. (English)

Torack RM, Lynch RG. Cytochemistry of brain amyloid in adult dementia. *Acta Neuropathol (Berl).* 1981;53:189-96. (English)

The following abstract is reprinted by permission of Springer-Verlag, (c) Copyright 1982, from the following source:

Tantam D, Kalucy R, Brown DG. Sleep, scratching and dreams in eczema: a new approach to alexithymia. *Psychother Psychosom.* 1982;37:26-35. (English)

The following abstracts are reprinted by permission of Bailliere Tindall, from the following sources:

Lord A, Sutton RN, Baker AA, Hussein SA. Serological studies in the elderly. *Age Ageing.* 1978;7:116-22. (English)

Martin JM, Kellett JM, Kahn J. Aneuploidy in cultured human lymphocytes; II--A comparison between senescence and dementia. *Age Ageing.* 1981;10:24-8. (English)

Mayer PP, Chughtai MA, Cape RD. An immunological approach to dementia in the elderly. *Age Ageing.* 1976;5:164-70. (English)

Snowden PR, Woodrow JC, Copeland JR. HLA antigens in senile dementia and multiple infarct dementia. *Age Ageing.* 1981;10:259-63. (English)

Author Index

Note: The numbers in this index refer to abstract numbers, not page numbers. Readers are also advised that authors' names have been recorded exactly as they appear in the original abstract; thus, the same author may be listed under two slightly different names.

A-Wahid F 354
Aarons RD 306
Abdel-Monem MM 481
Abe T 72
Abegg A 997
Abeioff MD 942
Abplanalp JM 614
Abraham AD 79
Abraham WC 19
Abrams DI 512
Abramsky O 952
Abramson HA 891
Abrass IB 1231
Achterberg J 27,576, 577,953,1316
Ackerman SH 889,890
Adams DB 260
Adelsberg BR 529
Ader R 908-910,912, 914,1305,1317-1321, 1341,1389
Agarawel RP 277
Agarwal K 778
Ago Y 779
Agreda VS 45
Ahlqvist J 80,1322
Ahmar H 780
Ahmed A 1425
Akerstedt T 647
Akiyama K 1105
Akkerman JW 252
Albrecht P 954,959
Alderson MR 1268
Alexander C 558
Alexander RW 313
Alexianu M 1232
Allalunis MJ 439
Allen JM 309
Allison IE 456
Allred SJ 324
Ally AI 1280
Altman EG 1060
Amdisen A 418
Amery W 979
Amkraut AA 596,648, 1313,1428,1429
Amorosi E 530
Anavi R 955,964,1120
Andersen HK 506
Anderson CF 1003
Anderson CL 311
Anderton BH 307
Andreev SM 1214
Angst J 997
Anisimov VN 103, 210,1233
Anisman H 680-682, 950,1323

Antel JP 1234
Antonaci S 451
Antonakopoulos C 788
Antonova LV 1214
Antonovsky A 1325
Antunes LJ 473
Aoki N 81
Appelboom T 232
Argentiero V 1107
Arkhangel'skaia SL 335
Arlazoroff A 1005
Armstrong-Esther CA 956
Arnason BG 273,281, 1234
Aronson M 1057
Arsene A 1232
Artenstein MS 138
Arthur RJ 567
Asaka A 1149
Asato T 624,625
Asch RH 432
Ashkenazi A 957,958
Askenase PW 235,236, 289,290,452,459,488
Assicot M 457
Athanassenas G 1154
Atkins RW 416
Atkinson JP 453
Aubert C 2
Aulakh GS 959
Aulakh HS 959
Aurigemma GP 516
Axelrod J 1278
Axford JS 307
Ayuso Gutierrez JL 960
Azarova MA 103

Babaian NG 961, 962,1044
Bach JF 84,149,1326
Bach MA 1326
Baehner RL 309
Bageley C 868
Bahl OMP 151
Bahnson CB 510, 578,579,1327,1328
Bahnson MB 510
Baida NA 1230
Bakal DA 1329
Baker AA 1256
Baker GA 355
Bakshi K 1330
Balazovich K 363
Baldwin JA 963
Balish E 636
Balitskii KP 356
Ballardin S 413

Bammer K 661, 1331,1332
Ban M 337
Bandini G 425
Bandyk MG 414
Bangs JD 173
Bankhurst AD 415
Barber TX 918
Barchas J 1345
Barchas PR 1345
Bardana EJ 1205
Bardin CW 1330
Bardos P 3,4
Barker W 357
Barkla DH 302
Barland P 889
Barnes J 338,339
Barnes P 237
Barocci S 1150
Baron M 955,964
Baron S 46
Barot L 1292
Barrois R 105
Barry RA 692
Bartoli M 1236
Bartos Z 1273
Bartrop RW 630
Barzens K 339,478
Bassett JR 691
Batson JW 522
Battner WA 382
Bauer DC 54
Baum J 522
Baxter JD 192
Bayley PM 58
Beadle E 999
Beall GN 297
Beck-Nielsen H 82
Becker B 83
Becker H 724
Beckmann H 1122, 1151,1155-1159
Behan P 17
Behan PO 1201
Beisel WR 1270
Belfer ML 138
Bell DA 1192
Bell IR 965,1333
Bellodi L 344,358, 1136,1137,1184,1185
Belmaker RH 533
Belokrylov GA 56
Belousova OI 649
Ben-Assuly S 777
Ben-Zvi A 454
Benedetto A 486
Benjamin S 781,782
Bennahum DA 1167

Bennie EH 397
Benotzen K 455
Bensman A 84
Benson H 239, 240,687,870
Beran M 441
Berchou R 420
Berczi I 32,33
Beregi E 1235
Berenbaum MC 85,456
Berenyi F 359
Bergen JR 966
Berger D 783
Bernacka K 431
Bernard H 1182,1183
Bernhard D 1273
Bernheim JL 141
Berry LJ 144
Bertagna SY 211
Berti N 1237
Besedovsky H 1389
Besedovsky HO 5,6, 86-89,317,1334
Besser GM 226
Betts RF 520
Betz BJ 711
Bhathena SJ 193
Bialek J 1022
Biales B 180
Bianchi C 1236,1237
Bianchi E 155
Bidart JM 457
Bieber J 844
Bieliauskas L 869, 882,1335
Biesbrouck M 979
Bigelow LB 1171
Biggar RJ 506
Bilder GE 1238
Bindler J 1183
Biondi M 581,631
Biriukov VD 169
Birnbaum JE 1379
Biro J 1235
Bishopric NJ 308
Bistrian BR 1271
Biziere K 3,4,41
Bjerkenstedt L 994
Bjerre-Christensen C 82
Bjune G 90
Blackwell B 1306
Blaha GC 199
Blalock JE 91,92, 124,228
Blecha F 692
Blevins RD 360
Blichert-Toft M 1239,1240
Blizard PJ 745
Blohmke M 510
Blomback M 646
Bloom B 93
Bloom FE 214
Bloom J 162
Bloom JR 1336,1337
Bloom V 1242
Blumenstein J 355
Bochenek C 923
Bock E 967,1135,1338
Bock KD 310
Bock OA 507
Bodner AC 774
Bogdanova ED 968,985,1074
Bohuon C 457
Bokos P 409
Bonara P 1137

Bonartsev PD 961, 969,970,1027
Bond PA 971
Bondiolotti GP 317
Bonfils S 1272
Bonica J 1345
Bonnyns M 709
Book JA 1058
Boone E 954
Boranic M 7,693,725
Borel Y 137
Borkowsky W 361, 362,429,430
Borresen T 238
Borysenko J 239,240, 687,694,870,871,1339
Borysenko M 239, 240,687,694,870
Borzecki M 923
Boss GR 458
Bosse K 892
Bottazzo GF 225
Bourguignon LY 363
Boushey HA 1340
Bovbjerg D 912,914
Boxer LA 309
Boyce WT 598
Boyd GW 546
Boyd S 1360
Boyd SC 949
Boyse EA 487
Braceland BM 177
Bradford JW 1138
Brainsky LS 726
Bramhall JS 145
Brandt MR 423
Brannon WL 1110
Brasla N 1232
Braunwald E 313
Bray J 364
Breier S 403, 972,1039,1040,1043
Brenner JK 257
Bresnihan B 1202
Brightman VJ 518,863
Brightwell DR 884
Britten AZ 145
Brodde O-E 310
Brodzicki S 47
Brollo A 1236
Bromberg S 635
Brooks WH 8, 12-14,42,43
Brouet JC 57
Brown DG 1106
Brown EL 803,973
Brown GM 632
Brown GW 563
Brown J 181
Brown M 237
Brown MR 219
Brown RS 872
Brown WA 615
Brusick D 1330
Bruto V 682
Bryant TN 956
Bryson YJ 365
Buchan A 433
Buckley JM 893
Budnevich RI 1092
Buescher EL 138
Buga G 79
Buimovici-Klein E 519
Bulloch K 9,10
Bullock L 1330
Bundick RV 85
Bunimovich LA 1034

Bunney W Jr 1341
Bunney WE 949,1025
Buravlev VM 969
Burbaeva GSH 65,1023,1115,1441
Burchfield SR 662
Bursztajn S 235,459
Burzzi P 343
Busch DF 516
Busse E 1241
Busse WW 280,311, 312,472
Bykova AA 660
Byrne DG 784
Byron JW 1342
Byrum RD 526

Cadie M 1203
Calamandrei G 425
Caldesi-Valeri V 50
Calhoun LG 534
Callard RE 1257
Calvanico NJ 1380
Camerino MS 26,48
Camerlain M 769
Campbell DG 58
Campbell J 1273
Campillo F 1124
Canoso RT 366
Cantell K 627,1204,1289
Canton T 267
Canuto RA 1274
Caparulo BK 1121
Cape RD 1192,1261
Cappel R 974
Carlson EC 1273
Carnaud C 1326
Carney DN 221
Carpenter CB 495,496,916
Carpenter WT 1110
Carr RI 1205
Carroll BJ 860,1128
Carroll RM 580
Carruba G 486
Carter J 94
Carty TJ 319
Caruso J 196
Casali R 417
Casimiro San Segundo C 960
Caspary EA 1201
Cassel J 939
Cassel JC 598
Cattaneo R 95
Cautela JR 913
Cazzullo CL 1137,1184
Cermak T 822
Cerny C 218
Chai H 1226
Chalmers RJ 397
Chandra RK 1343
Chang BH 785
Chang KJ 212, 213,215-217
Chang RJ 171
Chansouria JPN 684
Charles E 585
Chauhan NS 712
Chavapil M 1273
Chebotariov VF 1344
Cheido MA 243,258
Chelmicka-Schorr E 273
Chermeneva LI 649
Chervenick PA 392
Chess S 817
Cheung R 380
Childers SR 229

Mind and Immunity: Behavioral Immunology

Chirigos M 700
Chirigos MA 367
Chobotova Z 786
Chouraqui P 1166
Chretien PB 96
Christensen NJ 238
Christensen V 1239
Christie JE 1199
Christie KE 97
Christoffersen T 503
Chughtai MA 1261
Ciampor F 1041
Ciaranello R 1345
Cipriani R 605
Clayton B 179
Clemens LE 171
Clement-Jones V 226
Clements PJ 304
Cleve H 1191
Clutter WE 114
Clyman RI 463
Coban A 975
Cobb S 508,940,941
Cockrell JR 1358
Coffey RG 460
Cogburn LA 11
Cogen R 509
Cohen D 1190,
1242-1245,1249
Cohen DJ 1121
Cohen GH 1367
Cohen HJ 308
Cohen J 1346
Cohen JJ 253,713
Cohen MH 96,594
Cohen MM 1347
Cohen N 908,909,
912,914,1317
Cohen SI 1348,1349
Cohen-Cole S 509
Cohn DA 98
Cohn P 307
Coleman DL 516
Colle E 118
Collector MI 652,699
Collerain I 953
Collet H 342
Collier AM 598
Collins A 620
Colp C 529
Colten HR 257
Colucci WS 313
Comstock GW 551,739
Conant MA 512
Conn DL 147
Connelly M 264,
336,348,1255
Conolly ME 314,315
Conran P 406
Conti C 581,631
Cooke T 194
Cooley B 663
Cooper AF 740
Cooper DA 99
Cooper KD 532
Cooper WC 1276
Cope WA 85
Copeland JR 1197
Copenhagen 1134
Coppen A 1001,1025
Copperman SM 1206
Corbett WT 1004
Corder R 226
Cordoba CS 1359
Corenblum B 616
Cornia C 787
Cornia G 787

Costa D 975
Costantini M 1150
Cotton CU 331
Cotzias CG 461
Couch R 144
Coupek J 991
Cove-Smith JR 100
Cox T 1273,1307,1442
Coyas A 788
Coyne L 727
Crabtree GR 112,113
Craig JW 599,600
Craig P 953
Cramer I 510
Cramer RT 1276
Crapper DR 1246
Crary B 239,240
Crawford ML 1100
Creighton J 1427
Crisp AH 956
Crispens CC Jr 664
Crnic LS 713
Crockett G 397
Crook WG 1207
Crosby LO 1292
Cross RJ 8,12-14,42,43
Crow TJ 976
Crowe RR 1152
Crowley B 1225
Cruchaud A 350,502
Cryer PE 114,347
Csaba G 195
Cuatrecasas P 202,
203,212,213,215-217
Cullen BF 369
Cullen JW 1346,1350,1351
Cundall RL 971
Cunnane SC 15,1280
Cunningham AJ 1352,1353
Cunningham J 59
Curran JF 1102
Curtis GC 1354
Curtis JJ 101
Czubalski K
511,789,894,923

D'Onofrio CN 1355
D'Osualdo E 1236
Da Prada M 5
Dadhich AP 703
Dahlem NW 790,791,
818,819,944
Dalchau R 60
Daleva M 1356
Dancey JT 419
Daniel N 954
Daniels GE 1378
Danion JM 1182,1183
Dann JA 16
Dardenne M 84,1326
Darg C 1199
Darling S 418
Darnell BJ 432
Dattore PJ 727,728,734
Dausset J 1160
David JR 467,655-657
Davidson RJ 644
Davies AO 316
Davis DI 895
Davis J 1341
Davis JB 792
Day SB 1440
De Genne D 3
De Prada M 317
De Vere-Tyndall A 59
DeGaudio AR 417
DeLisi LE 977,978,1170

DeStefano MJ 422
Dean LM 704
Deberdt R 979
Deboni U 1246
Debray-Ritzen P 1160
Degenne D 4
Del Campo FJS 45
Del Mese A 417
Del Rey A 5,86,87,317
Del Vecchio M 1125
Delespesse G 342
Delgado Garcia G 980-983
Delpech B 1086
Dembinski S 860
Dement WC 965
Denckla WD 1238,1247
Dennis M 162
Depelchin A 241,242
Derman RM 449
Derogatis LR 942
Devoino LV 243-245
Dhar U 712
Dianzani MU 1274
Dichter MA 180
Dickson C 170
Diebold K 984
Dilman VM 103,1248
Dimitriu A 104
Dimsdale JE 617,618
Dirks DL 896
Dirks JF 793-803,
818-821,841,896
Distenfeld A 530
Dixon LK 713
Dmitrenko NP 462
Dobozy O 195
Docherty JP 379,949
Dolgov ON 1072
Doll R 729
Dollery C 237
Domashneva IV 968,
985-989,1024,1025,1153
Doniach D 225
Donofrio S 526
Doran TJ 1129
Dorian BJ 632
Dosch HM 368,380,381
Dostoevskaia LP 169,633
Douglas RG 520
Douglas WW 230
Dragutoiu N 1232
Drew WL 512,516
Dubay L 990
Dubey D 1312
Dubin N 526
Dubs R 997
Duckett M 99
Dulis BH 318
Dumic MP 360
Dumitrescu A 1232
Dumont F 105
Duncan PG 369
Dunleavy RA 1208
Dunn CD 772
Dupont B 1200
Duque del Rio M 1124
Durack DT 513
Duriseti L 325,327
Durrant B 1053
Dusel F 364
Duszynski DR 582
Duszynski KR 540
Dutz W 547
Duwe AK 1265
Dvorakova M 991,992,
1008,1131,1147,1148,1194

Dvorzhakova M 1146
Dwyer DS 993
Dynesius RA 655
Dyregrov A 730

Eaton L 326
Ebbesen P 506
Ebstein R 533
Eckstein B 185
Edelman JS 1282
Edelman R 1270
Edgerton MT 357
Edlich RF 357
Edwards EA 704,705
Efstratopoulos AD 142
Egan RW 471
Egberg N 646
Ehrnst A 994
Eicher W 1191
Eikelenboom P 1017
Eisdorfer C 1190,
1242-1245,1249
Eisen AZ 482
Eisenberg L 514
Eisenberg S 775
Elich MS 662
Eliseeva LS 243,246
Elosuo R 1204
Elwood TW 1368
Emory LE 1002
Engel EK 247
Engel G 310
Engel GL 1308
Englander T 1033,1048
Engle GL 515
Engquist A 1239
Enlow RW 529
Ensel WM 947
Enstrom JE 1275
Erbe C 940
Erbe RW 458
Eremina O 243
Eriksson B 106
Ershova NV 248
Erwin WJ 770
Eskola J 634
Eskra JD 319
Esmann V 279
Esterhay RJ 673
Etzkorn J 107
Evans AS 525
Evans NW 793,797
Eversmann T 619
Ewald RW 1151,1157,1159
Extein I 995
Exton-Smith AN 1257

Faber R 1126
Faber-Vestergaard B 1104
Fabio G 344,435,1137,1185
Fabre JW 60
Fabris N 1357
Fairbank DT 548
Faktor MI 962,1093
Falek A 409
Falloon IR 971
Famacy J-P 232
Farmer AE 1173,1174
Farzati B 1125
Fauci AS 108-110,
120,123,150
Faulk WP 1358
Fava AO 804
Febres F 171
Fedorova NV 248
Fedosejew GB 805
Fedotova MI 649

Fehlmann U 390
Feiguine RJ 973
Fekete B 470
Feldman JD 214
Felix D 6
Felsl I 619
Felten DL 53,54
Feo F 1274
Ferguson RM 370,371
Fernandes G 111,1267,1276
Fernandez LA 372,373
Ferrara A 817
Ferrario C 1345
Ferreia GG 320
Ferrier IN 976
Festimanni F 417
Fetisova TK 996
Fey F 447
Fickova E 806
Fieve RR 1139
Filippow WL 805
Fittingoff D 348
FitzGerald G 237
Fitzmaurice MA 162,
1417-1420
Fitzpatrick R 772
Flachi S 417
Flannery GR 917
Flink R 1152
Flood C 1143,1378
Floor E 644
Fobair P 1359
Fog-Moller F 1239
Fohlin L 1065,1066
Foker JE 481,500
Foley R 209
Follansbee SE 516
Folts JD 311
Fomenko AM 303
Fontaine C 1086
Fontan M 1162,1163
Fontana A 997
Foon KA 249
Fornasa CV 605,804
Forsum U 128
Forth MW 924
Fossan GO 374
Fossett NG 251
Fottrell PF 1097
Fox BH 375,583,
949,998,1360-1365
Fox RA 372
Franchi P 425
Frangos E 1154
Frank SJ 731
Frankenhaeuser M 620
Fraser CM 321
Fraser J 322
Fraumeni FJ Jr 382
Frazier CA 858
Frederick JF 549
Freed D 1053
Freel BJ 1047
Freedman HJ 465
Freeman A 509
Freeman WR 517
Frelinger JA 77
Freund J 376
Fricks CM 206
Friedenberg WR 377
Friedman AH 517
Friedman E 518
Friedman SB 673,1415
Friedman-Kien AE
519,526
Fritz GK 807,843
Froberg J 627,646

Fross KH 793-795,
798,799,802
Fu T-K 378
Fuccillo DA 999
Fuentenebro de
Diego F 1124
Fugiwara H 1254
Fugner A 323
Fujimoto S 340
Fujita S 61
Fujiwara H 250
Fukuda T 474
Fukuhara JT 973
Funahashi T 1119
Funder JW 192

Gaitan E 509
Gajdusek DC 1366
Gal J 306
Galant SP 324-327
Gale AE 1209
Galkin OM 1214
Gall JH 101
Gallimore P 433
Gallin JI 463
Gallison D 277
Galvao-Teles A 226
Gammond GD 379
Ganguly P 251
Garaci E 486
Garcea R 1274
Garcia JL 45
Garcia Landa J 980
Garcia-Calderon JV 1298
Garcia-Calderon PA 1298
Gardiner BM 771
Gardiner P 1056
Gardner LI 602,603
Garfinkel PE 632
Garfinkel R 1250
Garovoy MR 200,201
Garrity TF 550,714,715
Garron D 869
Garron DC 882
Gastpar M 1000,1025
Gathmann P 822
Gattaz WF 1122,
1151,1155-1159
Gausset PW 342
Gauthier Y 808
Gayrard P 897
Gazdan A 193
Gazdar AF 221
Geha RS 394
Gelfand EW 368,380,381
George D 194
George K 299
Geraghty SM 1097
Gergely P 468-470
Gerlach U 231
Gerner-Beurle E 1195
Gerritsen SM 252
Gershon ES 1140
Gershon MD 235,459
Gershon RK 235,236,
289,290,459,488
Ghani M 1047
Ghayur T 1280
Ghose K 1001
Giammarruto R 787
Gildow J 666
Gillis B 112
Gillis S 113
Gilman SC 214
Ginat Y 957
Gindilis VM 1153,1186

Ginsberg AM 114
Ginsberg BI 656,657
Girstenbrey W 584
Glasser L 115
Glick B 11
Godhwani JL 703
Goedert JJ 382
Goel Z 329
Goeringer GC 1287
Goetz CG 1210
Goldberg EL 551
Goldberg SJ 464
Goldney RD 1211
Goldstein AL 116,125,
330,1002,1367,1369,
1370,1425
Goldstein G 487
Goldstone AH 1257
Golikov AP 248
Golikov PP 248
Golla JA 1003
Golse B 1160
Golub ES 62
Golubeva NN 349
Good IJ 637
Good RA 111,1276
Goode DJ 1004
Goodrum KJ 144
Goodwin FK 995
Goodwin JS 117,383,635
Gorden P 204
Gordon D 409
Gordon MA 253,333
Gorizontov PD 649
Gormus R 294
Goroshnikova TV 462
Gorray KC 37
Gorzynski JG 732,733
Gotlieb-Stematsky T 1005
Gottschalk GH 1213
Gottsmann M 619
Goudemand J 1161-1164
Goudemand M 1161-1164
Goudemand-Joubert C
1161,1163,1164
Goudos B 171
Govaerts A 232,1127,1178
Gowdy JM 1006
Gower S 479
Gozes Y 196
Grabczewska E 254,
271,328
Granacher RP Jr 770
Grandi G 1237
Granstrom M 627
Gravitz MA 919
Gray HE 19
Gray J 107
Grayzel AI 889
Greden J 860
Green LA 180
Green LW 1368
Green N 914
Greenacre JK 314
Greenberg JH 386
Greenberg LJ 1267
Greenberg RP 734
Greene MH 382
Greene WA 520
Greer HS 751
Greer S 735,873,
874,876,878
Gregoire F 974
Greineder DK 283
Grieco MH 329
Griffiths K 194

Grigorev VA 18
Grigoriu M 1232
Grillione G 670,671
Grinspoon L 966
Grob PJ 997
Groen JJ 809
Gross RL 1277
Gross WB 706
Grossarth-Maticek R 521,
736,943
Grossman CJ 197-199
Grota LJ 908
Groundwater JR 512
Gruchow HW 255
Gruemer HD 442
Grumet FC 1123
Grunberger J 822
Grunwald P 1195
Gu TS 1007
Gueibe R 907
Guida L 1125
Guillaumin JM 41,161
Guilleminault C 965
Gul'iants ES 1116
Gullet J 516
Gullett JG 512
Gunn RA 414
Gunn T 118
Gupta BK 420
Gupta P 119
Gurtoo HL 465
Gushchin GV 256
Guthrow CE 352
Gutterman JU 441
Guttormsen S 1143
Gyenes L 161

Haaijman JJ 1251
Haak A 1262
Haas H 6
Haas S 1151
Hackett TP 921
Hadden EM 460
Hadden JW 460
Hadley WK 516
Haemmerli M 1413
Hafez H 379
Haga S 1010
Hain J 509
Haines RF 1128
Halberg D 1290
Halberg F 111,1303
Hall AK 477
Hall N 1389
Hall NR 19,20,
330,1369-1371
Hall R 444
Halonen P 606,
1078,1079,1422
Halperin B 957
Hamashima Y 334
Hambling MH 1196
Hamilton JB 98
Hamilton S 406
Handel AD 636
Haney CA 737
Hanifin JM 466,532
Hanna WT 772
Hansen MA 1276
Hansen O 810,915
Hanson PG 311
Hanson RP 688
Hara C 650,707
Harbeck R 698,
701,1205
Harden TK 331
Harley C 433

Harper L 433
Harrell EH 27
Harris R 928
Hart DA 387
Hartnett JA 449
Hartung M-L 811
Hastings D 380,381
Hasto J 403
Hastrup JL 528
Hatcher J 1002
Hauptmann G 1182,1183
Havens MB 465
Haynes BF 120
Haynes SG 552
Hazum E 213,215-217
Headley DB 738
Hedfors E 106
Hegstrand LR 306
Heim O 300
Heisel JS 639,640
Hekkens WTJM 1372
Helderman JH 121,174,
200,201
Heller AS 818
Hellstrom I 674
Hellstrom KE 674
Helmholz M 1241
Helsing KJ 739
Heltberg J 1025
Hendler N 1212
Hengst K 231
Heninger G 615
Henoch MJ 522
Henry JP 663,705,1373
Henschke PJ 1192
Heppner GH 401
Herberman RB 1374
Herd A 1341
Herha J 408
Herlin T 279
Herman JJ 257
Herxheimer H 898
Herzog P 992,1008
Heustis DW 115
Heyberger K 991
Hicks JT 954
Higashi S 1009
Higgins TJ 467
Hijmans W 1251
Hillary I 1224
Hilliard J 843
Hinterberger W 218
Hippius H 1025
Hirata F 1278
Hirata-Hibi M 1009,1105
Hirschhorn R 361
Hisada T 625
Ho WK 388
Hoecherl B 1025
Hoffman A 701,1205
Hoffman SA 1205
Hoffmann F 887
Hoigne R 390
Holdeman LV 637
Holland J 733,879,880
Holland JC 732,1375
Holm G 1279,1289
Holman BL 313
Holmes J 1138
Holmes TH 564,568,
569,859
Holzman RS 362
Homma M 72
Hong KM 716
Hooper JA 1367
Hopkins P 107

Hopwood MA 716
Horne RL 523
Horrobin DF 15,389,1280
Hors J 1160
Horton DJ 790,798,899
Horvat J 63,64,67-70,
73,74,391,1012-1016
Horwitz DA 263
Hough RL 548
Hoyer D 310
Hrbka A 990
Hryszko S 431
Hu S-K 330
Huang ES 512
Huang SW 654
Huberman R 544
Huddlestone JR 122
Huff JC 613
Hughes EC 1213
Hughson AVM 740
Hull D 553
Hummer L 1240
Humphrey LJ 148
Humphrey PA 148
Hunecke P 892
Hunninghake GW 123
Hunt GE 1129
Hunziker T 390
Hurdle AD 1001
Hurni H 1413
Hurst MW 554,572,640
Hussa RO 151
Hussein SA 1256
Hyde RT 750

Idar D 957
Idova GV 243,258
Igari T 259
Ignatov SA 65,1115,1441
Ikemi Y 779
Ikemori K 474
Iker HP 520
Imada Y 707
Inbar M 189
Ingbar SH 107,208
Inoue S 779
Insel PA 140,276,325,327
Irvine WJ 126
Isakovic K 21-23,66
Ishihara T 340
Ishii T 1010
Ishii Y 51
Ishikawa B 1149
Ismailov NV 1011
Isom GE 354
Issidorides MR 1096
Ito M 332
Ivanyi D 1165
Ivanyi P 1165

Jaaskelainen J 749
Jackson M 812,924
Jacobs S 202,203,555
Jacobs TJ 585
Jaffe BM 486
Jakoubkova J 136
Jakulic S 1012-1016
James NM 1128
Jandova A 991
Janiaud P 2
Jankovic BD 21-24,
35,63,64,66-70,73,74,
391,1012-1016
Jarvik LF 378
Javierre MQ 320
Jebaily GC 573
Jedrzecjzak WW 1425

Jehle W 619
Jemmott JB 559
Jenkins CD 554,572
Jenner C 741
Jenner FA 1294
Jensen EW 598
Jensen J 601,861,862
Jerrett I 830
Jezkova Z 653
Joasoo A 695
John R 397
Johnson A 1170,1172
Johnson DL 333
Johnson F 1213
Johnson GF 1129,1130
Johnson HM 124
Johnson PC 638
Johnson SB 524
Johnson WT 1121
Johnstone EC 976
Jones EH 274
Jones HJ 904
Jones JF 115
Jones NF 795,796,798,
799,813,819,820,842
Jones WO 260
Jonker C 1017
Jonsson J 994
Jose DC 1276
Joseph JG 1376
Joshua H 1033,1048
Jovanova K 24
Jovicic A 1018
Joyce RA 392
Juhlin L 1281
Juji T 1149
Julien RA 1166

Kabler P 100
Kahn A 421
Kahn J 1260
Kaiser N 1282
Kakad PP 1052
Kalian M 957
Kaliner M 293,321
Kalisnik M 665,1377
Kalmar L 468-470
Kalucy R 1106
Kamenskii AA 1214
Kammerer W 773
Kane C 830
Kang K 532
Kapfer MT 1183
Kaplan GW 1019
Kapotes C 900
Karasawa T 1054
Karasek E 298
Karasu TB 830,925
Karlsson CG 627,646
Karmali RA 1280
Karol C 814
Karpatkin S 530
Karush A 1378
Kasahara K 334
Kashima T 474
Kasl SV 490,508,525
Kasper S 1158,1159
Kasprisin DO 261
Kaszubowski PA 635
Katcher AH 518,863
Kater L 125
Katzman R 1057
Kavai M 359
Kay MMB 1252
Kay SR 1091
Kazimierczak W 1087

Keegan DL 815
Kehlet H 423,1239
Keirns JJ 1379
Keliger JH 797
Keller AJ 126
Keller HH 5
Keller M 156
Keller RH 1380
Keller SE 25,26,
696,697,1434-1437
Kellerman J 742
Kellett JM 1260
Kellner R 1167
Kellum RE 816
Kelly H 672,685
Kelly JP 453
Kelly KW 692
Kemali D 1125
Kemper T 30
Kenady DE 96
Kennedy L 1138
Kennedy S 482
Kenny JF 127
Kent JR 190
Kent S 1253
Keystone E 632
Khaitov RM 649
Khamidov D KH 262
Khatri S 684
Khavinson VK 103,
210,1233
Kholodkovskaia GV 395
Kidd KK 1132
Kielholz P 1025
Kiff J 599
Kikuchi K 51
Kil'gol'ts P 1024
Killian A 213
Kiloh LG 630
Kim KS 519
Kim SP 817
Kimball CP 562
Kimzey SL 638
Kinast H 218
King CL 414
King DS 1215
King S 1141
Kinnell HG 1020,1181
Kinsman RA 790,
791,796,798-801,
803,813,818-820,
841,842,899,944
Kirk K 509
Kirkley J 60
Kirkwood E 1020
Kirtland HH 263
Kishimoto S 1254
Kishimoto T 480
Kitamura J 61
Kjosen B 97
Klareskog L 128
Klawans HL 1210
Klebe JG 82
Kleiger JH 800,821
Kleinman JE 959,1171
Klimenko VM 1381
Kmet J 393
Knapp MS 100
Knapp PH 926
Kneier AW 945
Knezevic Z 21,23
Knight JG 1021
Knox AJ 129
Kobasa SC 556
Kobayashi H 146
Kocisova M 1039,1041
Kocur J 1022

Mougey EH 138
Mount CD 211
Mozes T 1005
Mucha V 1042
Mudge GH Jr 313
Mue S 340
Mueller J 156
Mulder JH 159
Mullen B 575
Mullen JL 1292
Muller W 1000
Multer MM 141
Munck A 209
Munitz H 1033,1048
Munson AE 402
Munster AM 645
Murgo AJ 220,223
Murken JD 1191
Murphy DL 384
Murphy E 563
Murray AB 1288
Murray C 382
Murray JB 877,1311
Murray MJ 1288
Murrell TG 784
Myhal D 769

Nachman RL 275
Nadeau J 322
Nadel C 775
Naess A 1062
Nagao T 1105
Nagata I 81
Nagata S 779
Nagy E 32,33
Nakasheva E 1356
Nakazawa T 1119
Namura I 1149
Nandkumar VK 838,839
Nasr SJ 416,1060
Nasrallah HA 1077
Nathan P 197-199
Nauss K 1270
Navarrete M 670,671
Nazarian KB 1115
Neal JF 635
Neckers LM 977,978,1171
Nedelcu A 1232
Negri F 358,435,1137
Neifeld JP 207
Neighbour PA 1057
Nekam K 468
Nelson AM 147
Nemeth G 1404
Neuland CY 382
Newberne PM 1277
Newberry BH 666-669,
1331,1332,1405,1406
Newby LG 542
Nicholson WE 211
Nieburgs HE 670,671
Niederman JC 490,525
Nielsen TT 82
Niemi T 749
Nies AS 306
Nigam A 840
Nijmeijer B 252
Nikic SM 1018
Nishanbaev KN 262
Nishimoto H 146
Nishimura T 146
Nishmi M 1079
Noel GL 626
Noeva K 1061
Noguchi T 78,1119
Nolte D 783
Nomura S 1119

Norberg R 1066,1289
Nordberg J 476
Norman GR 527
Novelli GP 417
Nowinski RC 76
Nye FJ 1203
Nyland H 1062

O'Connor JF 1378
O'Connor P 282
O'Connor R 484
O'Shaughnessy MV 464
O'Shea JA 1219
Obara K 259
Obe G 408
Ochitill HN 520
Ochs HD 1295
Oettinger L Jr 1213
Offenkrantz W 895
Ogawa K 337
Ogawa N 650,707
Ohara J 480
Ohmi T 340
Oifa AI 1063
Oka M 1280
Okazaki Y 1149
Okouchi E 34
Oldham RK 384
Oldstone MBA 122
Oleinik AV 1089
Olgaard K 1239
Olhagen B 604
On A 777
Ono S 259
Ookawara S 272
Oosterom R 125
Oppenheim JJ 249
Or A 957
Oreland L 1426
Orellana J 517
Orgel HA 1019
Orlova EN 1037
Orth DN 211
Osband M 277
Oskolkova SN 1064
Ostfeld A 555,869
Ostfeld AM 882
Ostroumova MN 103
Othmer E 884
Otsuki S 1105
Overall JB 1002
Overbeck A 932
Overbeck G 932
Owen JJT 295,345
Owens DGC 976

Paegelow I 278
Paffenbarger RA Jr 1403
Paffenbarger RS 750,1407
Paigen B 465
Pajntar M 665,1377
Palaxzynski E 1370
Paley A 794,802
Palit J 455
Palmberg PF 83
Palmblad J 627,646,647,
1065,1066,1262,1279,
1289-1291,1297, 1408
Palmer GC 153
Palmgren N 238
Palo J 1198
Panagis DM 1409
Pancheri P 581,631
Pang EJ 261
Pangburn PC 127
Panides WC 828
Pankaskie MC 481

Pankova R 867
Panoussopoulos DG 148
Panteleeva GP 987
Papamichail M 438
Papiernik M 149
Parfitt DN 1067
Parillo JE 150
Parker CW 453,482,
492,497,498,1410
Parker KL 498
Parker NB 465
Parodi GB 343
Parquet PJ 1161-1164
Parrott DM 332
Parry RP 976
Pashutova EK 1088
Pasqua F 787
Patel V 684
Patsakova EK 233,234
Patterson R 341
Pattillo RA 151
Paul O 869,882
Paunovic VR 35
Pavlidis N 700
Pawlikowski M 298
Peacock J 1273
Pedernera E 152
Pedersen EB 418
Pedersen O 82
Peduto VA 417
Pekkarinen A 629
Pelletier KR 1411
Pennel RB 966
Penny R 99,630
Pepper MD 1196
Perez-Cruet J 419
Pericic D 693
Perini GI 605,804
Perkins JP 331
Perrin MH 219
Perris AD 145,477
Perris C 1133,1180
Persad E 1143
Pert CB 221,1068
Pertschuk MJ 1292
Pesserico R 605
Peszke MA 490
Peters LJ 672,1412
Peterson CS 279
Peterson MR 1110,1111
Peterson PA 128
Peterson RD 153
Peterson RG 54
Peto R 729
Petranyi G 468-470
Petrich J 564
Petrini B 647
Petrov RV 154
Petrovic S 35
Pettengill OS 211
Pettingale KW 751,
873,876,878
Petts V 99
Petz R 653
Peutherer JF 1199
Pfeiffer SE 479
Pfitzner R 717
Phan T 267,398,440
Philalithis A 751
Phillips JL 1293
Piazza EU 933
Picard RS 523
Piccione M 864
Pickard N 442
Pieraccioli E 417
Pierloot RA 531

Pierpaoli W 36,155-158,
222,1394,1413,1414
Pietzcker A 408
Pilc A 1087
Pinals RS 426
Pinderis GM 752
Piperova D 1356
Piscitelli P 417
Pistiner M 829
Pitlik S 829
Pivovarova AI 1069,1070
Plantey F 1071
Platt R 1263
Plaut M 285
Plaut SM 654,673,1415
Pline M 409
Plotnikoff NP 220,
223,224
Plumb M 879
Plumb MM 880
Plutchik R 830
Pochet R 342
Pogady J 1039-1043
Pohl RB 420
Pointer H 218
Poletaev AB 1072
Polgar P 483
Poljak-Blazi M 693
Pollack M 365
Ponassi A 343
Ponten J 1416
Popova NN 1073
Popp DM 1264
Porter SF 1219
Post RM 1110
Potkin SG 978
Poupland A 225
Pownall R 100
Pozza G 95
Pozzan T 413
Prasad R 684
Pratt KR 108
Presley AP 421
Preston D 407
Prilipko LL 961,962,
968,985,1027-1031,
1045,1074,1075
Psychochemistry
Institute 1134
Puhakka P 1078
Pulkkinen E 1076,1204
Pullan PT 226
Purschel W 831
Purves EC 456
Pyle HM 966

Quay WB 37
Quimby F 687
Quint'ans J 273

Rabinovitch M 422
Rabkin JG 565
Racy J 566
Rada RT 1167
Radvila A 775
Rafaelsen OJ 1025,1135
Rahe RH 567-569,705
Raina A 481
Rajah SM 1173,1196
Rajcani J 1041
Rajcevic M 66
Ramey CT 598
Rampen FHJ 159
Rapp DJ 1220
Rapp F 119
Raq A 684
Rasmussen EO 532

Rassidakis NC 753
Ratnoff OD 776
Rauscher FP 1077
Rauste von Wright M 620
Raynor WJ 869,882
Recant L 193
Rechenberger HG 832
Rechenberger I 833,834
Rechsman F 775
Reddihough DS 904
Reddy BS 1300,1301
Reece ER 118
Reed CE 133,280,472
Reed SE 599,600
Rees AM 226
Rees LH 226
Rees WL 570,835
Reese RL 666
Regan DH 532
Reich P 655-658,
916,1312
Reichlin S 1393
Reichman ME 160
Reid KBM 58
Reilly FD 38,39
Reindell A 773
Reite M 698,701
Rella W 40
Rem J 423
Renieri-Livieratou N 1154
Rennke HG 657
Renoux G 3,4,41,161,424
Renoux M 41,161,424
Renvoize EB 1196
Resele L 358
Resnikoff P 813
Reynolds MT 1097
Ricci P 425
Richardson RL 384
Richman DP 281
Richter HE 754
Richter K 1191
Richter R 810
Rickards WS 904
Riley J 612
Riley V 162,593,594,
674-679,683,1417-1421
Rimer B 1368
Rimon R 533,
606,1078,1079,1422
Ring J 282,484
Rippere V 1080
Ritter M 163
Ritts RE Jr 184
Ritzmann SE 638
Rivier JE 219
Robbins CL 537
Roberts DF 446,1144,
1145,1181
Roberts M 341
Roberts NJ Jr 227
Robertson D 322
Robertson S 1129
Robinson LA 1221
Robinson SK 896
Roccatagliata G 1150
Rocklin RE 283,284
Rodenheaver GT 357
Roder JC 1265
Rodriguez Perdomo E 981
Rogentine GN Jr 949,1360
Rogentine N 1140,
1170,1172
Rogers MP 655-658,
916,1312
Rogers P 164
Roitt IV 225

Romain PL 529
Roman E 1232
Roman G 1180
Romano GS 449,450
Romano M 152
Roos M 1182,1183
Roppel RM 1081,1222
Rosch PJ 571
Rose RM 554,572,
614,628,1423
Rosen F 102
Rosenberg JC 165
Rosenberg NE 75
Rosenblatt JE 949,1171
Rosenfeld J 829
Rosenstreich DL 249
Rosenthal D 999
Roskowski W 285
Ross M 560
Ross RD 1336,1348
Ross T 516
Ross-Smith P 1294
Rossio J 1002
Rossio JL 116,1367
Rossipal E 547
Rossner S 1290
Roszkowski-Sliz W 485
Roszman TL 8,12-14,
42,43
Roth J 204,205
Rothschild AM 286
Rothwell TLW 260
Rougier P 1272
Row VV 129
Rowland JH 1375
Roy R 527
Royal College of
General Practitioners 166
Rubin AL 16
Rubin R 1428
Rubin RL 1223
Rubin RT 648,1429
Rubinstein P 519
Rude RE 313
Rudin DO 1082-1085
Rudzki E 789,894
Rugarli C 344
Runge LA 426
Rusnak SA 338,339,478
Russel A 454
Rutenburg AM 483
Ruuskanen O 634
Ryder LP 1135
Ryzewski J 254,271,
328,485

Sabbadini-Villa MG 1137
Sacchetti C 343
Sacchetti E 344,358,
1137,1184,1185
Saibene V 95
Saillant C 1086
Sainz Ruiz J 960
Saksena NK 756-758
Salmela K 1078
Samoilova NA 1214
Samuelson DC 573
Sandler JA 463
Sandwisch D 614
Sansaricq C 361
Santalo R 355
Santisteban G 162
Santisteban GA 593,679
Santonastaso P 804
Santoro MG 486
Saron C 644
Sarsfield MJ 1097

Sasazuki T 1123
Saso R 391
Sassine WA 320
Satake T 337
Sato JL 75
Sauer J 836
Saunders ME 386
Savchenko VP 1089
Savic V 70
Saxena RK 167
Saykaly RJ 101
Scarf M 934
Scarpace PJ 1231
Schayer RW 1087
Schecter GP 193
Scheer P 837
Scheid MP 487
Scherg H 510
Schey HM 1004
Schiavi RC 48
Schimpff RD 19
Schlager SI 168
Schleifer SJ 25,26,
696,697,1434-1437
Schleimer R 287
Schlewinski E 689,690
Schmale AH 1424
Schmedtje JF 54
Schmidtke JR 370,371
Schmutzler W 288
Schnaper N 673
Schnetzer M 836
Schoenfeld M 775
Schonfield J 881
Schraa JC 803
Schroeter H 408
Schuld D 766,767
Schultz RM 367
Schultze P 300
Schum R 813
Schuman SH 573
Schuurman RK 368
Schwartz A 236,289,
290,488
Schwartz JM 214
Scorza-Smeraldi R 344,
435,1137,1185
Scott DJ 527
Scurry MT 755
Seales CM 330
Sedvall G 620
Seegmiller JE 489
Sega E 631
Sega FM 631
Segal J 107,208
Seifter E 594
Selby JW 534
Seligman ME 686
Sell KW 1425
Selling K 418
Selner JC 338,339
Selye H 595,1440
Semenov SF 1088
Sengbusch L 667
Sensenbrenner LL 1425
Seslavina LS 349
Seth M 756-758
Sethi JP 778
Sevdalian DA 654
Sever JL 999
Seville RH 611
Shafer DA 409
Shaffer JW 540,582
Shah SD 114
Shalaby MR 151
Shamoon H 346

Shanfield SB 759
Shankariah K 1303
Shanon J 865
Shapiro A 1341
Shapiro HM 291
Shapiro IUA 1153
Shapiro R 25
Shapiro RW 1135
Shaposhnikov VS
1089,1090
Sharkis SJ 1425
Sharma S 838,839
Sharma VN 703
Sharp JT 142
Sharpington C 685
Shaskan EG BA 1121
Shea PA 54
Sheehan DV 920
Sheehan TF 760
Shekelle RB 869,882
Sheldrake P 535
Shelhamer JH 293
Shen FW 176
Shen L 307
Shenkman L 361,362,
429,430
Sheppard JR 294,500
Sherman J 26
Sherstnev VV 1072
Sherwin RS 346
Shields R 194
Shields WD 365
Shier DH 83
Shigekawa BL 77
Shiling DJ 978
Shimogawara A 51
Shinefeld LA 75
Shkhinek EK 169,256,
633,1381
Shneyour A 454
Shohmori T 1105
Sholiton LJ 197-199
Shontz FC 727
Shopsin B 361,362,
429,430
Shore A 381
Shreier MH 489
Shucard DW 1205
Shuval JT 536
Shyamala G 170
Siadak AW 76
Siani V 787
Siedlecki B 670,671
Siegal F 361
Siegel I 329
Siegel JN 236
Siegel PB 706
Siegrist J 574
Sierakowski S 431
Sigal M 1005
Siiteri PK 171
Silberfarb PM 1216
Siletskii OIA 1116,1117
Silva EN 473
Silva J 860
Silverman AY 432
Simeone RS 947
Simionescu N 1232
Simmons RL 370,371
Simon RH 44
Simonton OC 576,935,
936,1316,1427
Sinanan K 1224
Singer G 917
Singer L 1182,1183
Singh MM 1091
Singh SB 840

Singh U 295,296,345,491
Singhal SK 1265
Singman H 529
Sise HS 366
Sisenbaev SK 1092
Siskind M 886
Sitkovski MV 349
Sixma JJ 252
Siziakina LP 1116
Skinner GR 433
Sklar LS 680-682,
950,1323
Skodacek I 1041
Skoven I 434
Skovsted L 1239
Skyler J 601
Sless F 332
Smeraldi E 344,358,435,
1136,1137,1184,1185
Smeraldi RS 358
Smith AH 598
Smith BR 179,444
Smith CC 995
Smith CG 432
Smith EM 91,92,124,228
Smith KA 112,113
Smith PA 345
Smith RT 19,20
Smithwick E 361
Smouse PE 1128
Snider DE Jr 492
Snowden PR 1197
Snyder SH 229
Snyderman R 351,493
Snyderman S 361
Sohn RJ 30
Sokol WN 297
Solberg CO 97
Solntseva EI 1093,
1094,1186
Solokangas RK 948
Solomon GF 596,648,
1313,1389,1428-1431
Solomon JG 1095
Solomon S 1095
Soltes S 70
Soman VR 346
Somes GW 550,714
Sonkoly I 359
Soppi E 634
Sorenson GD 211
Soriano FM 45
Sorkin E 5,6,86-89,
317,1334,1413
Soucek K 1146-1148
Souhrada J 899
Soustek Z 905
South MA 1225
Southern DL 1102
Spackman DH 162,593,
674,675,679,683,1417-1420
Spalter L 777
Spangelo B 1370
Sparks TF 935
Spector NH 46,1432
Spector SL 841,899,944
Spengler H 390
Sperlingova I 1382
Spiers AS 537
Spigland I 519,529
Spiro HM 883
Spitzer G 441
Spoljar M 1191
Sporn MB 172
Sprake S 307
Spratt JS Jr 1401

Sprecher S 974
Srebro Z 47
Srivastava JR 840
Stachowiak J 1022
Stahl R 519
Stahle J 538
Stamm T 436
Stancek D 390,1020
Stancer HC 1143
Stangel-Rutkowski S 119
Stankova L 1273
Starr MB 517
Staszak C 635
Staub RA 977
Staudenmayer H 800,
841,842,906,944
Stavropoulou-
Ghioka E 1154
Stavrou J 788
Stefanesku E 1232
Stefanis C 437,1096
Stefanovich LE 246
Stein G 1138
Stein M 25,26,
48,49,696,697,1314,
1345,1434-1438
Steiner H 843
Steinhausen HC 937
Stember RH 1139
Stephens CG 493
Stephens PM 663,
705,1373
Stepien H 298
Stern M 964
Stevens A 509
Stevens FM 1097
Stevens JS 319
Stewart RB 464
Stierlin H 887
Stites D 171
Stoikova M 1032
Stolc V 494
Stoll BA 762,1439
Stone MG 685
Stone SP 816
Storck U 997
Storey P 1203
Strahilevitz M 1098,1099
Straker N 844
Strander H 627,1289
Strandman E 1133
Strausser HR 651
Strax P 671
Strayhorn G 951
Streiner DL 527
Strom T 1389
Strom TB 121,173-175,
196,200,201,291,
299,495,496,916
Strong DM 382
Struening EL 565
Strunk RC 901
Stubbs EG 1100,1101
Stubbs G 1187
Studt HH 845
Stunkard A 1341
Stunzner D 1039
Stutman O 176
Stuttgen G 846
Suda WL 899
Sudar F 195
Sugerman AA 1102
Suh SH 1004
Suleski P 361
Sulkava R 1198
Sullivan JL 1295

Sullivan TJ 453,497,498
Suls J 575
Sunblad L 1289
Suominen J 1204
Surawicz FG 884,885
Suskind RM 1270
Suszko IM 341
Sutherland DC 240
Sutherland JC 673
Sutter JM 1166
Sutton RN 1256
Sutton SL 290
Suzuki A 146
Suzuki T 1119
Svejgaard A 1135
Swahn CG 620
Swartz C 1103
Swenson WM 539
Swierenga SHH 177
Swinburne LM 1056
Sydow G 447
Sylvester-Jrgensen O 1104
Syme SL 1376
Syromiatnikova ED 248
Syvalahti E 629
Szabolosi M 359
Szegedi G 359
Szekely AG 1005
Szentwanyi A 300

Tache J 1440
Tachibana T 1009,1105
Tait NN 691
Takeda M 259
Takishima T 340
Talaban I 1232
Talal N 178
Tallman J 995
Talwar GP 167
Tamura G 340
Tanaka S 334
Tang LC 461
Tantam D 1106
Targum SD 1140
Tasini MF 921
Taunton OD 129?
Tavolato B 1107
Taylor BB 198
Taylor E 1227
Taylor G 654
Taylor WM 1108
Tee DE 751,878
Teiraamaa E 847-854
Teirstein A 671
Temme PB 1211
Teng CS 179
Tengerdy RP 1296
Terzic G 66
Teshima H 702,779
Theoharides TC 230
Thiry L 974
Thode J 1239
Thomas CB 540,541,
582,711,866
Thompson HC 901
Thompson JS 1152
Thormann J 421
Thurman GB 116,
1002,1367
Thurn A 855
Tick NT 330
Timoshenko LV 301
Ting JP 77
Tischler AS 180
Toben H 57
Todaro GJ 172
Todd PB 745

Toguchi T 72
Tohmeh JF 347
Tomar RH 426
Tomasi TB Jr 1003,1380
Tomaszek D 44
Tomino S 1254
Tongio MM 1182,1183
Tonney DC 207
Torack RM 1109
Torres BA 124
Torrey EF 933,938,
1088-1091,1149,1151
Torrielli MV 1274
Totman R 599,600
Trag KH 218
Trail G 127
Trainin N 454
Trang L 1297
Traxel WL 1228
Trentham DE 655-658
Trestcot AM 19
Tribukait B 994
Trichopoulos D 181
Trites R 1229
Trivers GE 116
Trotter JL 247
Troup GM 1167
Trubnikov VI 1186
Trung PH 499
Tryphonas H 1229
Tsaneva N 1356
Tsirkin SI 987
Tsokos G 438
Tsoneva M 1032
Tsuda A 659
Tsukada Y 78,1119
Tsutsul'kovskaia MIA
1024,1025,1029
Tuck ML 264,
336,348,1255
Tudor S 1232
Tudorache B 1232
Tur C 267
Turesky S 687
Turner AR 364,439
Turner WJ 1141,
1142,1200
Turns D 542
Tutton PJM 302
Tvenier P 1017
Twarog FJ 394
Twomey JJ 1299
Tyan ML 182
Tyano S 1033,1048
Tyroler HA 552
Tyrrell DAJ 976,1114

Uchiyama Y 272,1054
Udelman DL 888
Udelman HD 888
Uden AM 1297
Udupa KN 684
Uede T 51
Ueno K 625
Uhlich E 619
Ujhazyova D 1039
Underwood S 325,327
Unger P 627
Urbaniak SJ 1199
Uzan A 267,398,440

Vaillant GE 543
Valleteau deMouillac J 84
Valverde E 1298
Van Den Brenk HA 685
Van Eerdewegh M 1140
Van Hooren J 979

Van Kammen DP 949, 1110,1360
Vanley GT 544
Vardanian IK 349
Varma AO 449
Vartanian F 1025
Vartanian ME 1115,1441
Vasil'eva EF 335
Vaughan M 463
Vedernikova LV 65
Vedrenne C 1086
Veilleux F 763
Vejlsgaard-Goldschmidt V 1104
Vendysova E 867
Venizelos N 1297
Venter JC 321
Vera JC 483
Verbanck P 1127,1178
Verma DS 441
Verns GP 764
Verrill HL 442
Vessel K 547
Vestergaard BF 506
Vetoshkin AV 303
Vich JM 1298
Vievskaia GA 1230
Vievskii AN 1230
Vifrenko AE 1089
Vilkov GA 1116,1117
Villard HP 763
Villee CA 160
Vinarova E 1148
Vinglerova M 991
Visani G 425
Visintainer MA 686
Vitaliano PP 1242
Viukari M 606
Vogel PG 718
Volberding P 512
Volcho LS 1117
Vollhardt BR 889,890
Volpe R 129,183,607
Volpicelli JR 686
Von Gaudeceker B 1266
Von Westarp C 129
Von Wright J 620
Vostrikova SA 985,1074
Voth HM 765
Vraspir-Porenta C 1377
Vraspir-Porenta O 665
Vuia O 1118
Vurgrin D 733
Wachtel SS 16
Waddell CC 1299
Wadel G 1426
Wadler S 362,430
Wagner H 231
Wahl SM 249
Wahlby L 1180
Wakisaka G 81
Waldmann TA 489
Waldo GL 331
Walford RL 1190
Wallace AL 71
Wallace WW 1019
Wallen WC 382
Walsh DA 475
Waltman SR 83
Walton B 443
Wang T 481,500
Wangaard C 841
Wareheim LE 654,673
Warejcka DJ 52
Wasserman J 647
Watanabe M 78,1119

Watanabe N 1009,1105
Watanabe T 489
Watson ALM 1303
Watson CG 766,767
Watson KC 446
Watson M 876
Wayner EA 917
Wayner L 1442
Webel ML 184
Weber F 310
Weber G 887
Weetman AP 444
Weinberger B 1152
Weinberger DR 978, 1170-1172
Weiner H 1315,1443-1447
Weiner LP 77
Weinhold M 510
Weinrick M 1234
Weinstein Y 185-187,501
Weinstock C 768
Weisbart R 1255
Weisburger JH 1300,1301
Weisenbeck H 1120
Weiss J 670,671,696,697
Weiss JH 612
Weissman M 1341
Weitkamp LR 1143
Weksler BB 275
Weldy P 1273
Welscher HD 350,502
Weltzel WD 884
Wenner FC 719
Wentzel J 446,1144,1145
Wenzel SE 19
Werb Z 188,209
Werth GR 856
Wessels JM 445
Weston WL 613
Whalen G 108
Whalley LJ 446,1144, 1145,1199
Whitaker M 616
White CR Jr 532
White J 252
Whitlock FA 886, 1448-1450
Whitsett C 1200
Wiedermann V 403,1043
Wiernik PH 673
Wiesel FA 994
Wijsenbeek H 1033
Wikstrom J 1198
Wilckens A 810
Wilcox CB 1201
William DC 526
Williams AF 58
Williams CC 407
Williams GH 313
Williams GM 1300,1301
Williams JM 50,51
Williams LT 351
Williams MH Jr 830
Williams RC Jr 117, 415,545
Williams RM 189,640
Williams RS 352
Williamson N 421
Wilson IB 253,318
Wilson WR 1003
Winchester RJ 529
Winchurch RA 353
Winfrey CJ 1112
Wing AI 750
Wingerson L 938
Wirsching B 887
Wirsching M 887

Wirt RD 716
Wisloff F 503
Witkop CJ 252
Witz IP 955,964,1120
Wofsy CB 516
Wogan J 666
Wolf S 55
Wolf SG 1451
Wood AJJ 322
Woodford SY 101
Woodie B 1004
Woodrow JC 1197
Woods SC 662
Wright AF 1145
Wright R 1097
Wullieimier F 907
Wunderlich J 1452
Wunderlich V 447
Wyatt RJ 959,977,978, 1077,1170-1172,1341
Wybran J 232
Wyle FA 190
Wynder EL 1300-1302
Wynne J 313
Wysenbeek H 1048

Xanthou M 438

Yamamoto T 191
Yamamura Y 480
Yamasaki H 191
Yelenosky R 139
Yellin AM 716
Yen F-S 378
Yen SS 30
Yoda K 448
Yokono S 448
Yolken RH 1112
Yonace AH 1174
Youdale T 177
Young JG 1121
Yu DT 304
Yunis EJ 111,1267, 1276,1303,1395

Zaborwski A 1087
Zaccolin GP 413
Zaks AS 660
Zaloman S 1170
Zaloman SJ 977
Zander AR 441
Zanussi C 1137
Zaretskyaya IUM 1188
Zarrabi MH 449,450
Zatz MM 1453
Zawisza E 511,923
Zee HJ 597
Zeitlin DJ 608
Zeleny A 1382
Zemek P 1146,1148, 1165,1189
Zhikharev SS 305,504
Zhirnova IG 1059
Ziegler JL 512
Zierden E 231
Ziller RC 828
Zlatich D 857
Zolla-Pazner S 519
Zonis J 1005
Zorc M 665,1377
Zornetzer SF 19,20
Zozulia AA 233,234,303
Zucker S 449,450
Zukoski C 1273
Zumoff B 1304
Zvolsky P 991,992,1008, 1131,1146-1148,1194

Subject Index

Note: The numbers in this index refer to abstract numbers, not page numbers.

Acetylcholine 10,247,250,254,271,274,280,281,291,299,328,468,473,475, 503,504,660

Acetylcholinesterase 10,280

ACTH (see also Adrenocorticotropic hormone) 92,227,228,602,672,1240

Adaptation (see also Coping ability) 4,106,552,575,612,620,628,642,646, 682,779,817,849,852,1208,1315,1384

Adenylate cyclase 215,233,234,262,316,324,331,336,345,351,380,429,445, 453,457,461,462,476,483,492-494,1255

Adrenal cortex 86,259,627,678,683

Adrenal gland 659,1116

Adrenal medulla 78,276,621

Adrenalectomy 5,672,685,709

Adrenergic responses 38,39,53,107,114,134,216,222,264,276,279,280,293, 295-297,306,308,310,312-314,316,318-321,323-325,327,329,331-333, 335-339,341,342,344,346-348,350-353,457,466,472,474,478,484,493, 501,502,685,995,1231,1255

Adrenocorticotropic hormone (see also ACTH) 92,211,222,225-228,492,602,672,1240

Ageing 84,265,583,724,773,1057,1090,1190,1197,1198,1231-1267,1303,1312, 1357,1383,1395,1413,1416

Allergic response 94,283,288,321,390,394,427,448,511,702,778,779,809,810, 817,81387

Alpha-adrenergic agents (see also Receptors, alpha-adrenergic) 279,293, 321,329,353,466,685

Alzheimer's disease (see also Dementia) 1010,1017,1057,1107,1190,1192, 1195,1196,1198,1199,1201,1237,1246,1257

Amphetamine 19,526

Anaesthesia 20,44,345,357,369,371,391,399,413,417,422,423,438,443,448, 616,619,1239

Anaphylaxis 25,49,274,283,293,323,448,1286

Androgen (see also Hormones, sex) 98,159,197,206,207

Anger 520,541,637,736,827,868,871,874,876,878,915,944

Anorexia nervosa 956,1003,1065,1066,1104,1292,1304

Antagonists, opiate 44,91,213,214,223,232,388,409,417

Antibodies (see also Immunoglobulins) 3,15,19,20,32-34,40,46,54,56,60,64, 65,68,177,179,183,202,222,243,251,263,273,293,321,330,334,341,344, 354,366,99,108,118,123,124,126,127,139,154,158,164,168,169, 374,382,395,397,401-403,411,421,424,435,438,442,446,449,451,456, 470,480,501, 503,512,516,519,520,525,606,630,634,639,660, 703-707,774,863,908,914,917,954,956,964,966,974,978,986,990,994,997, 999-1001,1005,1020,1021,1034-1037,1039,1041-1043,1053,1056,1059, 1064,1070,1078 1080,1088,1093,1097,1101,1102,1104,1107,1110,1112, 1115,1116,1119,1169,1199,1205,1224,1233,1235,1243,1251,1256,1257, 1261,1265,1276,1289,1372,1422

  anti-receptor 183,202,354

  antinuclear 366,421,446,449,1000,1001,1243,1261

Antigenic competition 86

Antigens 6,10,20,22,25,26,32,33,40,56,58,60,63,65-67,69-73,75-78,83,86, 89,92,111-113,127,128,136,137,142,143,149,156-158,164,169,177, 183,186,200,201,222,242,250,269,273,283,284,288,293,295,323,330, 335,344,353,354,358,377,382,384,399,411,427,428,433,434,442,446,459, 479,501,512,532,607, 636,695,702-706,890,908, 914,917,956,964,990,991,1016,1032,1036,1040,1041,1073,1078,1084- 1086,1088,1115,1119,1122,1125,1127-1131,1133-1135, 1137-1140,1145- 1152,1154-1167,1170-1180,1182-1185,1187-1192,1194, 1197-1201,1205,1257,1264,1265,1276,1279,1292,1299

HLA 83,136,173,358,434,435,446,519,532,604,890,1122,1124-1141, 1143- 1152,1154-1157,1159-1167,1170-1175,1177-1180,1182-1185,1187, 1188,1190,1192,1194,1196-1201

  Ly 176

  T-independent 137

  Thy-1 3,58,71,78,163,176,186,295,479,487,637,1119,1141

  immune-associated 77,128

Antinuclear antibodies 366,421,446,449,1000,1001,1243,1261

Antipsychotic drugs 222,413,447,449,693,975,992,1004,1008,1009,1021, 1022,1055,1062,1077,1091,1131,1162,1171,1194

Anxiety 402,509,541,639,674,675,678,730,733,745,758,772,775,778,780,797, 800,803,804,818,819,838,841,845,850,861,864,867,871,876,887,890,902, 906, 1203,1242,1417,1419

Arachidonic acid 389,471,497,1278

Arthritis 32,33,147,166,259,389,426,522,533,604,606,608,655-658,769,771, 889,890,941,1108,1280,1297,1430,1446

Arthus reaction 391,1016,1040

Asthma 237,305,314,315,321,339,340,348,389,394,416,448,454,472,474,478, 504,609,610,612,778,779,781-787,790-803,805,806,808,809,812-814,817- 821,823-828,830,835,836,838-845,847-854,857,891,893,895-904, 906,907,915,924,926,932,933,937,944,973,1060,1208,1226,1250,1340, 1438,1444

Autism 958,1100,1101,1104,1121,1187

Autoantibodies 126,263,321,397,630,964,1000,1021,1088,1107,1235,1243

Autoimmunity 1,53,65,71,80,116,179,183,202,263,389,530,546,596,605,607, 608,655-658,660,750,861,909,952,964,966,997,1018, 1021,1022, 1032, 1068,1072,1082,1115,1157,1205,1267,1276,1280,1303,1326,1387, 1430

Autonomic agents 5,10,48,280,321,329,330,605,628,788

Autonomic nervous system 5,48,330,788

Aversive stimulation 681,917

B lymphocytes 15,26,51,56,63,69,72,74,77,105,108,109,121,127,129,154, 162,186,200,214,245,258,263,267,283,285,291,299,304,307,308,320,342, 347,370,381,394,409,412,432,440,442,476,480,487-489,501,607,630,649, 679,988,992,1008,1049,1235,1251,1254,1265,1276

  suppressor 245,1265

Behavior 10,48,55,331,389,401,412,437,483,536,555,562,565,572,590,641, 673,675,680,694,698,713,733,736,737,748,761,770,791,796,801,809,813, 814,817,827,868,871,874,884,887,895,909,912,913,916,917,920,937,944, 945,965,1045,1084,1143,1205,1208,1214,1217,1244,1249,1272,1319,1320, 1323,1339,1340,1349,1351,1353,1362,1363,1368,1371,1374,1375,1386, 1388,1390,1399,1400,1403,1405,1417-1419,1435,1436,1438,1443,1451, 1452

Bereavement 49,555,602,603,605,630,701,860,1315

Beta-adrenergic agents (see also Receptors, beta-adrenergic) 107,114, 134,264,276,279,280,293,295,297,306,308,310,312-314,316,318,319,321, 323-325,327,331-333,335-338,341,342,346-348,350-353,472,474,484,501, 502,685,995,1231,1255

Beta-adrenergic agonists 313

Beta-adrenergic antagonists 279,306,307,309

Biogenic amines (see also specific biogenic amines) 292,302,437,1211,1230

Blood cells, white 19,409,432,991,1044,1292

Bombesin 221

Bone marrow 19,20,22,56,69,75,76,109,116,139,154,186,188,245,246,252, 258,262,304,342,347,476,487,488,649,713,1251,1265

Bradykinin 219,250,278

Granulocytes 19,20,60,97,115,147,188,218,249,257,261,262,268,279,280,
288,309,311,312,316,318,322,324,325,327,373,377,392,423,425,441,
445,453,493,494,509,647,649,971,984,1065,1239,1262,1290,1291
Granulopoiesis 441,1324
Graves' disease 81,129,179,183,602,603,607,775,1445
Graves' lymphocytes 129
Growth hormone 34,174,204,205,490,509,614,615,622,624-626,629,630,762

HLA antigens 83,136,173,358,434,435,446,519,532,604,890,1122,1124-1141,
1143-1152,1154-1157,1159-1167,1170-1175,1177-1180,1182-
1185,1187,1188, 1190,1192,1194,1196-1201
Haematopoietic system 39,62,75,649,1342,1425
Haloperidol (see also Antipsychotic drugs) 222,292,401,402,427,447,693,
1171,1194
Handling effects 427,593,656,657,671,678,679,690,850
Happiness 863
Hepatitis 390,519,1042,1315
Herpes simplex virus 119,360,433,529,606,863,954,974,1005,1043,
1078,1079,1104
Histamine 53,117,134,153,191,219,230,236,237,248-250,257,260,269,270,
274,277,282-290,293,295,311,323,329,488,492-494,497,498,501,503,660,
788,841,899,905,1077,1087,1278,1293
Hodgkin's disease 15,359,750
Homosexuality 382,506,512,513,516,517,519,526,529,530,532,537,544
Hormones 6,7,10,13,14,20-23,34,37,41,48,56,79,80,82,84,86,88,89,91,92,95,
96,104,106,107,113,114,116,119,121,124,125,128,135,136,138,140,141,
152-158,161-163,168,172-175,177,178,180,183,188,190,192,196,200-205,
207,209,215-217,222,225,226,228,231,264,265,276,288,294,295,324,330,
336,417,423,424,483,487,490,495,509,572,579,583,585,593,596,601,602,
605,614-616,620-622,624-630,632,654,660,665,667,672,678,681,
683,685,697,709,710,725,737,738,751,762,768,773,871,1050,1082,1084,
1103,1188,1231,1233,1238,1239,1247,1267,1271,1304,1311,1312,1314,
1322,1326,1330,1334,1354,1357,1367,1370,1371,1387,1388,1394,1414,
1423,1425,1436
adrenal 86,423,621,678,683
sex 79,92,94,98,102,126,127,130,133,141,145,146,152,155,158-160,170,
171,181,185-187,190,194,197-199,204,206,207,209,222,465,477,509,616,
624,626,630,762,975,1004,1304,1380
steroid 13,14,83,85-87,97,99,101,102,104-106,108-110,112,113,115,117,
118,120,123,126,132-134,137-139,141-147,149,150,152,153,160,162-165,
168-170,176,178,182,184,186,188,190,191,197-199,206,207,209,237,248,
259,268,280,285,288,316,367,419,423,471,472,474,477,509,530,602,614,
620,625,630,632,641,654,672,674,675,678,679,683,684,688,691,700,703,
706,733,762,796-799,830,842,849,871,908,910,944,1238,1239,1264,1282,
1354,1391,1453
thymic 41,56,84,96,116,125,135,330,487,1050,1326,1367,1370,1425
thyroid 34,81,107,114,177,195,208,630,1238
Humoral immunity 10,48,54,137,143,168,169,183,292,401,708,862,912,
1011,1089,1267,1276
Hydrocortisone 86,97,99,105,106,108,109,117,118,120,123,142,143,168,176,
182,367
6-Hydroxydopamine 5,54,273,330,334
5-Hydroxytryptamine 235,246,252,260,278,459,616,1169
5-Hydroxytryptophan 222,243
Hypersensitivity 26,32,142,235,274,284,292,306,321,383,391,399,401,424,
427,428,452,459,488,529,601,630,692,774,861,862,1014,1016,1040,1210,
1284,1292
delayed-type 32,142,235,284,292,383,391,401,424,427,428,459,488,529,
601,630,692,861,862,1016,1040,1292
Hyperthyroidism 179,352,607
Hypophysectomy 12,32,709,1238
Hypophysis 22,34,155,1240
Hypothalamus (see also Posterior, Medial hypothalamus, Dorso- and
Ventromedial nuclei) 6-8,10,12-14,16,18-20,24-27,30,35,42,43,46-49,
52,78,89,101,156,169,187,243,397,603,605,621,725,733,762,903,1233,
1314,1413,1434,1435,1437
Hypothyroidism 420,1238

Immune system 4,6,10,12,20,25,41,48,52,54,86,88,89,93,116,154,224,232,
263,287,326,330,354,367,372,380,389,412,428,489,490,505,590,596,605,
630,632,639,641,690,697,702,713,724,751,861,913,915,1002,1003,1038,
1246,1247,1252,1258,1267,1270,1295,1307,1312,1314,1365,1369,1434
Immune tolerance 82,89,156,158,313,354,1281
Immunity 1,7,10,36,48,50,80,94,100,116,142,143,148,154-158,175,183,
222,236,260,265,288,292,367,377,389,396,399,400,404,412,426,451,495,
501,520,590,596,613,632,636,639-643,657,660,684,692,694,696,697,860,
871,919,974,991,1003,1011-1014,1016,1023,1033,1048,1049,1086,1088,
1089,1115,1233,1267,1276,1279,1292,1296,1303,1312,1326,1331,1358,
1441,1442,1452
cell-mediated 10,48,94,100,109,113,142,236,292,426,427,451,501,519,
590,607,613,636,640,641,647,692,697,860,871,909,974,991,1003,
1012-1014,1016,1033,1048,1267,1276,1279

humoral 10,48,54,137,143,168,169,183,292,401,708,862,912,1011,1089,
1267,1276
Immunodeficiency 32,33,116,154,269,361,367,429,517,529,544,613,650,707,
921
Immunoglobulin A 558,644,862,878,965,976,978,1047,1061,1076,1093,
1099,1102,1242,1244,1245,1289
Immunoglobulin D 1102
Immunoglobulin E 274,282,288,293,323,341,466,484,498,878,1019,
1102,1286,1289
Immunoglobulin G 98,99,120,129,139,147,243,251,258,263,275,374,415,
424,498,502,512,530,532,635,751,862,878,966,978,997,1010,1035,
1042,1061,1076,1078,1102,1110,1120,1193,1244,1245,1251,1254,
1286,1289
Immunoglobulin M 98,120,243,258,366,381,415,449,450,502,512,751,862,
878,967,978,997,1035,1061,1076,1093,1102,1107,1112,1242,1244,1245,
1254,1286,1289
Immunoglobulins 11,51,58,65,98,99,105,118,120,126,129,139,147,179,225,
235,243,251,258,263,274,275,282,283,288,293,304,321,323,341,354,361,
366,374,375,381,397,415,424,442,444,449,450,466,484,498,502,512,519,
530,532,558,602,603,607,630,635,644,708,751,862,878,962,964-
967,976,978,988,997,1000,1006,1010,1011,1017,1019,1021,1035,
1042,1047,1049,1052,1057,1059,1061,1076,1078,1086,1088,1093,1099,
1102,1107,1109,1110,1112,1115,1118, 1120,1121,1193,1232,1235,1242-
1245,1249,1251,1254,1261,1278,1286,1289, 1441
human thyroid-stimulating 129
thyroid-stimulating 129,179,602,603
Immunomodulation 8,12,36,42,43,547,1432
Immunosuppression 40,86,101,104,110,112,113,123,132,143,165,171,
190,283, 292,367,382,402,406,456,495,506,532,559,590,641,642,644,
645,650-652,674,908,909,912,914,916,917,1083,1380
Immunosurveillance 183,265,367,602,603,607,700,1247
Indoleamines (see also Serotonin) 1108
Infancy 701
Infectious disease (see also specific diseases) 7,255,490,862,1038,1065,
1263,1415
Infectious mononucleosis 292,490,525,1203,1206,1211,1212,1223
Inflammatory responses 80,94,109,110,140,147,188,249,288,361,389,411,
428,453,456,466,471,497,660,685,691,918,1273,1387
Influenza 365,414,433,520,954,956,1224
Innervation 9,10,38,39,53,54,238
Insulin 82,95,106,121,168,173,174,196,200-203,205,216,601,629,654,660,
768,773,1239,1271
Interferons 46,91-93,117,122,228,367,403,441,464,486,520,627,700,1039,
1041,1057,1084,1204,1289
human leukocyte 91,92,228,441
Interpersonal factors 608,838
Isoproterenol 107,117,133,264,279,283,285,293,296,311,312,314,318,319,
322-324,329,335-337,340,341,345,347,348,350-353,381,394,465,467,472,
473,479,482,493,494,502,503,995,1241,1255

Job loss 508
Juvenile diabetes (see also Diabetes) 524,773
Juvenile rheumatoid arthritis (see also Arthritis) 522,533,606

Kaposi's sarcoma 382,512,513,516,519,526,532

Learning, taste aversion 908-910,914,917
Leukemia (see also Cancer) 57,75,103,223,447,476,483,640,673,733,879,975
Leukocyte migration inhibition factor 142,957
Leukotrienes 451,471
Life change stress 520,527,550,559,560,564,567-569,574,581,587,588,632,
640,714-716,775,859,948
Limbic system 8,12,737,952,1082-1085,1314
Lipids (see also Nutritional factors) 168,376,1274,1287,1290
Lipopolysaccharide 40,105,143,186,214,242,330,370,371,412,652,700,914,
1265
Lithium 15,361,362,364,368,372,373,377,380,381,384,385,387,389,392,397,
404,405,407,415,416,418-421,425,429-431,433,434,436,439,441,444-446,
992,1001,1008,1125,1131,1137,1146,1148,1194,1324
Locus coeruleus 19,20
Luteinizing hormone (see also Hormones, sex) 92
Luteotropic hormone (see also Hormones, sex) 155
Lymph nodes 76,149,162,186,243,245,254,258,271,278,283,328,387,501,519,
679,912,949,1251,1264
Lymphatic system 7,8,11,13-15,20,22,23,26,31,34,38,40,42,43,49,51-53,56,
57,59,60,63,66,69,71,72,74-77,79-81,83-85,87-90,95,99-101,103-106,108,
109,111-113,116,118,120-123,126,129,133-135,141-143,145-147,149,
151-154,156,162-165,173-175,183,184,186,188,190,194-196,198,200,201,
204,205,207,214,217,218,220,223,228,232-235,239,240,243,245,246,248-
250,253,254,256,258,262-265,267,269,271,277,278,280,281,283-
286,288,289, 291,294,296,298-300,303-308,310,312-314,316,320,322,326,

About the authors:

Steven E. Locke, M.D., is a graduate of Columbia University College of Physicians and Surgeons. He completed a psychiatric residency at McLean Hospital at the Harvard Medical School, and was trained in psychosomatic medicine and biobehavioral science research at Boston University School of Medicine.

Dr. Locke was the primary psychiatric consultant to the medical and surgical oncology units at Boston's University Hospital, where he conducted research on the relationship of personality and life-change stress to human immune function.

In 1980, Dr. Locke joined the staff at Boston's Beth Israel Hospital where he established the hospital's Stress Disorders Program and the Clinical Psychophysiology Unit and also served as the Acting Director of the Psychiatry Consultation Service.

At present, Dr. Locke is a member of the faculty of Harvard Medical School, and is engaged in research consulting, and writing in the area of behavioral medicine and psychiatry. He maintains a private psychiatric practice in Newton, Massachusetts, specializing in behavioral medicine and diseases related to disorders of the immune system: cancer, allergy and auto immunity.

Dr. Locke is an editor of the forthcoming collection *Classics in Psychoneuroimmunology,* scheduled for publication in December 1983, by Aldine Press.

Mady Hornig-Rohan, M.A., received her degree in psychology from the Graduate Faculty of the New School for Social Research.

She has worked as a Research Assistant in basic immunology at both the Dana-Farber Cancer Institute (Harvard Medical School) and the University of Massachusetts Medical School.

About the Institute:

The Institute for the Advancement of Health was established in 1983 to further the scientific understanding of how mind/body connections affect health and disease.

The Institute's programs include publications, conferences, and support for research.

For further information write:

Institute for the Advancement of Health
16 East 53 Street, New York, N.Y. 10022

We would appreciate receiving your comments on the edition of **Mind and Immunity**. They will be helpful in preparing future supplements and other related publications. (If you recommend any citation, please include author's full article title, full journal name (or other sources), volume, inclusive page numbers, and date.

Institute for the Advancement of Health
16 East 53rd Street
New York, N.Y. 10022

Author's Permission Form

I, _____,
give permission to the Institute for the Advancement of Health and its assigns to reprint the abstract(s) of the paper(s) listed below in future editions of **Mind and Immunity: Behavioral Immunology (1976-1982)** or future annotated bibliographies on related topics contingent upon the approval of the respective publisher(s). I understand that a full acknowledgment of the source will accompany the reprinted abstract. No fee will be due to the authors for this reprinting right.

_____
Signature

_____
Print full name

_____
Institution

_____
Department

_____
Address

_____
City, State, Zip Code, Country

Please list any citations for possible inclusion below (authors, full title, full journal name or source, year, volume, pages [inclusive]):

Institute for the Advancement of Health
16 East 53rd Street
New York, N.Y. 10022